DeVita, Hellman, and Rosenberg's

CANCER

Principles & Practice of Oncology Review

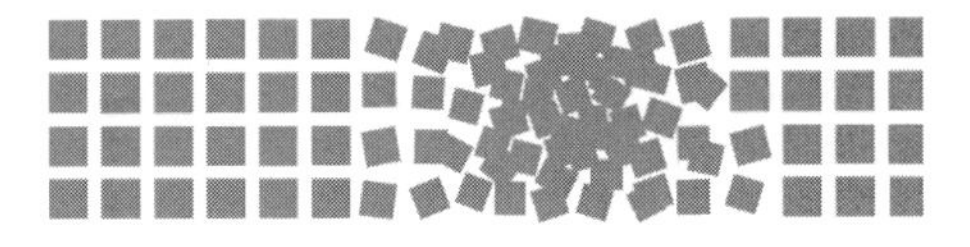

DeVita, Hellman, and Rosenberg's

CANCER

Principles & Practice of Oncology Review

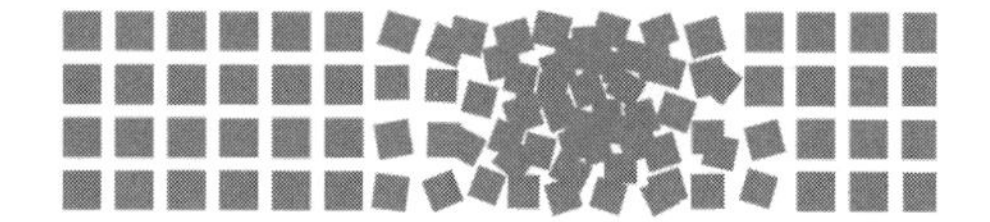

EDITOR

Ramaswamy Govindan, MD

Associate Professor

Department of Medicine

Division of Medical Oncology

Washington University School of Medicine

St. Louis, Missouri

LIPPINCOTT WILLIAMS & WILKINS

A **Wolters Kluwer** Company

Philadelphia • Baltimore • New York • London

Buenos Aires • Hong Kong • Sydney • Tokyo

Acquisitions Editor: Jonathan Pine
Developmental Editor: Kathleen Scogna
Project Manager: Nicole Walz
Senior Manufacturing Manager: Ben Rivera
Senior Marketing Manager: Adam Glazer
Creative Director: Doug Smock
Cover Designer: Karen Klinedinst
Production Services: Laserwords Private Limited
Printer: Edwards Brothers

530 Walnut Street
Philadelphia, PA 19106

Printed in the United States

Library of Congress Cataloging-in-Publication Data

Devita, Hellman, and Rosenberg's Cancer, principles & practice of oncology review / editor, Ramaswamy Govindan.— 1st ed.
p. ; cm.
Based on: Cancer : principles & practice of oncology / edited by Vincent T. Devita, Samuel Hellman, Steven A. Rosenberg. 7th ed. c2005.
Includes index.
ISBN 0-7817-5278-7
1. Cancer—Examinations, questions, etc. I. Govindan, Ramaswamy. II. Cancer. III. Title: Cancer, principles & practice of oncology review. IV. Title. [DNLM: 1. Neoplasms—Examination Questions. QZ 18.2 D496 2005]
RC266.5.D485 2005
616.99'4'0076—dc22

2005005874

Care has been taken to confirm the accuracy of the information presented and to describe generally accepted practices. However, the authors, editors, and publisher are not responsible for errors or omissions or for any consequences from application of the information in this book and make no warranty, expressed or implied, with respect to the currency, completeness, or accuracy of the contents of the publication. Application of this information in a particular situation remains the professional responsibility of the practitioner.

The authors, editors, and publisher have exerted every effort to ensure that drug selection and dosage set forth in this text are in accordance with current recommendations and practice at the time of publication. However, in view of ongoing research, changes in government regulations, and the constant flow of information relating to drug therapy and drug reactions, the reader is urged to check the package insert for each drug for any change in indications and dosage and for added warnings and precautions. This is particularly important when the recommended agent is a new or infrequently employed drug.

Some drugs and medical devices presented in this publication have Food and Drug Administration (FDA) clearance for limited use in restricted research settings. It is the responsibility of health care providers to ascertain the FDA status of each drug or device planned for use in their clinical practice.

The publishers have made every effort to trace copyright holders for borrowed material. If they have inadvertently overlooked any, they will be pleased to make the necessary arrangements at the first opportunity.

To purchase additional copies of this book, call our customer service department at (800) 638-3030 or fax orders to (301) 824-7390. Lippincott Williams & Wilkins customer service representatives are available from 8:30 am to 6:30 pm, EST, Monday through Friday, for telephone access. Visit Lippincott Williams & Wilkins on the Internet: http://www.lww.com.

10 9 8 7 6 5 4 3 2 1

Preface

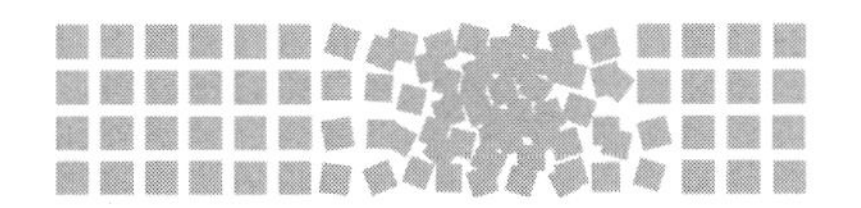

These are exciting and challenging times for those practicing oncology. While the significant advances made in understanding the molecular basis of cancer and new emerging targeted therapies are certainly exciting, the enormous information overload has presented a challenge. *Cancer: Principles & Practice of Oncology* has been an invaluable resource text for oncologists in training and practice. We felt that a review book that brings out the key points in each chapter would be a useful complement to the textbook. The corresponding chapters from the PPO text have been identified in each chapter in the review book. We have made an attempt to include real-life, case-based practice problems whenever possible. The carefully chosen contributors are well-known experts in their fields. In all, this review book has well over 900 questions. We hope this book will help prepare trainees for board examinations and drive home the key points for practising oncologists.

Ramaswamy Govindan

Acknowledgments

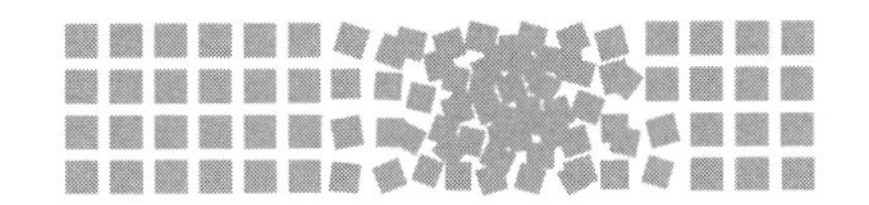

As is always the case, several individuals make publication of a book like this possible. I am grateful to the editors of *Cancer: Principles & Practice of Oncology* for supporting this project. Jonathan Pine, the editor of oncology, led the effort at Lippincott Williams & Wilkins. Jonathan was a pleasure to work with. I am thankful to Kathleen Scogna at Lippincott who was quite patient with me despite the fact that I missed many of her deadlines. Eileen Muse was instrumental in contacting the contributors and ensuring smooth flow of the manuscript to the editor. I am indebted to the authors for their contributions. I am grateful to my wife, Prabha, and two adorable children, Ashwin and Akshay, for tolerating my absence during family time as I was often away with my laptop working on this book.

Ramaswamy Govindan

Contributors

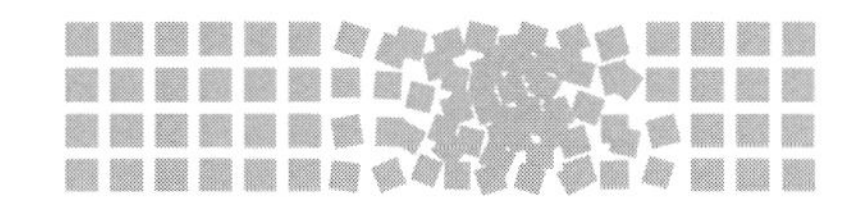

Alex A. Adjei, MD, PhD
Professor
Department of Oncology
Mayo Clinic College of Medicine
Consultant in Oncology
Department of Oncology
Mayo Clinic
Rochester, Minnesota

Rebecca L. Aft, MD, PhD
Assistant Professor
Department of Surgery
Washington University School of Medicine
Surgeon
Department of Surgery
Barnes-Jewish Hospital
St. Louis, Missouri

Clay M. Anderson, MD
Associate Professor of Clinical Medicine
Department of Internal Medicine
University of Missouri School of Medicine
Director of Clinical Services
Ellis Fischel Cancer Center
University of Missouri Health Care
Columbia, Missouri

Jordan D. Berlin, MD
Associate Professor
Department of Medicine
Division of Hematology/Oncology
Vanderbilt University
Clinical Director
GI Oncology
Vanderbilt Ingram Cancer Center
Vanderbilt University Medical Center
Nashville, Tennessee

Sanjeev Bhalla, MD
Assistant Professor
Mallinckrodt Institute of Radiology
Washington University School of Medicine
Co-Director
Department of Body CT and Emergency Radiology
Barnes-Jewish Hospital
St. Louis, Missouri

Julie R. Brahmer, MD
Assistant Professor
Department of Oncology
Johns Hopkins University
Assistant Professor
Department of Oncology
The Johns Hopkins Medical Institute
Baltimore, Maryland

Daniel B. Brown, MD
Assistant Professor
Department of Radiology and Surgery
Washington University
Barnes-Jewish Hospital
St. Louis, Missouri

Leanne S. Budde, MD
Fellow
Division of Hematology/Oncology
Indiana University School of Medicine
Indianapolis, Indiana

J. Andrew Carlson, MD, FRCPC
Associate Professor
Department of Pathology
Albany Medical College
Albany, New York

L. Chinsoo Cho, MD, MS
Associate Professor
Department of Radiation Oncology
University of Texas
Southwestern Medical Center
Dallas, Texas

Hak Choy, MD
Chairman
Department of Radiation Oncology
University of Texas
Southwestern Medical Center
Dallas, Texas

Ezra E. W. Cohen, MD FRCPS (C)
Assistant Professor
Department of Medicine
Section of Hematology/Oncology
University of Chicago
Chicago, Illinois

Lynn A. Cornelius
Associate Professor
Division of Dermatopathology
Washington University School of Medicine
St. Louis, Missouri

Alex E. Denes, MD
Associate Professor of Clinical Medicine
Department of Medical Oncology
Washington University School of Medicine
St. Louis, Missouri

John F. DiPersio MD, PhD
Professor of Medicine/
Pathology/Immunology
Chief, Division of Oncology
Washington University School of Medicine
St. Louis, Missouri

Martin J. Edelman, MD
Associate Professor
Department of Medicine
University of Maryland
Greenebaum Cancer Center
Baltimore, Maryland

David S. Ettinger, MD
Alex Grass Professor
Department of Oncology
Johns Hopkins University School
of Medicine
Act Staff Full Time
Department of Oncology
Kimmel Comprehensive Cancer Center
The Johns Hopkins Medical Institute
Baltimore, Maryland

Gini F. Fleming, MD
Associate Professor
Department of Medicine
University of Chicago
Chicago, Illinois

Sharlene Gill, MD, MPH
Assistant Professor of Medicine
Department of Medical Oncology
University of British Columbia
Medical Oncologist
GI Systemic Therapy
British Columbia Cancer Agency
Vancouver, Canada

Richard M. Goldberg, MD
Professor and Chief of Hematology
and Oncology
Associate Director Lineberger
Comprehensive Cancer Center
University of North Carolina
Chapel Hill, North Carolina

Ramaswamy Govindan, MD
Associate Professor
Department of Medicine
Division of Medical Oncology
Washington University School of Medicine
St. Louis, Missouri

David Gustin, MD
Assistant Professor
Hematology/Oncology Section
Department of Medicine
University of Chicago Hospital
Chicago, Illinois

Mouhammed Amir Habra, MD
Fellow
Department of Endocrine
Neoplasia/Hormonal Disorders
University of Texas
M.D. Anderson Cancer Center
Houston, Texas

Nasser Hanna, MD
Assistant Professor
Department of Medicine
Indiana University
Indianapolis, Indiana

J. William Harbour, MD
Associate Professor
Department of Ophthalmology
and Visual Sciences
Washington University School of Medicine
St. Louis, Missouri

Kristin L. Hennenfent, Pharm D, MBA
Assistant Professor
Department of Pharmacy Practice
St. Louis College of Pharmacy
St. Louis, Missouri

Philip C. Hoffman, MD
Professor
Department of Medicine
Section of Hematology/Oncology
University of Chicago
Attending Physician
Department of Medicine
Section of Hematology/Oncology
University of Chicago Hospitals
Chicago, Illinois

David H. Ilson, MD, PhD
Associate Professor
Department of Medicine
Weill Cornell Medical College
Associate Attending
Department of Medicine
Memorial Sloan-Kettering Cancer Center
New York, New York

William S. Jonas, MD
Fellow
Winship Cancer Institute
Emory University School of Medicine
Atlanta, Georgia

Fadlo R. Khuri, MD
Professor of Hematology, Oncology,
Medicine, Pharmacology and
Otolaryngology
Blomeyer Chair in Translational Cancer
Research
Associate Director of Clinical and
Translational Research
Chief Medical Officer
Hematology/Oncology
Winship Cancer Institute
Emory University School of Medicine
Attending Physician
Department of Hematology/Oncology
Emory University Hospital
Grady Memorial Hospital
Crawford W. Long Hospital
Veterans Affairs Medical Center
Atlanta, Georgia

Robert A. Kratzke, MD
Associate Professor of Medicine
Department of Medicine
Section of Hematology/
Oncology/Transplant
University of Minnesota
Minneapolis, Minnesota

Janessa J. Laskin, MD, FRCPC
Assistant Professor
Department of Medical Oncology
University of British Columbia
Medical Oncologist
British Columbia Cancer Agency
Vancouver, Canada

J. Jack Lee, PhD, DDS
Professor
Biostatistics and Applied Mathematics
MD Anderson Cancer Center
University of Texas
Houston, Texas

Susan B. LeGrand, MD, FACP
Director of Education
The Harry R. Horvitz Center
for Palliative Medicine
The Taussig Cancer Center Cleveland
Clinic Foundation
Cleveland, Ohio

William T. Leslie, MD
Assistant Professor
Department of Medicine
Rush University Medical Center
Chicago, Illinois

Gerald P. Linette, MD, PhD
Assistant Professor
Division of Oncology
Washington University School of Medicine

Member
Siteman Cancer Center
Barnes-Jewish Hospital
St. Louis, Missouri

Mary-Ellen Mazuryk, BScN, MD
Assistant Clinical Professor
Department of Medicine
University of California
Medical Oncologist
Department of Medicine
Rebecca and John Moores UCSD Cancer Center
San Diego, California

Kathy D. Miller, MD
Assistant Professor, Sheila D. Ward Scholar
Division of Hematology and Oncology
Indiana University
Indianapolis, Indiana

Julian R. Molina, MD
Assistant Professor
Department of Oncology
Mayo Clinic
Rochester, Minnesota

Daniel Morgensztern, MD
Instructor of Medicine
Department of Internal Medicine
Division of Oncology
Washington University School of Medicine
Staff Physician
Department of Medicine
Section of Hematology/Oncology
St. Louis Veterans Affairs Medical Center
St. Louis, Missouri

Joanne E. Mortimer, MD
Professor of Clinical Medicine
Department of Medicine
University of California
Deputy Director for Clinical Affairs
Moores UCSD Cancer Center
San Diego, California

David G. Mutch, MD
Ira and Juchy Gall Professor of Gynecologic Oncology
Director
Department of Obstetrics/Gynecology
Washington University School of Medicine
Attending Physician
Department of Obstetrics/Gynecology
Barnes-Jewish Hospital
St. Louis, Missouri

Bruno Nervi, MD
Hematology/Oncology Fellow
Department of Medicine
Washington University School of Medicine
Hematology/Oncology Fellow
Division of Oncology
Barnes-Jewish Hospital
St. Louis, Missouri

Susan O'Brien, MD
Professor of Medicine
Department of Leukemia
UTMD Anderson Cancer Center
Houston, Texas

Michel Panisset, MD
Associate Professor
Department of Medicine
University of Montreal
Co-Director
André-Barbeau Movement disorders clinic
Hôtel-Dieu – CHUM
Montreal, Canada

Michael C. Perry, MD, FACP
Professor of Hematology/Oncology
Nellie B. Smith Chair of Oncology
University of Missouri
Division Director
Ellis Fischel Cancer Center
Columbia, Missouri

Giancarlo Pillot, MD
Clinical Research Fellow
Division of Hematology/Oncology
Washington University School of Medicine
St. Louis, Missouri

Lee Ratner, MD, PhD
Professor
Medicine and Molecular Microbiology
Washington University School of Medicine
St. Louis, Missouri

William L. Read, MD
Assistant Professor
Department of Hematology/Oncology
University of California
San Diego, California

Alan B. Sandler, MD
Associate Professor of Medicine
Medical Director, Thorasic Oncology
Department of Medicine
Section of Hematology/Oncology
Vanderbilt University Medical Center
Director
Vanderbilt-Ingram Cancer Center
Affiliate Network Program
Nashville, Tennessee

Shalini Shenoy, MD
Assistant Professor of Pediatrics and Clinical Laboratories
Department of Pediatric Hematology/Oncology
Washington University School of Medicine
Associate Director, Stem Cell Transplant
Medical Director, SLCH Blood Bank
St. Louis Children's Hospital
St. Louis, Missouri

Walter M. Stadler, MD, FACP
Associate Professor
Department of Medicine
Section of Hematology/Oncology
University of Chicago
Chicago, Illinois

Roger Stupp, MD
Privat-docent
University of Lausanne
Senior Attending physician
Multidisciplinary Oncology Center
University of Lausanne Hospitals
Lausanne, Switzerland

Janakiraman Subramanian, MD
Resident
Department of Internal Medicine
St. Luke's Roosevelt Medical Center
St. Louis, Missouri

Benjamin R. Tan, MD
Assistant Professor
Department of Medicine
Washington University School of Medicine
St. Louis, Missouri

Gauri R. Varadhachary, MD
Assistant Professor
Department of Gastrointestinal Medical Oncology
University of Texas
MD Anderson Cancer Center
Houston, Texas

Nirmal K. Veeramachaneni, MD
Resident in Surgery
Department of Surgery
Barnes-Jewish Hospital
Washington University School of Medicine
St. Louis, Missouri

Parameswaran Venugopal, MD
Samuel G. Taylor III MD Professor of Oncology
Associate Professor of Medicine
Rush University Medical Center
Chicago, Illinois

Ravi Vij, MD
Assistant Professor
Section of BMT and Leukemia
Washington University School of Medicine
St. Louis, Missouri

James W. Watters, PhD
Instructor of Medicine
Department of Medicine
Washington University School of Medicine
St. Louis, Missouri

Megan E. Wren, MD
Assistant Professor
Department of Internal Medicine
Washington University School of Medicine
Chief, Shatz-Strauss Firm
Department of Internal Medicine
Barnes-Jewish Hospital
St. Louis, Missouri

Contents

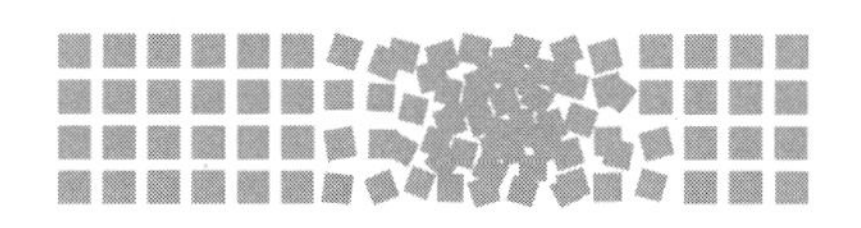

CHAPTER 1

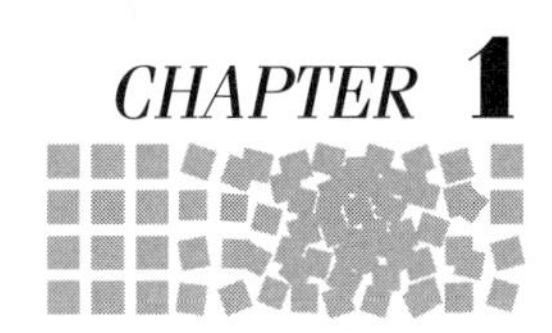

Molecular Methods in Oncology

ROBERT A. KRATZKE

Directions Each of the numbered items below is followed by lettered answers. Select the ONE lettered answer that is BEST in each case unless instructed otherwise.

QUESTIONS

Question 1.1. **The best example of a technology that may be useful to monitor minimal residual disease in chronic myelogenous leukemia (CML) is**

A. comparative genomic hybridization (CGH)
B. complementary DNA (cDNA) microarray analysis
C. polymerase chain reaction (PCR)
D. laser capture microdissection (LCM)
E. all of the above

Question 1.2. **The specificity of methylation-specific PCR in detecting methylated deoxyribonucleic acid (DNA) depends on the chemical conversion of cytosine to which of the following.**

A. Thymine.
B. Uracil.
C. Adenine.
D. Guanine.
E. Inosine.

Question 1.3. **Hypermethylation of cytosine residues in the vicinity of gene promoter sequences is frequently associated in cancers with**

A. silencing of tumor suppressor genes
B. overexpression of matrix metalloproteinases
C. activation of oncogenes
D. mutation of cytosine to uracil
E. gene amplification

Question 1.4. **The technology of CGH is ideal for studying**

A. single nucleotide polymorphisms
B. gene amplification of Her2/neu
C. chemosensitivity of tumors prior to treatment
D. genome wide allele loss or gain
E. differential gene expression between tissues

Corresponding Chapters in *Cancer: Principles & Practice of Oncology*, Seventh Edition: 1 (Molecular Methods in Oncology) and 2 (Genomics and Proteomics).

Question 1.5. **Ribonucleic acid (RNA) interference (RNAi) is a technique that involves**

A. silencing of gene expression using double-stranded RNA
B. a defensive mechanism for certain species of plants
C. a process dependent on introduction of exogenous nucleic acid into cells
D. useful for targeting specific acquired gene lesions in malignant cells
E. all of the above

Question 1.6. **Which of the following is least critical in using RNAi technology to "knock down" gene expression in cancer cells?**

A. Identifying a permissive cancer cell type that will allow vector delivery.
B. Creating double-stranded RNA that targets specific gene sequence.
C. Using an effective delivery technology (transfection).
D. Monitoring expression of the gene target after delivery of double-stranded RNA.

Question 1.7. **Which of the following is an example of how cDNA microarray analysis may identify genome wide profiles and regulation?**

A. Detection of amplified gene elements such as Her2/neu in breast cancer.
B. Identification of expressed messenger RNA (mRNA) transcript profiles, which correlates with prognosis in adenocarcinoma of the lung.
C. Measuring prostate specific antigen (PSA) levels in prostate cancer.
D. Detection of BCR-ABL fusion genes in CML in order to monitor residual disease.
E. Detection of *ras* family mutations in colon cancer.

Question 1.8. **Gene expression profiling by cDNA microarray may identify gene specific alterations in cancers in which of the following situations.**

A. Differentiating between mutations in breast cancer of either the BRCA1 or BRCA2 cancer susceptibility genes.
B. Gene amplification of *myc* in small cell lung cancer.
C. Alterations in dinucleotide repeats in colon cancer.
D. Detection of specific mutations of the RET gene in familial medullary thyroid cancer.

Question 1.9. **Barriers to routine use of expression array technologies include**

A. adequate sample size of biopsy
B. tumor specimen handling to ensure RNA stability
C. identifying pure tumor populations in biopsy samples
D. standardization of specimen processing and assay procedure
E. all of the above

Question 1.10. **Tissue microarray (TMA) technology is best suited for identifying**

A. p53 mutations in lung cancer
B. Her2/neu amplification using fluorescent *in situ* hybridization (FISH) in breast cancer specimens
C. chromagen based antibody detection of antigens such as cytokeratin by immunohistochemistry
D. expression of specific gene mRNA in tumor samples

Question 1.11. **Human chromosomes normally have two arms, designated "p" and "q." Which of the following statements is true regarding the "p" arm of chromosomes?**

A. It is always longer than the "q" arm.
B. It is roughly equivalent in length to the "q" arm since the chromosome is divided by a centrally located centromere.
C. It is always shorter than the "q" arm.
D. It is more likely to be rearranged in leukemia.

Question 1.12. **All of the following statements are true regarding heterochromatin EXCEPT**

A. it represents the darkly staining portion of chromosomes
B. it occurs as both facultative and constitutive forms
C. heterochromatin DNA is largely condensed
D. heterochromatin is primarily found in the centromere

Question 1.13. **The "Hayflick phenomenon," which is the name given to the limited replicative potential of cells, is thought to arise from which of the following.**

A. The sequential loss of genetic material from the ends of chromosomes (telomeres) with each round of division.
B. The gradual accumulation of uncorrected genetic defects passed on during division leading to senescence or malignancy.
C. The activation of telomerase in aging cells leading to enzymatic loss of genetic material from telomeres.
D. Dividing eukaryotic cells outgrowing their vascular supply.

Question 1.14. **Which of the following statements is NOT accurate regarding telomerase?**

A. It has both an RNA and protein component.
B. It is a DNA polymerase.
C. Overexpression of telomerase is found in all cancer specimens.
D. Telomerase protects the integrity of the chromosomal ends.
E. None of the above.

Question 1.15. **Which of the following is NOT a standard application of FISH?**

A. Revealing gene amplification of Her2/neu in breast cancer.
B. Detection of specific commonly observed chromosomal translocations.
C. Determining degree of engraftment following sex-mismatched bone marrow and cord blood transplants.
D. Identification of tumor specific mutations of p53 in ovarian cancer.
E. None of the above.

Question 1.16. **Which of the following characterizes metacentric chromosomes?**

A. Equal or almost equal size of the "p" and "q" arms.
B. More than one centromere.
C. Present only in myeloid malignancies.
D. Possessing extremely short "p" arms.
E. B and D.

Question 1.17. **Which of the following is an example of gene amplification found in cancer?**

A. N-*myc* amplification in neuroblastoma.
B. C-*myc* amplification in small cell lung cancer.
C. Her2/neu amplification in breast cancer.
D. All of the above.
E. None of the above.

Question 1.18. **Which of the following characterizes cytogenetic abnormalities in most human cancers?**

A. Universal (monoclonal) population of cells containing identical cytogenetic abnormalities.
B. Completely normal karyotype.
C. Heterogenous complex karyotypes.
D. Complete loss of X or Y chromosomes.

Question 1.19. **Homogenously staining regions in chromosomes are**

A. associated with gene amplification
B. more genetically stable than double minutes circular DNA
C. a laboratory artifact requiring a repeat cytogenetic test
D. found exclusively in undifferentiated stem cells
E. A and B
F. B and C

Question 1.20. **The primary Internet tool for identifying homologous gene sequences is**

A. caCORE (http://ncicb.nci.nih.gov/core)
B. Enterprise Vocabulary Services (EVS) (http://ncicb/nci/nih/gov/core)
C. Basic local alignment search tool (BLAST) (http://www.ncbi.nlm.nih.gov/BLAST)
D. Biomedical Informatics Grid (caBIG) (http://caBIG/nci.nih.gov)
E. B and D
F. none of the above

Question 1.21. **The primary curator of public genomic information in the United States is which of the following agencies.**

A. The National Institute of Technology and Standards.
B. Lawrence Livermore Laboratories.
C. The National Center of Biotechnology Information.
D. The Centers for Disease Control.
E. None of the above.

Question 1.22. **Which of the following is an example of an epigenetic molecular process?**

A. Gene amplification.
B. Histone deacetylation (HDAC).
C. Missense mutation.
D. DNA methylation.
E. A and C.
F. B and D.

Question 1.23. **Expression of wild-type p53 induces expression of which of the following cyclin-dependent kinases (CDK).**

A. CDKN2 ($p16^{INK4a}$).
B. p21/CIP1 (waf1).
C. p27.
D. A and C.
E. A and B.
F. All of the above.

Question 1.24. **Which of the following viral tumor antigens are causative agents in cervical cancer?**

A. Simian virus 40 (SV40) large T antigen.
B. Adenovirus E1a and E1b antigens.
C. Human papilloma virus (HPV) E6 and E7 antigens.
D. All of the above.

Question 1.25. **Bcl-2 gene overexpression is associated with which of the following.**

A. Inhibition of apoptosis.
B. Translocations of chromosome 8 and 14.
C. Tumor development in murine models.
D. Enhanced sensitivity to chemotherapy.
E. All of the above.

Question 1.26. **A newborn infant is found to have bilateral retinoblastoma. In addition to bilateral involvement, the disease shows multiple tumor foci on both retinae. The tumors will most likely demonstrate which of the following genetic lesions.**

A. Missense mutation of the retinoblastoma susceptibility gene (*Rb*).
B. Activating translocation involving the 13q14 locus.
C. Deletion of both alleles of the *Rb* gene.
D. Overexpression of pRb protein.

Question 1.27. **Mutations in the PTEN gene are associated with which of the following familial cancer syndromes.**

A. Li–Fraumeni syndrome.
B. Cowden syndrome.
C. Familial medullary thyroid cancer.
D. Familial adult polyposis.
E. von Hippel–Lindau syndrome.

Question 1.28. **Completion of the Human Genome Project has revealed that human cells have a repertoire of genes of which approximate number?**

A. 4,000 genes.
B. 40,000 genes.
C. 100,000 genes.
D. 1,000,000 genes.

Question 1.29. **At colonoscopy, a 49-year-old man is found to have colon cancer after a routine screening evaluation demonstrated iron deficiency anemia. He had a single tumor in the ascending colon. His brother and father have had colon cancer as well. In which of the following genes is the likely germline mutation present in this patient?**

A. p53.
B. APC.
C. BRCA2.
D. $p16^{INK4a}$.
E. MSH2.

Question 1.30. **Which of the following is a direct capability of laser capture microdissection?**

A. Harvesting of nucleic acid from individual cancer cells in tissue samples free of associated adjacent tissues.
B. Tumor-specific analysis of gene expression profiles.
C. Two-dimensional gel analysis of expressed proteins.
D. All of the above.
E. None of the above.

Question 1.31. **The term *oncogene* is applied to genetic elements that have which of the following characteristics.**

A. Germline deletion in patients with familial cancer syndromes.
B. Reexpression that suppresses the malignant phenotype.
C. Activation or overexpression leading to the transformed phenotype.
D. Binding to cognate receptors that activates growth pathways through tyrosine kinase activation.
E. None of the above.

Question 1.32. **Which of the following statements regarding chromatin remodeling is NOT true?**

A. HDAC is associated with gene silencing.
B. Overexpression of core binding protein (CBP/p300) plays a role in silencing tumor suppressor genes in certain cancers such as leukemia.
C. Novel agents inactivating HDAC should aid in gene reexpression of silenced gene elements.
D. Acetylated histones are associated with enhanced gene expression.

Question 1.33. **All of the following are receptor tyrosine kinases EXCEPT**

A. Met
B. platelet-derived growth factor receptor
C. insulinlike growth factor receptor 1
D. Kit
E. Akt

Question 1.34. **All of the following genes are inactivated in a known familial cancer syndrome EXCEPT**

A. *Rb*
B. PTCH
C. Ret
D. DCC
E. MLH1

Question 1.35. **Abnormalities of the Tal-1/SCL transcription factor in T-cell leukemia include which of the following.**

A. Deletion of both alleles of the Tal-1/SCL locus.
B. Epigenetic silencing of Tal-1/SCL expression following DNA hypermethylation.
C. The presence of activating missense mutations.
D. Expression of Tal-1/SCL in an inappropriate cell lineage.
E. None of the above.

Question 1.36. **Which of the following best describes the term *protooncogene*?**

A. A normal cellular gene that has been transduced by a retrovirus that is then mutated following viral replication.
B. A homologue of a known oncogenic element identified in prehistoric specimens.
C. A transforming viral gene that can cause malignant transformation in fibroblasts *in vitro*.
D. The first oncogene discovered to be associated with human cancer.
E. A viral oncogene that, following infection, is the direct causative agent of human cancer.

Question 1.37. **The presence of mutations in p53 has been associated with which of the following properties on cells.**

A. Loss of the G2 checkpoint following treatment with DNA damaging agents.
B. Enhanced capacity to undergo apoptosis following exposure to radiation.
C. Increased capacity for DNA amplification.
D. Loss of viability in transgenic murine models.
E. A and C.
F. B and D.

Question 1.38. **The proteome is which of the following.**

A. The set of all expressed gene products at a given time.
B. The proteins expressed preferentially in malignant cells.
C. The set of all proteins potentially expressed by the genome.
D. The set of protonated peptides subject to matrix-assisted laser desorption ionization-time of flight (MALDI-TOF) analysis.

ANSWERS

Answer 1.1. **The answer is C.**

PCR technology allows for the detection of extremely small quantities of specific genetic sequences and is well suited for identification of otherwise undetectable residual disease. PCR has the dual benefits of being able to detect both specific and minute quantities of a target sequence. However, because of its exquisite sensitivity, PCR can be susceptible to false-positive results in the case of incidental contamination or inappropriate hybridization of primers. In CML the presence of the specific BCR-ABL fusion gene is ideal for application of PCR since the joining of the BCR and ABL elements results in a unique DNA sequence that can be identified with both high specificity and sensitivity. Multiplex PCR allows for simultaneous detection of multiple gene targets. "Real-time" PCR is a technology that detects the presence of genes in a quantitative manner. Both CGH and cDNA microarray technologies are powerful tools for detecting genome wide alterations but lack both the specificity to conveniently detect a single gene sequence and the ease of use of PCR. LCM allows for sampling of individual cancer cells but cannot be easily used to detect isolated rare cancer cells.

Answer 1.2. **The answer is B.**

Methylation of cytosine residues is an important mechanism of gene regulation leading to altered expression of the methylated gene. Detection of DNA methylation has been made easier by the development of methylation specific PCR, which relies on the capacity of sodium bisulfite to deaminate unmethylated cytosine to uracil. This chemical reaction can only occur if the cytosine residue is unmethylated. Following this conversion, the gene sequence can be analyzed by PCR with primers designed to detect the new sequence. This technology is being used increasingly to detect epigenetic modification of DNA by methylation that is seen in almost all cancers.

Answer 1.3. **The answer is A.**

Methylation of cytosine is increasingly known to be an important regulatory mechanism. Although loss of methylation leading to aberrant gene expression is recognized as a mechanism of regulation in many cellular events, its importance in most cancers is either limited or remains to be fully appreciated. On the other hand, hypermethylation occurs frequently in cancers and is often associated with silencing of tumor suppressor genes. The chemical conversion of cytosine residues to uracil is part of methylation specific PCR, which is a technology to detect the methylation of cytosines in malignant cells. Gene amplification is primarily a genetic event with critical gene elements being duplicated.

Answer 1.4. **The answer is D.**

CGH is a useful research tool to identify genomic areas of gain or loss of genetic material. This can identify the location of previously unknown genes that are dysregulated in cancer. Specific gene rearrangements, such as Her2/neu gene amplification, can be more easily identified with gene specific technologies such as FISH. Genome wide identification of specific genes can best be detected with array-based technologies such as microarray or single nucleotide polymorphism (SNP) chip analysis.

Answer 1.5. **The answer is C.**

RNAi is a powerful technology for silencing specific genes in a research setting. It relies on the generation of specific double-stranded RNA that is then introduced into cells by transfection. Since the double-stranded RNA is matched precisely with the target in sequence, the specificity for the "knocking down" or silencing expression of a particular gene is quite high. The presence of RNAi was first identified in plants and is thought to be a defense mechanism for plants.

Answer 1.6. **The answer is A.**

The technology of RNAi is an extremely useful new technology that can silence selected genes in cancer cells *in vitro.* Currently, clinical use is not available but remains an area of intense interest. One of the more remarkable things about RNAi is how universally adaptable it is in silencing a wide spectrum of genes in virtually any type of cell. The success of an RNAi experiment can only be measured by looking at expression of the targeted gene RNA or consequent protein, so detection methods that can monitor whether gene silencing is successful is critical.

Answer 1.7. **The answer is B.**

Profiling of cancer cells using cDNA microarray has proven to be a powerful investigational tool in cancer research. Array technology allows for genome wide analysis of messenger RNA levels of thousands of genes in a single experiment. The results of a microarray experiment can lead to finding increased or decreased expression of specific mRNA in a wide variety of cancers. However, cDNA microarray technology will only detect alterations in gene transcript expression levels. Cancer specific single nucleotide mutations such as *ras* mutations in colon cancer can be best detected with gene specific hybridization or PCR techniques. Similarly, rearrangements or amplifications of specific genes are best detected by techniques that examine genomic DNA sequences. The measurement of secreted extracellular proteins such as PSA requires antibody directed tools such as enzyme linked immunosorbent assay (ELISA).

Answer 1.8. **The answer is A.**

Although cDNA array experiments are based on detecting genome wide alterations in expression, the resulting profiles could potentially be used to identify and classify cancers dependent on mutations of specific genes. A promising example of this application is identifying gene profiles that correspond to either BRCA1 or BRCA2 mutation dependent cancers. Identifying mutations in these genes by conventional DNA sequencing is cumbersome due to the size of the gene's open reading frame and the plethora of possible mutations. A common profile found in expression arrays will facilitate identifying patients who warrant further detailed analysis of the BRCA family genes. A similar approach could be developed for identifying patients at risk for familial medullary thyroid cancer, but strong family history and serum calcitonin screening easily identify patients at risk who should be further studied with DNA sequencing. Gene amplification and dinucleotide repeats are best analyzed by studies of genomic DNA.

The use of identifying common cDNA array or proteomic profiles is one of the more promising concepts in development. In the case discussed here, a profile has been proposed to detect the presence of inactivating mutations in a single gene. As an example of alternative use of this technology, similar concepts have been proposed and are in development to identify unique profiles that predict for response to a drug or class of drugs. This could prove useful for not only tailoring clinical care but in deriving new uses for existing drugs that result in identical profiles to known agents. Also, profile grouping is in development for predicting relapse, patterns of relapse, prognosis, and a variety of clinical parameters.

Answer 1.9. **The answer is E.**

Numerous barriers exist to routine use of cDNA array technologies in clinical practice. Although techniques of RNA amplification exist, they can introduce bias in the final profile results. Samples from needle aspirates are often inadequate for expression array use. In addition, most tumor biopsies are a mixture of benign and malignant tissues. Ideally, pure tumor tissues should be used, although mixed tissues may give alternative useful information. Laser capture microscopy can potentially help this situation but is a technology not widely available in clinical practice. Finally, to obtain high quality RNA, fresh frozen tissue is ideal, requiring immediate freezing and storage capabilities. All of these problems will likely be solved by developing technologies but currently are keeping expression profiling as largely a research tool for molecular target and profile identification.

Answer 1.10. **The answer is C.**

TMAs are proving very useful in analyzing large numbers of samples of formalin-fixed tumors while minimizing cutting of paraffin embedded blocks. Because developing tissue-based arrays uses fixed tissues, it is most ideal for studying proteins that can be detected with standard immunohistochemistry. A number of techniques are being developed to retrieve DNA and RNA from such samples, and these techniques work with varying success. Sometimes antibody-based tests can strongly indicate the presence of tumor-specific mutations in genes such as p53. Most, but not all, mutations of p53 result in protein stabilization and increased expression when examined by immunohistochemistry. However, such a test is rarely considered either adequately sensitive or specific when compared to gene sequencing.

Answer 1.11. **The answer is C.**

The shorter (smaller) arm of all human chromosomes is designated "p," deriving from the French word "petit." The longer arm is always called "q," which merely was chosen as a label since it is the next letter in the alphabet. Although chromosomes have a centralized structure that serves as a division between the "p" and "q" arms identified as the centromere, it does not necessarily divide the chromosome evenly into two arms. Vital genes that are targeted in the development of cancers are contained on both "p" and "q" arms of chromosomes.

Answer 1.12. **The answer is D.**

Chromosomal DNA is largely segregated into heterochromatin and euchromatin. Heterochromatin refers to the darker staining banded DNA that is more condensed. The darker pattern results from the more densely concentrated DNA picking up greater staining. Constitutive heterochromatin remains condensed, while facultative heterochromatin has the capacity to switch between condensed and decondensed states. Heterochromatin exists along both arms of all chromosomes and is not the primary component of the centromere.

Answer 1.13. **The answer is A.**

Hayflick and Moorehead documented a landmark finding of cell biology when they observed that normal eukaryotic cells would only replicate approximately 50 to 100 times before dying. This limited replicative capacity of nontransformed cells is called the "Hayflick phenomenon." It is now known that the ends of the chromosomes, called telomeres, gradually shorten, losing 25 to 200 base pairs with each round of division. After 50 to 100 rounds of division, the telomeres reach a critically shortened length, triggering cell senescence. Telomeres can be maintained by the enzymatic activity of telomerase, which function to restore and maintain telomeres at their full length. Activation of telomerase is a key mechanism by which some cells, such as cancer cells, evade senescence. Although gene defects occur spontaneously in cells and will lead to programmed cell death, this usually occurs in the immediate generation after the defect is established. Tumor growth does require neovascularization, but the "Hayflick phenomenon" applies to programmed senescence in nontransformed cells.

Answer 1.14. **The answer is C.**

Telomerase is the DNA polymerase that synthesizes the repeating six base pair motif (TTAGGG) that comprises the ends of all chromosomes. It is a nucleoprotein with both a protein and RNA component. With cell division, the telomere ends become progressively shorter until a critical length is reached and programmed cell death is initiated. Synthesizing and repairing the ends of the shortening telomeres allows cells to maintain the integrity of the chromosomal ends and is important for cells that need to divide without reaching senescence such as cancer cells. In light of this, it is not surprising that the majority of cancer cells overexpress telomerase, but there are cancers that appear to have invoked alternative mechanisms to repair telomeres. Indeed, telomerase-deficient (deleted) mice can be induced to develop tumors.

Answer 1.15. **The answer is D.**

FISH is a very useful technique to identify specific known gene rearrangements. It is dependent on DNA probes for previously identified common genetic markers such as BCR-ABL in CML and Her2/neu amplification in breast cancer. Also, probes designed to detect specific chromosomal markers can aid in the identification of grafted cells in transplanted patients. Given the large spectrum of mutations found in p53 in cancers, generating specific probes for all the common mutations of p53 combined with their minute size (single base pair) makes FISH less useful for this application.

Answer 1.16. **The answer is A.**

A metacentric chromosome is characterized by arms nearly equal in size. A number of normal human chromosomes are commonly metacentric, and this morphologic classification has no relevance to the identification of cancer cells except as a descriptive term to aid in karyotyping. Chromosomes that have extremely short arms are acrocentric. Multiple centromeres in a chromosome, an abnormal state resulting from translocations, are described as dicentric (two) or polycentric (multiple).

Answer 1.17. **The answer is D.**

Gene amplification as a mechanism resulting in overexpression of gene products involved in tumorigenesis or tumor progression has been reported in a number of cancers. It is known that N-*myc* amplification in neuroblastoma can be a useful prognostic factor aiding in designing therapy. In small cell lung cancer, c-*myc* amplification has been identified in up to 10% of specimens, a percentage that may rise after treatment. Her2/neu amplification occurs in up to 30% of breast cancers and is useful in predicting response to Her2/neu targeted therapy.

Answer 1.18. **The answer is C.**

Human cancers are largely characterized by complex karyotypes with multiple different populations. In particular, solid tumors such as lung and colon cancer exhibit great heterogeneity that is likely the result of the high level of genomic instability found in cancers. Some less common malignancies such as CML are characterized by the relatively uniform presence of an abnormal karyotype, often with a limited number of detectable breakpoints and translocations. In fact, the presence of a uniform karyotypic abnormality raises the possibility of a germline cytogenetic defect that may be further evaluated by examining the karyotype of noncancerous circulating lymphocytes from the same patient. The absence of any karyotypic abnormality in cancer cell populations is less common but can occur. For example, the presence of a normal karyotype is a well-recognized observation in acute myelogenous leukemia and gives important clinical information conferring an intermediate prognosis. The loss of a single X or Y chromosome is a normal variant commonly observed in older patients. It carries little clinical significance.

Answer 1.19. **The answer is E.**

Homogenously stained regions are found in chromosomes and represented repeated (amplified) genetic elements that are grossly demonstrating a repetitive banding pattern, as may be expected by a repeating genetic sequence. They are found to be more stable than the extrachromosomal circular pieces of DNA called "double minutes." Double minutes lack a centromere and fail to segregate properly with daughter nuclei at meiosis. Homogenously stained regions are commonly identified in cancers and often are associated with amplification of cancer specific genes.

Answer 1.20. **The answer is C.**

The BLAST search engine is the most commonly used Internet tool to identify gene sequences. The BLAST search engine provides a researcher with the capacity to quickly and easily align unknown or known nucleic acid or amino acid sequences with the complete library of catalogued sequences in all reading frames. The caBIG is a tool in development that will allow a wide variety of interactive data sources and services to facilitate both clinical and bench cancer research. In contrast, the cancer Common Ontologic Reference Environment (caCORE) is the existing knowledge "stack" through which the National Cancer Institute supports and translates cancer-related data for the research community. The EVS translates the cancer research overlapping terminologies for caCORE.

Answer 1.21. **The answer is C.**

Using the ENTREZ retrieval system (http://www.ncbi.nlm.nih.gov/Entrez), a user can access a wide variety of publicly held genomic data including GenBank, PubMed, and the BLAST genomic search and alignment tool. A number of other interesting resources are also available at this site, including chromosome maps and information on selected genetic loci associated with disease.

Answer 1.22. **The answer is F.**

Modification of gene expression can occur at many levels. Epigenetic changes are defined as those that are not associated with direct changes in the genetic sequence. Gene amplification, the process by which a specific sequence is repeated abnormally, and missense mutations, in which coding base nucleotides are mis-substituted, are examples of genetic changes. Extra genetic modification of DNA, such as aberrant methylation of DNA or modification of chromosomal histone proteins by unregulated deacetylation, are common examples of epigenetic modifications seen in cancer.

Answer 1.23. **The answer is B.**

Several research groups exploring different aspects of cell cycle control identified p21, a cyclin-dependent kinase inhibitor, independently. One research group used a p53 inducible cell system to identify proteins that were overexpressed in the presence of wild-type (normal) p53. Among the family of cyclin-dependent kinase inhibitors, p21 targets several cyclin-dependent kinases, and its induced expression is a powerful signal to inhibit cell proliferation. This is an important aspect of p53-induced inhibition of cell growth, particularly in the presumed role of p53 as "guardian of the genome."

Answer 1.24. **The answer is C.**

DNA tumor viruses have been known to possess the capacity to transform cells in tissue culture. Following the identification of the *Rb* and p53 tumor suppressor genes, it was found that certain viral antigens bound to these regulatory proteins and inactivated them. For example, the large T antigen of the SV40 virus binds to both wild-type p53 and *Rb* gene products and inactivates them. In a similar manner, the E6 and E7 antigens of HPV (primarily but not exclusively HPV types 16 and 18) inactivate p53 and *Rb* proteins respectively. This is particularly important in cervical cancer where the vast majority of tumors show evidence of HPV16 infection with expression of the E6 and E7 antigens. As evidence of the viral inactivation of these tumor suppressor genes, mutations in p53 and *Rb* are rarely detected in cervical cancer. This is quite different from carcinogen-induced cancers such as lung cancer, where these two tumor suppressor genes are commonly mutated as the mechanism of inactivation. The adenovirus E1a and E1b antigens inactivate the *Rb* and p53 gene products respectively but play no role in cervical cancer.

Answer 1.25. **The answer is A.**

Bcl-2 was identified as the element on chromosome 18 that is overexpressed following translocation with the antibody heavy chain enhancer elements from chromosome 14. This rearrangement of Bcl-2 was first identified in B cell leukemia and B cell lymphomas from which Bcl-2 derives its name. Bcl-2 expression is particularly common among follicular lymphomas but has been identified in a wide spectrum of both solid and liquid tumors. Bcl-2 expression inhibits apoptosis, a property that may allow for perpetuation of malignant clones and relative resistance to cytotoxic therapies. Unlike many oncogenic proteins, overexpression of Bcl-2 is not associated with tumors in transgenic animal models. Translocations of chromosomes 8 and 14 are typical for some aggressive lymphomas but do not directly involve Bcl-2.

Answer 1.26. **The answer is C.**

The disease of retinoblastoma occurs in two forms, hereditary and sporadic. This child demonstrates hereditary retinoblastoma, although there may be no family history of the disease. Hereditary retinoblastoma occurs when the patient inherits an allele from one of the parents that is deleted at the 13q14 locus. This results in the patient having a field defect with all somatic cells missing one locus of the *Rb* gene. The patient then loses the remaining allele in the developing retinal tumor, consequently losing all expression of the pRb protein, leading to unregulated cell growth. Why the developing retina is particularly unstable in the other allele is not completely understood. Because of the field defect nature of hereditary disease, the tumors are usually multifocal in nature, a general phenotype seen in other inherited cancer syndromes. Although this patient certainly has a germline loss of 13q14 in one of the parental alleles, many such cases arise in patients without a family history of the disease. On the other hand, sporadic retinoblastoma is commonly unifocal and arises from the sequential loss of both previously intact 13q14 loci.

Following his studies on the genetics of retinoblastoma, Knudson predicted the nature of the loss of these two alleles in 1971. Based on these studies, he hypothesized that the development of retinoblastoma required the loss of two discrete genetic elements, the so-called "two hit hypothesis." Following the identification of the *Rb* gene, studies involving its deletion in retinoblastoma made it clear that the two events were the losses of both alleles of the *Rb* gene ("two hits"). This two-hit paradigm has become the model for silencing of tumor suppressor genes in both hereditary and spontaneous tumors. A variety of mechanisms, including deletion, mutation, methylation, and viral inactivation, have been found in cancers as methods of inactivating and silencing both alleles of tumor suppressor genes. In retinoblastoma, deletion of the 13q14 locus with associated absence of any protein is by far the most common mechanism of *Rb* silencing. Inactivating missense mutations of *Rb* occur rarely in retinoblastoma, although they are seen in other solid tumors. When present in retinoblastoma, inactivating mutations of *Rb* are often incomplete in their inactivation and result in a syndrome of incomplete penetrance.

Answer 1.27. **The answer is B.**

Germline mutations in PTEN, a phosphatase, account for the relatively rare heritable cancer syndrome called Cowden disease. However, as is often the case with germline mutations associated with hereditary cancer syndromes, tumor specific mutations (not in the germline) of PTEN have been identified in a wide variety of cancers as well. The function of PTEN as a phosphatase targets several phosphorylated molecules for deactivation, most notably Akt and its associated pathway. Li-Fraumeni syndrome, associated with breast cancer and sarcomas, among other cancers, is associated with germline p53 mutations. Mutations in the Ret gene account for familial medullary thyroid cancer, while germline mutations in the APC gene are found in familial adult polyposis syndrome. Familial renal cancers associated with blood vessel proliferation are found in the von Hippel-Lindau syndrome and are caused by mutations in the VHL gene.

Answer 1.28. **The answer is B.**

One of the surprising findings of analysis of the sequenced human genome is the presence of only about 30,000 to 40,000 expressed genes in human cells. However, only a few thousand of these seem to be expressed at any given time. Previous estimates, based on the known approximate size of human chromosomes, were that there were up to 100,000 or more individual genes expressed in human cells.

Answer 1.29. **The answer is E.**

All of genes listed above fulfill the definition of tumor suppressor genes and are associated with familial cancer syndromes. This patient has a standard presentation of hereditary nonpolyposis colon cancer syndrome (HNPCC). These patients generally have germline mutations in one of the DNA mismatch repair genes associated with this syndrome (MSH2, MSH3, MSH6, MLH1, PMS1, or PMS2). MSH2 is one of the most commonly mutated genes in HNPCC. As in many familial cancer syndromes, HNPCC tumors often appear at a relatively young age. The standard criteria for this syndrome include identification of at least two first-degree relatives with the syndrome as well. The tumors are usually in the ascending (proximal) colon. The less common familial adult polyposis cancer syndrome is associated with germline mutation in the APC gene and is associated with multiple polypoid lesions in the colon. Mutations in p53 are associated with Li-Fraumeni syndrome that is manifested by hereditary breast cancer and sarcomas. BRCA2 is mutated in certain familial breast cancer cohorts, while $p16^{INK4a}$ germline mutations are associated with certain forms of familial melanoma.

Answer 1.30. **The answer is A.**

LCM is a powerful tool allowing for identification and selection of individual cells or clusters of cells for harvesting of nucleic acids and potentially other molecules. The power of LCM lies in its exquisite capacity to hone in on specific cells in a tissue section. Samples harvested this way can then be used for analysis utilizing other high throughput technologies such as cDNA microarray (gene expression profiling) and potentially for proteomic analysis by MALDI-TOF combined with two-dimensional gel analysis.

Answer 1.31. **The answer is C.**

The term *oncogene* has been applied to genes that directly mediate cell transformation and proliferation. This can be accomplished through several mechanisms including gene amplification leading to overexpression, mutation to constitutively active forms, or gene rearrangement resulting in increased expression. Loss of function leading to malignancy is a hallmark of tumor suppressor genes. This can occur through several mechanisms as well, including inactivating mutations, chromosomal deletions, and DNA hypermethylation. Replacement or reexpression of tumor suppressor gene function should also reverse the transformed phenotype. The capability of ligands to activate cell growth or migration upon binding to transmembrane receptors is a characteristic of cytokines and growth factors.

Answer 1.32. **The answer is B.**

Chromatin remodeling is an important level of regulation for gene expression. In general, histone acetylation mediated by histone acetyl transferases such as CBP/p300 results in less avid histone wrapping and increased expression. Conversely, HDAC results in gene silencing and appears to be an important level of epigenetic regulation in cancer. In order to exploit this characteristic of many cancers, novel agents, such as depsipeptide (FR901228), that inhibit HDAC inhibitors are now in clinical testing.

Answer 1.33. **The answer is E.**

Phosphorylation of tyrosine residues by tyrosine kinases is an important signal for cell stimulation and cancer growth. Each transmembrane tyrosine kinase is activated by its associated ligand. Increasingly, tyrosine kinases are an important target for novel therapeutics as well. Examples of this class of agents already in common use include both imatinib mesylate (Gleevec) and gefitinib (Iressa). All of the examples listed above are receptor tyrosine kinases except for Akt. Akt is a threonine/serine kinase and a key component of the downstream phosphatidylinositol 3 kinase-signaling pathway through which many of the tyrosine kinases transmit their signaling.

Answer 1.34. **The answer is D.**

Many of the tumor suppressor genes identified have been found to be associated with familial cancer syndromes. The first tumor suppressor gene identified as such, *Rb*, was found to be inactivated in both alleles of tumors found in hereditary retinoblastoma, thus fulfilling Knudson's "two-hit" hypothesis. This same phenomenon has been seen in other familial cancer syndromes such as familial nevoid basal cell carcinoma (PTCH), familial medullary thyroid cancer (Ret), and hereditary non-polyposis colorectal cancer (MLH1). DCC (deleted in colon cancer), on the other hand, has not been identified as being deleted or mutated in germline DNA of familial colon cancer patients. DCC appears to fulfill most of the criteria of a tumor suppressor gene, although its role in the development of colon cancer has been questioned. Nonetheless, many colon cancer tumors have lost expression of DCC, and DCC reexpression appears to inhibit colon cancer cell growth *in vitro.*

Answer 1.35. **The answer is D.**

The Tal-1/SCL gene product is a transcription factor that mediates multilineage hematopoiesis. Inappropriate expression of wild-type Tal-1/SCL is found in T cell acute lymphocytic leukemia. Tal-1/SCL is normally expressed in erythroid and myeloid precursors, but not in T-cells. Tal-1/SCL is an example of a normally occurring transcription factor expressed in an inappropriate context leading to malignancy. In the T-cell leukemias, this mechanism of inappropriate expression of non-mutated transcription factor is the prevailing paradigm for molecular oncogenesis. Gene silencing following allelic deletion or epigenetic silencing is characteristic of tumor suppressor gene inactivation. Activating mutations, such as seen in a variety of cancer-related genes (e.g., *ras* family members, EGFR, Met), are not a characteristic of Tal-1/SCL mediated transformation.

Answer 1.36. **The answer is A.**

It has been known for almost a century that certain viruses can cause malignant transformation. The responsible genetic elements identified in the viral genomes are called viral oncogenes (v-oncogenes). It was found that homologues of these viral oncogenes existed in the eukaryotic genome from which they had likely originated. These normal human genetic elements were given the name protooncogene. One of the first of these, *src,* was identified in the avian Rous sarcoma virus that had been studied as a transforming virus decades earlier. In most human cancers, mutations or aberrant expression of oncogenes have been identified.

Answer 1.37. **The answer is E.**

Mutations of p53 are among the most commonly identified in human cancers. Wild-type p53 has a function in signaling cells with damaged DNA to undergo programmed cell death (apoptosis). In the presence of an inactivating mutation of p53, commonly used genotoxic agents, such as radiation and chemotherapy, may prove less effective with the intact p53 signal. This has been demonstrated in preclinical models and correlates with some human clinical trial data. It must be noted, however, that many common malignancies harboring p53 mutations, such as small cell lung cancer and ovarian cancer, are quite sensitive to chemotherapy and radiation. The capacity of p53 to trigger apoptosis is associated with the cell cycle checkpoints that have been identified as critical nodal moments at which the cell may "choose" to continue to divide or, if sufficiently damaged, progress down a path to cell death and deletion of the potentially damaged clone. Interestingly, p53 mutant transgenic mice are viable and develop normally. However, they have an accelerated rate of tumor formation under certain tumorigenic stimuli.

Answer 1.38. **The answer is C.**

The term *proteome* is generally taken to refer to all potentially expressed proteins encoded by the genome. However, many operational definitions specify only those proteins expressed at a given time or under certain conditions, so answer "A" denotes a relatively common usage of the term as well. Increasingly, the term *proteome* is used in conjunction with a modifier such as "serum," cellular," or even "malignant" to denote a more limited set of conditions. Protonation is a preparative step prior to proteomic evaluation by current means. Most proteomic analyses require cleavage of the proteins in the samples followed by protonation of the resulting peptides prior to MALDI-TOF analysis.

CHAPTER **2**

Molecular Targets in Oncology

JAMES W. WATTERS

Directions Each of the numbered items below is followed by lettered answers. Select the ONE lettered answer that is BEST in each case unless instructed otherwise.

QUESTIONS

Question 2.1. **The correct order of the four phases of the cell cycle is**

A. G_1, G_2, S, M
B. S, G_1, M, G_2
C. G_1, S, G_2, M
D. S, M, G_1, G_2
E. G_1, S, M, G_2

Question 2.2. **D-type cyclins regulate the cell cycle by**

A. activating Cdk2, leading to the initiation of deoxyribonucleic acid (DNA) replication
B. activating Cdk1, causing cells to enter mitosis
C. activating Cdk4/6, allowing progression into S phase
D. inhibiting Cdk1, preventing premature entry into S phase
E. inhibiting Cdk4/6, preventing entry into mitosis

Question 2.3. **E-type cyclins regulate the cell cycle by**

A. activating Cdk2, facilitating entry into S phase
B. activating Cdk1, facilitating entry into M phase
C. activating Cdk4/6, facilitating entry into S phase
D. activating Cdk4/6, facilitating entry into M phase
E. activating Cdk1, facilitating entry into S phase

Question 2.4. **Modes of cyclin-dependent kinase (Cdk) regulation include**

A. temporal expression patterns of activating cyclins
B. activating phosphorylation on the T-loop
C. activation of Cdk activity through binding to INK4 family proteins
D. all of the above
E. A and B only

Corresponding Chapters in *Cancer: Principles & Practice of Oncology,* Seventh Edition: 3 (Molecular Targets in Oncology), 4 (Invasion and Metastases), and 5 (Angiogenesis).

Question 2.5. **One mechanism by which p53 regulates the G_1 DNA damage checkpoint is**

A. p53 is degraded in response to DNA damage, resulting in entry into S phase
B. p53 activates Cdk1 through repression of GADD45
C. p53 inhibits Cdk2 activity by increasing transcription of $p21^{Cip1}$
D. p53 ubiquitinates D-type cyclins in response to DNA damage
E. p53 activates cyclin E1, resulting in rapid progression into S phase

Question 2.6. **The restriction point of the cell cycle occurs in**

A. G_1
B. S
C. G_2
D. metaphase
E. anaphase

Question 2.7. **The retinoblastoma protein, pRb, regulates cell cycle progression by**

A. phosphorylating D-type cyclins, leading to increased cyclin activity
B. forming repression complexes with transcription factors that are critical for S phase entry and progression
C. binding to and inhibiting Ras GTPases, leading to reduced signaling through PI3 kinase
D. ubiquitinating the anaphase inhibitor securin
E. none of the above

Question 2.8. **Which of the following best describes the role of telomerase in cell senescence?**

A. Telomerase gradually degrades the ends of chromosomes (telomeres), leading to progressive telomere shortening and permanent G_1 arrest.
B. Telomerase activates INK4 family proteins, leading to Cdk inhibition and permanent G_1 arrest.
C. Telomerase plays no role in cell senescence.
D. Telomerase replicates the ends of chromosomes, preventing progressive telomere shortening and permanent G_1 arrest.
E. Telomerase activates the anaphase inhibitor securing, preventing progression through M phase.

Question 2.9. **The anaphase promoting complex/cyclosome (APC/C) facilitates the metaphase-anaphase transition by**

A. ubiquitinating anaphase inhibitors, such as securin, targeting them for degradation
B. phosphorylating pRb, inactivating its negative regulatory function, allowing progression into anaphase
C. cleaving INK4 proteins, causing activation of Cdk4/6 and progression into anaphase
D. sequestering cyclin B-Cdk1 in the cytoplasm, preventing premature phosphorylation of anaphase inhibitors
E. activating the kinases Wee1 and Myt1, leading to negative regulatory phosphorylation of Ckd1, preventing premature phosphorylation of anaphase inhibitors

Question 2.10. **Apoptosis is a term used to describe**

A. a genetically programmed and regulated process of cell death
B. the tightly regulated progression through the five phases of mitosis
C. the process of differentiation from a stem cell into a daughter cell
D. necrotic cell death
E. none of the above

Question 2.11. **BAX and BAK function in apoptosis by**

A. sequestering antiapoptotic "BH3-only" proteins in the cytosol, preventing them from inserting into the mitochondrial outer membrane (MOM)
B. phosphorylating and inactivating the proapoptotic protein BAD
C. forming oligomers and inserting into the MOM, resulting in the release of inter membrane space (IMS) proteins such as cytochrome *c*
D. cleaving BID at an unstructured loop, resulting in BID myristoylation and translocation to the mitochondrial membrane
E. none of the above

Question 2.12. **The activity of the BH3-only protein BAD is regulated by**

A. phosphorylation of serine 136 by AKT
B. phosphorylation of serine 112 by PKA
C. sequestration of phosphorylated BAD by 14-3-3
D. dephosphorylation upon exposure to a death stimulus such as the deprivation of survival factors
E. all of the above

Question 2.13. **The BH3-only protein BID regulates apoptosis in the following way.**

A. In response to survival factors, BID is activated via phosphorylation, resulting in the activation of the proapoptotic proteins BAX and BAK.
B. Following cellular exposure to TNFα of FasL, BID targets BCL-2 for destruction via ubiquitination.
C. Following cellular exposure to interleukin-1β, BID targets BCL-2 for destruction via ubiquitination.
D. Following cellular exposure to interleukin-1β, BID is activated via phosphorylation, resulting in the activation of the proapoptotic proteins BAX and BAK.
E. Following cellular exposure to TNFα of FasL, BID is activated by myristoylation, resulting in the activation of the proapoptotic proteins BAX and BAK.

Question 2.14. **FADD recruits __________ to activated Fas, resulting in the activation of effector caspases.**

A. caspase-8
B. TRADD
C. caspase-3
D. c-FLIP
E. TRAIL

Question 2.15. **In addition to the mitochondria, which other cellular organelle(s) serves as an important control point in the intrinsic apoptotic pathway?**

A. Golgi apparatus.
B. Vacuoles.
C. Endoplasmic reticulum.
D. Nucleolus.
E. None of the above.

Question 2.16. **A promising strategy for therapeutic intervention involving apoptosis in cancer is**

A. inhibition of TRAIL signaling via small molecule inhibitors or antagonistic antibodies
B. infusion of TNFα to induce apoptosis in tumors
C. inhibition of signaling through Fas via the administration of an antagonistic antibody
D. inhibition of BCL-2 and other family members via antisense oligonucleotides or small molecule inhibitors
E. inhibition of BAX/BAK activity via small molecule inhibitors or inactivating antibodies

Question 2.17. **In normal somatic human cells, telomeres**

A. prevent the ends of linear chromosomal DNA from being recognized as double-strand DNA breaks
B. serve as attachment points for microtubules during the metaphase-anaphase transition of mitosis
C. serve as a cellular mitotic clock that limits cellular life span via progressive shortening during cell division
D. are synthesized by the telomerase ribonucleoprotein complex in order to solve the "end-replication problem"
E. both A and C

Question 2.18. **Telomere shortening can facilitate carcinogenesis by**

A. Telomere shortening never facilitates carcinogenesis.
B. preventing the occurrence of oncogenic mutations in telomeric repeat sequences
C. facilitating numerous genetic changes necessary for carcinogenesis in early stage cancers that have inactivated telomere checkpoint responses
D. removing binding sites for telomere binding proteins, such as the INK4 family proteins, that are required for cell cycle inhibition
E. none of the above

Question 2.19. **One limitation of small molecules that inhibit the reverse transcriptase (RT) activity of telomerase as cancer therapy is**

A. the rarity of natural compounds and small molecules that have inhibitory activity against the RT activity of telomerase
B. the many off-target effects of all such small molecules identified to date
C. the stabilizing effect of these molecules on the hTERC component of telomerase
D. the significant lag time between inhibition of telomerase activity and cancer cell death
E. the lack of understanding of how such molecules lead to cancer cell death

Question 2.20. **The TRAP assay for hTERT expression is a useful biomarker for cancer because**

A. telomerase activity shows a typical cyclical expression pattern in most cancers
B. normal differentiated cells never express telomerase
C. telomerase activity is detected in 80% to 90% of the most common cancers
D. the high specificity of this test has been sufficiently evaluated for clinical use
E. hTERT activates alternative lengthening of telomeres (ALT) that is typical of most cancers

Question 2.21. **Which of the following strategies for targeting telomeres/telomerase in cancer does NOT exhibit a long lag time between therapeutic intervention and effect on tumor cells?**

A. Hammerhead ribozymes that target the hTERC RNA.
B. Small molecule inhibitors of telomerase RT activity.
C. Compounds that stabilize the formation of the G-quadruplex structure of the telomere.
D. Chemically modified antisense oligonucleotides against hTERC.
E. None of the above.

Question 2.22. **Metastasis is**

A. the process of transformation from normal to malignant cell
B. the spread of cancer cells from primary tumor to distant sites in the patient's body
C. the genetically regulated suicide of premalignant cells that have developed oncogenic mutations
D. reduction of tumor volume caused by high-dose chemotherapy
E. the dedifferentiation of stromal cells into pluripotent stem cells

Question 2.23. **The clonal dominance model of cancer metastasis suggests that**

A. neoplastic cells with metastatic capacity arise within the primary tumor through a process analogous to darwinian selection aided by genetic instability
B. metastases arise from rare, highly metastatic variants within the primary tumor that do not have a selective growth advantage within the primary tumor
C. subclones within primary tumors become dominant due to their ability to recruit angiogenic factors
D. metastases arise from a small number of metastatic variants within the primary tumor that have a selective growth advantage within the primary tumor
E. subclones within primary tumors become metastatic based on anatomic location within the primary tumor

Question 2.24. **Autotaxin is involved in which aspect of metastasis?**

A. Tumor cell motility.
B. Invasion of the basement membrane.
C. Cell-cell adhesion.
D. Cell-matrix interaction.
E. Remodeling of the extracellular matrix (ECM).

Question 2.25. **A mutation in E-cadherin would affect the metastatic process in what way?**

A. By increasing the activity of autocrine motility factor (AMF), conferring tumor cell motility.
B. By preventing degradation of the ECM, inhibiting invasion through the basement membrane.
C. By disrupting cell-cell adhesions, increasing metastatic potential.
D. By increasing expression of CD44, increasing metastatic potential.
E. By decreasing recruitment of angiogenic factors, reducing metastatic potential.

Question 2.26. **One function of the glycogen-synthetase kinase 3β (GSK-3β) is to**

A. phosphorylate E-cadherin, resulting in Ca^{2+} binding and the formation of cell-cell interactions
B. phosphorylate β-catenin, facilitating degradation of β-catenin via the ubiquitin-proteasome pathway
C. phosphorylate the frizzled and disheveled gene products, resulting in their degradation via the ubiquitin-proteasome pathway
D. phosphorylate factors that bind to VCAM-1, resulting in a loss of cell-cell adhesion
E. phosphorylate factors that bind to the cyclin B prompter, repressing its transcription

Question 2.27. **VLA-4 facilitates tumor metastasis by**

A. interacting with free β-catenin, resulting in the binding of β-catenin to the promoter of c-MYC and cyclin D1, causing malignant transformation
B. participating in the degradation of the ECM, leading to invasion through the basement membrane
C. decreasing transcription of cellular integrins, resulting in a loss of cell-cell adhesion and an increase in tumor cell motility
D. participating in tumor cell extravasation via the interaction of circulating tumor cells with endothelial cells expressing VCAM-1
E. both A and C

Question 2.28. **Which of the following best describes the action of focal adhesion kinase (FAK) in regulating tumor invasiveness?**

A. Autophosphorylation of FAK results in the activation of the ERK/MAP kinase signaling pathway, which is linked to the induction of cell migration.
B. FAK phosphorylates the tumor suppressor PTEN, resulting in the downregulation of ERK/MAP kinase signaling.
C. FAK phosphorylates free β-catenin, resulting in its degradation by the ubiquitin-proteasome pathway and a decrease in tumor invasiveness.
D. FAK directly binds to the promoters of c-MYC and cyclin D1, increasing tumor invasiveness.
E. None of the above.

Question 2.29. **The loss of PTEN function would most likely result in**

A. a decreased level of FAK phosphorylation
B. a decreased level of PIP_3 phosphorylation
C. an increased level of cellular phosphatase activity
D. an increased level of FAK and PIP_3 phosphorylation
E. both A and C

Question 2.30. **What is the most likely result of overexpressing MMP-2 in cancer cell lines?**

A. Enhancing metastatic potential via the degradation of PTEN.
B. Enhancing metastatic potential via degradation of basement membrane collagen type IV.
C. Decreasing metastatic potential via degradation of INK4 family proteins.
D. Decreasing metastatic potential via degradation of phosphorylated β-catenin.
E. Enhancing metastatic potential via degradation of phosphorylated β-catenin.

Question 2.31. **The most likely explanation listed below for the ineffectiveness of synthetic MMP inhibitors as a strategy for cancer therapy is**

A. lack of preclinical data supporting the notion that MMPs are involved in the metastatic process
B. the ability of TIMPs to substitute for MMPs when such inhibitors are used
C. MMPs have effects other than the removal of structural barriers to invasion
D. inhibition of MMPs induces an autocrine signaling loop that leads to increased telomerase expression
E. the slow nature of reaction kinetics limits the usefulness of current synthetic inhibitors

Question 2.32. **Angiogenesis is**

A. the process of establishing blood supply
B. the process of forming differentiated daughter cells from pluripotent stem cells
C. the process of malignant transformation from normal cells
D. the cell-cycle dependent production of cyclins to regulate Cdk activity at various phases of the cell cycle
E. none of the above

Question 2.33. **Vascular endothelial growth factor (VEGF) is**

A. an angiogenic molecule secreted by tumor cells that induces neovascularization
B. a molecule secreted by normal stromal cells that results in an increase in the thickness of the endothelial layer
C. an intracellular angiogenic transcription factor that induces the expression of growth-promoting genes in endothelial cells
D. an intracellular protease that cleaves inhibitors of endothelial differentiation
E. a molecule secreted by tumor cells that degrades cadherins

Question 2.34. **Which of the following best describes the relationship between Ang-1, Ang-2, and Tie-2?**

A. The angiogenic molecule Tie-2 can bind to either of the receptor tyrosine kinases Ang-1 or Ang-2.
B. The angiogenic molecule Ang-2 is sequestered in the cytoplasm by Tie-2, preventing binding to the receptor tyrosine kinase Ang-1.
C. The angiogenic molecule Ang-1 is sequestered in the cytoplasm by Tie-2, preventing binding to the receptor tyrosine kinase Ang-2.
D. Ang-1, Ang-2, and Tie-2 are all secreted glycoproteins that act in concert to inhibit angiogenesis.
E. None of the above.

Question 2.35. **A reduction of MMP-2 and MMP-9 in tumor cells and epithelial cells would most likely have which effect on neoplastic angiogenesis?**

A. Increase, as expression of MMP-2 and MMP-9 inhibit angiogenesis.
B. Decrease, as expression of MMP-2 and MMP-9 is associated with active neovascularization.
C. No effect, as MMP-2 and MMP-9 have not been linked to angiogenesis.
D. No effect, as MMP-2 and MMP-9 have antagonistic effects in the regulation of angiogenesis.
E. None of the above.

Question 2.36. **Agents that inhibit the tyrosine kinase activity of the VEGF receptor are attractive cancer therapies because**

A. VEGF receptor is expressed almost exclusively on endothelial cells
B. VEGF receptor is upregulated on tumor endothelium compared to surrounding normal epithelium
C. these agents also demonstrate some activity against other receptors such as EGF receptor or PDGF receptor
D. agents targeting the VEGF ligand/receptor system have shown relatively little toxicity in clinical trials
E. all of the above

ANSWERS

Answer 2.1. **The answer is C.**

The correct order of the cell cycle is GAP1 (G_1), synthetic phase (S), GAP2 (G_2), and mitosis (M). DNA synthesis occurs in a discrete interval called "synthetic phase," or S phase; the preceding phase is known as GAP1, or G_1, and the subsequent phase prior to cell division is known as GAP2, or G_2. Mitosis, or M phase, the most visibly dynamic interval of the cell cycle, occurs after G_2. G_1 follows M and the cycle begins anew.

Answer 2.2. **The answer is C.**

Cyclins are positive regulatory subunits of Cyclin-dependent kinases (Cdks). D-type cyclins activate Cdk4/6 at mid-to late-G_1, resulting in the phosphorylation of pRb, p107, and p130. The phosphorylation of these cell cycle inhibitory proteins by cyclinD-Cdk4/6 results in a loss of their negative regulatory function, allowing progression into S phase.

Answer 2.3. **The answer is A.**

Again, cyclins are positive regulatory subunits of Cdks. E-type cyclins are expressed with high cell cycle periodicity (accumulating in late G_1), and activate Cdk2. Premature expression of cyclin E1 leads to accelerated entry into S phase, demonstrating that E-type cyclins function to facilitate the G_1-S transition. Cyclin A appears to serve a redundant function to E-type cyclins, as cyclin A also accumulates in late G_1 and also activates Cdk2.

Answer 2.4. **The answer is E.**

Temporal expression of activating cyclins and phosphorylation of the T-loop are both mechanisms of regulating Cdk activity. However, binding to INK4 family proteins leads to inhibition of Cdk4/6 activity (not activation) by constraining them in an inactive confirmation. Therefore, A and B are correct but C is incorrect.

Answer 2.5. **The answer is C.**

p53 is a transcription factor that is both activated and stabilized in response to DNA damage. In the context of the G_1 checkpoint, the major transcriptional target of p53 is $p21^{Cip1}$. $p21^{Cip1}$ is a Cdk inhibitor that blocks Cdk2 and possibly Cdk4/6 activity, leading to G_1 arrest. p53 is activated in response to DNA damage. Therefore, C is correct.

Answer 2.6. **The answer is A.**

The restriction point occurs in the G_1 phase in cells that are deprived of an essential nutrient or growth factor. Cells that have passed the restriction point complete the current cell cycle and arrest in the subsequent G_1 interval. While the molecular mechanisms underlying the restriction point are not clear, most malignant cells lack a functional restriction point.

Answer 2.7. **The answer is B.**

pRb is a tumor suppressor that is inactivated via phosphorylation by activated Cdk4/6. pRb forms potent repression complexes with transcription factors that are critical for S phase entry and progression, most notably the E2F family of transcription factors. The E2F binding sequence is found in the promoters of many genes required for DNA replication. Therefore, inhibition of E2F and other transcription factors by pRb effectively blocks S phase entry and progression.

Answer 2.8. **The answer is D.**

Cells are normally restricted to a finite number of cell divisions. Due to the topology of telomeres, progressive telomere shortening occurs with each cell cycle in somatic cells. When sufficient telomere shortening has removed telomere sequences, cells enter into a chronic checkpoint response, characterized by the accumulation of Cdk inhibitors and permanent G_1 arrest. Germline cells express telomerase, which is a specialized replicase that replicates the ends of chromosomes, thereby preventing progressive telomere shortening and preventing senescence.

Answer 2.9. **The answer is A.**

The APC/C is a large complex, consisting of 12 core subunits and two specificity factors (Cdc20 and Cdh1), that acts as a ubiquitin ligase. The APC/C ubiquitinates targets substrates for ubiquitination depending on specificity factor activity. APC^{Cdc20} is active from metaphase until the end of mitosis, whereas APC^{Cdh1} is active during the subsequent G_1 interval. One important target of the APC/C complex is the anaphase inhibitor securin. The ubiquitination of securin targets it for degradation, facilitating the metaphase-anaphase transition.

Answer 2.10. **The answer is A.**

Apoptosis is a highly organized and carefully regulated mechanism of cell suicide utilized to craft development and maintain cellular homeostasis. Apoptosis is characterized by distinct ultrastructural features involving plasma membrane blebbing, volume contraction, nuclear condensation, and endonucleolytic cleavage of DNA. Such features are consistent with an active, regulated process of cell death, unlike necrotic cell death.

Answer 2.11. **The answer is C.**

The multidomain proapoptotic proteins BAX and BAK are critical regulators of the intrinsic pathway of apoptosis operating at the mitochondria and ER. Upon activation by BH3-only proteins, BAX translocates from the cytosol to the mitochondrion and inserts into the MOM, where its oligomerization and permeabilization of the MOM results in the release of proteins such as cytochrome *c* from the IMS. BAK resides in the MOM in viable cells, but is activated following death signals, resulting in oligomerization and release of IMS proteins including cytochrome *c*.

Answer 2.12. **The answer is E.**

The proapoptotic BH3-only molecule BAD is regulated by all of the above mechanisms. Phosphorylation on serines 112 (by PKA) and 136 (by AKT) results in an inactive BAD, which can be bound and sequestered by 14-3-3. In addition, upon exposure to a death stimulus (including the deprivation of survival factors), BAD is dephosphorylated, resulting in the interaction of its BH3 domain with the pocket of antiapoptotic BCL-2/ $BCL\text{-}X_L$. Thus, this single apoptotic molecule has multiple signal transduction pathways regulating its activity.

Answer 2.13. **The answer is E.**

BID connects the death signal through the TNF receptor or Fas to downstream cell death effectors. BID exists in the cytoplasm as an inactive protein. Upon cellular exposure to TNFα or FasL, BID is cleaved in an unstructured loop to expose a new myristoylation site. Myristoylation facilitates the translocation of BID to the mitochondrial membrane, resulting in the activation of the multidomain proteins BAX and BAK. BAX and BAK activation results in the release of cytochrome *c* from the mitochondria and induction of apoptosis.

Answer 2.14. **The answer is A.**

FADD (Fas-Associated DD protein) is an adaptor protein that interacts with activated Fas via the death domain (DD) present on both FADD and Fas. FADD recruits caspase-8 by way of interaction via its death effector domain (DED) in order to activate it, resulting in cleavage of downstream substrates, including effector caspases such as caspase-3.

Answer 2.15. **The answer is C.**

The endoplasmic reticulum (ER) serves as a second gateway for apoptosis, as both antiapoptotic BCL-2 and proapoptotic BAX/BAK can localize to the ER. Ca^{+2} levels appears to be the important factor regulated by these molecules at the ER, as certain death signals rely on an ER Ca^{+2} gateway (i.e., Ca^{+2}-dependent lipid second messengers and pathologic oxidative stress). Many death stimuli engage both the ER and mitochondrial gateways to apoptosis.

Answer 2.16. **The answer is D.**

The activation of apoptosis in cancer cells in an attractive strategy for therapeutic intervention. Inhibition of TRAIL, Fas, or BAX/BAK would all lead to reduced apoptosis. While infusion of TNFα may induce apoptosis in tumors, TNFα infusion has been shown to cause a lethal inflammatory response resembling septic shock. However, inhibitors of BCL-2 and other family members [such as the antisense oligonucleotide G3139 (Genta, San Diego, CA)] have shown encouraging results in animal models and represent a promising approach for the development of cancer therapeutics.

Answer 2.17. **The answer is E.**

Telomeres are specialized nucleoprotein complexes at the ends of linear chromosomes. Telomeres form complex secondary structures involving DNA-DNA, DNA-protein, and protein-protein interactions and serve as a capping structure, preventing the ends of linear chromosomes from being recognized as double-strand breaks. However, DNA polymerase requires an RNA primer for reverse-strand DNA synthesis during S-phase of the cell cycle, resulting in incomplete DNA replication of telomeres during each cell division. This progressive shortening functions as a mitotic clock in normal cells, limiting the number of cell divisions. While telomeres are replicated by telomerase in cells of the germline and in many cancers, telomerase activity is not sufficient to maintain telomeres in normal somatic human cells.

Answer 2.18. **The answer is C.**

Telomere shortening is usually a mechanism to limit the number of cell divisions by forcing cells into telomere-based crisis. However, many early stage cancers deactivate pathways essential for telomere checkpoint responses. Thus, if somatic mutations have inactivated Rb/INK4a/p53-dependent senescence checkpoints, continued growth beyond the Hayflick limit further drives telomere erosion, culminating in cellular crisis with attendant genomic instability. The rare transformed cells that emerge from this process with reactivated telomerase are able to stabilize the genome to a level compatible with cell viability, allowing initiated neoplasms to progress toward a fully malignant phenotype. Thus, telomere shortening serves as a barrier to cancer development in the presence of intact checkpoint response and as a facilitator of carcinogenesis in the absence of checkpoint response pathways.

Answer 2.19. **The answer is D.**

Many natural compounds and small molecules have been identified that have inhibitory activity against the RT function of telomerase. However, for all such compounds, there is a significant lag time (months) between inhibition of RT activity and the time telomeres are sufficiently shortened to achieve a reduction in tumor growth. This lag time could pose economic and logistical challenges for clinical development of these compounds and represent a hurdle to therapy as the median survival of some epithelial tumors is short.

Answer 2.20. **The answer is C.**

The PCR-based TRAP assay telomerase activity is detected in 80% to 90% of human cancers. Therefore, it is a near-universal marker of human cancer, with low or absent expression in most normal somatic cells. In addition, in some cancers in which telomerase activity is upregulated during cancer progression, telomerase activity also correlates with patient prognosis. However, some normal differentiated cells and stem cells in various organ compartments also express telomerase. Therefore, the specificity of this test must be more fully evaluated before wide application in the clinical diagnostic field is likely.

Answer 2.21. **The answer is D.**

Answers A, B, and C all exhibit long lag times between intervention and effect on tumor cell growth. However, second generation antisense oligonucleotides against hTERC, chemically modified to activate the cellular RnaseL system, have been shown to induce apoptosis in telomerase-positive cancer cells within 3 to 6 days. One possible explanation is that this treatment may cause degradation of the core telomerase enzyme, which appears to participate in the capping of telomeres, in addition to its enzymatic activity.

Answer 2.22. **The answer is B.**

Metastasis formation is the spread of cancer cells from a primary tumor to vital organs and distant sites within the cancer patient's body. This process is the result of a complex series of genetic alterations, epigenetic events, and host responses. Metastasis has significant prognostic and therapeutic implications, and targeting the metastatic process is a major focus of development for anticancer therapies.

Answer 2.23. **The answer is D.**

The clonal dominance model of Kerbel suggests that both the clonal progression and metastatic variant models are relevant to the evolution of metastatic tumor cells and are not mutually exclusive. In this model, rare metastatic variants exist within the primary tumor. In addition, cells within the primary tumor with metastatic potential also have a selective growth advantage. Clones with metastatic potential thus overgrow the primary tumor mass and produce metastases. Answer A describes the clonal progression model and answer B describes the metastatic variant model.

Answer 2.24. **The answer is A.**

Autotaxin is a stimulator of tumor cell motility. Autotaxin is a 125-kDa glycoprotein that elicits chemotactic and chemokinetic responses at picomolar to nanomolar concentrations in human tumor cells. Studies suggest that autotaxin has multiple enzymatic activities.

Answer 2.25. **The answer is C.**

E-cadherin is a cell-adhesion molecule that mediates homotypic cell adhesion in epithelial cells. E-cadherin is a single-pass transmembrane protein that is physically anchored to the actin cytoskeleton by cytoplasmic proteins called catenins. Any disruption of the intracellular E-cadherin/catenin complex results in a loss of cell adhesion and an increased likelihood of metastatic disease. E-cadherin function is frequently lost during progression of many cancers, and E-cadherin germline mutations in familial gastric carcinomas predispose individuals to develop malignant cancer.

Answer 2.26. **The answer is B.**

Glycogen-synthetase kinase 3β (GSK-3β) phosphorylates free β-catenin that is released from intracellular adhesion complexes when cell-cell interactions are disrupted. This phosphorylation and interaction with the tumor suppressor protein APC leads to β-catenin degradation via the ubiquitin-proteasome pathway. When APC is inactivated, free β-catenin translocates to the nucleus, where it complexes with transcription factors and upregulates expression of c-Myc and cyclin D1. Thus, GSK-3 β phosphorylation of free β-catenin functions to prevent neoplastic transformation.

Answer 2.27. **The answer is D.**

VLA-4 is an integrin that is normally expressed on leukocytes and functions in mediating the attachment of leukocytes to endothelial cells. VLA-4 is also found on tumor cells in malignant melanoma and metastatic carcinoma, but not in adenocarcinomas. VCAM-1 is a cytokine-inducible receptor for VLA-4 that is expressed on endothelial cells. It is thought that VLA-4 facilitates the interaction of circulating tumor cells with the endothelium prior to tumor cell extravasation by interacting with VCAM-1 that is expressed on the surface of endothelial cells. Therefore, while cell-cell interactions can function to inhibit metastasis, they can also facilitate metastasis in the case of circulating tumor cell extravasation.

Answer 2.28. **The answer is A.**

Autophosphorylation of FAK was one of the first integrin-mediated signaling events to be identified. This autophosphorylation event results in the activation of ERK/MAP kinase signaling via multiple mechanisms, and the activation of this signaling pathway is linked to the induction of cell migration.

Answer 2.29. **The answer is D.**

PTEN is a phosphatase that interacts directly with FAK and modulates its function via dephosphorylation. PTEN is a dual specificity phosphatase that is also capable of dephosphorylating the lipid phosphoinositol 3,4,5 triphosphate (PIP_3). Therefore, loss of PTEN function results in increased phosphorylation and integrin-mediated FAK and PIP_3 signaling, which results in a migratory and invasive tumor phenotype. As PTEN is a phosphatase, only answer D can be correct.

Answer 2.30. **The answer is B.**

Matrix metalloproteinase 2 (MMP-2) was the first MMP to be identified. MMPs participate in the metastatic process via proteolytic remodeling of the ECM, an event that is essential for tumor cell invasion. MMP-2 was identified as an MMP that is secreted from tumor cells that is able to degrade basement membrane collagen type IV (in addition to other proteins, such as the $\gamma 2$ chain of laminin-5, a structural protein in basement membrane). Thus, the overexpression of MMP-2 would be expected to lead to increased degradation of the basement membrane, enhancing invasiveness and metastatic potential.

Answer 2.31. **The answer is C.**

MMPs have been shown to have effects other than the removal of structural barriers to invasion. MMPs can act on other proteins to reveal hidden activities. For example, MMPs can process monocyte chemoattractant 3 (MCP-3), resulting in the conversion of MCP-3 into an agonist that blocks inflammatory cell recruitment. In addition, MMPs have been shown to degrade plasminogen into angiostatin, an inhibitor of angiogenesis. These examples demonstrate that MMPs can have diverse functions beyond ECM remodeling, and these functions may result in a reduction of overall metastatic potential.

Answer 2.32. **The answer is A.**

Angiogenesis is the process of establishing blood supply. The progressive growth of neoplasms and the production of metastasis is dependent on this process. Angiogenesis consists of multiple, sequential, and interdependent steps, involving degradation of local basement membrane and invasion of the surrounding stroma by the underlying endothelial cells in the direction of the angiogenic stimulus.

Answer 2.33. **The answer is A.**

The angiogenic molecule VEGF was initially discovered as a factor secreted by tumor cells into tissue culture medium or ascites fluid *in vivo*. Subsequently, VEGF was isolated as a secreted protein that had selective mitogenic activity for cultured endothelial cells. VEGF is a homodimeric heparin-binding glycoprotein that exists in multiple alternative splice forms and potently induces vascular permeability. The induction of permeability by VEGF allows for the diffusion of proteins into the interstitium on which endothelial cells migrate.

Answer 2.34. **The answer is E.**

Ang-1 and Ang-2 are members of a family of endothelial-cell specific molecules known as angiopoietins. Ang-1 and Ang-2 bind to the tyrosine kinase receptor Tie-2 on endothelial cells. Ang-1 acts as an agonist and is involved in endothelial cell differentiation and inhibition of endothelial cell death. Ang-2 also binds to Tie-2, but this binding event blocks the binding of Ang-1, leading to endothelial cell death and vascular regression. Ang-1 and Ang-2 therefore both bind to Tie-2 but have antagonistic mechanisms of action.

Answer 2.35. **The answer is B.**

High levels of matrix metalloproteinase (MMP-2 and MMP-9) in tissues have been associated with active neovascularization. Inhibitors of MMPs, such as TIMP-2, have been shown to inhibit *in vitro* proliferation and tube formation by endothelial cells. Both TIMP-1 and TIMP-2 have also been shown to suppress *in vivo* angiogenesis. Finally, tumor cells injected into nude mice that lack MMP-9 show decreased angiogenesis. These data indicate that deficiencies in MMP-2 and MMP-9 would lead to reduced neoplastic angiogenesis, and targeting these molecules may be an effective approach to controlling angiogenesis and inhibiting tumor growth.

Answer 2.36. **The answer is E.**

All of the above reasons make targeted inhibition of the VEGF ligand/receptor system an attractive strategy for cancer therapy. The endothelial-specific expression and tumor upregulation make VEGF receptor an attractive target in terms of specificity. The off-target effects of EGF receptor or PDGF receptor (while less than the effect on VEGF receptor) can aid in angiogenesis inhibition, as these molecules can also play a role in angiogenesis. Finally, these agents have shown little toxicity in clinical trials compared to conventional chemotherapy. However, adverse effects have included hypertension, headaches, nausea, proteinuria, and thrombotic events.

CHAPTER 3

Etiology of Cancer

WILLIAM S. JONAS AND FADLO R. KHURI

Directions Each of the numbered items below is followed by lettered answers. Select the ONE lettered answer that is BEST in each case unless instructed otherwise.

QUESTIONS

Question 3.1. **Which of the following is NOT a ribonucleic acid (RNA) virus associated with the development of malignancy?**

A. Human T-lymphotropic virus (HTLV).
B. Human immunodeficiency virus (HIV).
C. Hepatitis C virus (HCV).
D. Hepatitis B virus (HBV).

Question 3.2. **The following are major mechanisms by which retroviruses may participate in the malignant transformation process. Which of the following is the mechanism by which HTLV-1 causes cancer?**

A. Insertional mutagenesis.
B. Protooncogene capture.
C. Control of cell growth via viral proteins that act in *trans.*
D. None of the above.

Question 3.3. **Which of the following is NOT a known transmission route for HTLV-1?**

A. Cell-free blood products.
B. Needle sharing.
C. Breast-feeding.
D. Sexual intercourse.

Question 3.4. **Of the following, which is/are characteristic of adult T-cell leukemia (ATL)?**

A. Hypercalcemia.
B. Lytic bone lesions.
C. Lymphadenopathy.
D. All of the above.

Corresponding Chapters in *Cancer: Principles & Practice of Oncology,* Seventh Edition: 7 (Etiology of Cancer: Viruses), 8 (Etiology of Cancer: Chemical Factors), 9 (Etiology of Cancer: Tobacco Use), and 10 (Etiology of Cancer: Physical Factors).

Question 3.5. **Which of the following malignancies has HIV been found to directly cause?**

A. Kaposi sarcoma (KS).
B. Primary central nervous system (CNS) lymphoma.
C. A and B.
D. None of the above.

Question 3.6. **What percentage of people chronically infected with HCV go on to develop hepatocellular carcinoma (HCC)?**

A. 0.3%.
B. 3%.
C. 10%.
D. 30%.

Question 3.7. **Of those infected with HBV, how many go on to develop chronic infection and viremia?**

A. 5%.
B. 15%.
C. 25%.
D. 40%.

Question 3.8. **Papilloma viruses express their full productive cycle only in squamous epithelial cells.**

A. True.
B. False.

Question 3.9. **Human papillomavirus (HPV) is associated with which cancer?**

A. Liver cancer.
B. Stomach cancer.
C. Cervical cancer.
D. Colorectal cancer.

Question 3.10. **Most people have Epstein–Barr virus (EBV) specific antibody.**

A. True.
B. False.

Question 3.11. **What virus is the cause of oral hairy leukoplakia?**

A. EBV.
B. Herpes simplex virus (HSV).
C. HTLV.
D. HPV.

Question 3.12. **KS is NOT associated with which of the following groups.**

A. Elderly men of Japanese background.
B. Individuals from equatorial Africa.
C. Immunosuppressed organ transplant recipients.
D. Acquired immuno deficiency syndrome (AIDS) patients.

Question 3.13. **The risk for developing KS is equal among all HIV-infected patients.**

A. True.
B. False.

Question 3.14. **KS-associated herpesvirus (KSHV) has been associated with which of the following lymphoproliferative conditions.**

A. Primary effusion lymphoma (PEL).
B. Multicentric Castleman disease.
C. Both of the above.
D. None of the above.

Question 3.15. **Which statement about the development of cancer is NOT correct?**

A. Genetic factors dictate a very high cancer risk for a large percentage of people.
B. The general population carries hereditary susceptibility genes that increase the risk of developing cancer for certain exposures.
C. Most cases of cancer are not single-handedly genetically determined sequela of aging.
D. Cancer is the manifestation of personal and cultural behaviors combined with individually determined hereditary susceptibility genes.

Question 3.16. **Chemicals causing cancer were determined by which of the following.**

A. Documentation of differing organ-specific cancer rates among geographically distinct populations.
B. Changes in cancer frequency among migrating ethnic groups.
C. High cancer rates among specific occupations.
D. All of the above.

Question 3.17. **What is the most likely target for carcinogens?**

A. Cell surface.
B. RNA.
C. DNA.
D. Ribosomes.

Question 3.18. **What is the carcinogen produced by overcooking of meat, poultry, or fish at high temperatures?**

A. Aryl aromatic amines.
B. Aminoazodyes.
C. Heterocyclic aromatic amines.
D. Polycyclic aromatic hydrocarbons (PAHs).

Question 3.19. **Carcinogen targeting of DNA is random.**

A. True.
B. False.

Question 3.20. **Many chemical carcinogens are not able to be demonstrated to be genotoxic.**

A. True.
B. False.

Question 3.21. **Which of the following statements is/are considered fundamental principles underlying current studies of molecular epidemiology?**

A. Carcinogenesis is a multistage process where behind each stage are stages of numerous genetic events.
B. There is a wide variation among individuals in response to carcinogen exposure.
C. A and B.
D. None of the above.

Question 3.22. **A highly penetrant cancer susceptibility gene best describes which one of the following cases.**

A. A sporadic common cancer.
B. A sporadic rare cancer.
C. A familial cancer.
D. An infectious-derived cancer.

Question 3.23. **Which of the following is NOT a carcinogen contained in tobacco smoke?**

A. Polycyclic aromatic hydrocarbons.
B. N-nitrosamines.
C. Aromatic amines.
D. Ethylene glycol.

Question 3.24. **Which of the following industries or agents are suspected of being associated with lung cancer?**

A. Rubber industry.
B. Smoked foods.
C. Aluminum production.
D. Pickled foods.

Question 3.25. **Which of the following is associated with adenocarcinoma of the colon?**

A. Aflatoxin.
B. Asbestos.
C. Cadmium.
D. Tobacco smoke.

Question 3.26. **Which of the following genetic polymorphisms in connection with ethanol is associated with breast cancer?**

A. CYP2A6.
B. Nitroquinone oxoreductase.
C. Alcohol dehydrogenase.
D. Aldehyde dehydrogenase.

Question 3.27. **In the United States, tobacco is responsible for approximately how many deaths each year?**

A. 40,000.
B. 157,000.
C. 440,000.
D. 4,000,000.

Question 3.28. **Which of the following has a causal link to second-hand smoking related deaths?**

A. Infant deaths during pregnancy.
B. Residential fire victims.
C. Drunk driving.
D. A and B.
E. B and C.

Question 3.29. **In which of the following organs is the development of cancer NOT believed to be related to tobacco?**

A. Breast.
B. Kidney.
C. Pancreas.
D. Bladder.

Question 3.30. **At which of the following organ sites is smoking believed to have a protective effect?**

A. Brain.
B. Endometrium.
C. Breast.
D. Ovary.

Question 3.31. **Which of the following hematologic malignancies is most related to smoking?**

A. Acute lymphoblastic leukemia (ALL).
B. Chronic lymphocytic leukemia (CLL).
C. Acute myeloid leukemia (AML).
D. Multiple myeloma.

Question 3.32. **Which of the following ethnic groups have been found to have the highest rate of smoking?**

A. Alaskan natives and American Indians.
B. Asians and Hispanics.
C. Blacks.
D. Whites.

Question 3.33. **Of the following, which is associated with a higher rate of smoking?**

A. Government employee.
B. College education.
C. White-collar career.
D. Lower income status.

Question 3.34. **Which of the following is NOT a usual withdrawal symptom for those quitting smoking?**

A. Depression.
B. Headache.
C. Increased energy.
D. Increased appetite.

Question 3.35. **The acronym that the US Public Health Service has issued regarding the treatment of nicotine dependence is known as which of the following.**

A. CAGE.
B. The 5 A's.
C. MONA.
D. APLES.

Question 3.36. **Which of the following is a useful strategy for tobacco control?**

A. Increased tax on tobacco purchases.
B. Mass media antitobacco campaigns.
C. Reduced costs of smoking-cessation programs.
D. Workplace smoking restrictions.
E. All of the above.

Question 3.37. **Which of the following is NOT known to increase risk of cancer for an individual?**

A. Cell phones.
B. Ionizing radiation.
C. UV light.
D. Asbestos.

Question 3.38. **Ionizing radiation comes from which of the following sources.**

A. Naturally occurring from plants and soils.
B. Building materials derived from naturally occurring rocks.
C. Cosmic rays.
D. Diagnostic imaging procedures.
E. All of the above.

Question 3.39. **Radiation has been used to treat which of the following.**

A. Enlarged thymus glands.
B. Enlarged tonsils.
C. Tinea capitis.
D. All of the above.

Question 3.40. **Which of the following cancers has NOT been linked to increased risk following radiation exposure?**

A. ALL.
B. AML.
C. Chronic myelogenous leukemia (CML).
D. CLL.

Question 3.41. **What is the expected latent period for the development of leukemia following radiation exposure?**

A. 2 years.
B. 4 to 8 years.
C. 5 to 10 years.
D. 20 years.

Question 3.42. **What group of patients has been found to be at an increased risk of radiation-induced cancer?**

A. Women undergoing screening mammographies.
B. Women undergoing a single diagnostic mammographic procedure.
C. Children undergoing computer tomography (CT) scans.
D. Elderly smokers undergoing CT scans.

Question 3.43. **The risk of cancer as a result of radiation is greatest in which of the following.**

A. A single acute high level exposure such as a WWII A-bomb survivor.
B. Exposure accumulated over many years, such as a radiologist.

Question 3.44. **Individuals exposed to radon are at an increased risk for which of the following cancers.**

A. Lung cancer.
B. Stomach cancer.
C. Liver cancer.
D. All of the above.

Question 3.45. **The common link among individuals who are at higher risk for spontaneous cancer based on genetic susceptibility is the finding of having defects in known tumor suppressor genes.**

A. True.
B. False.

Question 3.46. **In examining secondary cancers after radiotherapy of the prostate, the highest level of observed increased risk was in which of the following.**

A. Sarcomas.
B. CLL.
C. Lung cancer.
D. AML.

Question 3.47. **The risk of secondary leukemia in long-term survivors of Hodgkin disease appears mainly associated with which of the following.**

A. Chemotherapy.
B. Radiation.
C. Age of the patient.
D. All of the above.

Question 3.48. **What is the annual approximate incidence of skin cancer?**

A. 10,000.
B. 100,000.
C. 500,000.
D. 1,000,000.

Question 3.49. **Which of the following is NOT considered a risk factor in developing skin cancer?**

A. Location where living.
B. Dark pigmentation.
C. Occupation.
D. Inability to tan.

Question 3.50. **People with xeroderma pigmentosum have a higher risk of skin cancer because they are defective in nucleotide excision repair (NER).**

A. True.
B. False.

Question 3.51. **There is an increased risk of skin cancer when exposure to UV radiation is followed by ionizing radiation.**

A. True.
B. False.

ANSWERS

Answer 3.1. **The answer is D.**

HTLV and HIV are both RNA retroviruses. HTLV appears to directly contribute to the development of ATL, while HIV and HCV, a flavivirus, likely contribute to the development of malignancy in a more indirect manner. In HIV-infected persons, non-Hodgkin lymphoma (Burkitt, immunoblastic, and primary CNS), KS, and cervical cancer are all AIDS-defining illnesses. HCV and HBV, which is a DNA virus, are risk factors for the development of HCC.

Answer 3.2. **The answer is C.**

Slowly transforming viruses alter gene expression by random integration of a provirus within or adjacent to cellular protooncogenes (insertional mutagenesis). Direct physical disruption of a gene or effects of viral promoters and enhancers on cellular gene expression can lead to a malignant phenotype in infected cells; however, most proviral integrations have no effect on the phenotype of the infected cell and, with the exception of rare cases of T-cell malignancy that appear to involve a monoclonal expansion of an HIV-1–infected cell, have not been shown to cause malignancy in humans. Acutely transforming retroviruses have incorporated into their genomes viral oncogenes derived from cellular protooncogenes (protooncogene capture) and subsequently transferred these altered or deregulated oncogenes into newly infected cells, thus leading to development of a malignant phenotype; however, there are no known acutely transforming human retroviruses. Finally, *trans*-acting retroviruses alter cellular gene expression and function and, consequently, the control of cell growth and differentiation genes. This is illustrated by HTLV-1, the only human retrovirus known to directly cause cancer. Given the fact that the sites of proviral insertion are random for HTLV-1 and that the virus does not appear to encode a host-derived oncogene, tumorigenesis, which appears to be a multistep process, is implicated with the Tax protein being central to transformation. Tax is a transregulating protein which promotes viral gene expression by indirectly activating the viral promoter in the long terminal repeat (LTR) via interaction with cellular transcription proteins. Tax also appears to play a critical role by direct interaction with cellular proteins involved with (in addition to transcription) cell cycle regulation, cell proliferation, and apoptosis.

Answer 3.3. **The answer is A.**

HTLV-1 is known to cause ATL. Transmission occurs by needle sharing, breast-feeding, sexual intercourse, and blood transfusion, but not cell-free blood products. HTLV-1 carriers have an estimated lifetime risk of developing ATL of around 3% to 5% with a latency period from time of infection to development of malignancy of 30 to 50 years. Therefore, it appears simple infection is insufficient to cause malignancy and other factors are necessary for transformation. The average age of onset is 58 years old with a slight male predominance of 1.4:1. Tumor cells are known to aggressively infiltrate multiple organs including the lymph nodes, liver, spleen, skin, and lungs. Either a leukemic or a non-Hodgkin T-cell lymphoma presentation may predominate with leukemic cells presenting with characteristic lobulated ("flower") nuclei morphology.

Answer 3.4. **The answer is D.**

Characteristics of ATL may include hypercalcemia, elevated lactate dehydrogenase levels, cutaneous leukemic infiltrates, lytic bone lesions, lymphadenopathy, and liver or spleen lesions. Laboratory characteristics include HTLV-1 sero-positivity, negative TdT staining, and CD4 positivity.

Answer 3.5. **The answer is D.**

HIV is unique in that it can infect nondividing cells. It also has extreme genetic variability because of the lack of proofreading ability of reverse transcriptase during reverse transcription, resulting in a high mutation rate. There is little evidence, however, that HIV is directly oncogenic. There are reports of insertional mutagenesis resulting in T-cell lymphoma; however, this disease does not occur disproportionately in HIV-infected individuals. In HIV-infected persons, non-Hodgkin lymphoma (Burkitts, immunoblastic, and primary CNS), KS, and cervical cancer are all AIDS-defining illnesses. In addition, anal squamous cell carcinoma is commonly seen in AIDS patients. Many of the cancers common to AIDS patients are associated with infection by DNA viruses; these include the associations of KS with human herpesvirus-8, non-Hodgkin lymphoma and EBV, and cervical and anal squamous cell carcinoma with human papilloma virus.

Answer 3.6. **The answer is B.**

HCV infection is a well-established risk factor for the development of HCC; however, its role in oncogenesis is likely indirect. HCV is transmitted by blood transfusions, contaminated needles, perinatally, sexual routes, and unknown in about 10% of cases. It is estimated that there are 3 million people chronically infected in the United States. HCV is associated with HCC in 50% to 70% of cases in Italy, Spain, and Japan compared with only 30% of cases in the United States. Following initial infection, about 25% of patients develop acute clinical hepatitis. HCV infection is chronic in 50% to 80% of cases; 60% to 70% of these will develop chronic hepatitis. From this group, 20% will progress to cirrhosis. Of patients with chronic HCV, approximately 1% to 5% will develop HCC. Of those with cirrhosis, 1% to 4% are expected to develop HCC each year. After initial HCV infection, there is an approximate 10- to 20-year period prior to the development of cirrhosis and a 20- to 30-year period prior to the development of HCC. It appears HCC largely develops indirectly as a result of the cellular turnover occurring during the inflammatory responses that lead to hepatocyte destruction, regeneration, and fibrosis characteristic of cirrhosis. This is supported by the observation that alcohol consumption or co-infection with HBV greatly increases the relative risk for developing HCC. There are no proven effective screening methods for HCC, and the only curative therapies include resection of tumors or liver transplantation.

Answer 3.7. **The answer is A.**

HBV is a DNA virus classified as a member of the hepadnavirus family. Primary HBV infection produces either a subclinical infection or acute liver injury, but irrespective of the clinical manifestations, 95% of infections resolve, with clearance of virus and the induction of lasting immunity. Five percent have chronic infection, in which most cases of HBV-associated HCC fall. In fact, patients with the highest levels of viremia display the highest risk of HCC. This is consistent with the finding that HCC largely develops as a result of the cellular turnover during the inflammatory response. Proliferation increases the opportunities for replicative errors. HCC risk is increased in every condition that provokes chronic liver injury. There are implications from laboratory research to suggest a role for a direct genetic contribution to HCC by HBV.

Answer 3.8. **The answer is A.**

The papilloma viruses induce squamous epithelial and fibroepithelial tumors in their natural hosts. These viruses have a specific tropism for keratinocytes and express their full productive cycle only in squamous epithelium. In squamous epithelium, the basal cell is the only cell normally capable of supporting cellular DNA synthesis and cellular division and, therefore, the virus must infect the basal cell in order to induce a lesion that can persist.

Answer 3.9. **The answer is C.**

Worldwide, there are approximately 500,000 cases of cervical cancer diagnosed a year with 250,000 attributed deaths. In the United States, because of effective screening, there are about 12,000 new cases a year with approximately 4,000 deaths. Risk factors include sexual promiscuity, an early age of onset of sexual activity, poor sexual hygienic conditions, and women whose partners have had multiple sexual partners. In studies, HPV-16 and HPV-18 have been demonstrated in approximately 70% of cervical carcinomas. There are around 25 different HPVs associated with genital tract lesions, and a causal role for HPV infections has been documented; the association is present in virtually all cervical cancer cases worldwide. It is clear, however, that HPV infection is not alone sufficient for the development of cervical cancer. Only a small fraction of those individuals infected by a specific HPV will eventually develop cancer, and the latency interval between infection and invasive cancer can be several decades. The recognition that other factors are involved in the development of cervical cancer suggests that HPV may work synergistically with other factors of which smoking is one. Research is ongoing regarding HPV and cancers in other squamous epithelium due to HPV's predilection for squamous epithelium.

Answer 3.10. **The answer is A.**

Most people have EBV-specific antibody. However, Africans with Burkitt lymphoma (BL), Chinese with anaplastic nasopharyngeal carcinoma, and people from the United States, Europe, and South America with Hodgkin disease frequently have higher EBV antibody titers. The role of EBV in malignancies was identified through a series of observations including posttransplant patients on high levels of immunosuppression who developed primary EBV infection that sometimes progressed to fatal EBV-infected B-lymphoproliferative disease; children with X-linked, severe combined immunodeficiency (SCID), or sporadic immune deficiencies also were found to develop EBV-positive malignant lymphoproliferative diseases (LPD).

Answer 3.11. **The answer is A.**

EBV is the cause of oral hairy leukoplakia, a wartlike lesion found on the tongue of HIV infected people or transplant patients. The lesions disappear in response to suppression with acyclovir.

Answer 3.12. **The answer is A.**

KS has long been known as an uncommon and indolent tumor of elderly Mediterranean and African men. The KS associated with these groups does not have an associated immune deficiency. More recently, KS has been recognized to occur at higher frequency in immunosuppressed organ transplant recipients and AIDS patients.

Answer 3.13. **The answer is B.**

KS risk is highest in homosexual men with untreated AIDS. Of these individuals, 20% to 30% will develop KS in the course of their disease if they remain untreated. Patients who contracted AIDS through blood transfusions, however, will have a 1% to 2% chance of developing KS, and it is even smaller in pediatric AIDS patients. This is what led to the search for a sexually transmitted cofactor and the virus known as KS-associated herpesvirus (KSHV) or human herpesvirus 8. KSHV sequences are present in virtually all KS tumors regardless of HIV status. The presence of KSHV, however, is not believed sufficient for KS development as, for example, 5% to 7% of the United States population is infected with KSHV.

Answer 3.14. **The answer is C.**

KSHV/HHV 8 has been associated with the rare B cell lymphoma known as PEL and with multicentric Castleman disease. PEL presents often as ascites and tumors in the pleural and peritoneal cavities often without clinically evident lymphadenopathy or bone marrow involvement. PEL cells are uniformly latently infected with KSHV. Castleman disease is a poorly understood lymphoproliferative syndrome that can occur in both HIV-positive and HIV-negative patients. The HIV-positive forms always appear associated with KSHV, while only about half of the HIV negative forms appear associated with KSHV.

Answer 3.15. **The answer is A.**

Genetic factors dictate a very high risk of developing cancer for those with hereditary cancer syndromes; however, this is only for a small group. Genetics are a factor for the development of cancer influenced by personal and cultural behavior. Such behaviors include tobacco use; occupation and associated work exposures such as vinyl chloride, aromatic amines, and benzene; and diets including overcooked meat and high quantities of fish.

Answer 3.16. **The answer is D.**

The extent to which chemical exposures contribute to the incidence of cancer was not well defined until population-based studies examined differing cancer rates among geographically distinct populations, changing cancer frequency among migrating ethnic groups, and high cancer rates among specific occupations. These results have been used to modify risk by limiting lifestyle, environmental, and work exposures.

Answer 3.17. **The answer is C.**

Genotoxic carcinogens have high chemical reactivity or can be metabolized to highly reactive intermediates. They form covalent adducts with macromolecules and target DNA in the nucleus and mitochondria. Genotoxic carcinogens may transfer simple alkyl or complexed (aryl) alkyl groups to specific sites on DNA bases, of which the following are examples: N-nitroso compounds, aliphatic epoxides, aflatoxins, polycyclic aromatic hydrocarbons and other combustible products of fossil fuels, and vegetable matter. Aryl aromatic amines, aminoazodyes, and heterocyclic aromatic amines transfer arylamine residues to DNA.

Answer 3.18. **The answer is C.**

Heterocyclic aromatic amines are produced by overcooking meat, poultry, or fish at high temperatures. They have been associated with breast and colon cancer. Individuals are exposed to PAHs from tobacco smoking. Dye workers and tobacco smokers are exposed to aryl aromatic amines; these have been associated with bladder cancer.

Answer 3.19. **The answer is B.**

The targeting of carcinogens to particular sites in DNA is determined by nucleotide sequence, by host cell, and by selective DNA repair processes putting some genetic material at greater risk than others.

Answer 3.20. **The answer is A.**

A number of chemicals, most noticeably pesticides and herbicides, have not been demonstrated to be genotoxic but have been demonstrated to cause cancer at high doses and for a prolonged exposure. The mechanisms by which these chemicals cause cancers are controversial.

Answer 3.21. **The answer is C.**

These two statements are fundamental principles which must be understood to comprehend current studies of molecular epidemiology. The first is that carcinogenesis is a multistage process involving numerous genetic events. Considering the presence of multiple genetic insults, a specific risk factor is difficult to isolate and limits statistical power. Second, predicting individual response is difficult given that models can only hope to approximate a mean of a population among which there are expected susceptible and resistant groups.

Answer 3.22. **The answer is C.**

The study of gene-environment interactions is complicated by a wide variability in risk largely influenced by its penetrance. A highly penetrant cancer susceptibility gene can cause familial cancers and accounts for less than 1% of all cancers. Low penetrant genes cause common sporadic cancers. A genetic polymorphism is a genetic variant present in at least 1% of the population.

Answer 3.23. **The answer is D.**

PAHs, N-nitrosamines, aromatic amines, ethylene oxide, and 1,3-butadiene are among the more than 20 carcinogens among the 3,500 chemicals contained in tobacco smoke.

Answer 3.24. **The answer is C.**

Smoked, pickled, and salted foods are all associated with gastric adenocarcinoma cancer. Exposures in the rubber industry are also associated with gastric adenocarcinoma cancer as well as leukemia and lymphoma. Aluminum production, coal gasification, hematite mining, and paint are all examples of industrial causes of lung cancer. Tobacco, arsenic, asbestos, crystalline silica, benzo(a)pyrene, beryllium, bis(chloro)methyl ether, 1,3-butadiene, chromium VI compounds, coal tar and pitch, nickel compounds, soots, and mustard gas are known agents believed associated with lung cancer as well.

Answer 3.25. **The answer is B.**

Asbestos and heterocyclic amines are suspected carcinogens associated with colon cancer. Aflatoxin, vinyl chloride, tobacco smoke, alcoholic beverages, and thorium dioxide are suspected carcinogens associated with HCC and hemangiosarcoma. Cadmium is associated with adenocarcinoma of the prostate.

Answer 3.26. **The answer is C.**

There is a growing list of genetic polymorphisms, defined as a genetic variant present in at least 1% of the population, that confer a higher rate of carcinoma in conjunction with various substrates. Alcohol dehydrogenase, in the presence of ethanol, is associated with oral cavity, liver, and breast cancer. Currently, there are two polymorphisms that are known that determine detoxification of alcoholic beverages. The other is aldehyde dehydrogenase, which has only been associated with liver cancer. CYP2A6, when combined with the tobacco smoke N-nitrosamines, is associated with lung cancer. Nitroquinone oxoreductase is a functional polymorphism which is found to be linked with leukemia in those exposed to benzene.

Answer 3.27. **The answer is C.**

In the United States, tobacco, chiefly through cigarette smoking but also through smoking pipes and cigars and smokeless tobacco, is responsible for an approximate death toll of around 440,000. Not all of these deaths are attributable to cancer as a full one third are linked to cardiovascular disease. The number of cases linked to secondhand smoke is around 40,000. The number 157,000 represents the annual mortality related to lung cancer. Worldwide, the World Health Organization estimated the number of deaths linked to tobacco was 4,000,000 in 1998.

Answer 3.28. **The answer is D.**

There are approximately 40,000 deaths annually of nonsmokers attributed to smoking. Secondhand smoke accounts for 38,000 deaths. There are an additional 1,000 infant deaths related to smoking during pregnancy and a further 1,000 deaths as a result of residential fires attributed to smoking.

Answer 3.29. **The answer is A.**

Tobacco is currently linked to the development of eight organ site cancers including oropharyngeal, laryngeal, esophageal, lung, stomach, pancreatic, kidney, and bladder. Recently, data support that tobacco is associated with cervical cancer, colorectal cancer, liver cancer, and acute leukemia. Additional sites suspected, but not enough data are present, include cancer of the adrenal gland, gall bladder, genitals, nasal cavity, and sinuses. Tobacco has not been demonstrated to be related to the following cancers: brain, breast, ovary, skin, and testicular, in addition to soft tissue sarcomas, childhood malignancies, and Hodgkin disease.

Answer 3.30. **The answer is B.**

Smoking has been found to have a small protective effect from the development of endometrial cancer. This is believed due to the fact that smokers are thinner and have lower serum estrogen levels than nonsmokers. Tobacco has not been found to have an effect on the development of cancers of the brain, breast, or ovary. Smokers have also been found to have slightly lower cases of thyroid cancer, for which the mechanism remains unclear.

Answer 3.31. **The answer is C.**

Smokers have been found to have a 30% to 50% increased risk of AML. Benzene, a chemical found in cigarettes, is believed to be the culprit. Smoking has not been demonstrated to increase the risk for ALL, CLL, or multiple myeloma.

Answer 3.32. **The answer is A.**

According to the National Health Interview Survey for 2000, Alaskan natives and American Indians had the highest rate of smoking at 36%, followed by whites, 24%; blacks, 23%; Hispanics, 19%; and Asians, 14%.

Answer 3.33. **The answer is D.**

Controlled for gender and race, people of lower income are more likely to smoke. When looking at education, women who have not completed high school are three times more likely to smoke than women with a college education. The gap in smoking rate is believed to be widening between white-collar and blue-collar workers, with a higher rate for the blue-collar workers.

Answer 3.34. **The answer is C.**

Withdrawal symptoms often reported include cravings, depression, irritability, fatigue, sleeping difficulties, headache, and increased appetite. Increased appetite can lead to weight gain, which is a reason often cited as to why women are less successful in quitting than men.

Answer 3.35. **The answer is B.**

The 5 A's include: ask (identify smokers), advise patients to quit, assess whether they are willing to try, assist with a plan to quit, and arrange follow-up. The three forms of treatment available, which are beneficial in combination, include (a) counseling, not just by the doctor, but also in group sessions; (b) nicotine replacement, available in the following approved 5 forms: gum, patch, lozenge, inhaler, and nasal spray; and (c) the antidepressant bupropion. The CAGE questions are helpful in identifying those who abuse alcohol. Morphine, oxygen, nitroglycerine, and asprin (MONA) is an acronym for the treatment of chest pain, and APLES is used to assist with the International Prognostic Index, which is used to further clarify lymphoma staging.

Answer 3.36. **The answer is E.**

All of the above have been demonstrated to be effective in smoking cessation as well as smoking prevention.

Answer 3.37. **The answer is A.**

Ionizing radiation, UV light, and asbestos are all agents for which there is clear evidence that exposure will lead to an increased risk of cancer. The amount of exposure required to increase risk is important as forms of the above are frequently encountered. Cell phones are being investigated for posing a risk for brain cancer, although a link has not been clearly established.

Answer 3.38. **The answer is E.**

Background exposure refers to the naturally occurring radiation we are all exposed to, which varies depending on where we live. There is a greater level of exposure to cosmic rays at higher altitudes and closer to the equator. Plants, soils, and rocks contain naturally occurring radioisotopes of which one is radon. In the northeastern United States, radon is often tested for when buying a new home. Building materials contain these radioisotopes. The most significant man-made exposure occurs in medical procedures, including diagnostic imaging, nuclear medicine, and therapeutic procedures.

Answer 3.39. **The answer is D.**

Radiation has been used to treat enlarged thymus glands, enlarged tonsils, tinea capitis, ankylosing spondylitis, and peptic ulcers. The patients in these groups have been studied to help determine the quantification of risk as a function of dose. Patients treated with radiation for these disorders have been observed to develop leukemia, thyroid cancer, breast cancer, and stomach cancer.

Answer 3.40. **The answer is D.**

Acute lymphocytic leukemia, acute myelogenous leukemia, and chronic myelogenous leukemia are sensitive to the effects of ionizing radiation, whereas the link does not exist between ionizing radiation and chronic lymphocytic leukemia or Hodgkin disease.

Among solid tumors, cancers of the thyroid gland, female breast, and lung cancer are the most sensitive. Evidence also suggests an increased link exists for the development of cancers of the salivary glands, colon, stomach, liver, ovary, bladder, esophagus, and CNS. Skin cancer is also in this category of risk, most of them being basal cancers, with less evidence for a dose-related increase in squamous cell skin cancer or malignant melanoma.

Answer 3.41. **The answer is B.**

Depending on dose, leukemia can develop as early as 2 years after exposure; however, the peak incidence is between 4 and 8 years. After 11 years, the risk of leukemia returns close to baseline. Solid tumors undergo a much longer latency period. While it is possible for solid tumors to appear after 5 years, most do not appear until at least 10 years have passed, and it is not uncommon for the latent period to exceed 20 years. It is also not established that the exposed patient's risk ever returns to baseline; therefore, it is prudent to assume the individual remains at increased risk for the remainder of his or her lifetime.

Answer 3.42. **The answer is C.**

Currently, the risk associated with mammograms is not well defined, and it is believed the low dose from a single procedure is below the level for which direct-linked risks can be established. Pediatric CTs, however, expose the patient to an estimated radiation dose of 10 to 15 times the dose of a mammogram, putting this procedure in the level where there is evidence for an increased risk of cancer. The higher doses combined with evidence that children are more sensitive to radiation-induced cancer (estimates suggest young children may be 10 to 15 times more sensitive than middle-aged adults) is the leading thought for reconsidering the need for procedures as there is evidence for a small, but significant increase in the rate of leukemia in children who undergo at least two CT scans. There is not enough data, however, to link screening mammography, CT scans in adults, or exposure from a single procedure with an increased risk of cancer.

Answer 3.43. **The answer is A.**

There are epidemiologic studies establishing a 2 times greater risk of developing cancer in those who received a single acute exposure compared with lower level exposure over the course of many years. In experimental models, at low doses of radiation, the risk appears to be a linear function, whereas at high levels the risk increases more rapidly as a function of the square of the dose. Extrapolations suggest that upon linear models there is a 10% increased risk over normal risk per Sv of exposure.

This means if a person's background risk were 10%, it would increase to 11% for a 1 Sv exposure. As an example, a screening mammogram has an approximate mean ionizing exposure of 0.003 Sv.

Answer 3.44. **The answer is A.**

Radon is a gas that comes from naturally occurring rocks and soil. The spontaneous decay of radon results in electrically charged particles that attach to dust particles that can be inhaled and deposited in the lung. Underground miners, who have been exposed to high levels of radon, have been observed to have a higher risk of lung cancer.

Answer 3.45. **The answer is A.**

Studies have demonstrated increased risks for radiation-induced osteosarcoma and soft tissue sarcoma in patients with the hereditary form of retinoblastoma. Patients with basal cell nevus carcinoma syndrome have been found to be at an increased risk for basal cell carcinoma and ovarian tumors in the irradiated field. Also, patients with Li-Fraumeni cancer syndrome appear to be at an increased risk for radiation-induced cancer. What these all have in common are defects in genes known to be tumor suppressor genes, the retinoblastoma gene, the human homologue of the patched gene, and the p53 gene, respectively.

Answer 3.46. **The answer is A.**

The highest risk was for the development of sarcomas and cancer of the bladder and rectum following local radiotherapy. After radiation, two groups of secondary cancer risks should be considered. First is the development of sarcomas in, or adjacent to, a heavily irradiated treatment field (the risk appears small in low-dose fields). Second is the development of carcinomas in tissues and organs at a distance from the treatment site. CLL is not associated with an increased risk following radiation.

Answer 3.47. **The answer is A.**

Chemotherapy appears to be the main risk in the development of secondary leukemia. While it is difficult to identify one causative drug, as patients receive combination chemotherapy to treat Hodgkin disease, it appears that the risk is conferred by alkylator therapy. The risk has decreased almost to normal with the switch from mechlorethamine, oncovin (vincristine), procarbazine, and prednisone (MOPP) therapy to the combination of adriamycin (doxorubicin), bleomycin, vinblastine, dacarbazine (ABVD) therapy. The role of radiation in the development of secondary leukemia in Hodgkin patients is controversial.

Answer 3.48. **The answer is D.**

There are in excess of 1,000,000 new cases of nonmelanoma skin cancers each year, of which 80% are basal cell carcinomas and 20% are squamous cell carcinomas. The mortality for nonmelanoma skin cancers is low. There were around 54,000 cases of malignant melanoma last year with over 7,000 of these resulting in death.

Answer 3.49. **The answer is B.**

Skin cancer is more frequent in regions with high ambient solar radiation (the closer to the equator one lives), and increased risk exists in the following: light pigmentation, inability to tan, propensity to burn, history of sunburns, and cumulative exposure to UV radiation. Malignant melanoma appears to be more related to a history of acute sunburn rather than accumulated dose. A history of five or more sunburns as an adolescent appears to double the risk for malignant melanoma.

Answer 3.50. **The answer is A.**

Individuals with xeroderma pigmentosum are extremely sensitive to sunlight and have a high risk of developing skin cancer. People with xeroderma pigmentosum have been found to have a defective mechanism of NER. NER is the repair pathway that removes cyclobutane pyrimidine dimers produced in DNA by exposure to UV light and repairs the damaged site.

Answer 3.51. **The answer is B.**

Studies and some epidemiologic data suggest that ionizing radiation can initiate skin cancers that can be subsequently promoted by chronic UV light exposure. The reverse as stated in the question does not hold true.

CHAPTER 4

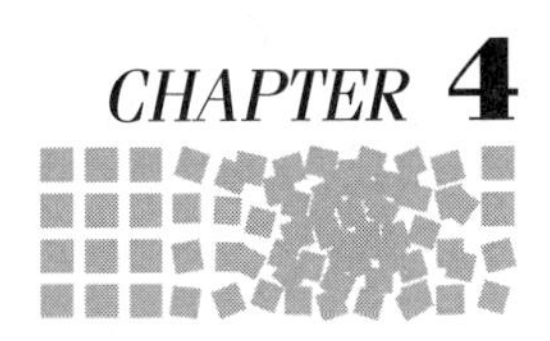

Epidemiology of Cancer

MARTIN J. EDELMAN

Directions Each of the numbered items below is followed by lettered answers. Select the ONE lettered answer that is BEST in each case unless instructed otherwise.

QUESTIONS

Question 4.1. **Epidemiologic studies can take which of the following basic forms?**

A. Observational studies.
B. Nutritional studies.
C. Experimental studies.
D. Developmental studies.
E. A and C.
F. None of the above.

Question 4.2. **Prevalence of a disease is**

A. the amount of a disease
B. the number of cases of a disease
C. the number of cases of a disease each decade divided by the total population
D. the number of cases of a disease in a specified period of time divided by the total population

Question 4.3. **Incidence of a disease is**

A. the amount of a disease
B. the number of cases of a disease
C. the number of new cases of a disease each decade divided by the total population
D. the number of new cases of a disease in a specified period of time divided by the total population

Corresponding Chapters in *Cancer: Principles & Practice of Oncology*, Seventh Edition: 11 (Epidemiology of Cancer).

Question 4.4. **Surveillance Epidemiology and End Results Program (SEER) provides data on new cancer cases in the United States. The SEER data base includes**

A. the entire US population
B. sites selected on the basis of demographics
C. sites selected on the ability to collect high quality population-based reporting systems as well as representation of epidemiologic significant subgroups
D. sites in representative states with appropriate demographic groups

Question 4.5. **Incidence rates of trends for diseases frequently have to be adjusted. Which of the following are reasons why comparing incidence rates of disease in different countries without adjustment could be misleading?**

A. Different numbers of men and women.
B. Different age structures.
C. Cohort effects.
D. All of the above.

Question 4.6. **The following types of studies utilize the individual rather than the population as the basis for analysis EXCEPT**

A. cross-sectional studies
B. cohort studies
C. case control studies
D. ecologic studies

Question 4.7. **Which of the following is a limitation of cross-sectional studies?**

A. Populations must be observed over time.
B. Assesses prevalent cases rather than incident cases.
C. Difficult to establish proper control groups.
D. Does not assess general health status of the population.

Question 4.8. **For many years it was thought that the San Francisco Bay area was an epicenter of breast cancer, and some proposed that there were particular environmental risks in that area. However, a more thorough analysis ultimately demonstrated that the population studied was at a higher risk for breast cancer as a result of known risk factors (parity, age at first pregnancy, age at menarche, etc.). What was the cause of the apparent increased risk?**

A. Information bias.
B. Selection bias.
C. Confounding variables.

Question 4.9. **Popular media frequently discuss the possibility that people have a certain percentage risk of developing cancer. This statistic, while of some use, has a significant problem in that it**

A. underestimates the risk for different ages
B. underestimates the risk for year of birth
C. overestimates the risk for individuals with risk factors
D. overestimates the risk for individuals without risk factors

Question 4.10. **An investigator in Minnesota wishes to evaluate the long-term effects of dietary fat intake on the risk of prostate cancer. To do so, he designs a trial that follows all the men in one city over a 20-year period. The men are periodically questioned regarding their health and prior to entry are screened for and excluded if they have elevated prostate specific antigen (PSA) or a prior history of prostate cancer. This is an example of a(n)**

A. case control study
B. interventional study
C. cohort study
D. prospective case control study

Question 4.11. **Advantages of case control studies over cohort studies include all the following EXCEPT**

A. cost
B. susceptibility to bias
C. speed

Question 4.12. **Dr. Bush wishes to determine the relationship between cancer and religious observance in the population of his city. He asks the members of his bible study class (consisting of other medical oncologists) to provide the number of patients in their practices with cancer who regularly attend services and those who do not. He then totals the numbers and finds that there are fewer patients with cancer amongst the observant patients than the nonobservant and concludes that religious observance results in a decrease in cancer risk. This is an example of**

A. selection bias
B. information bias
C. both
D. neither

Question 4.13. **There has been a growing interest in the use of computer tomography (CT) scans to screen for lung cancer. It is conceivable that "earlier detection" of lung cancer may not lead to improved outcomes. For example, a patient may undergo a scan and be diagnosed in 2004 and then dies in 2007. Alternatively, if he were not screened and developed symptomatic disease in 2006 and then died in 2007, there really would be no difference in outcome even though it would appear that survival had increased from 1 year to 3 years. This is an example of**

A. selection bias
B. length time bias
C. information bias
D. lead time bias

Question 4.14. **Dr. Ghoul in Transylvania is interested in the prevalence of vampirism. To screen for cases, he throws a party (at night, of course) and invites all the adults. He screens for cases by evaluating only those who avoid the shrimp scampi (lots of garlic). What problem does this study suffer from?**

A. Selection bias.
B. Lead time bias.
C. Information bias.
D. Length time bias.

Question 4.15. **Molecular biology has changed the nature of medical research, including epidemiology. In addition to the usual issues of study design and sample size, which of the following issues must also be addressed?**

A. Consent.
B. Storage procedures.
C. Assay standards.
D. All of the above.

ANSWERS

Answer 4.1. **The answer is E.**

Experimental studies evaluate the effects of various interventions on an outcome. One example is the influence of a program of smoking cessation on the occurrence of lung cancer. Observational studies do not involve any manipulation of the study population. They may focus on the distribution of a disease (descriptive), while analytical studies focus on the determinants of a disease.

Answer 4.2. **The answer is D.**

Prevalence describes the total number of cases of a disease in a population during a given period of time.

Answer 4.3. **The answer is D.**

Incidence describes the number of new cases that occurred in the population during a specified time period. The population is the population at risk. While this may include the entire population (i.e., the number of new cases of acquired immuno deficiency syndrome (AIDS) worldwide), it can also be defined as the population in a defined geographic area (e.g., the United States) or in a particular group (e.g., homosexuals).

Answer 4.4. **The answer is C.**

The SEER data base covers approximately 26% of the US population and is selected on the ability of sites to collect and report data as well as demographics.

Answer 4.5. **The answer is D.**

Sex and gender clearly influence the incidence of several nonsex specific diseases. For example, until recently women had a much lower incidence of lung cancer due to less tobacco use. After World War II, as smoking increased in women, the incidence of lung cancer increased as well. Cancer is a disease of aging, and populations with a younger population would appear to have a lower incidence of cancer unless adjusted. Cohort effects refer to the influence of year of birth rather than age on the occurrence of a disease.

Answer 4.6. **The answer is D.**

Ecologic studies utilize groups of people as the basis for analysis.

Answer 4.7. **The answer is B.**

The cross-sectional design provides a "snapshot" of the population. Therefore, it is good at assessing the general health status of the population. The assessment is done at a particular point in time. Control groups are not utilized in this type of analysis (case control design). The major limitation of this type of design is that it is poor for assessing etiology. For example, if a disease is rapidly fatal in most cases, the prevalent cases (which may be patients with indolent disease) may not be representative in terms of etiology as compared with the overall population with the disease.

Answer 4.8. **The answer is C.**

The result was appropriate for the population; no bias was introduced. However, there were confounding variables due to the nature of the population studied.

Answer 4.9. **The answer is D.**

The probability of developing cancer is estimated for the entire population. For cancers with clearly defined risk factors, this may severely overestimate the risk for people who do not have those risk factors and underestimate the risk for people with those specific factors. For example, mesothelioma is almost exclusively diagnosed in individuals with asbestos exposure. An individual who worked in an asbestos mine is at many times the risk of the population, while an individual with no known exposure has a far lower risk.

Answer 4.10. **The answer is C.**

A case control study would evaluate existing prostate cancer cases and controls without prostate cancer and evaluate dietary fat intake. A prospective case control study would enroll cases as they occur and then match to a control without the disease. A cohort study is a prospective design that follows a group of individuals without disease at the outset.

Answer 4.11. **The answer is B.**

Case control studies are inherently more susceptible to bias than cohort studies.

Answer 4.12. **The answer is C.**

The study described has several potential biases. First, the patients seen by these physicians may be inherently different from the population at large (selection bias). Second, the information was collected from the physicians, who may or may not be aware of their patients' actual level of observance (information bias).

Answer 4.13. **The answer is D.**

The earlier detection (lead time) did not change outcome. Selection and information bias refer to the selection of cases in studies. Length time bias results from the great opportunity to discover indolent tumors by screening than their more aggressive counterparts, resulting in an apparent survival advantage.

Answer 4.14. **The answer is A.**

The study suffers from possible misclassification of the variable (i.e., selection bias). It is quite possible that part of the local population simply does not like garlic but does not suffer from vampirism. Alternatively, it is conceivable that the vampire adheres to dietary restrictions prohibiting the consumption of shellfish.

Answer 4.15. **The answer is D.**

Studies of molecular epidemiology introduce a number of unique issues. First, consents must be properly worded. There are frequent regulatory requirements for patients to be allowed to "opt out" of such a study or to recover a specimen if they change their minds. In addition, specimens are frequently run after conclusion of accrual, an event that may occur years after collection. In addition, the specific methods of assay, including controls among other things, must be established.

CHAPTER 5

Principles of Surgical Oncology

REBECCA L. AFT AND NIRMAL K. VEERAMACHANENI

Directions Each of the numbered items below is followed by lettered answers. Select the ONE lettered answer that is BEST in each case unless instructed otherwise.

QUESTIONS

Question 5.1. **A 35-year-old female requires central venous access for chemotherapy. The best anesthetic choice for inserting a Port-a-Cath is**

A. topical anesthesia
B. local anesthesia
C. local anesthesia with a field block
D. peripheral nerve block

Question 5.2. **A 32-year-old man presents with a 2-year history of a lump on his left buttock. On examination, he has a firm nodule in his left buttock, approximately 4 cm in size. The mass appears to be in the subcutaneous tissue but is not freely mobile. The patient has no associated neurologic findings. The next appropriate step in management is**

A. obtain magnetic resonance imaging (MRI)
B. perform fine needle aspiration
C. perform core biopsy
D. perform incisional biopsy
E. perform excisional biopsy
F. perform complete excision with wide margin

Question 5.3. **Which of the following patients would most likely benefit from surgical resection?**

A. A 42-year-old woman has a sister with breast cancer diagnosed at age 38. The patient had a breast biopsy for abnormal mammographic finding which revealed lobular carcinoma *in situ* (LCIS).
B. A 52-year-old overweight man has a history of gastroesophageal reflux treated with proton pump inhibitors. Upper endoscopy was performed and revealed high-grade Barrett dysplasia.
C. A 46-year-old man was diagnosed with ulcerative colitis in his teens. The patient undergoes regular surveillance colonoscopy and has evidence of dysplasia on his last colonoscopy.
D. A 22-year-old woman whose father and great uncle were treated for medullary thyroid carcinoma.
E. All of the above.

Corresponding Chapters in *Cancer: Principles & Practice of Oncology*, Seventh Edition: 12 (Principles of Surgical Oncology).

Question 5.4. **An 87-year-old patient presents for right colon resection after evaluation for microcytic anemia revealed a 3-cm villous adenoma in his cecum. The adenoma was not able to be resected endoscopically, but biopsy revealed dysplastic changes. Computer tomography (CT) of the abdomen and chest x-ray did not provide evidence of metastatic disease. Which of the following statements is true?**

A. Surgery should be avoided in this patient due to the prohibitive morbidity and mortality in this octogenarian.
B. The patient's past medical history and physical examination are the best determinants of preoperative risk.
C. The patient requires a cardiac stress test and possible cardiac catheterization prior to surgical resection.
D. No additional testing besides routine labs is required.

Question 5.5. **A 45-year-old woman with previously diagnosed metastatic pancreatic adenocarcinoma presents with a 4-day history of nausea and nonbilious emesis. She has just initiated chemotherapy with gemcitabine. She has previously had a common bile duct stent placed. CT scan of the abdomen reveals dilated loops of bowel and possible transition point with nondilated bowel in the pelvis. There is a moderate amount of ascites in the abdomen. The appropriate management includes**

A. nasogastric tube decompression and IV hydration OR placement of percutaneous gastrostomy tube for palliation
B. open gastrostomy for palliation
C. exploration of the abdomen with possible bowel resection and bypass of the area of obstruction
D. exploration of the abdomen with possible bowel resection and bypass of the area of obstruction, as well as pancreaticojejunostomy and choledochojejunostomy

Question 5.6. **A 36-year-old woman with T3N1 rectal cancer is undergoing chemoradiation therapy treatment prior to definitive resection. A diverting colostomy with mucous fistula had been performed 6 weeks previously and is functional. The patient began chemotherapy 2 weeks ago and now presents with a fever of 38.9°C, nausea, and vague abdominal pain. Colostomy output had increased and is essentially liquid. On examination, the patient is thin, mildly tachycardic, with orthostatic change, and has decreased skin turgor. A right subclavian central venous catheter is present. The patient has no abdominal distension, but has right lower quadrant tenderness on palpation. The patient's clinical syndrome is most likely due to**

A. line infection
B. infectious diarrhea
C. abdominal viscous perforation
D. typhlitis

Question 5.7. **The benefits of laparoscopy are**

A. reduction in postoperative pain
B. decreased healing time
C. decreased adhesion formation
D. all of the above

Question 5.8. **The decrease in cardiac indices and ejection fraction observed in laparoscopic procedures is due to**

A. the increased requirement for anesthetic agents during laparoscopic types of procedures
B. vasodilation due to CO_2 in the pneumoperitoneum
C. decreased venous return and increased transmitted intrathoracic pressure

Question 5.9. **When compared with wound site recurrences observed with open surgery, port site recurrences in laparoscopic surgery for malignancy are**

A. significantly more
B. significantly less
C. almost the same
D. not known

Question 5.10. **A 55-year-old man with a several month history of hemoccult positive stools has recently been diagnosed with gastric cancer by upper endoscopy. Staging CT demonstrates no evidence of intraabdominal disease. You recommend a staging laparoscopy prior to definitive resection because**

A. CT has a high false-negative rate in the staging of some cancers
B. carcinomatosis and peritoneal seeding is more accurately diagnosed with laparoscopy
C. nontherapeutic laparotomies can be avoided in over 20% of patients after staging laparoscopy
D. biopsy techniques including percutaneous Tru-Cut, wedge biopsy, and cup forceps allow tissue to be easily obtained for pathologic analysis
E. all of the above

Question 5.11. **The most common cause of postoperative death following surgery for cancer is**

A. wound infection and sepsis
B. pulmonary complications
C. stroke
D. cardiac arrhythmia

Question 5.12. **When compared with younger patients, the postoperative mortality rate for elderly patients (over 70 years of age) is**

A. slightly higher
B. significantly higher
C. significantly lesser
D. no change

ANSWERS

Answer 5.1. **The answer is C.**

Field block refers to injection of local anesthetic by circumscribing the operative field, which would be the most appropriate method to anesthetize the skin for a Port-a-Cath insertion. Topical anesthesia refers to the application of local anesthetics to the skin or mucous membranes. Local anesthesia involves injecting anesthetic agents directly into the operative field. Peripheral nerve block results from the deposition of a local anesthetic surrounding major nerve trunks.

Answer 5.2. **The answer is A.**

Sarcoma must be considered in the differential diagnosis of soft tissue masses. Imaging by MRI can provide information on size, tumor characteristics, and relationship to adjacent structures. Subsequent tissue sampling is essential to obtain a diagnosis.

Answer 5.3. **The answer is E.**

All four patients could be candidates for prophylactic surgery. The major risk factors for a woman to develop breast cancer include family history of breast or ovarian cancer, a personal history of breast tissue atypia, or prior diagnosis of LCIS. Prophylactic mastectomy is appropriate in patients with known genetic mutations or multiple risk factors. Indication for esophageal resection includes high-grade Barrett esophagus dysplasia. In patients with only Barrett metaplasia, antireflux surgical therapy may be indicated *if* reflux can be demonstrated. The indications for prophylactic surgery in ulcerative colitis include the presence of dysplasia or carcinoma. Germline mutations for MENIIa can be assessed by screening for *ret* oncogene mutations. In the event the genetic mutation is detected, prophylactic thyroidectomy and total parathyroidectomy with partial reimplantation outside the neck can be done.

Answer 5.4. **The answer is B.**

Given that physiologic age does not always correlate with chronologic age, surgery in the elderly population should be decided on a case-by-case basis. Approximately half of surgical morbidity is attributed to perioperative cardiac events. The American College of Cardiology has defined an algorithm to estimate risk and the need for preoperative testing. Risk is stratified based on the intrinsic risk of the procedure, the patient's cardiac history, and the exercise tolerance of the patient. High-risk procedures carry a risk of cardiac morbidity greater than 4% (noncarotid vascular surgery, thoracic procedures, abdominal procedures, major head and neck procedures, and emergent procedures). Intermediate risk procedures (1% to 4% risk of cardiac morbidity) include carotid surgery, radical prostatectomy, and orthopedic procedures. Low-risk procedures (<1% risk) include breast surgery and soft tissue biopsies. Patient risk factors include history of congestive heart failure (CHF), diabetes, prior myocardial infarction (MI), angina, and ventricular arrhythmia. These patients should undergo some form of preoperative risk assessment with cardiac stress testing prior to high-risk surgery.

Answer 5.5. **The answer is A.**

Palliative care versus aggressive therapy must be tempered by the understanding of the biology of the malignancy, the expected life expectancy of the patient, the time to recovery, and the risk of complication. This patient has a bowel obstruction most likely due to metastatic pancreatic cancer. The poor nutritional status and presence of ascites indicates a high risk of complication and probable prolonged recovery. The best method of palliation in this situation is placement of a nasogastric tube or percutaneous gastrostomy tube to prevent emesis with IV hydration.

Answer 5.6. **The answer is D.**

Neutropenic enterocolitis (typhlitis) is characterized by fever, diarrhea, and right lower quadrant pain. It is caused by a transmural inflammation of the cecum and often the ileum. While the exact etiology is unclear, neutropenia is often found. Predisposing conditions include mucosal injury due to cytotoxic agents and myelosuppression due to chemotherapy. The differential diagnosis does include infectious diarrhea and radiation-induced enteritis. CT imaging of the abdomen is the most sensitive and specific method for diagnosis. Treatment is nonoperative and comprised of bowel rest and broad spectrum antibiotics.

Answer 5.7. **The answer is D.**

All of the above are the beneficial effects of laparoscopy. This is attributed to the use of small incisions and lack of retractors holding the incision open. In addition, exposure to CO_2 contributes to a diminished acute phase systemic response, which likely leads to decreased inflammation and pain.

Answer 5.8. **The answer is C.**

During laparoscopic colectomies, the mean arterial pressure, central venous pressure, and systemic vascular resistance are found to increase significantly. Cardiac index and ejection fraction decease. In animal models, significant pressure gradients are found along the iliac veins and vena cava, which is a direct result of decreased venous return and increased transmitted intrathoracic pressure.

Answer 5.9. **The answer is C.**

Retrospective reviews have demonstrated a wound site recurrence rate of less than 1% in patients undergoing surgery for colon cancer. Port site recurrence rates for a similar population of patients have been reported to be approximately 1%. Port site metastases have been associated with aerosolization caused by the pneumoperitoneum, tumor manipulation, and the degree of tumor burden.

Answer 5.10. **The answer is E.**

One of the most important aspects of laparoscopic staging is the exclusion of patients from undergoing a major operation by identifying metastatic or unresectable disease, such as carcinomatosis, which is easily missed on imaging studies. Undetected metastatic disease has been found in 13% to 57% of patients initially staged with having no metastatic disease with conventional imaging. However, laparoscopy is not yet performed as a routine procedure since many patients are often symptomatic and require palliative resection.

Answer 5.11. **The answer is B.**

The five most common causes of death following surgery are bronchopneumonia, congestive heart failure, myocardial infarction, pulmonary embolism, and respiratory failure. Perioperative pulmonary complications are therefore a major threat.

Answer 5.12. **The answer is B.**

In a study of the postoperative mortality of 17,199 patients undergoing general surgical procedures, the overall mortality rate of patients younger than age 70 was 0.25%, as compared with 9.2% for patients older than 70. The operative mortality rate for emergency operations was even higher in elderly patients for elective surgical procedures (36.8% versus 7.8%). The four leading causes of operative mortality in this age group were pulmonary embolism, pneumonia, cardiovascular collapse, and the primary illness itself.

CHAPTER **6**

Principles of Radiation Oncology

HAK CHOY AND L. CHINSOO CHO

Directions Each of the numbered items below is followed by lettered answers. Select the ONE lettered answer that is BEST in each case unless instructed otherwise.

QUESTIONS

Question 6.1. **Which of the following is NOT true about ionizing events in tissues due to x-rays?**

A. Radiation dose describes the quantity of energy deposited per mass of tissue.
B. The fast electrons produced by high-energy x-ray photons can damage deoxyribonucleic acid (DNA) by a direct action.
C. Indirect action of ionizing radiation where hydroxyl radicals damage target tissues is not commonly seen.
D. The relative biological effectiveness (RBE) describes the ratio of doses required to yield an equivalent biologic event.

Question 6.2. **Which of the following statements describes the DNA damage from ionizing radiation?**

A. It is the single-stranded breaks of the DNA that is thought to represent the lethal event.
B. The majority of radiation-induced double-stranded breaks are rejoined in cells within 2 hours.
C. There is essentially no difference between double-stranded rejoining and DNA repair.
D. The efficiency of DNA rejoining is not related to the cell's ability to survive the standard radiotherapy (2 Gy).

Question 6.3. **Which of the following statements describes the dose-related cellular response to radiation?**

A. The term D_0 describes the slope of the exponential survival curve, and it represents a dose required to reduce the surviving fraction to 37%.
B. Both mammalian cells and bacterial cells display "shoulder" in the low-dose region.
C. In mammalian cells, there is generally a linear relationship between the cell killing and the dose given.
D. In general, postirradiation conditions that accelerate the cell division are the ones most favorable to repair of potentially lethal damage.

Corresponding Chapters in *Cancer: Principles & Practice of Oncology*, Seventh Edition: 13 (Principles of Radiation Oncology).

Question 6.4. **Which of the following statements is NOT true regarding molecular responses to radiation-induced cellular injury?**

A. The signaling/surveillance proteins ATM and ATR appear to have central roles in the response pathways.
B. Phosphorylation of p53 is predominantly ATM-dependent following radiation damage, whereas ATR performs it after UV-induced damage.
C. The protein p53 appears to have a minor role in activation of apoptosis and cell cycle arrest following DNA damage.
D. Ionizing radiation damage activates a number of signaling pathways that may contribute to lethality independent of DNA damage.
E. Irradiation leads to induction of tumor necrosis factor (TNF) α protein expression.

Question 6.5. **Nonirradiated cells can express all of the following responses after radiation damage to neighboring cells EXCEPT**

A. gene induction
B. induction of genomic instability
C. differentiation
D. changes in apoptotic potential
E. double-stranded breaks in DNA

Question 6.6. **Which of the following describes the specific pathways for the repair of double-strand DNA breaks?**

A. The repair may be by homologous recombination (HR) or nonhomologous end-joining (NHEJ) pathway.
B. The HR repair pathway functions by degrading the single strand at each side of the break and then annealing the two ends.
C. The nonhomologous end-joining pathway functions by replicating the missing genetic information from the homologous DNA template.
D. NHEJ is a minor component of mechanism for repair of double-stranded DNA breaks in mammalian cells.

Question 6.7. **Which of the following statements describes the role of oxygen in radiation effects?**

A. A greater dose of radiation is required for cell killing in an oxic condition compared to a hypoxic condition.
B. The oxygen enhancement ratio (OER) has more relevance on the exponential portion of the cell survival curve.
C. A randomized trial showed that epoetin β improved survival in patients with head and neck cancer.
D. Oxygen need not be present at the time of irradiation for oxygen enhancement of radiotherapy to occur.
E. Hyperbaric oxygen often shows a dramatic increase in curability with standard fractionated radiotherapy.

Question 6.8. **Which of the following statements describing interaction of chemotherapy and radiotherapy is FALSE?**

A. Radiation appears to increase the cellular uptake of platinum drugs and increase the number of platinum intermediates.
B. Hydroxyurea preferentially kills cells in the radio-resistant phase of the cell cycle (M phase).
C. Paclitaxel is thought to synchronize tumor cells in the G2/M phase.
D. Some chemotherapy can recall irradiated volumes by erythema on the skin or by producing pulmonary reactions.

Question 6.9. **Which of the following statements is NOT true regarding modulation of radiation by hyperthermia?**

A. Localized heat treatment can be delivered with microwaves, ultrasound, or radiofrequency sources of energy.
B. The temperature 42.5°C appears to be critical, with small increments above this temperature leading to a steep increase in lethality.
C. The lethality of hyperthermia is thought to be in part from denaturation of proteins.
D. Similar to radiation-induced kill, lethality from heat is most pronounced when cells are in the G2/M phase.

Question 6.10. **Which of the following statements is an INCORRECT description of the interaction of x-rays with biologic material?**

A. In photoelectric effect, an incoming x-ray transfers all its energy to an inner orbit electron, which is ejected from the atom. A photon is produced as an outer shell electron fills the vacant hole.
B. In Compton scattering, energy from the x-ray is both absorbed and scattered. The photon emerges with reduced energy and a change in direction.
C. In pair production, an electron and a positron are produced.
D. In modern treatment with greater than 4 MeV photons, photoelectric effect dominates the interaction.

Question 6.11. **Which of the following statements describes the depth dose characteristics of radiation?**

A. Higher energy photons deposit more dose to the skin surface.
B. Depth of maximum dose increases as the energy of the incident beam increases.
C. For a given energy, electrons generally penetrate deeper in tissue compared to photons.
D. Electron beams deposit less dose to the skin surface as the incident electron energy increases.

Question 6.12. **Which of the following best describes the modern linear accelerator?**

A. A modern linear accelerator (linac) can deliver energies up to 1 MeV.
B. The focal point of the gantry's rotation is called the *field edge.*
C. The ^{60}Cobalt teletherapy unit is a megavoltage machine that relies on radioactive cobalt to produce an electron beam.
D. Unlike the linacs, the ^{60}Cobalt unit is always "on" and must be kept in shielded position until the beam is needed for treatment.

Question 6.13. **The following statements describe proton beams and neutron beams used for therapy EXCEPT**

A. a neutron beam is notable for its characteristic *Bragg peak*
B. charged particles such as protons can be accelerated by an electric field
C. neutrons have no charge and interact in matter mainly by generating recoil protons
D. proton beams in the range of 50 to 500 MeV have been used

Question 6.14. **Which of the following best describes the treatment planning process?**

A. Immobilization is not important since it does not add to accuracy.
B. At the time of image acquisition for planning, tumor motion due to respiration must be determined.
C. 3D dose distribution in each patient is easily measured.
D. Intensity modulated radiation therapy (IMRT) cannot control the shaping of the dose distribution.

Question 6.15. **Which of the following statements is NOT true regarding brachytherapy?**

A. Relative to external beam energies, the emitted spectra are of low energy.
B. High doses can be delivered within a few centimeters of the source.
C. Isotopes with properties of very long half-lives and high energy are used for permanent implants.
D. Half-life is the time required for half of the initial number of nuclei to decay.

Question 6.16. **Which of following statements best describes the tissue effects from radiation?**

A. Early or acute effects typically occur within months following irradiation.
B. The frequencies of late effects depend very strongly on radiation fraction size.
C. Large α/β ratio has a small "shoulder" in the low-dose portion.
D. Typical human tumors and early-responding normal tissues have a small α/β ratio.

Question 6.17. **Which of the following statements is FALSE regarding independent events (4 R's) that occur during fractionated radiotherapy?**

A. Repair explains the shoulder of the radiation survival curve showing that cells can repair some of the radiation damage.
B. Redistribution explains migration of cells away from an irradiation source.
C. Repopulation refers to spontaneous repopulation and induced cell proliferation or recruitment of cells after irradiation.
D. Reoxygenation explains how the proportion of hypoxic cells present in a tumor return to preradiation level.

Question 6.18. **Which of the following best describes the concept of altered fractionation?**

A. Hyperfractionation refers to a radiotherapy schedule that utilizes multiple daily treatments more than 6 hours apart with reduced fraction size and increased number of fractions.
B. Accelerated fractionation does not reduce the overall treatment time.
C. A Radiation Therapy Oncology Group (RTOG) 9003 randomized trial showed that standard fractionation treatment was superior to hyperfractionation and accelerated fractionation with concomitant boost used for advanced head and neck squamous cell carcinomas.
D. Continuous hyperfractionated accelerated radiation therapy (CHART) gives a higher total dose than the standard fractionated treatment.

ANSWERS

Answer 6.1. **The answer is C.**

All other statements are true. The indirect effects of x-rays predominate the biologic effects seen with x-rays. The photons cause ejection of fast electrons. The ejected fast electrons can directly damage the DNA (direct action) or, more commonly, the fast electrons interact with plentiful water molecules to produce hydroxyl radicals (OH^-), which in turn can damage the biologic target (indirect action).

Answer 6.2. **The answer is B.**

Although single-stranded and double-stranded breaks are observed from ionizing radiation, it is the double-stranded breaks that are thought to represent the lethal event. Although the majority of the radiation-induced, double-stranded breaks are rejoined in cells within 2 hours after exposure, the process can continue for 24 hours. The DNA repair refers to the correction of the DNA to the original genetic codes, whereas the double-stranded rejoining refers to the joining of the DNA without regard to the original genetic sequence. The efficiency of rejoining of DNA after radiation exposure has been correlated with the portion of cells surviving treatment with 2 Gy.

Answer 6.3. **The answer is A.**

D_0 is related to the slope of the exponential survival curve, and it represents a dose that is required to reduce the surviving fraction to 0.37 or 37% of the original population. The smaller D_0 represents more radiosensitivity. Mammalian cell lines display a "shoulder" in the low dose region and the exponential relation at higher doses. The "shoulder" represents a reduced efficiency of cell killing. The linear quadratic model rather than the linear model best describes the cellular response to radiation. The postirradiation conditions that suppress the cell division are the ones most favorable to potentially lethal damage repair.

Answer 6.4. **The answer is C.**

Phosphorylation of p53 is predominantly ATM-dependent following radiation damage, whereas ATR performs it after UV-induced damage. The protein p53 appears to have a key role in activation of apoptosis and cell cycle arrest following DNA damage. The chemical inhibitor of p53, α-pifithrin, has been shown to protect mice from lethal doses of total body radiation. Ionizing radiation damage activates a number of signaling pathways that may contribute to lethality independent of DNA damage. An example includes activation of sphingomyelinase, which hydrolyzes plasma membrane derived sphingomyelin and produces ceramide. Ceramide can promote apoptosis. Radio resistance can be seen in cells that are sphingomyelinase deficient. Irradiation leads to a rapid activation of the TNFα receptor and induction of TNFα protein expression.

Answer 6.5. **The answer is E.**

The responses of nonirradiated cells appear to be cell-type dependent. This may be mediated by diffusible substances or by cell–cell contact. The doublestranded breaks are seen after cells are directly irradiated.

Answer 6.6. **The answer is A.**

There are two generally accepted mechanisms of repair. They are broadly known as the homologous recombination (HR) or nonhomologous end-joining (NHEJ). HR functions by replicating the missing genetic information from the homologous DNA template. NHEJ functions by degrading the single strand at each side of the break and then annealing the two ends in a region of microhomology. The NHEJ may result in loss or gain in genetic information and is mutation prone. Some have suggested that HR and NHEJ have overlapping complementary roles. NHEJ is a dominant mechanism for repairing double-stranded DNA breaks in mammalian cells. Several investigators have demonstrated enhanced radiosensitivity of human cell lines by inhibiting the proteins required for NHEJ.

Answer 6.7. **The answer is B.**

Greater doses of radiation are required for cell killing in hypoxic conditions. The oxygen enhancement is seen more readily during the exponential portion of the survival curve due to the reduced capacity for cells to repair sublethal damage under hypoxic conditions. Tumor cells growing in physiologic hypoxic condition have reduced capacity to repair sublethal damage. The OER is the ratio of dose required for equivalent cell killing in the absence of oxygen compared with the dose required in the presence of oxygen. The range of OER varies from 2.5 to 3.5. Oxygen must be present at the time of irradiation for oxygen enhancement of radiotherapy to occur. OER is more important for radiation that damages cells via hydroxyl radical intermediates. Hyperbaric oxygen often does not show a dramatic increase in curability with standard fractionated radiotherapy. However, hyperbaric oxygen appears to increase curability in a small number of fractions. A meta-analysis showed that hyperbaric oxygen improves the local control of solid tumors by about 10%. Unfortunately, a randomized trial published recently showed that epoetin β did not improve cancer control or survival in patients with head and neck cancer.

Answer 6.8. **The answer is B.**

Radiation appears to increase the cellular uptake of platinum drugs and increase the number of platinum intermediates. Hydroxyurea preferentially kills cells in the radio-resistant phase of the cell cycle (S phase). The G2/M phase of the cell cycle is the most radiosensitive portion of the cell cycle. Paclitaxel is thought to synchronize tumor cells in the G2/M phase, which is relatively radiosensitive. Some chemotherapy can recall irradiated volumes by erythema on the skin or by producing pulmonary reactions.

Answer 6.9. **The answer is D.**

Localized heat treatment can be delivered with microwaves, ultrasound, or radiofrequency sources of energy. The temperature 42.5°C appears to be critical, with small increments above this temperature leading to a steep increase in lethality. The lethality of hyperthermia is thought to be in part from denaturation of proteins. Unlike radiation-induced kill, lethality from heat is most pronounced when cells are in the radio-resistant S phase. When hyperthermia and radiation are combined *in vitro*, the net effect is greater than additive lethal effect. However, in a clinical setting, the effect appears to be additive or independent.

Answer 6.10. **The answer is D.**

The relative probabilities of photoelectric, Compton, and pair production interaction depends on the photon energy and the atomic number of the irradiated material. In modern treatment machines with greater than 4 MeV photons, the Compton interactions and pair productions are commonly seen. At diagnostic equipment energy range (25 kvp), photoelectric effect predominates. In photoelectric effect, an incoming x-ray transfers all its energy to an inner orbit electron, which is ejected from the atom. A photon is produced as an outer shell electron fills the vacant hole. In Compton scattering, energy from the x-ray is both absorbed and scattered. The photon emerges with reduced energy and a change in direction. In pair production, an electron and a positron are produced, which then deposit energy through collisions with other electrons. The threshold energy for pair production is 1.02 MeV.

Answer 6.11. **The answer is B.**

Higher energy photons deposit less dose to the skin surface. Thus, it is called the skin-sparing effect of high-energy photons. Depth of maximum dose increases as the energy of the incident beam increases. It is often desirable to use high energy photons (>10 MeV) to reach deeply located tumors. For a given energy, electrons do not penetrate deeper in tissue compared to photons. It is for this reason that electron beams are often used to treat superficially located tumors such as skin cancer. Electron beams, unlike photons, deposit more dose to the skin surface as the incident electron energy increases.

Answer 6.12. **The answer is D.**

A modern linear accelerator (linac) can deliver energies up to 25 MeV. The focal point of the gantry's rotation is called *the isocenter.* The ^{60}Cobalt teletherapy unit is a megavoltage machine that relies on radioactive cobalt to produce a photon beam. Unlike the linacs, the ^{60}Cobalt unit is always "on" and must be kept in shielded position until the beam is needed for treatment.

Answer 6.13. **The answer is A.**

A proton beam is notable for its characteristic *Bragg peak.* This describes a sharp rise in energy deposition at the end of the proton beam track. Charged particles such as protons can be accelerated by an electric field in the gap between the magnets. Neutrons have no charge and interact in matter mainly by generating recoil protons from hydrogen atoms and nuclear disintegrations. Proton beams in the range of 50 to 500 MeV have been used to treat cancer. The energy of the proton beam can be modulated so that the Bragg peak occurs at a specified depth.

Answer 6.14. **The answer is B.**

Immobilization is critically important since it adds to accuracy of daily setup and treatment. A planning computer tomography (CT) scan is obtained after immobilization has been completed. At the time of image acquisition for planning, tumor motion due to respiration must be determined. The planning volume must account for respiratory movement and uncertainty of tumor position. 3D dose distribution in each patient is not easily measured, and it must be predicted from computer calculation. IMRT can have a high degree of control on the shaping of the dose distribution. The computer determines the intensity profiles to achieve the desired dose distribution.

Answer 6.15. **The answer is C.**

Relative to external beam energies, the emitted spectra are of low energy, but high doses can be delivered within a few centimeters of the source. Isotopes with properties of very short half-lives and low energy are used for permanent implants such as for prostate cancer treatment with iodine-125 with half-life of 59.4 days and x-ray energy of 27 to 35 keV. Half-life is the time required for half of the initial number of nuclei to decay.

Answer 6.16. **The answer is B.**

Early or acute effects typically occur within weeks following irradiation. They often occur in tissues that have rapid turnover, and it is thought to result from the depletion of the clonogenic or stem cells within that tissue. The frequencies of late effects depend very strongly on radiation fraction size. There are fewer late effects with smaller fraction size. Large α/β ratio has a large "shoulder" in the low dose portion. The α/β ratio represents the dose at which the quadratic (β) and the linear α components of cell kill are equivalent. The dose response to radiation can be described by the formula $S = \exp(-\alpha D - \beta D^2)$, where S is surviving fraction and D represents dose. Typical human tumors and early-responding normal tissues have large α/β ratios (9 to 13 Gy).

Answer 6.17. **The answer is B.**

Repair explains the shoulder of the radiation survival curve showing that cells can repair some of the radiation damage. The majority of sublethal damage repair occurs within 6 hours following irradiation. Redistribution explains differences in cell cycle radiation sensitivity with the mitotic (M) phase being the most sensitive. Cells gradually increase in resistance as they proceed through the late G1 and S phases. Repopulation refers to spontaneous repopulation and induced cell proliferation or recruitment of cells after irradiation. This may occur in some tumors but occurs less than that in normal tissues. Reoxygenation explains how a proportion of hypoxic cells present in a tumor return to preradiation level. Some tumor cells may reoxygenate after radiotherapy, and the proportion of the hypoxic cells that was present prior to irradiation may be seen.

Answer 6.18. **The answer is A.**

Hyperfractionation refers to a radiotherapy schedule that utilizes multiple daily treatments more than 6 hours apart with reduced fraction size and increased number of fractions. A randomized trial performed by the European Organization for Research and Treatment of Cancer (EORTC) showed that a hyperfractionated regimen was significantly better than standard fractionation in improving local control. Accelerated fractionation reduces the overall treatment time. It delivers the same dose with same fraction size but in shorter overall treatment time. An RTOG 9003 randomized trial showed that standard fractionation treatment was *inferior* to hyperfractionation and accelerated fractionation with concomitant boost used for advanced head and neck squamous cell carcinomas. CHART as developed at Mt. Vernon Hospital in the United Kingdom gave a 54 Gy total dose, which is significantly lower than the standard fractionated treatment dose for lung cancer.

CHAPTER 7

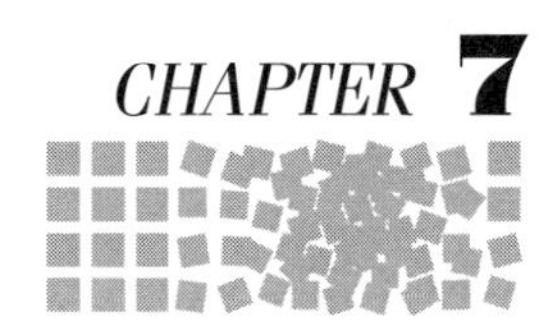

Principles of Medical Oncology

MICHAEL C. PERRY

Directions Each of the numbered items below is followed by lettered answers. Select the ONE lettered answer that is BEST in each case unless instructed otherwise.

QUESTIONS

Question 7.1. **Historically, what factors have been the major obstacles to the effectiveness of chemotherapy?**

A. Development of resistance.
B. Toxicity to normal tissues.
C. Both A and B.
D. None of the above.

Question 7.2. **Which of the following is/are among the first "targeted agents?"**

A. 5-fluorouracil.
B. Methotrexate.
C. Gemcitabine.
D. All of the above.

Question 7.3. **The goals of primary induction therapy are all but one of the following.**

A. Palliation of tumor-related symptoms.
B. Improve quality of life.
C. Prolong time to tumor progression and survival.
D. Cure in a majority of patients.

Question 7.4. **Cancers cured by chemotherapy include**

A. metastatic non-small cell lung cancer
B. metastatic breast cancer
C. metastatic colorectal cancer
D. Hodgkin disease

Question 7.5. **Pediatric cancers cured by chemotherapy include all but one of the following.**

A. Acute lymphoblastic leukemia.
B. Wilms tumor.
C. Burkitt lymphoma.
D. Ewing sarcoma.

Corresponding Chapters in *Cancer: Principles & Practice of Oncology*, Seventh Edition: 14 (Principles of Medical Oncology).

Question 7.6. **Neoadjuvant therapy has proven effective for**

A. anal cancer
B. endometrial cancer
C. renal cell carcinoma
D. pancreatic cancer

Question 7.7. **A woman with a 7-cm breast cancer and clinically palpable nodes would best be served by**

A. surgery
B. neoadjuvant chemotherapy
C. adjuvant chemotherapy
D. radiation therapy

Question 7.8. **The principles of adjuvant chemotherapy include all but which one of the following.**

A. All drugs must be active against the cancer.
B. All drugs should be given at the optimal dose and schedule.
C. Therapy should be for prolonged periods to kill every micrometastasis.
D. All drugs should be given at consistent intervals.

Question 7.9. **Which clinical end point is most important in determining the potential for cure of a chemotherapy program?**

A. Median survival.
B. Freedom from progression.
C. Median response duration.
D. Complete response rate.

Question 7.10. **Which of the following statements about neoadjuvant chemotherapy is NOT true?**

A. Permits determination of the effectiveness of the therapy in a given patient.
B. Allows determination of the lymph node status of the patient.
C. May compromise staging.
D. May compromise surgery since patients may refuse if their tumor responds well.

Question 7.11. **Adjuvant chemotherapy is routinely used for**

A. gall bladder cancer
B. colorectal cancer
C. pancreatic cancer
D. hepatoma

Question 7.12. **Resistance to chemotherapy is due to**

A. abnormal genetic machinery in the cancer cell
B. alterations in cell cycle checkpoint control
C. loss of p53 function
D. all of the above

Question 7.13. **Combination chemotherapy is the treatment of choice for**

A. chronic myelogenous leukemia
B. diffuse large B-cell lymphoma
C. melanoma
D. pancreatic cancer

Question 7.14. **Normal tissues commonly affected by chemotherapy include**

A. hair follicles, gastrointestinal mucosa, and bone marrow precursors
B. hair follicles, gastrointestinal mucosa, and hepatocytes
C. gastrointestinal mucosa, bone marrow precursors, and neurons
D. bone marrow precursors, Kupfer cells, and renal tubular cells

Question 7.15. **Which of the following is NOT a targeted agent?**

A. Trastuzumab (Herceptin).
B. Gefinitib (Iressa).
C. Rituximab (Rituxan).
D. Pentostatin (Nipent).

Question 7.16. **Which of the following hematologic malignancies is least likely to be cured by chemotherapy?**

A. Acute myelogenous leukemia.
B. Diffuse large B-cell lymphoma.
C. Childhood acute lymphoblastic leukemia.
D. Hodgkin disease.

Question 7.17. **Which of the following is NOT an approach to dose-dense delivery of chemotherapy?**

A. Dose escalation.
B. Combination chemotherapy.
C. Reduced cycle interval.
D. Sequential scheduling.

Question 7.18. **In the recent Phase III chemotherapy trial in adjuvant node-positive breast cancer, Citron et al. showed all but which one of the following from their dose dense arms?**

A. Improved disease free survival.
B. Improved overall survival.
C. Increased toxicity.
D. Equal toxicity.

Question 7.19. **Which of the following statements is/are true?**

A. Cytotoxic effects of chemotherapy or radiation therapy may be more pronounced in neoplastic cells than in normal tissues.
B. p53 mediates G_1 and G_2 arrest of the cell cycle following exposure to deoxyribonucleic acid (DNA) damage and induces apoptosis.
C. Mutations in the p53 gene occur in at least 50% of human tumors.
D. All of the above.

Question 7.20. **Which of the following statements is/are NOT true?**

A. Alternating combination chemotherapy programs result in improved responses and survival.
B. Reduction of dose levels in adjuvant chemotherapy does not compromise its effectiveness.
C. Inclusion of ineffective chemotherapeutic agents in combination therapy may still improve response rates and survival.
D. Combination chemotherapy is always better than single agent therapy.
E. All of the above.

Question 7.21. **The outcome of exposure of a cell to DNA damage depends upon**

A. the specific cytotoxic treatment
B. the conditions of treatment
C. p53 status
D. other cell-cycle regulatory elements
E. all of the above

Question 7.22. **Which of the following statements is/are true?**

A. Bcl-2 is a potent suppressor of apoptotic cell death.
B. Bcl-2 expression leads to repression of cell death triggered by chemotherapy.
C. Bcl-2 protein is overexpressed in non-Hodgkin lymphoma.
D. Antisense strategies targeting Bcl-2 may reverse chemoresistance.
E. All of the above.

Question 7.23. **Inhibition of the epidermal growth factor receptor (EGFR) tyrosine kimases gefinitib or erlotinib in non-small cell lung cancer may accomplish all of the following EXCEPT**

A. low objective response rates in non-small cell lung cancer
B. toxicities of rash and diarrhea
C. conversion of partial responses to complete responses
D. improved quality of life in some patients

ANSWERS

Answer 7.1. **The answer is C.**

Although chemotherapy often produces tumor shrinkage, the eventual development of resistance results in tumor regrowth and treatment failure. For many conventional chemotherapy drugs, the dose-limiting factor has been toxicity to normal tissues such as bone marrow or gastrointestinal tract mucosa.

Answer 7.2. **The answer is D.**

All three agents were "designed" to inhibit normal pathways of purine and pyrimidine metabolism, with secondary retardation of cell growth.

Answer 7.3. **The answer is D.**

At this time the most common metastatic solid tumors cannot be cured by chemotherapy, so the goal of therapy changes to palliation of symptoms produced by the tumor or its products, which often improves the quality of life and prolongs the period of time from diagnosis to recurrence. As an example, a woman with metastatic breast cancer and pain due to bone metastases is incurable, but chemotherapy may relieve her pain, improving and extending her life.

Answer 7.4. **The answer is D.**

The hematologic malignancies—acute lymphoblastic leukemia, Hodgkin disease, and some non-Hodgkin lymphomas—are frequently curable with combination chemotherapy, as are chronic myelogenous leukemia and hairy cell leukemia. The most frequently occurring solid tumors (lung cancer, colorectal cancer, breast cancer, and prostate cancer) are not curable once they are metastatic. This is the major challenge to oncologists today.

Answer 7.5. **The answer is D.**

The success rate of treatment of acute lymphoblastic leukemia is one of the milestones of oncology, and Burkitt lymphoma and Wilms tumor can also often be cured by chemotherapy.

Answer 7.6. **The answer is A.**

Neoadjuvant therapy for anal cancer with the combination of radiation therapy, 5-fluorouracil, and mitomycin has a high success rate. "Organ-sparing therapy" is also effective for laryngeal cancer, esophageal cancer, bladder cancer, breast cancer, osteogenic sarcoma, and locally advanced (stage III) non-small cell lung cancer. In most of these cancers, the radiation therapy and chemotherapy are given concurrently rather than sequentially.

Answer 7.7. **The answer is B.**

This patient has a locally advanced breast cancer and conventional therapy with either surgery, radiation therapy, or both will likely be unsuccessful due to both local recurrences and the development of distant metastases. While a response rate of 50% would be considered typical for therapy of established metastatic disease, response rates of 80% or better may be achieved with neoadjuvant therapy. This also provides an *in vivo* chemotherapy sensitivity test.

Answer 7.8. **The answer is C.**

The tenet of combination chemotherapy is the use of only agents active against the cancer in question, given at optimal dose and schedule that is not reduced because of overlapping toxicities. The interval between treatment cycles should be as short as possible for maximum effect. Prolonged therapy is unlikely to be more successful because of the development of drug resistance or end-organ toxicities.

Answer 7.9. **The answer is D.**

Although other measures of treatment effect such as median survival, median response duration, and freedom from progression are useful, only patients who achieve a complete response are candidates for cure.

Answer 7.10. **The answer is B.**

Successful therapy may produce a complete response in the primary and any (formerly) metastatic nodes.

Answer 7.11. **The answer is B.**

Adjuvant chemotherapy for stage III colorectal cancer can reduce the risk of recurrence by one third and reduce the risk of death by the same amount. Since there is no effective chemotherapy (as measured by improvements in response rates), the other three cancers are not candidates for adjuvant therapy.

Answer 7.12. **The answer is D.**

All three of the above mechanisms can lead to resistance to chemotherapeutic drugs and, thus, to treatment failure.

Answer 7.13. **The answer is B.**

Diffuse large B cell lymphoma is curable in at least 50% of patients with the combination of cyclophosphamide, doxorubicin, vincristine, and prednisone, with the recent addition of rituximab, a monoclonal antibody. Chronic myelogenous leukemia can be effectively treated with imatinib (Gleevec) and does not require combination therapy, while melanoma and pancreatic cancer remain major problems for oncologists.

Answer 7.14. **The answer is A.**

Tissues that rapidly reproduce themselves, such as hair follicles, the lining of the gastrointestinal tract, and bone marrow precursors are particularly sensitive to most chemotherapeutic agents, with resultant toxicities of alopecia, mucositis, and cytopenias the consequence. Hepatocytes, Kupffer cells, and renal tubular cells are not typically affected by chemotherapy.

Answer 7.15. **The answer is D.**

All three of the others are considered targeted agents, while pentostatin is an antimetabolite with several mechanisms of action.

Answer 7.16. **The answer is A.**

All three of the other malignancies have cure rates in excess of 50%, but acute myelogenous leukemia remains difficult to cure.

Answer 7.17. **The answer is B.**

While combination chemotherapy is certainly effective for many cancers, the other three choices indicate means of increasing dose density.

Answer 7.18. **The answer is C.**

Dose dense therapy, in this trial, resulted in improved outcomes with respect to disease-free and overall survival with equal toxicity.

Answer 7.19. **The answer is D.**

Answer 7.20. **The answer is E.**

While possessing great theoretical appeal, alternating chemotherapy combinations has not proved to be an improvement over conventional therapy. Reduction of dose levels in the adjuvant setting often compromises the effectiveness of therapy. Ineffective agents add only toxicity to combination chemotherapy programs. For some malignancies [chronic myelogenous leukemia treated with imatinib (Gleevec)], single-agent therapy is sufficient.

Answer 7.21. **The answer is E.**

Answer 7.22. **The answer is E.**

Answer 7.23. **The answer is C.**

The currently available EGFR TKIs (gefinitib, erlotinib) produce objective response rates of about 10% in non-small cell lung cancer, with another 40% of patients experiencing subjective benefit. The usual toxicities are rash and diarrhea. There is no evidence that either targeted agent can convert partial responses to complete responses.

CHAPTER **8**

Systemic Therapy for Cancer

CLAY M. ANDERSON

Directions Each of the numbered items below is followed by lettered answers. Select the ONE lettered answer that is BEST in each case unless instructed otherwise.

QUESTIONS

Question 8.1. **Among the following anticancer agents, the one that is synthetic and not derived from natural sources is**

A. Daunorubicin
B. Gemcitabine
C. Vincristine (VCR)
D. Paclitaxel
E. Bleomycin

Question 8.2. **A new experimental small molecule drug with a novel mechanism of action, specific to a certain intracellular receptor, is in development and being tested in early human trials. The dose chosen for further studies after phase I trials is most likely to be**

A. the maximum tolerated dose
B. one dose level below the maximum tolerated dose
C. the optimal biologic dose (minimal effective dose)
D. the minimal tolerated dose
E. the LD_{10} dose (dose that kills 10% of cohort)

Question 8.3. **A 55-year-old woman with metastatic breast cancer is initiating up-front systemic therapy. She is being started on cyclophosphamide/doxorubicin chemotherapy. The feature below that will limit her ability to receive doxorubicin is**

A. emphysema
B. malnutrition
C. renal insufficiency
D. jaundice
E. liver metastases

Corresponding Chapters in *Cancer: Principles & Practice of Oncology*, Seventh Edition: 15 (Pharmacology of Cancer Chemotherapy), 16 (Pharmacology of Cancer Biotherapeutics), and 17 (Pharmacology of Endocrine Manipulation).

Question 8.4. **The body surface area (BSA) is the mostly widely used dosing paradigm for cytotoxic drugs because**

A. flat doses of cytotoxic drugs have resulted in many patient deaths in the past
B. it is the best reflection of organ clearance related to body size, especially for the kidney and liver
C. it is known to be highly accurate in predicted drug metabolism
D. cytotoxic drugs can commonly accumulate in body fat and result in prolonged toxicities
E. it has been proven in large phase III clinical trials to be superior in terms of safety and efficacy to other methods of dosing correction for cytotoxic drugs in adults

Question 8.5. **A 66-year-old white man has metastatic colon cancer and is receiving 5-fluorouracil (5FU) and irinotecan chemotherapy. After his first cycle, his course is complicated by severe, prolonged neutropenia with fever, thrombocytopenia requiring platelet transfusion, and grade 4 stomatitis requiring parenteral opiates and several days of fluid resuscitation. What is the most appropriate future management of this patient?**

A. He should receive full doses of 5-fluorouracil in future cycles but can no longer receive irinotecan.
B. This is a hypersensitivity reaction and necessitates cessation of both agents for the life of the patient.
C. This is an inherited enzyme deficiency that impairs the metabolism of fluoropyrimidines, leading to excessive toxicity, and fluoropyrimidines are best avoided in the future.
D. Since the cause of this reaction is unknown, he should be challenged with full doses of both drugs again and watched carefully.

Question 8.6. **A 31-year-old woman is treated with mechlorethamine, vincristine, procarbazine, and prednisone for stage IV nodular sclerosing Hodgkin disease. She only has a partial response and then progresses after 4 months off therapy. She developed resistance to mechlorethamine and will likely be resistant to busulfan or cyclophosphamide because of**

A. upregulation of glutathione synthetase
B. upregulation of alkyl-guanine alkyl transferase
C. increased excision repair of deoxyribonucleic acid (DNA)
D. all of the above
E. none of the above

Question 8.7. **The same patient as in Question 8.6 received an autologous transplant with busulfan and cyclophosphamide for recurrent disease 9 months after diagnosis. Four years after diagnosis, she was noted to have moderate, progressive pancytopenia. A bone marrow aspiration and biopsy is most likely to reveal**

A. recurrent Hodgkin disease
B. multiple myeloma
C. autoimmune aplastic anemia
D. alkylator-associated myelodysplastic syndrome
E. hypocellular bone marrow without a specific diagnosis

Question 8.8. **A 55-year-old man with locally advanced oral cavity squamous cell carcinoma is receiving cisplatin 100 mg per m^2 every 21 days during 7 weeks of external beam radiation therapy to the head and neck. What are the most expected toxicities for the cisplatin regimen during this treatment?**

A. Myelosuppression and stomatitis.
B. Neuropathy and myelosuppression.
C. Renal toxicity and hearing deficit and stomatitis.
D. Alopecia and diarrhea.
E. Nausea, vomiting, and neuropathy.

Question 8.9. **Cisplatin and carboplatin have the same mechanism of action and similar spectra of activities but different pharmacologic properties and different dose-limiting and common toxicities. They are used interchangeably in many types of cancer, but only cisplatin should be used for curative treatment of**

A. non-small cell lung cancer
B. germ cell tumors
C. ovarian cancer
D. head and neck cancer
E. bladder cancer

Question 8.10. **Capecitabine may be more effective than 5-fluorouracil because**

A. it is a more potent inhibitor of thymidylate synthase
B. it inhibits a different enzyme than 5-fluorouracil does
C. it is a prodrug that is activated preferentially in tumor cells
D. it has direct cytotoxic effect on malignant cells of the gut lining as it is being absorbed
E. it crosses the blood-brain barrier effectively and is very potent against brain metastases

Question 8.11. **Antimetabolites are used more frequently than other cytotoxic drugs to treat nonmalignant conditions because**

A. they are more active against normal lymphocyte populations that cause autoimmune disease
B. they are less toxic and safer, including a lack of significant carcinogenic risk
C. they do not cause nausea or vomiting
D. they do not cause immunosuppression
E. all of the above

Question 8.12. **A 62-year-old man with extensive small cell lung cancer is receiving cisplatin and etoposide chemotherapy. He lives 2 hours away from his oncologist's clinic and infusion center. He wishes to only be at the infusion center for 1 day out of each cycle. He is given his cisplatin dose over 2 hours on day 1 and his etoposide dose of 100 mg per m^2 over 1 hour on day 1. To complete his total dose of etoposide for this cycle, he should**

A. return to the clinic, as etoposide can only be administered intravenously
B. change the etoposide to low dose oral administration for 14 more days
C. take oral etoposide at twice the IV dose for 2 more days
D. skip the further etoposide as it is unimportant to this regimen

Question 8.13. **Important predictors of irinotecan toxicity include(s)**

A. age
B. genetic polymorphisms of metabolic enzymes
C. gender
D. all of the above
E. none of the above

Question 8.14. **A 14-year-old boy with acute lymphoblastic lymphoma is receiving combination chemotherapy with an excellent clinical response. After 4 months on therapy, he develops numbness, tingling, and pain in his feet and fingertips. The best response to this toxicity of the vincristine in his curative combination chemotherapy regimen is to**

A. reduce the dose of vincristine, continue the regimen, and monitor the neuropathy closely
B. stop the vincristine immediately but continue the other drugs
C. continue the vincristine at full dose plus all other drugs and monitor
D. stop the whole regimen and start a salvage regimen
E. the neuropathy is not due to vincristine so the question is not pertinent

Question 8.15. **A 63-year-old woman has ER-negative, Her2/neu overexpressing metastatic breast cancer and is receiving weekly docetaxel/trastuzumab therapy. After 10 weeks of therapy, she developed mild-to-moderate ankle edema and worsening dyspnea. A chest radiograph revealed a new moderate left pleural effusion. The best management of this finding in this patient is**

A. cessation of docetaxel and substitution of a new cytotoxic with continued trastuzumab
B. tube thoracostomy and talc pleurodesis for a malignant pleural effusion
C. therapeutic and diagnostic thoracentesis and low-dose diuretics, followed by restaging studies and review of supportive measures
D. therapeutic thoracentesis and change to single-agent liposomal doxorubicin therapy
E. admission to the hospital for diuretic and inotropic medication for congestive heart failure

Question 8.16. **Which of the following statements is true regarding l-asparaginase?**

A. It is widely used in hematologic and solid neoplasms.
B. It is a microtubule active agent.
C. It is carcinogenic.
D. It is very active in acute lymphoblastic leukemia.
E. It is available as an oral capsule.

Question 8.17. **A 55-year-old man with metastatic gastrointestinal stromal tumor has been receiving imatinib mesylate therapy at a dose of 400 mg once a day. A follow-up evaluation after 3 months revealed partial response, which was maintained for 7 months. A follow-up computer tomography (CT) scan subsequently was done and revealed evidence of progressive disease. The best management option in this circumstance is**

A. continuation of the drug at the current dose as a clinical benefit is likely occurring
B. cessation of the drug and change to salvage cytotoxic chemotherapy
C. increasing the imatinib dosage to 600 mg a day with close monitoring for response and toxicity
D. open surgical biopsy to confirm the diagnosis
E. referral to hospice care

Question 8.18. **A 44-year-old man with stage III melanoma has completed his surgical treatment and has started a regimen of 1 year of high-dose interferon. He has completed 2 weeks of intravenous interferon-alpha at 20 million units per m^2 daily 5 days a week. On Monday, he is tired, achy, and has a temperature of 37.8°C. His serum glutamine oxalate transaminase (SGOT) is 80, his serum glutamine phenylalumine transaminase (SGPT) is 94, his white blood cells (WBC) is 3.3, Hb – 11.9, platelet count – 77K. The best response to this circumstance is to**

A. stop the interferon induction and wait for normalization before starting subcutaneous maintenance
B. hold the interferon for 1 week and resume at a 33% dose reduction
C. continue the interferon at the same dose and check lab parameters again in 1 week
D. stop the interferon permanently, as this patient will be unable to tolerate this therapy safely
E. stop the interferon and start GM-CSF therapy as a substitute

Question 8.19. **Five months later, this same patient complains of weight loss, lethargy, and depressed mood. The best set of interventions for this patient are**

A. cessation of interferon
B. reducing the dose of interferon by 33%
C. supportive psychotherapy
D. 1 week break, antidepressant, nutritional supplements, and activity counseling
E. change to melanoma vaccine therapy

Question 8.20. **Interleukin-2 can produce significant responses in a proportion of cases in certain solid tumors. Which of the following patients are most likely to respond to high-dose interleukin-2?**

A. A breast cancer patient with two small liver metastases.
B. A renal cell carcinoma patient with a grade 4 tumor and synchronous bone and brain metastases.
C. A renal cell carcinoma patient with prior nephrectomy and now liver and bone metastases with a Eastern Cooperative Oncology Group (ECOG) performance status of 2.
D. A melanoma patient with ECOG performance status of 0, normal lactate dehydrogenase (LDH) level, and lung metastases.
E. A melanoma patient with brain metastases only.

Question 8.21. **Interleukin-2 can be given in a variety of doses, routes, and schedules. Which of the following is the dose most likely to lead to a complete response in a 44-year-old man with lung metastases 4 years after nephrectomy for a grade II clear cell renal carcinoma?**

A. Subcutaneous interleukin-2, 9 million units per m^2 daily 5 days a week for 2 weeks out of 4.
B. Subcutaneous interleukin-2, 9 million units per m^2 daily 5 days a week for 4 weeks out of 6.
C. Intravenous interleukin-2, 720,000 units per kg 15 min infusion every 8 hours up to 14 doses, twice over 3 weeks, repeated once.
D. None of the above.

Question 8.22. **Histone deacetylase inhibitors target cancer cells by**

A. inhibiting methylation of DNA
B. inhibiting gene expression in malignant cells
C. inducing apoptosis in rapidly dividing cells
D. modulation of gene expression by enhancing acetylation of DNA-associated histone complexes
E. depriving cells of acetyl groups required for protein synthesis

Question 8.23. **Histone deacetylase inhibitors, when subjected to a wide range of clinic trials, should work well in**

A. hematologic malignancies only
B. solid tumors only
C. patients after failure of up-front chemotherapy only
D. breast cancer only due to the unique mechanism of action in breast cancer cells
E. in a variety of cancer types and settings, including synergy with other cytotoxic and targeted therapies

Question 8.24. **A 49-year-old woman with metastatic Her-2 overexpressing infiltrating ductal breast cancer is receiving trastuzumab single-agent therapy as second line after failure of docetaxel/capecitabine combination chemotherapy. Her disease does not progress for 8 months on the trastuzumab therapy. It is now decided that she needs second salvage chemotherapy because of documented progressive disease in the lungs. The best regimen for her from the list below is**

A. vinorelbine
B. gemcitabine
C. doxorubicin and trastuzumab
D. vinorelbine and trastuzumab
E. pemetrexed

Question 8.25. **A 71-year-old man has had grade I follicular lymphoma for 4 years. He was initially observed for 2 years. He developed evidence of progressive disease in the groin and axilla with no evidence of transformation. You would consider**

A. rituximab
B. HLA-identical sibling allogeneic stem cell transplant
C. high-dose chemotherapy with autologous transplant
D. high-dose Ara-C

Question 8.26. **A 44-year-old premenopausal woman has a new diagnosis of ER-positive T2N1M0 infiltrating ductal breast cancer. She is going to have lumpectomy, lymph node dissection, chemotherapy, breast irradiation, and 5 years of antiestrogen hormone therapy. The reason she will NOT receive an aromatase inhibitor as her hormonal treatment is that**

A. it is shown to be inferior adjuvant hormonal treatment for ER-positive breast cancer
B. aromatase inhibitors are only active in ER-negative breast cancer
C. aromatase inhibitors are only felt to be effective in postmenopausal women
D. her risk of recurrence is too low to have benefit from a hormonal intervention
E. she is at risk of moderate to severe bone toxicity from the aromatase inhibitor

Question 8.27. **A 77-year-old black man with metastatic prostate cancer has bone metastases, a prostate specific antigen (PSA) of 44 ng/ml that is rising, and moderate bone pain. He is on flutamide and goserelin. The rationale for stopping his flutamide is**

A. it is not working and thus should be removed from the regimen
B. its removal as an androgen antagonist, if it has become an agonist, may paradoxically result in antiandrogenic effect
C. it is never useful to use in combination with a luteinizing hormone-releasing hormone (LH-RH) agonist
D. it is not indicated for prostate cancer
E. none of the above

ANSWERS

Answer 8.1. **The answer is B.**

Many of our currently available cytotoxic agents have been isolated or derived from natural sources, including plants, fungi, and bacteria. More recently, though searches for natural agents continue, synthesis of small molecules, peptides, and proteins is leading to identification of agents with specific mechanisms and diminished toxicity. The number of new drugs developed through molecular targeting and combinatorial chemistry will probably exceed those isolated from nature with or without chemical modification. Gemcitabine is a synthetic purine nucleoside analog similar to cytarabine that acts as an antimetabolite to disrupt DNA synthesis and replication.

Answer 8.2. **The answer is C.**

For typical cytotoxic agents, the highest dose of the drug that allows survival of the host is the dose most likely to kill the most cancer cells. In human clinical trials, this is called the maximum tolerated dose. The dose selected for a phase II clinical trial is generally one dose level below the maximum tolerated dose. For targeted agents, the optimal dose may be at, above, or below the maximal tolerated dose, as the optimal level of the drug is the lowest dose that maximally blocks or inhibits the target pathway or protein. This is called the optimal biologic dose. For many of these agents, the optimal biologic dose is reached long before a maximum tolerated dose is identified, which is reflected by remarkably low toxicity for these targeted agents relative to typical cytotoxic agents.

Answer 8.3. **The answer is D.**

Only significant liver impairment, best reflected by an elevation of serum bilirubin even to a moderate degree, will dramatically increase the host toxicity of doxorubicin, leading to extreme mucositis, diarrhea, myelosuppression, and potential excess cardiotoxicity. Alkaline phosphatase level, transaminase level, and extent of liver involvement are less reliable predictors of diminished hepatic clearance of agents such as doxorubicin. Lung disease, heart disease, and kidney disease may affect her tolerance to the doxorubicin somewhat from the point of physiologic reserve to respond to stress, but not in the dramatic way that liver disease diminishing drug metabolism will do.

Answer 8.4. **The answer is B.**

There is actually only a moderately convincing body of evidence that the BSA is reflective of the expected metabolism and volume of distribution of pharmacologic agents. That being said, the BSA seems to be a better predictor for most drugs than weight or height. Still, it is far from perfect and over the years has been corrected for lean body weight or other adjustments. The routine use of BSA-based dosing of anticancer drugs has been heavily criticized, and fixed doses of drugs for patients of different sizes may be a more rational approach for a large number of oncology agents.

Answer 8.5. **The answer is C.**

Dihydropyrimidine dehydrogenase (DPD) is an enzyme that detoxifies halogenated pyrimidine cytotoxic drugs. Genetic alterations associated with DPD deficiency have been identified in rare cases of patients experiencing severe and fatal toxicity after treatment with standard doses of 5FU. Family members may have inherited the same allelic variant of DPD and thus may be at risk for the same toxicity should they require treatment with pyrimidine analogues.

Answer 8.6. **The answer is D.**

The modes by which cancer cells become resistant to alkylator drugs are multiple and include all of those listed above. Most importantly, alkylator drugs are generally not substrates for p-glycoprotein.

Answer 8.7. **The answer is D.**

Pancytopenia after chemotherapy has a multitude of causes, and the most likely cause relates to the chemotherapy used, the time after chemotherapy, and the unique features of the patient. In this case, pancytopenia 4 years after the use of alkylator drugs in a curable malignancy in a young patient makes recurrent or second malignancy less likely but myelodysplastic syndrome more likely. Autoimmune aplastic anemia is rare, with or without prior chemotherapy.

Answer 8.8. **The answer is E.**

Cisplatin, the prototypical platinating agent, is the oldest drug commonly used in this class. It has the reputation, mostly deserved, as a very effective cytotoxic drug with the greatest toxicity of all the drugs in this class. These toxicities are manageable in most patients but are different than those for other commonly used cytotoxic drugs. For instance, cisplatin causes marked nausea and vomiting without the use of 5 HT3 antagonists. Peripheral neuropathy is cumulative, although less common than with agents such as vinca alkaloids. This neuropathy is usually reversible, though recovery is often slow. A number of agents with the potential for protection from neuropathy have been developed, but none is yet used widely. On the other hand, alopecia and myelosuppression are mild, and diarrhea is uncommon.

Answer 8.9. **The answer is B.**

Germ cell tumors are readily curable with chemotherapy as the main treatment in the majority of cases. In this context, the substitution of a potentially less toxic but similarly active drug may be regarded as imprudent unless results of well-conducted clinical trials document true clinical equivalence. In fact, carboplatin has not yet convincingly been shown to be equivalent to cisplatin in this setting, and evidence to date suggests slight superiority in cure rate with cisplatin in non-seminomatous germ cell tumors.

Answer 8.10. **The answer is C.**

In contrast to 5FU, capecitabine is rapidly and extensively absorbed by the gut mucosa, with nearly 80% oral bioavailability. It is inactive in its parent form and must undergo enzymatic conversion via three successive steps. It is first hydrolyzed in the liver by a hepatic carboxylesterase to an intermediate, 5′-deoxy-5-fluorocytidine (5′-DFCR), which in turn is converted to 5′-deoxy-5-fluorouridine (5′-DFUR) by the enzyme cytidine deaminase. The third and final step occurs in tumor tissue and involves the conversion of 5′-DFUR to 5FU by the enzyme thymidine phosphorylase (TP). TP is expressed at significantly higher concentrations in tumors than in surrounding normal tissue, including cancers of the breast, colon and rectum, cervix, head and neck, and stomach. Clinical studies have shown that 5FU concentrations are nearly 3.5-fold higher in tumor tissue compared to normal tissue and are more than 20-fold higher in tumors than that measured in serum. Capecitabine and capecitabine metabolites are primarily excreted by the kidneys, and caution must be taken in the presence of renal dysfunction.

Answer 8.11. **The answer is B.**

Although antimetabolites *are* effective at reducing lymphocyte populations that are active in autoimmune disease, they are not more potent in this affect than other types of cytotoxic drugs, but they are safer and better tolerated in general than other classes of cytotoxic drugs such as alkylators.

Answer 8.12. **The answer is C.**

After oral administration, etoposide is rapidly absorbed with a relative bioavailability of 50% (range 24% to 137%) with high interpatient variability. Oral etoposide's bioavailability tends to decrease at absolute doses greater than 300 mg. Variability in etoposide absorption may be due in part to intestinal P-glycoprotein expression.

Answer 8.13. **The answer is B.**

After administration of irinotecan, the active metabolite, SN-38, is generated from irinotecan by the action of irinotecan-converting enzyme, predominantly in the liver. SN-38 is predominantly cleared via conjugation by liver uridine diphosphate glucuronosyl transferase (UGT) to form the inactive beta-glucuronidated derivative SN-38G (10-O-glucuronyl-SN-38). UGT mediated glucuronidation is the rate-limiting step in SN-38 clearance, and variability in its activity may contribute to interpatient differences in drug toxicity during irinotecan chemotherapy. The UGT1A1 isoform that catalyzes bilirubin glucuronidation is also the major enzyme responsible for glucuronidation of SN-38. Genetic testing for the UGT1A1*28 promoter region polymorphism associated with decreased glucuronidating activity is undergoing prospective evaluation in larger clinical studies of irinotecan based therapy.

Answer 8.14. **The answer is A.**

VCR principally induces neurotoxicity characterized by a peripheral, symmetric mixed sensory-motor, and autonomic polyneuropathy. In adults, neurotoxicity may be profound after cumulative doses of 15 to 20 mg. Children appear to be less susceptible than adults, but the elderly are particularly prone. Advanced age, hepatic dysfunction or obstructive liver disease, and antecedent neurologic disease are associated with increased risk of neurotoxicity. The only known treatment for VCR neurotoxicity is discontinuation of the drug or reduction of the dose or frequency of treatment. Although a number of antidotes, including thiamine, vitamin B_{12}, folinic acid, and pyridoxine, have been used, these treatments have not been clearly shown to be effective.

Answer 8.15. **The answer is C.**

In this case, it is uncertain whether the effusion is due to cancer progression, docetaxel or trastuzumab toxicity, or congestive heart failure (or another cause). It is incorrect to assume without appropriate diagnostic testing that this represents cancer progression. Similarly, heart failure for trastuzumab or underlying heart disease is unlikely without other accompanying signs, symptoms, or history. Fluid retention causing edema, pleural effusions, ascites, or pericardial effusion is a known and common side effect of docetaxel and partially ameliorated by corticosteroid therapy. Further reevaluation is necessary to rule out progression of the disease.

Answer 8.16. **The answer is D.**

This drug is an enzyme, isolated in highly purified form from bacteria. It is only bioavailable by the intravenous route. It cleaves the essential amino acid asparagines and is required for ongoing active cellular processes, primarily protein synthesis. Without adequate levels of asparagine, highly active leukemia cells cannot divide and are thus preferentially killed. Available as an unmodified molecule and as a longer acting pegylated form, the drug can cause hypersensitivity reactions, prolong clotting times, induce pancreatitis, and result in transient neurologic toxicity, but it is not myelosuppressive or carcinogenic.

Answer 8.17. **The answer is C.**

The optimal dose of imatinib in advanced gastrointestinal stromal tumor (GIST) remains uncertain. Although there were no documented benefits to the higher dose of 600 mg per day, in the US-Finland trial, there were a few patients who regained disease control when crossed over from the lower dose (400 mg daily) to the higher dose level. Therefore, there might be some marginal benefit to be obtained from modest dose escalation of imatinib in a subset of patients whose disease progresses despite continued imatinib therapy.

Answer 8.18. **The answer is C.**

This patient is experiencing fever, "transaminitis," and pancytopenia. These laboratory abnormalities are expected and nearly universal. They are slightly more marked at this point than is typical, but not yet overly concerning. It is recommended that full chemistries and blood counts be checked weekly during high-dose intravenous induction with interferon. If myelosuppression is severe, or transaminases are elevated to over 5 times normal, then the high-dose interferon should be stopped until the laboratory tests return to normal or near normal, and then resumed at a 33% dose reduction. If the laboratory tests do not meet this threshold, the interferon should be continued at full dose and the labs checked again 1 week later. With this monitoring and intervention, morbidity and mortality from high-dose interferon IV induction has been minimal.

Answer 8.19. **The answer is D.**

The above-mentioned toxicities are grade 1 to 2 and are expected from high-dose interferon-alpha. They are usually treatable without dose reduction. Each symptom has a potentially effective intervention. Antidepressants will lead to improvement in mood; nutritional supplements, appetite stimulants, or both will lead to weight stabilization or gain in most cases; and supervised physical activity and support for continuation of activities with energy conservation will improve the perception of lethargy or fatigue in many cases. In the meantime, a short break from interferon will allow rapid modest improvement. More severe toxicity or lack of improvement after intervention may lead to a need for dose reduction or cessation of therapy.

Answer 8.20. **The answer is D.**

Only patients with melanoma and renal cell carcinoma have demonstrated reliable dramatic responses to high-dose interleukin-2, or interleukin-2-base regimens. These favorable responses occur in less than 10% of cases in either disease. Patients with lower-grade tumors; longer history of disease or disease-free interval; good performance status; minimal symptoms; normal LDH level (for melanoma); and skin, lymph node, or lung involvement are more likely to respond to therapy. But those who are more ill, usually because of their cancer, are very likely to suffer significant morbidity and very unlikely to benefit, and thus should not be treated with interleukin-2.

Answer 8.21. **The answer is C.**

Only high-dose intravenous interleukin-2 has been shown to produce complete and durable responses in less than 10% of treated patients. Neither lower dose interleukin-2 nor interleukin-2 containing regimens have shown equivalent complete response rates or durations of complete response in renal cell carcinoma compared to high-dose interleukin-2, despite some clinical data suggesting some responses. Thus, other doses and schedules and regimens of interleukin-2 should only be used if high-dose interleukin-2 cannot be used for medical or practical reasons.

Answer 8.22. **The answer is D.**

This novel class of compounds exploits a phenomenon called epigenetic regulation, whereby gene expression is modified by enzymatic attachment of side chains to DNA or DNA-associated structural proteins. Methylation of DNA and acetylation of histone complexes are two examples of this phenomenon. Cancer cells lose the normal physiologic modulation in most cases, leading to decreased gene expression on the whole and subsequent dedifferentiation. Thus, this class of drugs attacks a common mechanism in many neoplasms and may work by upregulation of genes that control cell growth or inhibit invasive properties.

Answer 8.23. **The answer is E.**

Most cancer cells, including sensitive and resistant cell lines or tumors, have been found to have an altered histone acetylation state, namely hypoacetylation leading to decreased gene expression and presumed resultant primitive cell characteristics, including frequent mitosis and diminished responsiveness to external cues. Inhibiting the removal of acetyl groups from histone complexes should increase acetylation and increase gene expression, leading to diminished proliferation and reattainment of regulated cell processes. This should occur in many types of cancer in many clinical settings.

Answer 8.24. **The answer is D.**

There is a wealth of preclinical data suggesting that trastuzumab, a monoclonal antibody directed at the her2/neu cell surface growth factor receptor, is effective at blocking the her2/neu growth signal pathway in her2 overexpressing breast cancer cells, leading to cell death. This is an effective strategy clinically as a single modality and results in cytotoxic and clinical synergy when combined with certain cytotoxic chemotherapy agents. The clinical benefit from targeting the her2/neu overexpression may be beneficial with further chemotherapy even when progression occurs on single agent trastuzumab. Trastuzumab should not, however, be used with doxorubicin, as excess risk of cardiac toxicity has been documented in clinical trials.

Answer 8.25. **The answer is A.**

In this patient with indolent lymphoma, the goal is to control the disease with the least toxic therapy. In a study reported by Hainsworth et al., patients were administered rituximab 375 mg per m^2 IV each week for 4 consecutive weeks as initial therapy in patients with indolent lymphoma. Patients who did not progress received an additional 4-week course of rituximab every 6 months for 2 years. In 62 chemotherapy-naive patients, most of whom had stage III or IV disease, overall response rates at 6 weeks and at maximum response were 47% and 73%, with 7% and 37% complete remissions, respectively. At a median follow-up of 30 months, median progression-free survival was 34 months. Although maintenance therapy with rituximab appears to be safe, current ongoing studies will determine optimal duration of maintenance therapy and whether rituximab is associated with improved survival.

Answer 8.26. **The answer is C.**

This woman has a 30% to 40% risk of recurrence after locoregional treatment only. This risk can be reduced to about 20% to 25% (relative risk reduction of approximately 40%) by appropriate systemic adjuvant therapy, which should include at least 3 months of combination chemotherapy and 5 years of estrogen-antagonizing hormonal therapy. This therapy can be either estrogen blocking with drugs such as tamoxifen or inhibiting estrogen production, which is the mechanism of aromatase inhibitors. Aromatase inhibitors block the synthesis of peripheral estrogen production via androgens but do not block gonadal production. In a 44-year-old pre-menopausal woman, gonadal estrogen is still being produced, so an aromatase inhibitor is likely to block estrogen effects on breast cancer cells minimally, whereas tamoxifen should block most of the estrogenic effects on any residual breast cancer cells. Thus, tamoxifen, or another selective estrogen receptor modulator, is the preferred adjuvant hormonal treatment for premenopausal women with primary breast cancer.

Answer 8.27. **The answer is B.**

Antiandrogen agents, such as flutamide, can become functional androgen agonists over time if prostate cancer cells develop androgen receptor defects through mutation that modify the androgen binding sites. Clinically, this is manifest as a phenomenon called "antiandrogen withdrawal effect." A transient anti-tumor effect is seen following withdrawal of flutamide. This effect is unfortunately not durable. However, it can be used therapeutically for a period of weeks before salvage hormonal strategies or chemotherapy will be needed.

CHAPTER **9**

Design and Analysis of Clinical Trials

J. JACK LEE

Directions Each of the numbered items below is followed by lettered answers. Select the ONE lettered answer that is BEST in each case unless instructed otherwise.

QUESTIONS

Question 9.1. **Observational studies often yield more credible results because the sample size tends to be larger and the results are more applicable to general practice settings. Which one of the following describing the pros and cons of observational studies and clinical trials is NOT true?**

A. Clinical trials are prospectively planned and conducted under a controlled condition, meaning every key feature such as patient eligibility criteria, treatment modality, primary endpoint, and statistical design must be prespecified to govern the study conduct.
B. In studying the prognostic factor for rare diseases, it may not be feasible to conduct clinical trials. Observational studies can provide useful information in this setting.
C. Clinical trials are often expensive and time-consuming to run.
D. In an observational study, the investigators are passive observers.

Question 9.2. **Clinical trials require careful planning. Specifically, protocol is an operational menu for the conduct of clinical trials. Which one of the following items is NOT typically included in the protocol?**

A. Patient eligibility criteria.
B. Treatment plan.
C. Statistical considerations.
D. Cost of medication.
E. Informed consent.

Corresponding Chapters in *Cancer: Principles & Practice of Oncology*, Seventh Edition: 18 (Design and Analysis of Clinical Trials).

Question 9.3. **The primary objective of Phase I trials is to establish the toxicity profile, evaluate the pharmacokinetics, and define the maximum tolerated dose of a new agent. Regarding the phases of cancer clinical trials, which one of the following descriptions is NOT true?**

A. Phase II trials provide initial efficacy assessment of a new agent or combination. The goal of Phase II trials is to identify promising agents for further evaluation.
B. Typically, Phase III trials are large, randomized trials designed to compare the new agent with standard therapy. These are rigorously designed confirmatory trials, and the outcome may change clinical practice.
C. When a patient comes to a clinic, investigators should consider offering Phase I trials first. If the patient is not eligible for a Phase I trial, the patient can be considered for Phase II or Phase III trials subsequently.
D. "Window-of-opportunity design" is sometimes used in Phase II settings to allow previously untreated patients to receive one or more courses of experimental treatment, and then, switch to a standard treatment or a combination of standard treatment and experimental treatment.

Question 9.4. **Please choose one of the following that best describes Phase I trials.**

A. Phase I trials of new cytostatic drugs are designed to determine the maximum tolerated dose (MTD).
B. Accelerated titration design permits within-patient dose escalation and takes the grade of toxicity into consideration while modeling the dose-toxicity curve.
C. The conventional 3 per cohort design (3+3 design) provides a model-based approach, while the continual reassessment method (CRM) provides an algorithm-based approach in estimating the MTD.
D. Modified Fibonacci series provide an optimal solution in determining the dose levels in Phase I trials.
E. Phase I trials should be conducted in cohorts with a selected, homogeneous disease type to yield valid inference.

Question 9.5. **Please choose the answer that best describes the Simon's two-stage design for Phase II trials.**

A. The target activity level of interest, p_1, is often set at the activity level of the currently available treatments.
B. One attractive feature of the optimal two-stage design is that it minimizes the expected sample size under the alternative hypothesis.
C. The goal of the minimax design is to minimize the maximum sample size under the alternative hypothesis.
D. With $p_0 = 0.10$, $p_1 = 0.30$, and both type I and type II error rates under 10%, the optimal design requires 12 patients to be enrolled in the first stage. If two or more responses are observed, 23 more patients will be enrolled in the second stage.
E. With the same setting as in D above, the sample sizes for the minimax design will be smaller than the optimal design in both the first and second stages.

Question 9.6. **Which one of the following statements regarding computing the statistical power and sample size is NOT true?**

A. Type I error rate is the probability of rejecting the null hypothesis when it is true.
B. To limit the chance of making a false-positive conclusion, conventionally, type I error level is set at 5%. One should always respect the 5% level of significance and use it as a criterion to determine whether to publish papers.
C. Type II error is to accept the null hypothesis when it is not true. Power is defined as one minus the type II error rate.
D. Maintaining the overall type I error is important in interim analyses. Many stopping boundaries can be applied depending on the emphasis on the early or the later part of the trial.
E. When all other parameters are fixed, statistical power increases as sample size increases.

Question 9.7. **Which one of the following best describes clinical trials involving targeted cytostatic/biologic agents?**

A. Cytostatic agents may not cause tumor shrinkage; therefore, the time to progression is a more relevant endpoint than the response rate.
B. Randomized discontinuation trials can "enrich" the study population by randomizing only patients with stable diseases to either continue or stop the targeted agents.
C. Factorial design provides attractive design features for cytostatic agents. For example, most cytostatic agents have a mild toxicity profile and are suitable for combining with other agents. Factorial design also allows investigators to study the interaction between multiple agents.
D. Pertinent assays on biopsy material taken before and after treatment are the best ways to assess the modulation of targeted agents. When a biopsy is not feasible, surrogate tissues, such as peripheral blood mononuclear cells, skin, serum, buccal brush, or molecular imaging, can be considered.
E. All of the above.

Question 9.8. **Which one of the following statements about the statistical analysis is NOT true?**

A. Survival analysis methods such as the Kaplan-Meier estimates, logrank test, and Cox model are suitable for analyzing time-to-event data when censoring might happen.
B. Generally speaking, the chi-square test is preferred over the Fisher's exact test because it gives more significant P values.
C. Confidence intervals generally provide more information than significance testings. Both the magnitude and precision of the treatment effect can be estimated by confidence intervals.
D. Compared to the frequentists' methods, Bayesian approaches can offer more flexible and efficient study design and analysis. Proper choice of the prior distribution and available computing tools are the key to the successful implementation of Bayesian methods.
E. Unplanned subset analyses, multiple comparisons, or multiple interim analyses need to be treated with care because multiplicity can increase the overall type I error rate.

Question 9.9. **Which one of the following regarding clinical trial design, analysis, and conduct is not true?**

A. Intention-to-treat analysis includes all randomization and eligible patients in the analysis, hence it reduces the selection bias of arbitrarily removing certain patients in the analysis.
B. Futility analysis such as stochastic curtailment allows investigators to terminate the trial early when the interim data shows that the new agent is not promising. It saves resources and limits patients to be treated with ineffective agents.
C. When analyzing time-to-event endpoints, additional follow-up on selected, high-yield patients (such as the ones without follow-up for a long period of time) is recommended because it can increase the study power without committing a high cost to perform a comprehensive follow-up evaluation on the entire study sample.
D. An independent Data Monitoring Committee is important for Phase III studies because the committee can review unblinded interim safety and efficacy data, give advice to the study investigators, and preserve the study integrity.
E. Meta-analysis provides a quantitative summary of the results in, typically, randomized trials in a particular area of interest. It should not be considered as a substitute for a well-designed and conducted clinical trial.

ANSWERS

Answer 9.1. **The answer is A.**

Even though clinical trials can be expensive and time-consuming, prospectively planned, well controlled and conducted clinical trials provide a more rigorous foundation for valid results. Although observational studies can be large, many uncontrolled biases can easily settle in, which makes the results less generalizable.

Answer 9.2. **The answer is D.**

Although cost of medication and other study costs are important in planning a clinical trial, the cost component is not usually included in the protocol. All the other answers are essential parts of a protocol.

Answer 9.3. **The answer is D.**

Typically, Phase III agents are further developed with proven therapeutic efficacy. Prior untreated patients should be offered participation in Phase III trials first when possible. Most Phase II and particularly Phase I trials are reserved for patients who failed at least one standard therapy.

Answer 9.4. **The answer is B.**

Many of the cytostatic agents have excellent toxicity profiles and, typically, MTD is not reached in Phase I studies. MTD is more relevant for cytotoxic agents. The conventional 3+3 design is an algorithm-based method, while CRM is a model-based method. Although modified Fibonacci series are commonly used in Phase I studies, the choice of dose level is based on a reasonable, yet ad hoc rule. No optimality has been established for the modified Fibonacci series. Phase I studies typically enroll patients with heterogeneous disease types. The rationale is that drug toxicity is the primary endpoint for Phase I trials and should not differ much in patients with different disease types.

Answer 9.5. **The answer is D.**

The activity level of the currently available treatments is set as the *lower* activity level, p_0, and not the *targeted* activity level, p_1. Both B and C refer to the characteristics under the *null* hypothesis and not under the *alternative* hypothesis. In the setting specified in D, the sample sizes for the first and second stages are 12 and 13 for the optimal design and 16 and 9 for the minimax design. The minimax design minimizes the maximum sample size but, in the first stage, it often requires a larger sample size than the optimal design.

Answer 9.6. **The answer is B.**

The first sentence of answer B is correct, but the second is not. The 5% type I error rate should be used as a "guide" rather than a permanent, sacred, ordained, and unchangeable value to call for statistical significance. Using whether the results are statistically significant at a 5% level to publish the paper is definitely wrong.

Answer 9.7. **The answer is E.**

Targeted agent development is a rapidly progressing field. Modifications of traditional design are necessary due to the paradigm shift. A proper endpoint needs to be chosen according to the properties of the agents. Otherwise, one might miss an active agent by looking at the wrong things. For example, an effective cytostatic agent may prolong time to progression but has no effect on response rate. Because not everyone will respond to a targeted agent, enrichment design chooses the population with the best chance to allow the target agents to work. Randomized discontinuation design is such an example. Factorial design is useful in combining targeted agents with more traditional anticancer treatment such as chemotherapy and/or radiation. The use of surrogate tissues has gained more attention in targeted agent development because biopsies may not be feasible in many settings. With assays run on surrogate tissues, the investigators will be able to see if the targeted agents work via their intended mechanism.

Answer 9.8. **The answer is B.**

Statistical analysis is not an exercise of chasing after smallest P values. When sample size is large, the large sample approximation of the chi-square test works well. But, when sample size is small, an exact test such as Fisher's exact test should be considered.

Answer 9.9. **The answer is C.**

Selective follow-up is dangerous. A prespecified follow-up strategy on all patients should be stated and implemented to avoid bias. Intention-to-treat analysis should be used in general, and particularly in Phase III trials. Establishing an independent Data Monitoring Committee is now a standard practice for large-scale, multicenter, double-blind, randomized Phase III clinical trials. Meta-analysis can provide useful information and give an overview of the field. It alone, however, can never replace a clinical trial that is well designed and conducted.

CHAPTER 10

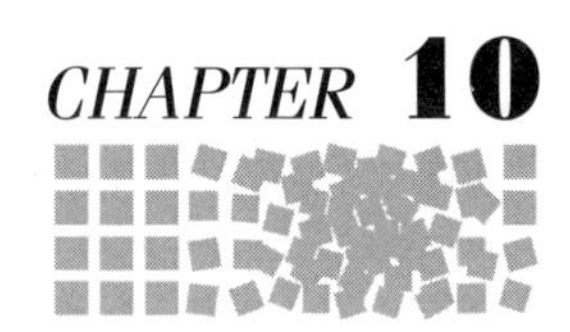

Cancer Prevention

DAVID GUSTIN

Directions Each of the numbered items below is followed by lettered answers. Select the ONE lettered answer that is BEST in each case unless instructed otherwise.

QUESTIONS

Question 10.1. **Which of the following chemicals in tobacco smoke is NOT a carcinogen?**

A. Polycyclic aromatic hydrocarbon (PAH).
B. N-nitrosamine.
C. Nicotine.
D. Benzo(a)pyrene (BaP).
E. 4-(methylnitrosamino)-1-(3-pyridyl)-1-butanone (NNK).

Question 10.2. **Which of the following statement(s) is/are true with regard to tobacco smoking?**

A. It causes approximately 30% of all deaths in the United States.
B. It is the leading cause of preventable death in the United States.
C. A and B.
D. None of the above.

Question 10.3. **The approximate percentage of adult smokers who start smoking by the age of 18 is**

A. close to 20%
B. close to 40%
C. close to 60%
D. close to 90%

Question 10.4. **Environmental tobacco smoke ("second-hand smoke") has been associated with which of the following.**

A. Increased lung cancer in partners of smoking husbands.
B. Increased deaths due to cardiovascular disease.
C. Increased respiratory problems including asthma and bronchitis.
D. All of the above.
E. None of the above.

Corresponding Chapters in *Cancer: Principles & Practice of Oncology*, Seventh Edition: 19 (Cancer Prevention: Preventing Tobacco-Related Cancers), 20 (Cancer Prevention: Diet and Chemopreventive Agents), and 21 (Cancer Prevention: Role of Surgery in Cancer Prevention).

Question 10.5. **Which of the following statement(s) is/are true regarding the 46 to 47 million smokers in the United States?**

A. Less than 50% would like to quit.
B. Less than 30% have made at least one serious attempt at quitting.
C. Of those who attempt to quit, around 30% are successful.
D. All of the above.
E. None of the above.

Question 10.6. **Which of the following statements is true with regard to smoking cessation practices?**

A. There is no evidence to suggest that providing a brief physician intervention to all smokers could increase annual quit rates.
B. There is no evidence to suggest that more intense interventions lead to more effective long-term abstinence from tobacco.
C. The success of an intervention is maximized by proper training and education of physicians and medical students, by increasing the number of modalities used and the number of professionals involved, and by the creation of office-based systems.
D. There is no clear role for nicotine replacement therapy and other pharmacologic interventions such as the use of sustained-release bupropion.

Question 10.7. **Which of the following statements is true regarding fat intake and cancer?**

A. There is a well-defined effect of dietary fat intake on cancer risk which is independent from total caloric intake.
B. The total amount of dietary fat consumed independent of source (vegetable, animal) increases the risk of breast cancer in women.
C. Well-conducted randomized prevention studies have clearly documented a chemopreventive effect of dietary restriction of fat intake on colorectal cancer.
D. There exists a strong association between animal fat consumption and risk of prostate cancer, particularly the aggressive form of this disease.

Question 10.8. **All the following statements are true EXCEPT**

A. fiber is amenable to hydrolysis by the digestive enzymes in humans
B. fiber is fermented by the luminal bacteria in the colon
C. fiber's bulking effect may mediate its postulated chemopreventive effect
D. fiber is capable of inducing apoptosis *in vitro*
E. fiber may aid in producing short-chained fatty acids that may be directly anticarcinogenic

Question 10.9. **All the following statements are true EXCEPT**

A. case–control data support an inverse association between dietary fiber and colon cancer, which for the most part has not been confirmed by prospective cohort studies
B. results of randomized clinical trials have confirmed a protective effect of dietary fiber against colon adenomas
C. despite initial evidence from case-control studies suggesting a strong protective effect of fiber against breast cancer, most prospective studies have failed to confirm these findings
D. the observational data presently available do not indicate an important role of dietary fiber in the prevention of cancer

Question 10.10. **Which one of the following statements about carotenoids is NOT true?**

A. Carotenoids have been linked to cancer protection in case-control studies.
B. Carotenoids are natural antioxidants that in the laboratory have been shown to enhance cell-to-cell communication, promote cell differentiation, and modulate immune response.
C. Randomized clinical trials have clearly demonstrated a protective effect of beta-carotene against lung malignancies.
D. Randomized clinical trials have failed to demonstrate a protective effect of beta-carotene against lung malignancies.

Question 10.11. **Which of the following statements about chemoprevention as a modality is true?**

A. It is defined as a pharmacologic intervention with specific nutrients or other chemicals to suppress or reverse carcinogenesis and to prevent the development of invasive cancer.
B. It is based on two basic concepts supporting this cancer control strategy—multi-step and field carcinogenesis.
C. It is premised on the notion that one can intervene (and suppress) at many steps in the carcinogenic process and over a many-year period.
D. All of the above.
E. None of the above.

Question 10.12. **Which of the following statements about retinoid receptors is true?**

A. Retinoid receptors are active both as dimers and monomers.
B. Two retinoid receptor dimer types have been identified: RAR/RXR heterodimers and RXR/RXR homodimers (RAR/RAR homodimers have not been identified).
C. Two retinoid receptor dimer types have been identified: RAR/RXR heterodimers and RAR/RAR homodimers (RXR/RXR homodimers have not been identified).
D. Retinoid receptors are not part of the steroid superfamily and none of its members can bind other receptors within this family such as the vitamin D and the thyroid hormone receptor.

Question 10.13. **Which one of the following statements regarding oral premalignancy is true?**

A. Small hyperplastic leukoplakia lesions have a 5% to 10% spontaneous regression rate and more than a 25% risk of malignant transformation.
B. Erythroleukoplakia and dysplastic leukoplakia lesions are associated with a high rate of spontaneous regression.
C. Molecular markers [e.g., aneuploidy and loss of heterozygosity (LOH)] recently have been shown to potently predict cancer risk.
D. Oral premalignant lesions are not markers of field carcinogenesis since patients with oral premalignancy may develop squamous cancers at the site of the lesions but do not usually develop cancers at distant sites within the upper aerodigestive tract.
E. High-risk, diffuse, and multifocal disease, accounting for 10% to 15% of all oral premalignant lesions, is often controlled adequately by local therapy.

Question 10.14. **Which one of the following statement(s) is/are true with regard to randomized clinical studies with retinoid compounds in chemoprevention?**

A. Treatment with high-dose retinoid compounds induces significant regression of oral premalignant lesions but at the expense of high toxicity and with high recurrence rates after treatment discontinuation.
B. Treatment with high-dose retinoids is capable of preventing second primary tumors of the head and neck but at the expense of very significant toxicity.
C. Treatment with low-dose retinoids was ineffective in preventing second primary tumors of the head and neck.
D. All of the above.
E. None of the above.

Question 10.15. **Which one of the following statements about retinoids is true?**

A. The retinamide fenretinide, when administered for 5 years, prevented contralateral breast cancer in women with a history of resected early breast cancer and no prior adjuvant therapy.
B. High doses of retinoid treatment prevent skin cancers in certain high-risk groups, whereas low doses seem not to have a preventive effect, highlighting the importance of retinoid dose, biologic timing of intervention, and target histopathology.
C. Most randomized studies with a variety of retinoid compounds in cervical dysplasia have shown significant chemopreventive effects.
D. Retinoids and beta-carotene have been clearly shown to decrease the incidence of large bowel adenomas in placebo-controlled trials.

Question 10.16. **In reference to dietary carcinogens, which one of the following statements is correct?**

A. Food additives are the most prevalent class of carcinogens encountered in food.
B. Synthetic pesticides and environmental contaminants are by far the most common source of carcinogens encountered in food.
C. Although chemicals such as food additives, synthetic pesticides, and environmental contaminants have received considerable research and public attention, these agents comprise less than 1% of all carcinogens found in food.
D. Naturally occurring substances, such as toxins produced by plants for protection, mycotoxins produced by molds in food, or substances produced during food preparation, represent less than 1% of all carcinogens encountered in food.

Question 10.17. **Which of the following statements highlight limitations associated with our understanding of human risk associated with naturally occurring carcinogens?**

A. For many potentially carcinogenic constituents of foods, concentration data do not exist.
B. Determining human exposure levels is difficult and sometimes inconclusive.
C. Dietary assessment tools are subjective, often biased, and the food levels of some substances can vary widely.
D. All of the above.
E. None of the above.

Question 10.18. **Which one of the following compounds is a mycotoxin that has been clearly proven to be genotoxic and carcinogenic to humans?**

A. Aflatoxin B1.
B. Heterocyclic aromatic amines.
C. Polycyclic aromatic hydrocarbons.
D. N-nitroso compounds.
E. Ochratoxin A.

Question 10.19. **Select the statement that is NOT true about nonsteroidal anti-inflammatory drugs (NSAIDs) and colorectal cancer chemoprevention.**

A. Epidemiological data have consistently demonstrated a protective association of approximately 30% to 50%.
B. Randomized clinical trials have demonstrated that adenomatous polyp recurrence is significantly suppressed by aspirin and by sulindac when given to patients with prior adenomatous polyps or individuals previously treated for early colorectal malignancies.
C. Sulindac and celecoxib are the only agents proven by randomized clinical studies to be of benefit to familial adenomatous polyposis (FAP) patients.
D. Piroxicam at reasonable clinical doses is unable to reach rectal mucosal levels that are sufficient to inhibit prostaglandin E2 (PGE2).

Question 10.20. **With regard to physical activity and cancer, which one of the following statements is NOT true?**

A. Epidemiologic data have not been able to disclose an association between physical activity and colon cancer.
B. Current data suggest the strongest protective association against colorectal and breast malignancies.
C. The proposed mechanism of colorectal cancer protection includes modulation of insulin resistance and of specific prostaglandins.
D. Proposed mechanisms of breast cancer prevention include modulation of hormonal levels.
E. Occupational activity may be more important than leisure-time activity given its stability over time.

Question 10.21. **Which one of the following statements is true with regard to medullary thyroid cancer?**

A. It has been associated with multiple endocrine neoplasia (MEN) 2A but not MEN 2B.
B. It has been associated with mutations of the RET protooncogene.
C. It may occur as an inherited disorder, but there are no data to support the use of prophylactic thyroidectomy in kindred with the inherited forms of the disease who are identified at risk on the basis of genetic testing.
D. In its familial form, it represents over 50% of all medullary thyroid malignancies.

Question 10.22. **Which one of the following statements about Barrett esophagus is NOT correct?**

A. The presence and degree of dysplasia is the most important predictor of progression to adenocarcinoma.
B. Intestinal metaplasia can be detected in the mucosa adjacent to virtually all cases of adenocarcinoma of the esophagus and in most cases of adenocarcinoma of the gastric cardia.
C. Surgical resection is usually indicated in healthy individuals with Barrett esophagus and severe dysplasia.
D. Medical treatment with H2 blockers or proton pump inhibitors has been shown to have a chemopreventive effect against progression to adenocarcinoma.

Question 10.23. **Which one of the following statements about hereditary diffuse gastric cancer is correct?**

A. A specific germline mutation has not yet been identified.
B. Germline mutations in the E-cadherin gene (CDH1) have been associated with this disorder.
C. Hereditary diffuse gastric cancer follows an autosomic recessive pattern of inheritance.
D. Endoscopic screening for diffuse gastric cancer is appropriate because early abnormalities are usually visible as masses, and these tumors rarely spread along the submucosa.

ANSWERS

Answer 10.1. **The answer is C.**

Tobacco and tobacco smoke contain at least 4,000 chemicals, of which 55 are known carcinogens identified by the International Agency for Research on Cancer. The most notable carcinogen classes include polycyclic aromatic hydrocarbons (PAHs), N-nitrosamines, and miscellaneous organic compounds. Of the PAHs, benzo(a)pyrene (BaP) is the most extensively studied lung carcinogen. Of the N-nitrosamines, 4(methylnitrosamino)-1-(3-pyridyl)-1-butanone (NNK) is best known. Metabolic activation of these agents can incite DNA adduct formation, gene mutations, and a sequence of events that can lead to cancer. The balance between detoxification and metabolic activation determines, in part, the susceptibility of smokers to cancer. Although nicotine does not cause cancer, addiction to nicotine exposes the user to carcinogens.

Answer 10.2. **The answer is C.**

Tobacco use causes approximately 30% of all deaths and more than 440,000 deaths annually. It is the leading cause of preventable death in this country. Tobacco use kills more Americans each year than do alcohol, cocaine, heroin, homicide, suicide, car accidents, firearms, and the acquired immunodeficiency syndrome (AIDS) combined.

Answer 10.3. **The answer is D.**

Tobacco use qualifies as a pediatric disease. The 2001 Youth Risk Behavior Survey indicated smoking rates for girls and boys as 61.6% and 66.3% respectively for lifetime cigarette use and 27.7% and 29.2% respectively for current cigarette use. Nearly 90% of adult smokers begin smoking by the age of 18 years. Even by grade 9, 58.4% of children have experimented with cigarettes. It is estimated that of nearly 3,000 young people who start smoking each day, 1 in 3 will die prematurely. At least 3 million American teenagers smoke regularly.

Answer 10.4. **The answer is D.**

The 1986 U.S. Surgeon General's report defined environmental tobacco smoke (ETS), also called secondhand smoke, as the combination of sidestream smoke (released from a burning cigarette between puffs) and the fraction of mainstream smoke exhaled by the smoker. Those at greatest risk for harm from ETS are those who live with smokers in homes. An increasing number of studies has documented the health risks of the nonsmoker exposed to ETS. In 1992, the U.S. Environmental Protection Agency (EPA), in the most thoroughly documented analysis ever undertaken of the effects of exposure to ETS, concluded that secondhand smoke can cause lung cancer in nonsmoking adults and can impair the respiratory systems of children. The EPA report and other ETS studies now attribute approximately 3,000 deaths a year in the United States to lung cancer, up to 62,000 deaths to ischemic heart disease, and up to 2,700 deaths to sudden infant death syndrome. The 1997 California Environmental Protection Agency report also notes that ETS is responsible for new cases of low-birth-weight infants, new cases of childhood asthma, exacerbation of childhood asthma, and bronchitis or pneumonia in children aged 18 months and younger.

Answer 10.5. **The answer is E.**

Each year, approximately 20 million (of the 46 to 47 million smokers in the United States) try to quit smoking. In addition, 77% of smokers would like to quit, and 65% have made at least one serious attempt at quitting. Yet, studies indicate that one-third relapse after 24 hours and another third relapse after 48 hours. Of all smokers who attempt to quit each year, fewer than 10% are successful. Cigarette smokers who have successfully quit required on average seven serious attempts before achieving abstinence.

Answer 10.6. **The answer is C.**

Physicians and health professionals should view smoking cessation as a cornerstone of their practice. Providing a brief physician intervention to all smokers could more than double annual quit rates. Seventy percent of smokers see their doctors at least once annually, thereby granting physicians ample opportunity for smoking-cessation counseling. If only one half of all U.S. physicians gave brief advice to their patients regarding smoking cessation leading to success in 10%, clinician intervention would account for 2 million new nonsmokers in the United States each year. The 1996 Agency for Health Care Policy and Research (AHCPR) and 2000 Public Health Services (PHS) smoking cessation guidelines also describe that a dose-response relationship exists between the intensity and duration of treatment and its effectiveness. In general, more intense intervention leads to more effective long-term abstinence from tobacco. The success of an intervention also is maximized by proper training and education of physicians and medical students, by increasing the number of modalities used and the number of professionals involved, and by the creation of office-based systems. Three particularly effective elements of smoking cessation treatment are (1) nicotine replacement therapy (NRT), (2) social support (clinician-provided encouragement and assistance), and (3) skills training and problem-solving techniques for achieving and maintaining abstinence. Other pharmacologic interventions such as the use of sustained-release bupropion have shown promise.

Answer 10.7. **The answer is D.**

Based largely on the results of animal studies, international correlations, and a few case-control studies, great enthusiasm developed in the 1980s that modest reductions in total fat intake would have a major impact on breast cancer incidence. However, as the findings from large prospective studies have become available, support for this relationship has greatly weakened. A vast literature on dietary fat and cancer in animals has accumulated. Dietary fat has a clear effect on tumor incidence in many models; however, it is not yet clear whether this is independent of the effect of total energy intake. Although recent evidence suggests that high intake of animal fat early in adult life may increase risk of premenopausal breast cancer, this is not likely to be due to fat per se because vegetable fat was not related to risk. For colon cancer, the associations seen with animal fat internationally have been supported in numerous case-control and cohort studies, but this also appears to be explained by factors in red meat other than simply its fat content. Further, the importance of physical activity and leanness as protective factors against colon cancer indicates that international correlations probably overstate the contribution of diet to differences in colon cancer incidence. No definitive randomized studies have demonstrated a clear beneficial effect of dietary restriction of fat on the occurrence of colorectal cancer. At present the available evidence most strongly suggests an association between animal fat consumption and risk of prostate cancer, particularly the aggressive form of this disease. As with colon cancer, the possibility remains that other factors in animal products contribute to risk.

Answer 10.8. **The answer is A.**

Dietary fiber is defined as "all plant polysaccharides and lignin which are resistant to hydrolysis by the digestive enzymes of men." Fiber, both soluble and insoluble, is fermented by the luminal bacteria of the colon. Among the properties of fiber that make it a candidate for cancer prevention are its "bulking" effect, which reduces colonic transit time and the binding of potentially carcinogenic luminal chemicals. Fiber may also aid in producing short-chained fatty acids that may be directly anticarcinogenic, and fiber may induce apoptosis.

Answer 10.9. **The answer is B.**

A combined analysis of 13 case-control studies as well as a meta-analysis of 16 case-control studies indicated an inverse association between fiber intake and colorectal cancer. Inclusion of studies was selective, however, and effect estimates unadjusted for potential confounders were used for most studies. Moreover, recall bias is a severe threat to the validity of retrospective case-control studies of fiber intake and any disease outcome. Data generated through prospective cohort studies have largely failed to support the inverse association between dietary fiber and colorectal cancer incidence found in retrospective studies. Evidence from at least ten prospective studies is currently available. A number of randomized clinical trials have explored the effect of fiber supplementation on colorectal adenoma recurrence. Evidence has consistently indicated no effect of fiber intake. It has been speculated that dietary fiber decreases the risk of breast cancer by reducing intestinal absorption of estrogens excreted via the biliary system, by down-modulation of serum estrogen levels, and by lowering insulin sensitivity. Relatively few epidemiologic studies have examined the association between fiber intake and breast cancer. In a meta-analysis of ten case-control studies, a significant inverse association was observed. Results from at least six prospective cohort studies of the association between fiber intake and breast cancer incidence have been reported, with most of them failing to reveal an inverse association between breast cancer incidence and dietary fiber. Overall, the observational data presently available do not indicate an important role of dietary fiber in the prevention of cancer.

Answer 10.10. **The answer is C.**

Carotenoids, prevalent in fruits and vegetables, are antioxidants, enhance cell-to-cell communication, promote cell differentiation, and modulate immune response. Some 20 years ago, epidemiologists speculated that beta-carotene may be a major player in cancer prevention and encouraged testing its anticarcinogenic properties. Indeed, subsequent observational studies supported a reduced cancer risk, in particular of lung cancer, with high intake of carotenoids. Randomized clinical trials of beta-carotene supplements, in contrast, have not revealed evidence of a protective effect of beta-carotene. In contrast, beta-carotene was found to increase the risk of lung cancer and total mortality among smokers in the Finnish Alpha-Tocopherol, Beta-Carotene Cancer Prevention Study. The discrepancy in evidence between epidemiologic studies and randomized clinical trials has been in part attributed to recall bias in case-control studies and to residual confounding.

Answer 10.11. **The answer is D.**

Cancer chemoprevention can be defined as pharmacologic intervention with specific nutrients or other chemicals to suppress or reverse carcinogenesis and to prevent the development of invasive cancer. Two basic concepts support this cancer control strategy—multistep and field carcinogenesis. Carcinogenesis is a chronic, multistep process characterized by the accumulation of specific genetic and phenotypic alterations that can evolve over a 10- to 20-year period from the first initiating event. The premise of human chemoprevention is that one can intervene (and suppress) at many steps in the carcinogenic process and over a many-year period. We now understand that the process of neoplastic evolution can involve mutations in key tumor-suppressor genes and/or oncogenes, epigenetic changes via aberrations of histone acetylation or DNA methylation, genetic instability, and defects in signal transduction, with clonal expansion and, remarkably, intraepithelial spread/metastasis of premalignant cells. Field carcinogenesis was first described in the early 1950s as "field cancerization" in the head and neck and subsequently was ascribed to many epithelial sites. The field concept is that patients at high risk for an epithelial cancer have a wide surface area of carcinogenic tissue change that can be detected at the gross (oral premalignant lesions, polyps), microscopic (metaplasia, dysplasia), and/or molecular (gene loss or amplification) levels. The implication of the field effect is that multifocal, genetically distinct, and clonally related premalignant lesions can progress over a broad tissue region. The essence of chemoprevention, then, is intervention within the multistep carcinogenic process and throughout a wide field.

Answer 10.12. **The answer is B.**

The term *retinoid* was redefined in 1985 by Sporn to include a substance that binds and activates one or more specific receptors, the latter producing a biologic response. The retinoid molecular mechanism of action is similar to that of steroid/thyroid hormones in that retinoid nuclear receptors are members of the steroid receptor superfamily. Research studies indicate that retinoid receptors are unique among other members of the steroid receptor family in that there are two receptor classes—retinoic acid receptors (RARs) and RXRs. Each receptor contains α, β, and γ subtypes, and several of these subclasses have multiple isoforms. These receptors are DNA-binding transcription factors that can activate or suppress the expression of many genes, the products of which mediate retinoid effects on cell growth, differentiation, and apoptosis. Different retinoids bind to the different receptor classes and subclasses with different affinities. This receptor complexity and great diversity in ligand-binding activation and receptor function has important preventive and therapeutic implications. As with other members of the steroid family, retinoid receptors are active only as dimers. Two retinoid receptor dimer types have been identified: RAR/RXR heterodimers and RXR/RXR homodimers (RAR/RAR homodimers have not been identified). Part of the retinoid receptor binds to the ligand, and part binds to specific DNA sequences (RARE or RXRE) and either induces or suppresses gene transcription. The best characterized pathway involves RAR/RXR heterodimers. RXRs recently have been shown to form heterodimers with other members of the steroid receptor family, including the vitamin D receptor and thyroid hormone receptor. RXRs and their ligands, therefore, can modulate the activities of other steroid hormones.

Answer 10.13. **The answer is C.**

Oral premalignant lesions include leukoplakias and erythroplakias. Small hyperplastic leukoplakia lesions have a 30% to 40% spontaneous regression rate and less than a 5% risk of malignant transformation. Erythroleukoplakia and dysplastic leukoplakia lesions, however, are associated with a low rate of spontaneous regression and a 30% to 40% long-term risk of oral cancer. Molecular markers [e.g., aneuploidy and loss of heterozygosity (LOH)] recently have been shown to potently predict cancer risk. High-risk, diffuse, and multifocal disease, accounting for 10% to 15% of all oral premalignant lesions, often is not controlled adequately by local therapy. Oral premalignant lesions are markers of field carcinogenesis since patients with oral premalignancy develop squamous cancers at the site of the lesions as well as at distant sites within the upper aerodigestive tract. Thus, regression of oral premalignant lesions has been used to screen agents that may have utility in the prevention of upper aerodigestive tract cancers.

Answer 10.14. **The answer is D.**

Retinoids have been studied extensively in the reversal of oral premalignant lesions. One of the first such trials, reported in 1986, was a 3-month placebo-controlled study of high-dose 13cRA. The complete plus partial response rate in the 44 evaluable patients was 67% in the retinoid arm and 10% in the placebo arm ($p = 0.0002$). The histopathologic improvement rate (e.g., reversal of dysplasia) was also higher in the retinoid arm (54% versus 10%, $p = 0.01$). There were two major problems, however, with this high-dose, short-term approach. First, high-dose 13cRA toxicity was substantial and not acceptable in this clinical setting. Second, over half of the responders recurred or developed new lesions within 3 months of stopping the intervention. High-dose 13cRA was also tested in 103 head and neck cancer patients. Following definitive local therapy with surgery and/or radiotherapy, patients were assigned randomly to 12 months of high-dose 13cRA (50-100 mg/m^2/d) or placebo. At a median follow-up of 32 months, there were no significant differences in primary disease recurrence (local, regional, or distant) or survival. The rate of second primary tumors, however, was significantly lower in the retinoid arm than in the placebo group, developing in 2 (4%) of the 13cRA-treated patients compared with 12 (24%) of the placebo-treated patients ($p = 0.005$). Side effects were substantial and included skin dryness and peeling, cheilitis, conjunctivitis, and hypertriglyceridemia. Approximately 30% of the retinoid-treated patients required dose reduction, and 18% did not complete the 12-month intervention because of toxicity. A large-scale National Cancer Institute (NCI) Intergroup phase III trial of low-dose, long-term 13cRA was launched in 1991 in stage I, II head and neck squamous cell carcinoma patients definitively treated with radiation therapy or surgery. Of 1,384 registered patients, 1,191 were eligible and randomized to receive either 13cRA or placebo for 3 years and were followed for 4 more years. There was no significant difference between the treatment and placebo arms in overall survival or second primary tumor (SPT)- or recurrence-free survival.

Answer 10.15. **The answer is B.**

The retinamide fenretinide is a potent apoptosis-inducing retinoid with retinoid receptor-dependent and -independent activities and accumulates in human breast tissue. Although preclinical data suggested a strong chemopreventive effect for the breast, a large-scale randomized trial of fenretinide (versus no treatment) for 5 years produced no significant overall effect. A randomized, placebo-controlled trial of the retinoid acitretin (30 mg per day for 6 months) was conducted in 38 renal transplant recipients. The retinoid group had significant reductions in (a) premalignant lesions ($p = 0.008$), (b) the number of patients with skin cancer ($p = 0.01$), and (c) the cumulative number of skin cancers ($p = 0.009$). Nine of the 19 placebo patients developed a total of 18 skin cancers, and 2 of the 19 retinoid patients developed skin cancer, one cancer each. There have been two other randomized acitretin trials in this setting, one significantly reducing skin squamous cell carcinoma and one significantly reducing actinic keratoses. Three large-scale randomized phase III trials of retinoids and skin cancer have been reported. A trial of very low-dose 13cRA (10 mg per day)) and one of retinol (25,000 IU) or 13cRA (5-10 mg per day) versus placebo in patients with prior skin cancers were negative. The third trial, involving retinol in patients with prior actinic keratoses, did see a significant reduction of squamous but not basal skin cancers in the retinoid arm. The contrasting results of the phase III retinoid trials in skin cancer chemoprevention suggest the importance of retinoid dose, biologic timing of intervention, and target histopathology. Many randomized chemoprevention studies have been conducted in cervical dysplasia. Only one of these trials, using topical all-trans-retonic acid (ATRA), found a significant treatment effect. However, more recent randomized retinoid studies involving topical ATRA and oral fenretinide, 13cRA, and 9cRA have all been negative. Several randomized trials aimed at the prevention of recurrent colorectal adenomas with supplemental beta-carotene have been completed, but none of them demonstrated a chemopreventive effect.

Answer 10.16. **The answer is C.**

The human diet is a highly complex and variable mixture of naturally occurring and synthetic compounds, including compounds that have been identified as carcinogens. Although chemicals such as food additives, synthetic pesticides, and environmental contaminants have received considerable research and public attention, these agents comprise less than 1% of all carcinogens found in food. The majority of dietary carcinogens are "natural pesticides," toxins produced by plants for protection, mycotoxins produced by molds in foods, or substances produced during food preparation.

Answer 10.17. **The answer is D.**

With regard to naturally occurring carcinogens, current knowledge is incomplete and does not allow reliable estimates of risk. For many potentially carcinogenic constituents of foods, concentration data do not exist. In addition, determining human exposure levels is difficult and sometimes inconclusive. Dietary assessment tools are subjective and often biased; the food levels of some substances can vary widely, and exposure to mixtures of substances at low doses might be more important than exposure to single agents. Determination of carcinogenic potential and potency is based on information obtained from epidemiologic observations, animal models, and *in vitro* systems. However, most food constituents have not undergone carcinogenic or toxicity testing. Further, extrapolation of the effects of the near-toxic doses used in animals to risk to humans consuming low concentrations of the same dietary constituents is difficult, particularly without a more complete understanding of the mechanisms of action of these compounds and of the level of human exposure.

Answer 10.18. **The answer is A.**

Mycotoxins are structurally diverse, toxic, fungal metabolites that are common contaminants of ingredients in animal feed and human food. To date, more than 300 mycotoxins have been identified. A group of mycotoxins have been shown to have carcinogenic potential in animals. Examples of these include aflatoxins (corn, peanuts, seed nuts, peanut butter), ochratoxin A (grains, green coffee beans), T-2 toxin (barley, maize, safflower seeds, cereals), zearalenone (feed grains, soybean, maize, wheat), fumonisins (corn), deoxynivalenol (wheat, maize) and nivalenol (wheat, maize, barley). However, only aflatoxin B_1 and naturally occurring mixtures of aflatoxins are known to be genotoxic and carcinogenic to humans (liver carcinogenicity). Food preparation and preservation are major alternative sources of dietary carcinogens. These include heterocyclic aromatic amines (HAAs), formed during frying, broiling, and grilling high-protein foods (more prevalent in well-done meats); polycyclic aromatic hydrocarbons (PAHs), formed during broiling and smoking food; acrylamide, formed during high-temperature cooking of starchy foods such as potato chips and french fries; and N-nitroso compounds (NOCs), formed in smoked, salted, and pickled foods cured with nitrate or nitrite. NOCs also form endogenously at sites such as the stomach from nitrites and amines in the diet.

Answer 10.19. **The answer is B.**

Although randomized clinical trials have proven that aspirin is capable of preventing the development of adenomatous polyps in patients with prior polyps and/or treated for early colorectal malignancies, studies in individuals with previous sporadic adenoma have found no evidence that sulindac suppressed adenoma recurrence. Most of the nearly 40 epidemiologic (nonrandomized) studies that have now examined the relationship between NSAID use and colon adenoma/cancer risk have found 30% to 50% lower risk of colorectal adenoma or cancer among people who regularly use NSAIDs. This finding is one of the strongest and most consistent associations seen in epidemiologic studies of colorectal cancer. Studies show that piroxicam administered at acceptable doses has failed to suppress PGE2 production in rectal mucosa. Several phase II or III randomized clinical trials have now established that two NSAIDs, the pro-NSAID sulindac and the selective COX-2 inhibitor celecoxib, effectively suppress the development of adenomatous polyps and cause regression of existing adenomas in FAP patients. Celecoxib has been formally approved by the Food and Drug Administration (FDA) as adjuvant therapy for patients with FAP. While randomized trials have now confirmed the efficacy of aspirin in preventing recurrent adenoma, they have not resolved questions about the optimal treatment regimen or the risk/benefit balance of administering prolonged treatment with NSAIDs prophylactically to healthy people. In general, questions about the safety of long-term NSAID prophylaxis and the efficacy of NSAIDs against cancers other than colon and rectum cancer currently limit their clinical application to FAP patients.

Answer 10.20. **The answer is A.**

The 1994 report of the U.S. Surgeon General concluded that lack of physical activity is causally related to increased risk of coronary heart disease, diabetes, and colon cancer. In 2002, the International Agency for Research on Cancer (IARC) published an updated report on weight control and physical activity concluding that the epidemiologic evidence for colon and breast cancer was convincing with suggested associations existing for endometrial, prostate, and lung cancers. Several biologic mechanisms have been proposed for the protective effect of physical activity against colorectal cancer reflecting changes in physiologic measures following physical activity. The role of insulin is increasingly seen as an important mechanism as abdominal obesity and low physical activity are independently related to insulin resistance. Across a gradient of physical activity, insulin sensitivity improves with exercise. Further, insulin is a strong growth factor for colon mucosal cells in laboratory studies and an animal model of colon cancer. Thus, it is possible that activity exerts its protective effect through reduced insulin levels. Another proposed mechanism is the effect of prostaglandins on colon cell proliferation. Physical activity produces an increase in prostaglandin F2 alpha, which increases intestinal motility and inhibits colonic cell proliferation. Activity also results in a decrease in prostaglandin E2 levels, which in cell culture can act to stimulate colon cell proliferation. Regular physical activity has been hypothesized to prevent breast cancer, largely by reducing circulating levels of sex hormones. The mechanisms by which physical activity reduces exposure to hormones vary by period of life. Young girls participating in strenuous athletic training such as running and ballet dancing have delayed menarche, which is known to reduce risk of breast cancer, and even moderate-intensity physical activity may also delay menstruation. A later menarche is associated with a later onset of regular ovulatory cycles as well as lower serum estrogen concentrations during adolescence. Once menstruation has been established, anovulatory and irregular menstrual cycles may be more frequent among moderately and strenuously active women than among inactive women, although there is disagreement regarding the degree to which the intensity of physical activity influences menstrual abnormalities. Among older women, levels of past and current physical activity influence fat stores, which after menopause are the locus of conversion of androstenedione to estrogen. Epidemiologic studies have measured activity in two ways: by occupation and by leisure time activities. These measures may represent somewhat different patterns of energy expenditure. Activity demanded by employment in a certain occupation may be relatively constant from week to week and year to year, whereas leisure-time activity is far more labile, changing from week to week, season to season, and year to year. Over the past century, occupational energy expenditure within any class of occupation has declined steadily as mechanization has increased. Leisure time activity, on the other hand, varies substantially from season to season with a high in the summer months and a low during winter. In the epidemiologic study of chronic diseases like colon cancer, long-term patterns of activity may be the relevant factor in determining disease risk. Therefore, occupational activity may be a better marker of cancer-determining activity level than is self-reported leisure-time activity.

Answer 10.21. **The answer is B.**

Multiple endocrine neoplasia (MEN) is characterized by the development of multiple tumors in endocrine organs in a patient and close relatives. The syndrome is divided into MEN 1, MEN 2A, and MEN 2B. MEN 2 is defined by the combination of tissues affected and the presence of developmental abnormalities and has been the focus of extensive genetic analysis. MEN 2A is associated with medullary carcinoma of the thyroid and hyperparathyroidism. Individuals with MEN 2B have medullary carcinoma of the thyroid, pheochromocytoma, and developmental abnormalities involving hyperplasia of intestinal autonomic nerve plexuses and growth of nerve axons in the lips, oral mucosa, and conjunctiva, which give rise to the characteristic facies. A syndrome related to MEN 2 is familial medullary thyroid carcinoma (FMTC) in which patients have only medullary carcinoma of the thyroid. MEN 2A, MEN 2B, and FMTC have an autosomal dominant pattern of inheritance and account for approximately 25% of all cases of medullary carcinoma of the thyroid. In 1993, it was established that mutations in the RET protooncogene were responsible for the hereditary predisposition to medullary thyroid cancer. This genetic breakthrough has allowed accurate identification of kindred at high risk for developing medullary carcinoma of the thyroid and has permitted families to consider the risks and benefit of prophylactic thyroidectomy. In 1994, Wells et al. reported the first experience with prophylactic thyroidectomy based on identification of RET protooncogene mutations. Thirteen patients were confirmed to carry a mutation in the RET protooncogene in association with MEN 2A and underwent immediate thyroidectomy. In each patient, the resected thyroid gland demonstrated C-cell hyperplasia. There were no metastases found in regional nodes, and all patients had normal post-operative stimulated plasma calcitonin levels. Subsequent reports have confirmed the validity of this approach, and prophylactic thyroidectomy is now recommended for these patients at about age 6.

Answer 10.22. **The answer is D.**

Barrett esophagus is a premalignant condition in which the stratified squamous epithelium in the distal esophagus is replaced to a variable extent by metaplastic columnar epithelium. This is significant from an oncologic perspective because of the close association between Barrett esophagus and the development of adenocarcinoma of the esophagus. In fact, intestinal metaplasia can be detected in the mucosa adjacent to virtually all cases of adenocarcinoma of the esophagus and in most cases of adenocarcinoma of the gastric cardia. Epithelial dysplasia is the best indicator of the risk of cancer and is an important clinical factor used to stratify patients with Barrett esophagus. Most patients with reflux are treated medically with weight reduction, head of bed elevation, and H2 receptor antagonists or protein pump inhibitors. The goal of therapy is symptomatic relief of gastroesophageal reflux. Although symptoms of reflux often improve with therapy, there is no evidence to suggest medical therapy will consistently induce regression of the metaplastic columnar epithelium. Most experts recommend that healthy patients with high-grade dysplasia undergo esophagectomy by an experienced surgeon. The pathologic diagnosis should be independently confirmed. However, since there is a wide spectrum of reported mortality following esophagectomy and because not all patients with high-grade dysplasia develop adenocarcinoma, some experts have made a case for aggressive surveillance for these patients.

Answer 10.23. **The answer is B.**

In 1998 Guilford reported that 3 germline mutations in the E-cadherin gene (CDH1)were found in kindred of Maori families from New Zealand who had early onset of poorly differentiated diffuse gastric cancer. Subsequently other CDH1 mutations have been found in other families with diffuse gastric cancer. It has become clear that a small percentage of gastric cancers (1% to 3%) arise as a result of this inherited syndrome. Germline mutations in the E-cadherin gene are inherited as autosomal dominants with high penetrance. It is estimated that affected individuals carry a lifetime risk of developing gastric cancer of approximately 70%, and patients with this syndrome have developed gastric cancer as early as age 18. The optimal management of patients with hereditary diffuse gastric cancer has not been defined. Endoscopic screening for diffuse gastric cancer is problematic because early abnormalities may not be visible as masses and these tumors tend to spread along the submucosa. Multiple reports suggest that prophylactic total gastrectomy may be effective in preventing gastric cancer.

CHAPTER **11**

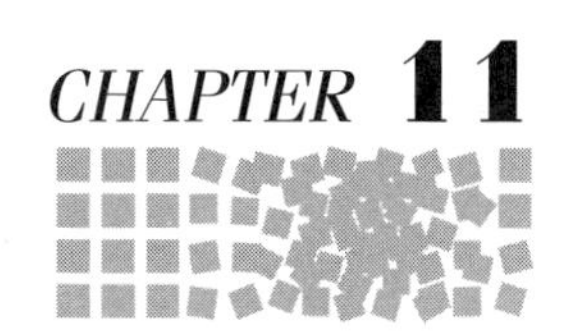

Cancer Screening

MEGAN E. WREN

Directions Each of the numbered items below is followed by lettered answers. Select the ONE lettered answer that is BEST in each case unless instructed otherwise.

QUESTIONS

Question 11.1. **You just read an article about a new laboratory test that has been proposed as a screening test for a certain disease. It reports a sensitivity of 99%, specificity of 95%, and a positive predictive value of 10%, with a disease prevalence of about 0.5% in the study population, which is similar in demographic characteristics to your clinic population. You order this test on one of your patients and the result is positive (abnormal). How would you interpret this test?**

A. There is a 1% chance that this represents a false-positive result.
B. There is a 5% chance that this represents a false-positive result.
C. There is a 9 in 10 chance that this represents a false-positive result.
D. You can be 99% sure that your patient has the disease.

Question 11.2. **Studies of screening for cancer are subject to several types of bias. If screening detects a cancer sooner (before it becomes symptomatic), but treatment has no effect on the course of the disease, the subject will seem to live longer than if he or she had presented symptomatically. (That is, the cancer is known for a longer period of time, but the time of death is not altered.) This type of bias is known as**

A. lead time bias
B. length bias
C. volunteer bias

Question 11.3. **The most important physician action to reduce lung cancer mortality is which one of the following.**

A. Annual chest x-ray for all smokers over age 50.
B. Annual low-dose helical computed tomographic (CT) scan for current or former smokers with a 20 pack-year history.
C. Chest x-ray and sputum cytology every 6 months for heavy smokers (>$\frac{1}{2}$ pack per day).
D. Aggressive efforts to help patients stop smoking and to prevent youths from starting to smoke.

Corresponding Chapters in *Cancer: Principles & Practice of Oncology*, Seventh Edition: 22 (Cancer Screening).

Question 11.4. **Almost all cervical cancers are associated with infection by sexually transmitted human papilloma virus (HPV). Of the following statements about HPV infection in young women (in their teens and 20s), which one is INCORRECT?**

A. HPV infection is common in young, sexually active women.
B. HPV infection is often transient in young women.
C. In young women, most cases of low-grade squamous intraepithelial lesion (LSIL) will regress without treatment.
D. HPV infection and LSIL are the earliest stages in the development of cervical cancer and require aggressive treatment.

Question 11.5. **For women who have had a hysterectomy, which one of the following is the most appropriate practice for screening for cervical cancer with Pap smears?**

A. Pap smears should be performed every 1 to 3 years indefinitely.
B. Pap smears should be performed every 1 to 3 years until age 65.
C. Women who have had a "simple" or supracervical hysterectomy do not need screening.
D. Women who have a history of cervical cancer can discontinue screening following a total abdominal hysterectomy.
E. Women who have had a total hysterectomy for benign conditions no longer need Pap smears.

Question 11.6. **Which one statement regarding screening for breast cancer is MOST true?**

A. Teaching women to perform a thorough breast self-exam (BSE) has been shown to have a small but measurable impact on breast cancer mortality rates.
B. The monthly BSE is a crucial component of breast cancer screening programs.
C. A high quality clinical breast exam (CBE) provides a small additional benefit in mortality reduction, beyond that achieved by mammographic screening alone.
D. The physician's clinical breast exam is redundant and is unnecessary for patients who receive annual mammograms.

Question 11.7. **The best evidence for a mortality benefit for mammography is in women aged**

A. 40 to 49 years
B. 50 to 69 years
C. 70 to 79 years

Question 11.8. **Regarding screening programs for prostate cancer, which one statement is LEAST true?**

A. Population-based screening has been proven to detect early stage disease and to decrease mortality from prostate cancer.
B. Many very elderly men die "with" rather than "of" prostate cancer. This raises concerns that studies may overestimate the benefits of screening (overdiagnosis bias).
C. Prostate cancer is the second leading cause of cancer deaths in men.
D. Testing for prostate specific antigen (PSA) has a low specificity, resulting in many false-positive tests.
E. PSA levels can be normal in men with localized prostate cancer.

Question 11.9. **The most important factor influencing people to be screened for cancer is**

A. physician recommendation
B. educational background
C. socioeconomic background
D. ethnicity

Question 11.10. **For which of the following cancers has screening been shown, in well-designed studies, to decrease mortality? (More than one answer is possible.)**

A. Lung cancer.
B. Prostate cancer.
C. Cervical cancer.
D. Breast cancer.
E. Colorectal cancer.
F. Ovarian cancer.

ANSWERS

Answer 11.1. **The answer is C.**

The sensitivity of a test reflects its ability to detect a known disease, and the specificity reflects the ability of a test to give a normal result when the disease is known to be absent. From the point of view of the clinician, the presence or absence of a disease is unknown, and the pertinent question is the accuracy of the test result. The positive predictive value (PPV or PV+) is an estimate of the accuracy of the test in predicting the presence of disease; the negative predictive value (NPV or PV–) is an estimate of the accuracy of the test in predicting the absence of disease. The positive predictive value represents the proportion of all positive tests that are true positives: TP/(TP+FP). A PPV of 10% means that 10% of positive test results are true positives, so 90% are false positives.

Answer 11.2. **The answer is A.**

Lead-time bias is the interval between the diagnosis of disease at screening and when it would have been detected due to the development of symptoms. Length bias is the overrepresentation among screen-detected cases of those with a long preclinical period (thus, less rapidly fatal), leading to the incorrect conclusion that screening was beneficial. Volunteers who choose to participate in screening programs are likely to be different from the general population in ways that affect survival. They may be more compliant or may have healthier habits. Conversely, they may volunteer because they feel they are at higher risk for disease.

Answer 11.3. **The answer is D.**

Randomized trials of chest x-rays with or without sputum cytology have failed to show any improvement in lung cancer mortality. The newer technique of low-dose helical CT scanning has no published randomized controlled trial (RCT) data regarding mortality. Prevention of smoking and smoking cessation remain the best tools for combating lung cancer.

Answer 11.4. **The answer is D.**

HPV infection is common in young, sexually active women, but is often transient: up to 70% of high-risk HPV infections will resolve spontaneously. Similarly, up to 90% of low-grade squamous intraepithelial lesions will regress without treatment. Concerns have been raised that screening young women could lead to overdiagnosis, aggressive treatment, and unnecessary harm from ablative surgical procedures.

Answer 11.5. **The answer is E.**

Women without a cervix are not at risk for cervical cancer unless there was a prior history of cervical cancer (then Pap smears are for follow-up of the cancer, not for screening). Vaginal cuff smears are unnecessary; they have an extremely low likelihood of detecting vaginal dysplasia, and the false-positive rate is high.

Answer 11.6. **The answer is C.**

Large trials of careful BSE instruction have failed to show any mortality benefit, so BSE is no longer a standard component of breast cancer screening programs (the American Cancer Society lists BSE as an option). The evidence suggests that a 5% to 20% additional benefit in mortality reduction can be achieved by the addition of a high quality clinical breast exam.

Answer 11.7. **The answer is B.**

Numerous randomized controlled trials have demonstrated a mortality benefit to mammographic screening of women aged 50 to 69. The benefit of screening women in their 40s is much more modest (estimated 1 to 2 lives saved per 1,000 women screened for 10 years), and recommendations have been the subject of much controversy. Too few women over age 70 have been enrolled in RCTs to provide definitive evidence.

Answer 11.8. **The answer is A.**

To date there is no definitive evidence that screening leads to reduction in prostate cancer mortality. Approximately one third of men with localized prostate cancer have normal PSA levels (false negative), while PSA elevations are common in noncancerous conditions, such as benign prostatic hyperplasia (false positive). Because prostate cancer is common in very elderly men and may be indolent, questions have been raised about overdiagnosis, lead time, and length biases.

Answer 11.9. **The answer is A.**

Physician recommendations are the most important factor in motivating people to be screened. Simple reminders and letters can increase compliance with screening programs.

Answer 11.10. **The answers are C, D, and E.**

RCT evidence supports the roles of mammography and clinical breast exam in reducing mortality from breast cancer (up to 20% to 30% reduction). Fecal occult blood testing has been shown in RCTs to reduce mortality from colorectal cancer. The effectiveness of flexible sigmoidoscopy has been supported by case-control studies, but RCT data has yet to be published. Colonoscopy and barium enema have been shown to have superior sensitivity and specificity but have not been shown to decrease mortality. Although no RCTs of cervical cancer screening have been conducted, there is strong supportive evidence from case-control studies and from observed trends in countries as screening programs are introduced. At this point, no rigorous studies have documented mortality reductions from screening programs for lung, prostate, or ovarian cancer.

CHAPTER 12

Advances in Diagnostics

SANJEEV BHALLA

Directions Each of the numbered items below is followed by lettered answers. Select the ONE lettered answer that is BEST in each case unless instructed otherwise.

QUESTIONS

Question 12.1. **Regarding percutaneous needle biopsy, which is NOT true?**

A. Needle biopsy may be useful in distinguishing infection versus tumor.
B. Core biopsies are often required in the diagnosis of lymphoma, thymoma, and sarcoma.
C. If lymphoma is suspected, cells are sent in Roswell Park Memorial Institute (RPMI) solution.
D. Intravenous contrast is necessary.
E. Even though procedures are image guided, prebiopsy imaging is key to procedural planning.

Question 12.2. **Regarding percutaneous lung needle biopsy, which is true?**

A. Computed tomography (CT) is faster than fluoroscopy.
B. Fluoroscopy is better for central (mediastinal) lesions.
C. Most common complications are pneumothorax and hemoptysis.
D. With appropriate image guidance, pneumothorax rates are less than 10%.

Question 12.3. **Regarding percutaneous abdominal and pelvic biopsies, which is NOT true?**

A. Pneumothorax is a well-known potential complication of adrenal biopsies.
B. Liver biopsies may need a core biopsy to distinguish well-differentiated neoplasms from benign lesions.
C. Fewer complications are sustained from crossing the transverse colon than the inferior vena cava when performing pancreatic biopsies.
D. Pelvic percutaneous biopsies are the preferred technique when ovarian cancer leads the differential diagnosis.
E. Pelvic sarcomas often require core biopsies.

Corresponding Chapters in *Cancer: Principles & Practice of Oncology*, Seventh Edition: 23 (Advanced Molecular Diagnostics), 24 (Advanced Imaging Methods), and 25 (Cancer Diagnosis: Endoscopy).

Question 12.4. **Regarding central venous access, which is NOT true?**

A. Image guidance reduces the risk of pneumothorax.
B. Internal jugular approach is contraindicated in patients with an ipsilateral axillary nodal dissection.
C. Subclavian access increases the risk of pneumothorax (compared with internal jugular access).
D. Subclavian access increases the rate of venous stasis and thrombosis (compared with internal jugular access).
E. Right internal jugular approach is preferred over left because of the shorter intravascular course of a right-sided catheter.

Question 12.5. **Regarding percutaneous gastrostomy tubes, which is NOT true?**

A. Requires less sedation than endoscopy-placed feeding tube.
B. May be placed for feeding or decompression.
C. Contraindicated in patients with prior gastrectomy.
D. Contraindicated in patients with ascites.
E. If in place over 4 weeks, no imaging guidance is required to reinsert the tube if it falls out.

Question 12.6. **Regarding percutaneous nephrostomy, which is NOT true?**

A. Treatment for pyonephrosis.
B. Useful for diverting urine proximally from a genitourinary fistula.
C. Requires preprocedural antibiotics.
D. Requires CT guidance to access the kidneys.

Question 12.7. **Regarding biliary procedures, which is NOT true?**

A. High strictures are usually treated by interventional radiology and low strictures are usually treated by gastroenterology.
B. The right biliary system is more likely to have isolated dilated segments from a central mass.
C. Biliary dilatation is the major indication for intervention.
D. Pruritus can be cured by draining just one segment.
E. Cholangitis may require multiple catheters to cure sepsis.

Question 12.8. **Regarding percutaneous transhepatic biliary drainage, which is NOT true?**

A. Preprocedural antibiotics are required.
B. Usually drainage is via a two-staged procedure: external drainage then internal drainage.
C. High biliary outputs warrant nutritional replenishment.
D. Contrast is usually used.
E. Liver function usually takes weeks to return to normal.

Question 12.9. **Regarding percutaneous cholecystostomy, which is NOT true?**

A. May be a diagnostic tool in unexplained sepsis.
B. May be a therapeutic tool in acute cholecystitis.
C. A transhepatic approach is preferred.
D. Distension of the gallbladder during cholecystography is avoided in the acute setting.
E. It usually avoids a future cholecystectomy.

Question 12.10. **Regarding malignant pleural effusions, which is true?**

A. Surgical pleurodesis offers a higher success rate in their management than chemical pleurodesis.
B. Usually transudates from tumor obstruction.
C. Usually asymptomatic.
D. Thoracentesis is the definitive treatment.
E. Large-bore tubes are better than small-bore catheters in their management.

Question 12.11. **Regarding superior vena cava obstruction, which is NOT true?**

A. Occlusion is a common consequence of thoracic malignancy.
B. Collateral vessels predispose to hemorrhage and require embolization.
C. Radiographic occlusion may be asymptomatic.
D. Angioplasty with stenting is better than radiation therapy for immediate symptomatic relief.
E. Recurrent obstruction may be treated with thrombolysis, balloon angioplasty, or repeat stenting.

Question 12.12. **Which is NOT an indication for an inferior vena cava filter?**

A. History of recurrent gastrointestinal hemorrhage.
B. Recurrent venous thrombus despite anticoagulation.
C. Propagating lower extremity thrombus.
D. Eccentric mural thrombus in inferior vena cava.
E. Planned surgery.

Question 12.13. **Regarding inferior vena cava filters, which is true?**

A. Femoral approach preferred for their deployment.
B. Symptomatic caval thrombosis is fairly rare complication.
C. It is permanent.
D. Jugular approach requires the patient to lie flat for 6 hours.
E. No role for inferior vena cavagram prior to deployment.

Question 12.14. **With respect to recurrent ascites, which is NOT true?**

A. Transjugular intrahepatic portosystemic shunt (TIPS) has been used to control ascites from portal hypertension.
B. TIPS is contraindicated in patients with hepatic encephalopathy.
C. Peritoneovenous shunting is an effective method of dealing with malignant ascites.
D. TIPS is more beneficial in dealing with ascites from portal hypertension than medical management alone.
E. Large-volume paracentesis is an effective method for obtaining symptomatic relief from malignant ascites.

Question 12.15. **Regarding percutaneous abscess drainage, which is true?**

A. Urinomas are readily distinguished from abscesses with routine imaging.
B. Transbowel approach is an acceptable route of drainage.
C. Bilomas do not require drainage as they are sterile.
D. Pancreatic leaks may be suspected because of high amylase.
E. Small bowel leaks require surgical intervention.

Question 12.16. **Regarding concepts of hepatic embolization, which is NOT true?**

A. Coils provide an effective hepatic embolization technique.
B. The hepatic artery provides greater blood supply to hepatic tumors than the portal vein.
C. Hypervascular lesions are more sensitive to ischemia than hypovascular lesions.
D. For neuroendocrine tumors, therapy is often aimed at symptomatic relief.
E. Postembolization symptoms are often self-limited.

Question 12.17. **Regarding hepatic tumor ablation, which is NOT true?**

A. Percutaneous ethanol injection (PEI) is not as useful for metastatic disease as it is for hepatocellular cancer.
B. Radiofrequency ablation (RFA) is limited when the tumor is near a vessel.
C. Acetic acid is an alternative to ethanol.
D. Combination therapy refers to a combination of intraarterial and percutaneous therapies.
E. RFA and PEI are usually reserved for larger tumors (>7 cm).

Question 12.18. **Regarding the variety of imaging modalities, which is NOT true?**

A. Bone magnetic resonance imaging (MRI) has essentially replaced radiography for the evaluation of osseous lesions.
B. Sonography may be used for the evaluation of chest lesions.
C. Multidetector computer tomography (MDCT) has resulted in improved temporal resolution in cross-sectional imaging.
D. MRI has the advantage of functional analysis.
E. Both MDCT and MRI allow for high-quality multiplanar imaging.

Question 12.19. **Regarding nuclear medicine studies, which is true?**

A. Increased number of images results in increased radiation dose.
B. Bone scintigraphy is a good screening for bone metastases from prostate cancer when the prostate specific antigen (PSA) is less than 5.
C. Sentinel node mapping is of no value in the staging of melanoma.
D. Positron emission tomography (PET)/CT relies on spiral CT for its attenuation correction.
E. Single photon emission computed tomography (SPECT) relies on injection of fluorodeoxyglucose (FDG) for diagnosis.

Question 12.20. **Regarding therapeutic response assessment, which is true?**

A. There are three categories of response: complete response, partial response, and disease progression.
B. Response evaluation criteria in solid tumors (RECIST) rely on bidirectional measurements.
C. Partial response represents less than 25% reduction in the sum of the tumor cross products.
D. One shortcoming of the RECIST is the lack of inclusion of bone marrow involvement by neoplasm.
E. There is no role in using perfusion techniques to assess tumor response.

Question 12.21. **Regarding brain neoplasms, which is true?**

A. Cross-sectional imaging is a highly specific way to distinguish recurrent tumor from radiation change.
B. MRI with contrast is superior to CT for the evaluation of sellar lesions.
C. CT plays no role in the presurgical evaluation when high-quality MRI is used.
D. Because of high spatial resolution, MRI does not require contrast to detect cerebral lesions.
E. Functional MRI is a great way to look at the behavior of small nodules and avoid overstaging a patient.

Question 12.22. **Regarding head and neck cancers, which is true?**

A. MRI is favored over CT when the lesion is in the upper aerodigestive tract near the skull base.
B. Neck CT with intravenous contrast is better than endoscopy in the evaluation of small mucosal lesions of the aerodigestive tract.
C. There is no role for PET/CT in head and neck cancers since intravenous contrast material is not used.
D. CT does not delineate bone involvement in paranasal sinus tumors.

Question 12.23. **Regarding lung cancer, which is true?**

A. Chest radiography screening results in improved mortality.
B. CT screening further improves mortality because smaller lesions are detected.
C. MDCT can accurately predict chest wall or mediastinal invasion in greater than 95% of patients.
D. MRI is useful in the evaluation of superior sulcus tumors.
E. PET/CT obviates the need for any additional imaging in the staging of clinically suspected metastatic non-small cell lung cancer (NSCLC).

Question 12.24. **Regarding lung cancer treatment planning, which is true?**

A. Adrenal lesion biopsy is no longer needed in the era of MRI and MDCT.
B. Routine imaging of the brain and bone in the absence of clinical suspicion of metastases is unwarranted.
C. CT of the chest requires intravenous contrast to exclude adrenal metastases.
D. Liver should be imaged in its entirety on an initial staging CT because of the high incidence of liver metastases.

Question 12.25. **Regarding lymphoma, which is true?**

A. Lymphangiography remains a highly sensitive and specific way to evaluate portal and mesenteric lymphadenopathy.
B. CT is an effective way to evaluate bone marrow involvement.
C. Routine MRI is equally as sensitive as CT for detection of lymphadenopathy in the chest, abdomen, or pelvis.
D. Gallium scintigraphy is better than PET in the detection of lymphadenopathy from lymphoma.
E. The added sensitivity of PET is its ability to adequately characterize bone marrow involvement by lymphoma.

Question 12.26. **Regarding breast cancer, which is true?**

A. Annual screening mammography should begin at age 50.
B. There is no role for early screening in high-risk patients.
C. Calcium is an indication of benign disease.
D. Final assessment on mammography is based on likelihood of malignancy.
E. Percutaneous biopsy of a potential cancer is contraindicated for fear of seeding the needle tract.

Question 12.27. **Regarding nonmammographic breast imaging, which is true?**

A. Sonography is not useful for the evaluation of dense breasts.
B. To distinguish cysts from solid masses, sonography should be used as a first-line tool.
C. Because of breast geometry, sonography cannot be used for needle biopsy guidance.
D. MRI is limited because of the inability to have MRI-guided biopsies.

Question 12.28. **Regarding breast cancer staging, which is NOT true?**

A. Lymphoscintigraphy is useful for the staging of large breast cancers (>5 cm).
B. Disease greater than one quadrant is known as multicentric disease.
C. Less than one focus of disease in the same quadrant is known as multifocal disease.
D. Sonography is limited in the detection of depicting carcinoma *in situ* (DCIS).
E. MRI is useful in the detection of infiltrating lobular cancer.

Question 12.29. **Regarding breast MRI, which is true?**

A. Not useful in the postoperative breast.
B. More specific than sensitive in neoplasm detection.
C. Intravenous contrast is not needed.
D. Obviates need for biopsy.
E. Impact on mortality has yet to be determined.

Question 12.30. **Regarding colorectal cancer, which is true?**

A. CT colography is limited by reliance on intravenous contrast.
B. Transrectal ultrasound (TRUS) is a useful way of evaluating the entire colon.
C. MDCT is an accurate way to evaluate the bowel wall tumor extension.
D. MRI is better than CT in the evaluation of distant metastasis.
E. MRI is a more sensitive way to assess localized disease extension than MDCT.

Question 12.31. **Regarding gynecologic malignancies, which is true?**

A. Transabdominal ultrasound is the first step in staging endometrial cancer.
B. CT is limited in the assessment of localized extension of cervical cancer.
C. MRI is less sensitive than MDCT for detecting myometrial invasion of cervical cancer.
D. MRI is much better than MDCT in detecting lymphadenopathy from gynecologic malignancies.

Question 12.32. **Regarding cervical cancer, which is true?**

A. Ultrasound is a highly effective way to stage cervical cancer.
B. MRI is a more effective technique for evaluating parametrial invasion than CT.
C. CT is an effective staging tool for localized disease.
D. No role for PET in the staging of cervical cancer.

Question 12.33. **Regarding ovarian cancer, which is NOT true?**

A. Ultrasound is an effective method for distinguishing ovarian from uterine lesions.
B. MRI is superior to ultrasound in determining whether an adnexal lesion is malignant.
C. CT and MRI are better than ultrasound for the detection of peritoneal disease.
D. MRI is better than CT for detection of lymphadenopathy from ovarian cancer.

Question 12.34. **Regarding prostate cancer, which is true?**

A. Imaging is key in its early detection.
B. MDCT is a useful way to localize a biopsy site.
C. CT is not useful for the detection of distant nodal disease.
D. The role of MRI is to determine whether the cancer is confined to the prostate.
E. The main role of MR spectroscopy is to determine whether a prostate nodule is malignant.

ANSWERS

Answer 12.1. **The answer is D.**

Percutaneous needle biopsy has become a very important tool in diagnosing new masses. Radiologists and referring physicians must be aware of the general technique in order for appropriate patients to be referred for this minimally invasive procedure. All of the choices given for this question are correct except the need for intravenous contrast. In fact, contrast is often not needed as it exits the bloodstream long before the biopsy ends. On occasion, contrast is administered in order to plan the part of the lesion that is most likely to yield a diagnosis (least necrotic and, therefore, most enhancing). Oftentimes, a contrast-enhanced scan has already been performed and so a repeat is not needed. The biopsy physician must review the preprocedural studies in order to determine the best route to the lesion and the lesion or part that will be biopsied. The differential will determine whether core biopsies must be performed (as in lymphoma, sarcoma, mesothelioma, thymoma), whether the solution must be in RPMI (lymphoma) or whether cultures must be sent (infection a consideration). As treatments based on molecular analysis of tumors continue to improve, percutaneous tissue sampling will surely increase. The physician's job is to make sure the correct patients are selected.

Answer 12.2. **The answer is C.**

Although many centers have converted all chest needle biopsies to CT guidance, fluoroscopy continues to be a safe and preferred method for lung needle biopsies. This comes, in part, because it is faster than CT as real-time visualization of the needle tip can be part of the procedure. Conventional fluoroscopy also has a significantly lower radiation dose than the newer CT fluoroscopy. The advantage of CT is that it allows for better resolution of smaller lung lesions and central lesions. Despite the use of small needles and appropriate planning, hemoptysis and pneumothorax remain fairly common complications of this procedure. Often times they are self-limiting. In most centers, pneumothorax rates approach one third of all patients undergoing lung biopsies. Those requiring chest tube placement fall below 10%.

Answer 12.3. **The answer is C.**

As with lung biopsies, preprocedural imaging is very important in determining the route of approach and type of needles to be used for percutaneous abdominal and pelvic biopsies. Certain organs, because of their most common locations, are associated with certain complications. The adrenal gland is one such organ. Because of its cranial location in the retroperitoneum, percutaneous biopsy may lead to pneumothorax. The pancreas is another such organ. It is often surrounded by bowel, precluding an unobstructed approach to a pancreatic mass. In such cases, a transcaval approach is preferred. The differential diagnosis from any preprocedural imaging will also dictate biopsy technique. While liver masses may represent well-differentiated neoplasm (e.g., fibrolamellar hepatocellular carcinoma), core biopsies are required to distinguish them from normal liver or benign lesions, such as focal nodular hyperplasia. Core biopsies are also valuable in diagnosing histology or retroperitoneal and pelvic masses that may be sarcomas. When ovarian cancer heads the differential diagnosis, alternatives to percutaneous biopsy should be sought. High risk of tract and peritoneal seeding make an open procedure the favored route of tissue sampling.

Answer 12.4. **The answer is B.**

Central venous access is crucial in patients with cancer, given the sclerosing effects of many chemotherapy regimens on small, peripheral veins. Image guidance allows for safe, reliable placement of access, usually in an outpatient setting. Proper placement can result in fewer complications, such as thrombosis or pneumothorax. Regarding placement, right internal jugular is the favored route, even when a tunneled catheter is to be placed. This selection is based on the shorter intravascular route of a right catheter versus a left catheter and the preferred placement within an internal jugular vein as compared to the subclavian vein. This preference stems from a decreased incidence of thrombosis and pneumothorax with an internal jugular approach as compared to a subclavian approach, even with image guidance. In patients with axillary nodal dissection, an ipsilateral subclavian approach is avoided because of the higher rate of venous stasis and symptomatic thrombosis; internal jugular vein, however, can be used safely.

Answer 12.5. **The answer is D.**

Percutaneous gastrostomy (also known as g-tube) is an alternative to an endoscopically placed gastrostomy tube that is beginning to gain acceptance as a method of providing nutrition or gastric decompression. It can be placed quickly with less sedation than required for its endoscopic counterpart. Percutaneous placement can be via a pull technique, where the catheter is advanced into the stomach and a snare is used to retrieve it through the skin, and in a push technique, where the catheter is pushed externally into the stomach via a tract that is serially dilated. The former method may allow for larger catheters to be placed, but the latter method may result in less seeding of the tract in aerodigestive malignancies. Contraindications to the percutaneous technique include uncorrectable coagulopathy, gastric varices, and previous gastrectomy. Ascites may hinder endoscopic placement because of the increased distance from stomach to skin and therefore decreased effectiveness of gastric translumination. It is not a contraindication for percutaneous placement. The presence of ascites may require gastropexy, whereby the stomach is affixed to the abdominal wall. When gastropexy has been performed or after a tract has been established (usually after 4 weeks of a gastrostomy tube in place), catheter replacement may be performed without image guidance.

Answer 12.6. **The answer is D.**

Percutaneous nephrostomy (referred to informally as a "perc" or "PCN") is a way of percutaneously draining a kidney that is usually hydronephrotic. Preprocedural imaging is key to identifying the site of obstruction and relevant information regarding the collecting system. It is performed as a way to treat an infected, hydronephrotic kidney (pyonephrosis), divert urine away from a fistula, or preserve renal function if the obstruction is temporary or treatable. Percutaneous nephrostomies are usually performed from a posterior or flank approach with fluoroscopic or ultrasound guidance and do not require CT guidance. Preprocedural antibiotics are used that target skin organisms to prevent infection from the procedure itself. Postprocedural antibiotics depend on the quality of the urine aspirated at the time of the procedure.

Answer 12.7. **The answer is C.**

Hepatobiliary drainage is one of the main procedures in most interventional radiology suites today. Bile duct obstructions can be divided into high and low obstructions—an important distinction as the former are usually referred to interventional radiologists while the latter are usually treated endoscopically by gastroenterologists. Isolated segments or isolated bile ducts occur when the duct is obstructed and no longer is communicating with the other ducts. These, too, usually fall to interventional radiologists for treatment. Because the right duct is shorter than the left, isolated right segments are more common than isolated left segments from a central mass. Percutaneous drains can only drain a portion of the liver but that may be all that is required to cure pruritus. For an infected biliary tree (cholangitis), multiple catheters may be required to cure sepsis. Because catheters may be in place for a long time and the remainder of a terminally ill patient's life, percutaneous drainage should be reserved for patients who are symptomatic or in whom clear benefit will be obtained. Biliary dilatation on its own is not an indication for drainage.

Answer 12.8. **The answer is E.**

Patients who are scheduled to undergo percutaneous biliary drainage receive prophylactic antibiotics targeting skin flora so as to avoid infection from the procedure. First, percutaneous transhepatic cholangiography (PTC) is performed to provide information about the biliary tree. This step provides invaluable information regarding the nature of an obstruction. Drainage is usually done as a two-step procedure. First, an external drain is used to cross a level of obstruction. If the patient can tolerate this catheter with side holes proximal and distal to the obstruction without any external drainage, the catheter is converted to an internal one. When external outputs are high, oral replenishment of electrolytes may be required. In a majority of patients, drainage can result in rapid recovery of hepatic function with decrease in liver enzymes and bilirubin.

Answer 12.9. **The answer is E.**

Percutaneous cholecystostomy is a safe procedure in the treatment of acute cholecystitis (calculus or acalculous) in patients who are unable to undergo cholecystectomy. Because of its few complications, it can be a useful diagnostic tool in patients with sepsis of unknown etiology. Usually ultrasound or CT is used for needle guidance. A transhepatic route is usually preferred to minimize intraperitoneal leakage and subsequent bile peritonitis. Although cholecystography can be a useful diagnostic tool, distension of the gallbladder in the acute setting is avoided to prevent rupture. In a majority of patients, the catheter will be left in place until the patient's condition improves, the tract is established (2 to 4 weeks), and the tube can be removed. In others, the tube will be left in place until the time of definitive treatment, which is usually a cholecystectomy. In certain high-risk patients, percutaneous stone removal can be performed via the cholecystostomy. Recurrent disease may be found in up to 50% of these patients within 5 years. This conservative approach is often reserved for patients with limited life expectancy. Most patients will undergo a future cholecystectomy after the acute illness has resolved because of the high incidence of recurrence of cholecystitis.

Answer 12.10. **The answer is A.**

Malignant pleural effusions are a common cause of chest pain, dyspnea, and cough in patients with metastatic cancer, usually breast carcinoma, lung carcinoma, and lymphoma. These effusions are usually symptomatic and exudates. Thoracentesis will result in immediate relief of symptoms but the majority of these effusions will recur. Definitive treatment requires tube drainage at first, which may be better accomplished via image guidance so that the tube rests in the location of the majority of the fluid. This is particularly true when the amount of fluid is small or if the effusion is loculated. Although surgical teaching suggests large bore catheters are required for successful drainage, recent data suggests that smaller bore catheters are equally as effective and may be associated with less pain and restriction of mobility. A majority of patients will not be adequately treated with chest tube drainage alone. In these patients, pleurodesis is performed to give better long-term results. Mechanical pleurodesis can be performed at surgery [usually video assisted thoracoscopic surgery (VATS)] and offers a slightly higher success rate than chemical pleurodesis (which relies on a sclerosing agent such as talc, doxycycline, or bleomycin). Though hospital stays are shorter with surgical pleurodesis, chemical pleurodesis is less invasive, less expensive, and has a lower morbidity. Another approach currently under investigation is the use of a long-term tunneled chest tube drainage catheter. Drainage can be performed in an outpatient setting. In this group, mechanical pleurodesis may be achieved in up to 50% of patients in 30 days.

Answer 12.11. **The answer is B.**

Superior vena cava (SVC) obstruction is a fairly common consequence of thoracic malignancy, usually lung cancer. Often, radiographic SVC occlusion is asymptomatic secondary to collateral formation throughout the mediastinum with diversion of blood to the azygous or inferior vena cava systems. These patients do not warrant any treatment. In others, no collateral vessels have formed, resulting in symptoms of head and neck swelling, headache, and mental status changes. In these symptomatic patients, radiation may be beneficial when the tumors are radiosensitive. This form of therapy usually works but may require therapy over weeks with symptomatic relief over days. An alternative therapy is balloon angioplasty with stent deployment. This technique (if the obstruction can be crossed intravascularly) results in immediate symptomatic relief. Recurrent symptoms may follow stent deployment and are usually related to tumor overgrowth, neointimal hyperplasia, and rarely stent migration. Recurrent occlusion may be treated with thrombolysis, angioplasty, or repeat stenting.

Answer 12.12. **The answer is D.**

The incidence of pulmonary embolism in cancer is three times that in the general population. The first-line treatment for pulmonary embolism or deep venous thrombosis is systemic anticoagulation. In patients in whom anticoagulation is contraindicated (brain metastases, gastrointestinal hemorrhage), an inferior vena cava (IVC) interruption filter should be considered. An IVC filter is also warranted when a deep venous thrombus continues to propagate or emboli continue to be observed despite anticoagulation or if surgery is planned. Free-floating clots within the inferior vena cava or a deep vein is also another relative indication for a filter as these types of thrombi tend to embolize. Eccentric, mural thrombi are usually chronic and are less likely to embolize. Their presence alone would initially warrant systemic anticoagulation.

Answer 12.13. **The answer is B.**

IVC filters can be deployed by a femoral or jugular approach. The latter is preferred because of a decreased chance of dislodging a clot in a deep femoral vein or the inferior vena cava, the ability to place a simultaneous venous line if needed, and the ability of the patient to sit upright in bed after the procedure. A femoral approach requires the patient to lie flat in bed for 4 hours after the procedure, which is less comfortable. The predeployment cavagram is important in excluding any congenital anomalies or IVC thrombus that may alter the site of deployment. Therefore, intravenous contrast is usually used for IVC filter placement. Complications of IVC filter placement are fairly uncommon and include symptomatic IVC thrombosis. Recent work suggests that this may be seen in less than 3% of patients with IVC filters. Recently, a retrievable filter has been approved for use in the United States. This filter can be left in place, however, if the need for it persists.

Answer 12.14. **The answer is C.**

Ascites is a common association with malignancy, either from malignant peritoneal deposits or from end-stage liver disease. In the latter group, refractory ascites may be managed by a portal vein bypass in the form of a percutaneous shunt known as a TIPS (transjugular intrahepatic portosystemic shunt). In this procedure, a stent is placed in the liver from the portal vein to the hepatic vein. Portal pressures are reduced and ascites resolves. Though TIPS has gained in its use in patients with portal hypertension, certain patients are not TIPS candidates: those with congestive heart failure and preexisting hepatic encephalopathy as the TIPS can exacerbate these underlying conditions. TIPS has been shown to be superior to medical therapy alone in patients with ascites. In patients with malignant ascites, large volume paracentesis is the most common means of managing their condition. While this technique allows for immediate, symptomatic relief, it is rarely definitive, and repeat treatments with all their associated risks are often required. Long-term catheters have been used with some degree of success. Another alternative is a peritoneovenous shunt (such as a Denver shunt). Their role in the management of malignant ascites remains unclear.

Answer 12.15. **The answer is D.**

Percutaneous techniques have dramatically changed the way postoperative abdominal fluid collections are managed. A majority can be drained without the need for reoperation. Postoperative leaks may result from urine leaks, bile leaks, bowel leaks, pancreatic leaks, or lymphatic obstruction. These may warrant drainage if infection is suspected, leak is suspected, mass effect is symptomatic, or the fluid requires further characterization. Cross-sectional imaging has made tremendous strides with recent advances in CT but does not always allow for adequate characterization of fluid collections with standard protocols. An example is a urinoma, which may be overlooked unless delayed images are obtained, and small bowel leaks, which may be confused with ascites if oral contrast is not administered. Bilomas can be another confusing fluid collection, which may be suspected in patients with a history of hepatobiliary surgery. Because of communication with the bowel via the bile ducts, these fluid collections can lead to peritonitis and should be drained. Pancreatic leaks should be suspected when the amylase is elevated (3 to 5 times serum levels).

Answer 12.16. **The answer is A.**

Hepatic tumor embolotherapy is a promising tool for the treatment of hepatic lesions. This therapy relies on the increased reliance of tumors on hepatic arterial perfusion compared to normal liver. The result is that a variety of agents can be used intraarterially to cause *in situ* tumor death. Hypervascular tumors are known to be sensitive to ischemia, which has given rise to hepatic particle embolization with very small particles. Because of their larger size, coils are not used for hepatic embolotherapy. In patients with hepatocellular carcinoma, the goal of embolization is to prolong survival. In patients with neuroendocrine tumor, the control of symptoms is the more common endpoint. When tumors are bulky, pain control may be the main goal of treatment. Occasionally, post embolization syndrome may be witnessed and is marked by pain, fever, nausea, and vomiting. Usually its course is self-limited.

Answer 12.17. **The answer is E.**

An alternative to embolotherapy is percutaneous tumor ablation. This is usually reserved for patients who are not surgical candidates. Whereby embolotherapy is the mainstay for patients with high volume disease, percutaneous ablation may be used in patients with limited disease (1 to 3 lesions). Percutaneous ethanol injection (PEI) and percutaneous acetic acid injection have been used in cirrhotic patients with hepatocellular carcinoma (HCC). The hard surrounding cirrhotic liver contains the injected material within the tumor and allows for uniform distribution of material within it. This therapy is reserved for tumors less than 5 cm as larger lesions preclude effective uniform distribution of ethanol and may cause ethanol toxicity from the increased volume of ethanol needed. More recently, radiofrequency ablation (RFA) has been used for small HCCs. RFA uses heat to cause cell death and requires a larger tract than PEI. Not all lesions are amenable to RFA, though it has been shown to be slightly more effective than PEI for treatment of small lesions. Like PEI, RFA is limited in larger lesions. When a lesion is near a vessel, the vessel can act as a "heat sink," precluding temperatures sufficient to cause cell death. In certain lesions, combination therapy may be warranted, which combines embolotherapy and percutaneous ablation.

Answer 12.18. **The answer is A.**

Recent years have seen great advances in anatomic imaging. Among these is faster scanning techniques with MRI and faster CT. The advent of multidetector CT (MDCT) has resulted in improved temporal resolution and the ability to scan a targeted region in many phases of enhancement. The improved spatial resolution of MDCT has resulted in improved reconstructions in both coronal and sagittal plains. Though acquired axially, these images can rival MRI in their depiction of complex nonaxial anatomy. MRI remains superior to CT in its ability to create functional images (spectroscopy, perfusion, and cine images). Ultrasound, too, has seen dramatic improvements with better probes and more sophisticated techniques of scanning (tissue harmonics, extended field of view). Though not traditionally used for thoracic imaging because of the air interface with normal lung, sonography may be useful for needle guidance in thoracentesis and peripheral lung lesion biopsy. Occasionally, a mass can be characterized by sonography by use of color Doppler. With all of the recent advances, it would be tempting to discount the role of conventional radiography. One area in which plain films are still of great value is bone radiography. The high spatial resolution of bone films allows for lesion characterization that is quite complementary to MRI. In fact, at Washington University, no bone MRI is interpreted without a comparison radiograph. Lack of a comparison bone film may result in benign disease being confused with malignancy.

Answer 12.19. **The answer is D.**

Nuclear medicine studies are a form of molecular imaging that have been around for a while but continue to occupy an important role in staging and diagnosis. This has become even more true in the era of positive emission tomography (PET) and PET/CT. Nuclear medicine studies rely on the administration of biologically active material (usually injected). Images are then obtained to document the biodistribution of the material. Though resolution of the images is somewhat limited, when viewed in conjunction with anatomic imaging, the studies can be enormously powerful. Since radioactivity is with the agent that is administered, radiation dose is completely independent of the number of images obtained, unlike CT, which increases the radiation dose with increased number of images. Bone scintigraphy represents one of the older techniques in which a tracer is injected that is taken up by osteoblasts. Tumors with a predisposition to osseous metastases are well imaged by this technique. However, it is very sensitive but not very specific, as any process resulting in increased bone turnover will result in increased tracer uptake. As a result, bone scintigraphy should be reserved for instances in which there is a reasonable likelihood of osseous metastasis. For example, in prostate cancer, a bone scan is recommended when serum prostate specific antigen (PSA) levels are greater than 10. Another technique that has been in use for a few years is sentinel node mapping. In this technique, radiotracer is injected into a tumor and the lymph node drainage pattern is mapped. The first or sentinel node that is seen can then be biopsied. This technique is useful when lymph node drainage patterns are unpredictable, such as melanoma or breast cancer. A recent major advance in nuclear medicine has been the increased use of PET in the diagnosis and staging of a variety of tumors. PET relies on the injection of a radiotracer [currently, usually fuorodeoxyglucose (FDG)], which is taken up by metabolically active tissues. These tissues may represent infection, inflammation, or neoplasm. When combined with CT (PET/CT), this has become a powerful tool in neoplasm detection and characterization. A major pitfall of anatomic imaging is that it relies on an abnormal mass or abnormal size of a normal structure before pathology is appreciated. PET/CT allows for normal-sized structures (e.g., lymph nodes) with disease to be imaged before they become enlarged. This has been quite helpful in accurately staging many different types of tumors. The advantage of using a simultaneous CT for attenuation correction is that areas of increased uptake can be more accurately localized. Another major advantage is that by using spiral CT for the transmission scan for attenuation correction, the entire process has become faster, which has resulted in improved patient satisfaction and throughput.

Answer 12.20. **The answer is D.**

A major role of imaging in oncology is to determine the effect of therapy on the clinical behavior of a tumor. To that end, a new study may show complete response to therapy, partial response (defined as >50% reduction in the sum of tumor cross products), and stability or progression (defined as 25% increase in the sum of one or more of the tumor deposits). In 1994, an attempt was made to create a more reliable method of assessing tumor response. These principles were published as the Response Evaluation Criteria in Solid Tumors (RECIST) guidelines. These RECIST principles relied on the same four categories of tumor response assessment and used unidimensional measurements to quantify tumor size. RECIST also more strictly defined disease progression. Major criticism of RECIST rests on the lack of universal application of one measurement to all tumors, which may vary in shape, and the lack of inclusion of bone or marrow involvement. Newer techniques may make measurement less important in assessing tumor response to therapy. These include PET, where altered FDG metabolism may be seen as a sign of response, and rapid perfusion techniques that may measure altered tissue perfusion, which may be another early sign of tissue response.

Answer 12.21. **The answer is B.**

Neuroimaging continues to be on the forefront of modern anatomic imaging. MRI with contrast has become the standard method for detecting and characterizing intracerebral masses. It is very helpful in diagnosing and planning surgery for brain masses, especially those near the brainstem, posterior fossa, pituitary region, and cerebellopontine angle. CT is limited in these regions secondary to beam hardening from adjacent bone. Though spatial resolution of MRI is higher than CT, intravenous contrast is still used. It can be very helpful in the detection of small lesions and meningeal lesions. CT with contrast is usually reserved for patients unable to undergo MRI or in some cases where it may help in refining a differential diagnosis by showing calcium or osseous destruction. Both techniques are limited in their ability to differentiate between tumor recurrence and radiation change. Newer techniques have recently been developed that may allow for improved performance in the MRI detection and characterization of brain lesions and in the presurgical planning. These include MR spectroscopy, perfusion, and diffusion weighted imaging. Spectroscopy, which relies on noninvasive measurements of brain tumor metabolites, is useful in guiding biopsy. It is limited, however, in small lesions (<2 cm) and in those adjacent to bone, fat, or cerebrospinal fluid (CSF).

Answer 12.22. **The answer is A.**

Head and neck cancers can be quite challenging to detect on imaging. Usually, CT or MRI is reserved once a lesion is detected by endoscopy. Endoscopy is far better than imaging for the detection of small mucosal lesions. The role of imaging is to evaluate any extension of disease. Both CT with contrast and MRI with contrast are used for staging of head and neck cancers. The preference seems to vary by institution. For upper aerodigestive malignancies, MRI is the favored technique because of less artifact from the skull base. PET/CT has become a valuable tool in the staging of head and neck cancer. Though CT with intravenous contrast is usually used initially, PET/CT with FDG but no intravenous contrast allows for quite a nice complement. This is particularly true in the postoperative neck, which can be quite confusing on routine CT or MRI. CT is usually favored when early cortical base erosion is suspected or if invasion of the orbital walls or paranasal sinus walls is the clinical question.

Answer 12.23. **The answer is D.**

Lung cancer is the most common cancer in both men and women, and its incidence is increasing. Screening, therefore, has been a topic of a great deal of discussion. Unfortunately, studies have not demonstrated any improvement in mortality from chest radiograph screening though lesions were detected at more favorable stages. Currently, studies are underway to determine whether CT with its ability to detect smaller lesions will be any better. It is still too early to tell whether detecting smaller lesions will impact mortality from this dreaded disease. Another role of imaging lung cancer is in the staging of disease. Despite improvements in spatial resolution, CT is still limited in its ability to detect chest wall and mediastinal invasion. MRI has shown greater promise in the evaluation of tumor extension, owing to its improved multiplanar capability and soft-tissue resolution. This is particularly true in the superior sulcus or lung apex where MRI can delineate tumor involvement of the subclavian vessels and brachial plexus better than CT. PET/CT is also useful in the staging of lung cancer. It is better than CT alone in the detection of mediastinal lymphadenopathy and quite sensitive for adrenal and bone metastases. Because of its high sensitivity, PET/CT may overstage patients with non-small cell lung cancer. Because of the high glucose uptake of normal brain, PET/CT with FDG is limited for the evaluation of brain metastases. If these are suspected clinically, further imaging with MRI may be indicated.

Answer 12.24. **The answer is B.**

Adrenal glands represent the most common site of abdominal metastases from lung cancer. For this reason, a routine chest CT should include the adrenal glands. Most adrenal nodules in patients with lung cancer will be adrenal adenomas. Because of their high lipid content, many (but not all) will be low attenuating on non-contrast CT examinations. If intravenous contrast is given, adenomas will enhance and may not be distinguishable from metastases. Many adrenal adenomas will show signal dropout on opposed phase gradient recalled echo imaging. PET may also be helpful in adrenal imaging in that metastases should have increased uptake when they are larger than 1 cm. Because of false positives with CT, PET, and MRI, any patient with isolated suspected adrenal metastasis should be biopsied to prevent false overstaging. Routine imaging of the brain, liver, and bone is not warranted in patients with lung cancer unless suspected metastasis has a clinical basis, because likelihood of disease is quite low.

Answer 12.25. **The answer is C.**

Lymphoma is a fairly common neoplasm that has seen dramatic change in its imaging in the era of cross-sectional imaging. In the past, lymphangiography was used for evaluation of paraaortic lymphadenopathy, but its role in lymphoma imaging has been replaced by CT, MRI, and PET. CT is an efficient way to evaluate nodal and solid organ involvement by lymphoma but is limited in the evaluation of bone marrow involvement. MRI is equally as effective as CT in the evaluation of nodal and solid organ involvement. MRI tends to take longer and is more expensive and often is performed in patients unable to undergo CT or in patients who cannot receive intravenous iodinated contrast. MRI is also useful in depicting bone marrow involvement. PET is highly accurate in the staging of lymphoma and with CT fusion is better than gallium scintigraphy for the staging of lymphoma. PET is limited in evaluating bone marrow involvement by lymphoma as increased uptake can be seen diffusely in reactive bone marrow, especially after chemotherapy and marrow-stimulating drugs.

Answer 12.26. **The answer is D.**

Mammography remains the standard of care for breast cancer screening. Annual screening is recommended beginning at 40 years. High-risk patients (those with personal or strong family history of breast cancer) should consult their physician regarding initiation of screening at an earlier age. In these patients, there may be a role for screening sonography or MRI. On mammography, screening is based on the detection of a spiculated mass, architectural distortion, or microcalcifications that may be indicative of *in situ* carcinoma. Each mammogram has a final assessment category defined by the American College of Radiology breast imaging reporting and data system (BI-RADS) lexicon based on the likelihood of malignancy (1 = normal; 5 = highly suggestive of malignancy). This standardized reporting format has gained wide acceptance and serves as a model for other screening imaging modalities. Imaging can provide guidance for biopsy of any suspicious lesion (by ultrasound, mammography, and, most recently, MRI). Unlike with ovarian cancer, there is no fear of seeding the needle tract. Percutaneous needle biopsy is faster, safer, and less expensive than surgical biopsy. Patients undergoing percutaneous needle biopsy are more likely to be treated with a single, definitive surgery than patients undergoing surgical biopsy.

Answer 12.27. **The answer is B.**

Breast sonography is an important adjunct to mammography in the detection of breast cancer. It is especially useful in patients with dense breasts but is not standard of care in breast cancer screening. It is a great first-line tool in the evaluation of a mass to determine whether it is cystic or solid and to guide intervention. It is faster and cheaper than breast MRI. The role of MRI of the breast is currently under study. Until recently, the role of MRI in screening has been limited because of the inability to biopsy lesions that were not palpable and only seen on MRI. MRI compatible biopsy devices have recently been developed. Studies are underway to determine what the makeup of these mammographically occult, sonographically occult, nonpalpable lesions are.

Answer 12.28. **The answer is A.**

Understanding breast cancer staging and potential therapy requires one to realize than more than one focus of breast cancer in one quadrant (multifocal disease) may warrant a wider excision and that disease in more than one quadrant (multicentric disease) may warrant mastectomy. Sonography is useful in depicting axillary adenopathy, which also affects staging, but sonography is limited in depicting *in situ* carcinoma (DCIS). MRI is sensitive in evaluating ipsilateral and contralateral breasts in women with cancer. It is particularly useful in depicting invasive lobular carcinoma and in finding an occult primary tumor in patients presenting with axillary lymphadenopathy. Nuclear medicine techniques may also be used for breast cancer staging. PET may play a role in depicting metastases and in showing tumor response to therapy. Lymphoscintigraphy has also become useful for lesions less than 5 cm and in some centers is considered the standard of care. For larger lesions, the results of lymphoscintigraphy may not be reliable for sentinel node mapping.

Answer 12.29. **The answer is E.**

As useful as breast MRI may be on a case-by-case basis, its impact on breast cancer mortality has yet to be determined. MRI is a very sensitive technique that is not as specific; consequently, biopsy of detected lesions may be needed. For this reason, MRI compatible biopsy instruments have been devised. MRI is still expensive and requires intravenous contrast for dynamic enhancement. In the postoperative breast, however, MRI can be very useful in separating recurrent tumor from postoperative change.

Answer 12.30. **The answer is E.**

Colorectal cancer is the most common gastrointestinal malignancy. As a result, many studies have been performed in order to determine an effective way of screening for this malignancy. Recently, MDCT has allowed for the propagation of CT colography, which shows early promise. This technique is relatively noninvasive and does not require intravenous contrast. In the initial staging of colorectal cancer, CT, MRI, and transrectal ultrasound (TRUS) are all commonly used. TRUS allows for clear visualization of the layers of the bowel wall and can allow for accurate depiction of tumor penetration. TRUS does not allow for visualization of the entire colon. CT is best used for assessing metastases and lymphadenopathy. Even MDCT does not allow for differentiation of the layers of the bowel wall. MRI, owing to its better soft-tissue resolution, is better than CT for localized staging. High-resolution sequences may allow for clearer depiction of extension into adjacent fat and organs. CT and MRI have similar sensitivity and specificity for the assessing nodal involvement.

Answer 12.31. **The answer is C.**

Imaging in endometrial and cervical cancer is usually performed after a diagnosis is clinically made. The main role of imaging is to determine the depth of myometrial invasion, endocervical tumor extension and lymphadenopathy with endometrial cancer, and the extent of parametrial extension and lymphadenopathy with cervical cancer. Imaging is also performed to evaluate for distant metastases. MRI is better than CT in delineating localized invasion of both tumors. CT is limited in depicting the extent of myometrial invasion from endometrial carcinoma and the extent of parametrial invasion from cervical cancer. MRI is about equal to CT in delineating lymphadenopathy from gynecologic malignancy. Though transabdominal sonography is often used to investigate the pelvis, it should not be routinely performed in endometrial cancer staging. Even transvaginal ultrasound is limited because of its limited field of view and lack of soft-tissue resolution.

Answer 12.32. **The answer is B.**

Imaging in cervical cancer is usually performed after a positive biopsy or PAP smear. The main role of imaging is to determine the extent of parametrial extension and lymphadenopathy. MRI is better than CT in delineating localized invasion. CT is limited in depicting the extent of parametrial invasion from cervical cancer. MRI is slightly better than CT in delineating lymphadenopathy from cervical cancer. Though transabdominal sonography is often used to investigate the pelvis, it should not be routinely performed in cervical cancer staging. Even transvaginal ultrasound is limited because of its limited field of view and lack of soft-tissue resolution.

Answer 12.33. **The answer is D.**

Imaging in adnexal masses is aimed at delineating the origin of the mass (ovarian or uterine), whether a mass is malignant, and whether distant metastases are present. Ultrasound is very effective at identifying the location of an adnexal tumor (bowel, ovarian, or uterine) and in distinguishing benign from malignant disease. When ultrasound is inconclusive, CT or MRI may be used. MRI is more accurate in separating malignant from benign ovarian pathology. Staging accuracy for MRI equals that of CT. Both are felt to be slightly more accurate than ultrasound, especially in the evaluation of peritoneal disease. CT is slightly better than MRI for the evaluation of lymphadenopathy. Both are equal in their depiction of hepatic metastases.

Answer 12.34. **The answer is D.**

Digital rectal examination and serum prostate specific antigen (PSA) are effective means for screening for prostate cancer. Imaging plays no role in prostate cancer detection. It is useful (usually by ultrasound) for guiding biopsy. CT does not allow adequate prostate resolution for cancer detection in an abnormal prostate. It is quite useful, however, for detection of metastases. MRI, especially with an endorectal coil, provides high quality imaging of the zones of the prostate. Its role is to determine whether the cancer is confined to the prostate. Spectroscopy is a relatively new technique that may improve tumor localization and detection of extracapsular spread. The role of spectroscopy is not in the characterization of a prostate nodule.

CHAPTER 13

Cancer of the Head and Neck

EZRA E. W. COHEN

Directions Each of the numbered items below is followed by lettered answers. Select the ONE lettered answer that is BEST in each case unless instructed otherwise.

QUESTIONS

Questions 13.1–13.3.

A 54-year-old man presents with a 2-month history of altered speech and odynophagia. He relates gradual onset of symptoms initially treated as an upper respiratory tract infection with amoxicillin without relief. Over this period, he has lost 5 kilograms due to decreased oral intake. Past medical history is noncontributory other than a 30 pack-year history of cigarette smoking. Examination reveals an indurated mass at the left base of the tongue. Tongue mobility is intact and there is no trismus. There is also evidence of a 4-cm left-sided cervical mass.

Question 13.1. **Which of the following should be part of this patient's management?**

A. Computed tomographic (CT) or magnetic resonance imaging (MRI) imaging of the neck.
B. Ear, nose, and throat (ENT) evaluation.
C. Chest CT.
D. All of the above.

Question 13.2. **Fine-needle aspiration of the cervical lymph node confirms squamous cell carcinoma. CT scanning of the head and neck reveals a 3-cm mass confined to the left base of the tongue with two ipsilateral lymph nodes, 4 cm and 2 cm in diameter, respectively. CT scanning of the chest is unremarkable. Examination under anesthesia and triple endoscopy confirm the CT scan findings. The correct TNM staging for this patient with the above information is**

A. T2N2A M0
B. T2N2B M0
C. T2N3 M1
D. T2N2B M1

Corresponding Chapters in *Cancer: Principles & Practice of Oncology*, Seventh Edition: 26 (Cancer of the Head and Neck).

Question 13.3. **This patient would benefit from which of the following.**

A. Speech and swallow evaluation.
B. Dental evaluation.
C. Nutrition counseling.
D. All of the above.

Question 13.4. **A 43-year-old man presents with a 3-month history of irritation on the right side of his tongue, which is exacerbated on drinking or eating acidic or spicy food. He denies difficulty swallowing or speaking. He is otherwise well and admits to using chewing tobacco for 13 years but quit 10 years ago. He denies heavy alcohol intake. Examination of the oral cavity reveals a 1-cm lesion of the right middle-third lateral tongue without ulceration, fixation, evidence of invasion of adjacent structures, or palpable lymphadenopathy. Biopsy of the lesions confirms invasive squamous cell carcinoma. The appropriate treatment is**

A. limited glossectomy
B. radical glossectomy

Question 13.5. **A 43-year-old man presents with a 3-month history of a painful left tongue lesion, difficulty moving the tongue, and left otalgia. Evaluation reveals a T3N1 squamous cell carcinoma of the right lateral tongue. The patient elects to undergo surgery consisting of hemiglossectomy and ipsilateral modified neck dissection. Pathology confirms a 4.2-cm primary tumor with 2 of 16 lymph nodes harboring metastatic disease. In addition, the larger lymph node measuring 2.5 cm has evidence of extracapsular extension. The appropriate treatment option is**

A. surgery followed by radiotherapy
B. chemoradiation
C. surgery followed by chemoradiation
D. all of the above

Question 13.6. **A 55-year-old female senior public relations executive presents with a 2-month history of hoarseness and sore throat. Examination including laryngoscopy reveals a mass of the right true vocal cord with fixation. CT scanning shows no evidence of cartilage invasion or lymphadenopathy. Pathology confirms squamous cell carcinoma. The patient states that normal speech is critical in her occupation and is very motivated to preserve function. The most appropriate treatment option for this patient is**

A. total laryngectomy
B. total laryngectomy followed by radiation
C. chemoradiation

Questions 13.7–13.9.

A 64-year-old man presents with progressively worsening sore throat accompanied by difficulty speaking and left otalgia. Recently he has increased difficulty opening his mouth. On examination the tongue is fixed with a tumor of the base of the tongue that extends across the midline and to the left tonsil and floor of the mouth. In addition, two ipsilateral cervical lymph nodes are palpable, 2.0 cm and 2.5 cm in size, respectively. CT scanning confirms a tongue base mass that invades the deep musculature of the tongue and the medial and lateral pterygoid muscles as well as the ipsilateral lymphadenopathy. CT scanning of the chest is unremarkable. Biopsy of the lesion confirms squamous cell carcinoma.

Question 13.7. **The most appropriate treatment option for this patient is**

A. chemoradiation
B. radiation alone
C. chemotherapy alone

Question 13.8. **The patient has completed treatment with concomitant chemoradiotherapy, achieving a complete clinical response. At 30-day follow-up visit, his mucositis and dermatitis are completely healed, and he is tolerating semisolid food very well. He lost a total of 10 kg during therapy, necessitating placement of a feeding gastrostomy tube, but has maintained his weight over the last 3 weeks. Which of the following imaging modalities would be the most appropriate to order?**

A. CT imaging of the neck.
B. Positron emission tomography (PET) imaging.
C. MRI imaging.
D. Any of the above.

Question 13.9. **One year after completing therapy, the patient returns to your office complaining of increasing dysphagia and pain. Examination and CT scanning reveals a localized recurrence at the primary tumor site without evidence of metastasis. Pathology confirms squamous cell carcinoma. Otherwise the patient has recovered well from therapy and is in good general health. The most appropriate option for therapy is**

A. salvage surgery
B. palliative chemotherapy
C. supportive care only

Question 13.10. **A 43-year-old Asian man presents with right-sided otitis media and is prescribed a 10-day course of amoxicillin. Eight weeks later he returns complaining of ongoing right otalgia and new onset diplopia and occipital headache. Examination at this time reveals bilateral cervical lymphadenopathy, all smaller than 6 cm without palpable supraclavicular lymph nodes. He is referred to an otolaryngologist who notes a mass on the right lateral wall of the nasopharynx that extends superiorly. MRI scanning confirms the physical findings and demonstrates invasion of the ipsilateral cavernous sinus. Pathologic examination of a biopsy specimen classifies the lesion as World Health Organization 3 undifferentiated carcinoma or lymphoepithelioma. The likely causative agent is**

A. tobacco
B. human immunodeficiency virus (HIV)
C. human papilloma virus (HPV)
D. Epstein-Barr virus (EBV)

Question 13.11. **A 55-year-old woman presents with a right facial mass near the angle of the jaw and ipsilateral peripheral facial nerve palsy. There is high suspicion for malignancy, and she undergoes superficial parotidectomy with sparing of the facial nerve. Pathology reveals a high-grade mucoepidermoid carcinoma with negative margins. The majority of the salivary gland tumors are**

A. benign
B. malignant

Question 13.12. **A 37-year-old female smoker presents with oral leukoplakia, which is successfully excised. She is aware that this could portend a risk for the subsequent development of oral cancer and inquires regarding prophylactic measures. What is the most appropriate recommendation?**

A. Celecoxib.
B. Gefitinib.
C. Low-dose retinoids.
D. Reassurance and close follow-up.

Question 13.13. **The following genes or proteins are commonly dysregulated in squamous cell carcinoma of the head and neck EXCEPT**

A. cyclin D1
B. signal transducer and activator of transcription (STAT3)
C. BRCA1
D. p63
E. epidermal growth factor receptor (EGFR)

Question 13.14. **Expression of which of the following tumor suppressor genes is commonly lost in squamous cell carcinoma of the head and neck?**

A. p53.
B. p16.
C. ARF.
D. c-kit.
E. All of the above.
F. A, B, and C only.

Question 13.15. **Which of the following is an early event in the progression of squamous cell carcinoma of the head and neck?**

A. Loss of 11q.
B. Loss of 9p and 3p.
C. Loss of 13q.
D. Loss of p27 protein.

Question 13.16. **The concept of field cancerization is important in cancers of the upper aerodigestive tract. Which of the following is the most accurate definition of cancerization?**

A. The theory that a mucosal field defect allows independent transformation of epithelial cells at a number of sites.
B. The theory that multiple cancers in related family members are caused by a single genetic defect.
C. The theory that multiple genetic events need to occur in a clonal cell population to allow progression from normal mucosa to cancer.
D. The theory that all acquired cancers are related to an infectious agent that causes DNA disruption.
E. The theory that cancer only occurs in individuals who played in fields as children.

Question 13.17. **All of the following characteristics are typical of HPV-associated squamous cell carcinoma of the head and neck EXCEPT**

A. younger age
B. oropharynx primary site
C. minimal tobacco use
D. mutated p53 protein
E. improved disease specific survival

ANSWERS

Answer 13.1. **The answer is D.**

This patient likely has a primary cancer of the left base of the tongue. Tobacco use is a contributory risk factor and is highly prevalent in this patient population. In this case pathologic diagnosis can be easily confirmed with fine needle aspiration of the cervical lymph node. Further staging should proceed with imaging of the head and neck usually with CT scanning or MRI. Referral should be made to an otolaryngologist for complete examination including laryngoscopy. Due to the relatively high incidence of metachronous primary cancers of the upper aerodigestive tract, many centers will perform triple endoscopy to include esophagoscopy and bronchoscopy as well as imaging of the chest, usually with CT scanning. CT scanning is the most commonly employed diagnostic imaging modality in patients with head and neck cancer in the United States. For most disease sites, CT scanning offers comparable positive predictive value compared with other modalities, is widely available, and offers better visualization of bone invasion than MRI. A nuclear total body bone scan is usually unnecessary in patients with locoregionally advanced disease unless symptoms or laboratory values raise suspicion for bone metastasis.

Answer 13.2. **The answer is B.**

According to American Joint Committee on Cancer (AJCC) Staging Criteria 6th edition, this patient has T2N2B M0, stage IVA, squamous cell carcinoma of the left base of the tongue. Note that patients with cancers of the head and neck can have stage IV disease without metastases. In fact, only 10% of patients with squamous cell carcinoma of the head and neck will present with metastatic disease initially (i.e., stage IVC), although up to 50% of patients with recurrent disease will have clinically apparent metastatic foci.

Answer 13.3. **The answer is D.**

This patient is at risk for long-term speech and swallowing difficulties because of the location of the primary tumor, the presence of symptoms and associated weight loss, and his subsequent treatment. Almost all patients with head and neck cancer, but especially those with tumors of the speech and swallowing organs, should undergo consultation and formal functional evaluation with a qualified therapist. Beyond providing baseline data pretherapy, the speech and swallow therapist can provide counseling, advise on dietary intake, and strategies to regain long-term function.

A dental specialist, prior to therapy, must also assess patients receiving radiotherapy. Any evidence of oral infection should be addressed, and patients with poor dentition should have extraction prior to initiating radiotherapy to prevent complications posttherapy. Several centers have made it common practice to also discuss patients with locoregionally advanced disease at a multidisciplinary tumor conference prior to initiating any therapy. This ensures that all necessary individuals and specialties are involved in the patient's comprehensive management.

Answer 13.4. **The answer is A.**

This gentleman has a stage I (T1N0 M0) squamous cell carcinoma of the tongue. After complete evaluation, treatment of these lesions usually consists of either surgery or radiotherapy with comparable cure rates. The advantages of surgery in early lesions like this one are low morbidity, the expectation of excellent functional outcome, and low likelihood of occult lymph node metastasis, obviating the need for neck dissection. Surgery will usually consist of a transoral limited glossectomy with primary closure for small, well-circumscribed lesions as in this case. If partial glossectomy is predicted to produce a significant degree of functional impairment, radiation therapy should be selected as the treatment of choice. In addition, larger lesions (T2 or T3) or those with clinically involved lymph nodes would likely benefit from initial radiotherapy with surgical salvage if necessary. With either modality, local control rates of 80% to 90% and 5-year cause specific survival rates of 60% to 70% are expected. Complications of surgery include orocutaneous fistula, flap necrosis, dysphagia, and damage to the lingual or the hypoglossal nerves.

Answer 13.5. **The answer is D.**

In contrast to the previous case, this patient has intermediate stage III disease that necessities a multimodality approach. Traditionally, this would have consisted of surgery followed by radiotherapy with more recent studies advocating chemoradiotherapy as initial management. In cancers of the larynx or hypopharynx, an organ preserving strategy, discussed below, is supported by phase III data. However, for cancers of the oral cavity, randomized trials comparing chemoradiotherapy to surgery followed by radiotherapy are lacking. Nevertheless, patients with high-risk features do appear to benefit from postoperative chemoradiotherapy over radiotherapy alone. Two recently reported randomized trials performed by the Radiation Therapy Oncology Group (RTOG) and the European Organization for Research and Treatment of Cancer (EORTC), respectively, have both shown an advantage to chemoradiotherapy in this setting. In both trials, high-risk was defined by pathologic features including positive resection margins, extracapsular nodal extension, or more than one involved lymph node. The EORTC trial also enrolled patients with pT3 or pT4 disease and perineural or vascular involvement. Both trials administered single-daily fractionated radiotherapy with or without cisplatin 100 mg per m^2 on days 1, 22, and 43. The EORTC trial reported higher locoregional control, disease-free survival, and overall survival in the combined treatment group. The RTOG trial also observed a benefit to concurrent chemoradiotherapy with respect to locoregional control and disease-free survival but not overall survival. Thus, the management of adequate performance status patients with intermediate stage disease and high-risk features should include postoperative chemoradiotherapy.

Answer 13.6. **The answer is C.**

This woman has a stage III (T3N0) squamous cell carcinoma of the larynx. Historically, her treatment would involve total laryngectomy followed by postoperative radiotherapy, which would make normal speech impossible. With a goal of maintaining laryngeal function, randomized trials were conducted to compare induction chemotherapy with cisplatin and 5-fluorouracil (5FU) followed by radiotherapy to surgery followed by radiotherapy. The largest trial conducted in patients with larynx cancer by the Department of Veterans Affairs Laryngeal Cancer Study Group demonstrated that the two approaches were equivalent with respect to survival but that 64% of subjects treated nonsurgically were able to preserve the organ. A parallel study was performed by the EORTC in subjects with hypopharynx cancer using identical treatment arms. In this disease site, 35% of subjects were able to retain larynx function. Thus, sequential chemoradiotherapy has become an acceptable alternative to surgery in these settings. Several questions still remained unanswered, including whether radiotherapy alone would achieve similar results or whether concomitant chemoradiotherapy could prove superior to sequentially administered chemoradiotherapy. Thus, an intergroup trial was undertaken to compare concomitant chemoradiotherapy, sequential chemoradiotherapy, and radiotherapy alone in resectable patients with stage III or IV (excluding T4) disease with a primary endpoint of larynx preservation.

Intergroup 91-11 revealed that concomitant was superior to sequential chemoradiotherapy and radiotherapy alone with respect to 2-year laryngeal preservation with similar rates of late toxicities and swallowing function at 2 years. There was no significant difference in overall survival rates between the three arms. Thus, it appears that concomitant chemoradiotherapy can be considered a standard of care in patients with cancer of the larynx and offers a validated nonsurgical treatment approach.

Answer 13.7. **The answer is A.**

This patient has stage IVb (T4bN2b) squamous cell carcinoma of the base of the tongue. Primary treatment in patients with advanced oropharynx and hypopharynx tumors usually consists of chemoradiotherapy because of the high risk of bilateral cervical lymphatic spread and because surgery involves greater functional disability. Radiotherapy can address occult lymphatic metastasis while also allowing organ preservation. In reality, however, patients with advanced primary tumors in this area are at high risk of long-term functional consequences, especially dysphagia. Thus, it is critical to engage the entire multidisciplinary team early in management to ensure a successful outcome. Historically, radiotherapy alone has offered disappointing long-term survival rates of 30% or less. Concurrent chemoradiotherapy was advanced in an effort to enhance locoregional control through radiosensitization and provide systemic antitumor activity. Recent randomized trials investigating the addition of chemotherapy concomitantly with radiotherapy have almost universally demonstrated a survival advantage in the chemoradiotherapy cohort. A meta-analysis of 63 randomized trials from 1965 to 1993 including 10,741 patients confirmed an absolute survival benefit of approximately 8% at 5 years with concomitant chemoradiotherapy compared with radiotherapy alone. Furthermore, recent trials utilizing combination chemotherapy (especially cisplatin and 5FU) have reported long-term survival rates of approximately 50% compared with radiotherapy alone. Although a standard regimen does not exist, single agent cisplatin given on days 1, 22, and 43 of single-daily fractionated radiotherapy at 80 to 100 mg per m^2 is widely used. It is noteworthy that analysis of the pattern of failure in concomitant chemoradiotherapy trials reveals that this approach appears to have a dramatic effect on locoregional control, but distant metastatic failure is becoming an increasing cause of mortality. Along with a survival advantage offered by concomitant chemoradiotherapy, all clinical trials have reported increased acute toxicities such as mucositis and dermatitis compared with radiotherapy alone. Long-term toxicities, however, appear to be similar between the two treatments. The acute toxicities have, nevertheless, often necessitated chemotherapeutic dose reductions or radiotherapy dose interruptions, which can theoretically diminish any benefit. Thus, it is important to provide adequate supportive care, especially with regards to analgesia and nutrition to these patients during therapy. Randomized trials of sequential (induction or neoadjuvant) chemotherapy have failed to demonstrate a survival advantage over local therapy alone despite the fact that combination regimens can result in complete and overall response rates of 30% and 80%, respectively. Nevertheless, a reduction in distant failure rates has been consistently observed in these trials. It is interesting to consider that the strategies of sequential and concomitant chemoradiotherapy can have complementary effects to reduce distant and local failure, respectively. Randomized trials to address this issue are underway.

Answer 13.8. **The answer is D.**

The management of this patient should now include radiographic and pathologic assessment of response in addition to swallowing evaluation. The most commonly utilized imaging modality remains CT scanning; however, it is often difficult to differentiate between posttherapy changes and residual or recurrent tumors. Many centers are beginning to incorporate PET scanning for surveillance after treatment. So long as PET scanning is performed 4 weeks or later after completion of radiotherapy, it appears to offer higher accuracy and predictive value compared to either CT or MRI. Addressing the clinically negative neck is controversial at this point, although several studies have demonstrated the safety of modified or selective neck dissection in the treated neck. The optimal period to perform surgery appears to be 6 to 12 weeks post-radiotherapy as healing is usually complete, radiation induced fibrosis is not yet apparent, and vascularization is adequate. Although not subjected to randomized trials, retrospective analyses demonstrate that neck dissection appears to improve local control rates but does not impact survival. Along with neck dissection, a primary tumor site biopsy is usually performed.

Commonly encountered sequelae of chemoradiotherapy will be xerostomia and neck fibrosis. The former can further impair swallowing and increases the risk for dental disease but can usually be managed with simple measures including mouthwash, sprays, gels, chewing gum, or prescription medications that increase salivary flow. Fibrosis is best addressed with regular range-of-motion exercises of the mouth, tongue, and neck, especially in the first 6 months following treatment.

Patients who receive radiation therapy should be evaluated for acute side effects and subsequently followed for the emergence of late-occurring complications. Functional speech and swallowing assessment in this patient is critical as he is at high risk for long-term difficulty. Behavioral therapy strategies are often very effective for speech articulation and swallowing deficits. Changes in head posture, use of feeding devices, and/or altered diet consistencies can improve swallowing.

Regular visits with the treating physicians, including close surgical surveillance, should proceed every 3 to 4 months for the first 3 years, as recurrences are most likely to occur over this period. Patients can be seen every 6 months for the fourth and fifth year and annually thereafter. It is important to perform thyroid function tests, usually a thyroid stimulation hormone level, at least annually as these patients are at risk of developing hypothyroidism. Radiographic imaging is usually done in conjunction with physician visits.

Answer 13.9. **The answer is A.**

This patient now presents with a localized recurrence and should be viewed as a surgical salvage candidate. His tumor can be managed with a wide local excision in an attempt to achieve negative margins. Unfortunately, 80% to 90% of patients with recurrent disease, even with surgical salvage, will succumb to their disease. In patients who are not surgical candidates or who have metastatic disease, palliative care is appropriate. Palliative chemotherapy has never been tested in randomized trials against best supportive care but is commonly utilized in patients with adequate performance status. The most widely tested regimen in these patients has been cisplatin and 5FU, resulting in response rates of approximately 30% and median survival of 6 to 8 months. More recent trials have incorporated a platinum/taxane combination without a demonstrable improvement in survival. In fact, doublet chemotherapy has not proven to offer a survival advantage over single agent regimens despite a higher response rate.

Answer 13.10. **The answer is D.**

This patient has a T4N2, stage IVa carcinoma of the nasopharynx. Nasopharyngeal cancer is endemic to the Far East and Mediterranean and is linked to EBV exposure. In fact, EBV titers are associated with tumor burden, have been linked with prognosis, and can be used in surveillance of patients after therapy. Due to rich lymphatic supply of the nasopharynx, 80% to 90% of patients have at least unilateral lymph node metastases, and 50% of patients have bilateral lymph node involvement at presentation. Since the location of the great majority of nasopharynx tumors renders complete surgical resection improbable, the preferred treatment is concurrent chemoradiotherapy, which has demonstrated improved survival compared to radiotherapy alone in randomized trials. It is important to note that the radiation fields required to treat a patient with nasopharyngeal cancer can encompass large volumes often involving the retropharynx, skull base, the parotid glands, and bilateral neck to the clavicles. This creates a high incidence of acute toxicities, especially mucositis, and places patients at risk for long-term sequelae including cranial neuropathies, optic neuritis, spinal cord injury, and trismus.

Answer 13.11. **The answer is A.**

Tumor of the salivary gland accounts for 3% to 4% of head and neck tumors and the majority are benign. Malignant tumors usually arise from the parotid or submandibular glands. There are several histologic subtypes, but the important distinction is between low-grade and high-grade features. The former are associated with an excellent prognosis and require only surgical resection. High-grade tumors carry an approximate incidence of 20% to 25% lymph node involvement at diagnosis, while the absence of adenopathy has been found to be the major predictor of disease-free survival. High-grade malignancies should be managed with total parotidectomy and dissection of node-positive necks.

Performing a selective (levels II–V) neck dissection for high-grade tumors should be considered. The local recurrence rate for operation alone is approximately 50% to 60% for high-grade tumors. Postoperative radiotherapy, therefore, is indicated for nearly all high-grade lesions, for low-grade neoplasms with close or positive margins, for tumors of the deep lobe, for perineural invasion, for recurrent tumors, and for multiple regional node metastases.

Answer 13.12. **The answer is D.**

Chemoprevention in squamous cell carcinoma of the head and neck has been attempted for patients with oral leukoplakia or erythroplakia and is based on the concept of field cancerization. However, the great majority of leukoplastic and erythroplastic lesions do not progress to malignancy, and histology is apparently a poor predictor of outcome. Clinical trials administering retinoic acid therapy have shown promise with high-dose therapy, although this is associated with often intolerable mucocutaneous toxicity and relapses if therapy is discontinued. Low-dose retinoids have not proven effective. Other strategies utilizing cyclooxegenase-2 inhibition, epidermal growth factor receptor inhibition, and Bowman-Birk inhibitor concentrate have preclinical support but have yet to be proven. At this time there is no standard screening procedure or preventative measure for patients at risk for squamous cell carcinoma of the head and neck.

Answer 13.13. **The answer is C.**

All the genes listed are thought to play a significant role in the development or growth of squamous cell carcinoma of the head and neck except for BRCA1, which appears to confer genetic susceptibility to other malignancies including breast and ovarian cancer. Amplification of the cyclin D1 locus at 11q13 has been noted in approximately 30% of squamous cell carcinomas of the head and neck, and appears to be independent of p16 inactivation. Amplification of 3q has also been noted in squamous cell carcinoma of the head and neck and evidence suggests that p63 may be the relevant oncogene at this locus. Recent studies have shown that p63 is indeed amplified, that p63 isotypes are overexpressed in squamous cell carcinoma of the head and neck, and that p63 enhances growth *in vitro* and *in vivo*. The exact function of p63 is not understood, but evidence suggests that it is an important regulator of β-catenin dependent transcription. The EGFR is a transmembrane tyrosine kinase receptor that, upon activation, regulates a number of cellular functions including proliferation, survival, invasion, metastasis, and angiogenesis. Squamous cell carcinomas of the head and neck express EGFR in 80% to 90% of specimens, and this expression has been linked to worsened prognosis. The EGFR is currently a target for therapy by both small molecule inhibitors and monoclonal antibodies, which have shown early promising activity. Recent evidence suggests that activation of signaling pathways downstream of EGFR are also critical in squamous cell carcinoma of the head and neck, and STAT3 has emerged as an important oncogene. Upon activation, the STAT proteins act as transcription factors regulating several key processes with ample evidence demonstrating their involvement in several types of cancer, including squamous cell carcinoma of the head and neck. STAT3 activation has been associated with carcinogenesis, cell growth, survival, and invasion.

Answer 13.14. **The answer is F.**

c-kit is a tyrosine kinase receptor that is an established protooncogene in several cancer types but not squamous cell carcinoma of the head and neck. High expression of c-kit has been noted in salivary gland cancers but activating mutations have not.

More than 50% of all primary squamous cell carcinomas of the head and neck harbor p53 mutations in the conserved region of the gene on chromosome 17p, and, in fact, inactivation of p53 represents the most common genetic change in all of human cancer. The p53 protein plays a critical role in cell cycle progression and response to DNA damage by regulating apoptosis. The most commonly deleted chromosomal region in squamous cell carcinoma of the head and neck, however, is located at chromosome 9p21-22. Loss of chromosome 9p21 appears to be an early event in carcinogenesis and occurs in the majority of invasive carcinomas. The p16 (*CDKN2*) gene is located within this locus and functions as a potent inhibitor of cyclin dependent kinase 4 and subsequent cell cycle progression. Mechanisms of p16 inactivation have been identified including homozygous deletion and methylation of the 5′ CpG region. Hypermethylation is a commonly described mechanism of p16 inactivation, which blocks transcription of the gene. It is believed that p16 inactivation is directly involved in the progression of primary tumors.

In addition to p16, a second tumor suppressor gene resides at 9p21, named ARF (alternate reading frame). ARF is an alternative RNA transcript for p16 that binds to MDM2, leading to a decrease in p53 degradation and a subsequent increase in p53 levels. Thus, loss of ARF, which occurs in approximately 30% of squamous cell carcinomas of the head and neck, would result in functional loss of p53.

Answer 13.15. **The answer is B.**

All the genetic events listed have been documented in squamous cell carcinomas of the head and neck, but loss of 9p and 3p have been consistently seen in dysplastic and neoplastic lesions, suggesting that this is an early alteration in carcinogenesis. It is interesting to note that early genetic changes do not necessarily correlate with histologic changes. In fact, loss of 3p or 9p is associated with extremely high rates of progression of nonmalignant oral cavity lesions despite normal appearing morphology.

The progression of squamous cell carcinoma of the head and neck involves dysregulation of several genes, and the process is by no means universal or consistent throughout all tumors. Nevertheless, some generalizations can be made. Chromosomes 9p and 3p appear to be lost early, closely followed by loss of 17p. Mutations of p53 are seen in the progression of the preinvasive to invasive lesions. Other specific genetic events, such as amplification of cyclin D1 and epigenetic inactivation of p16, have been tested predominantly in invasive lesions; thus, their order in the progression model cannot be fully determined. Loss of 11q, 13q, 14q, 18q, and p27 protein appear to occur later in progression.

Answer 13.16. **The answer is A.**

Slaughter, in 1953, originally described field cancerization as an environmentally related mucosal field defect that develops in tissues that are exposed to the same carcinogen, resulting in subsequent malignancies. The concept of field cancerization is an important one in squamous cell carcinoma of the head and neck as tobacco results in exposure of the entire upper aerodigestive tract. Field cancerization helps to explain the occurrence of metachronous, second, and occult primary tumors. Genetic evidence has shown that lesions that surround but are distinct from the original primary tumor appear to share the same genetic alterations. Ostensibly, a cell is transformed by a critical genetic event and begins to migrate through or repopulate the normal mucosa. Additional genetic events eventually result in the primary. Direct molecular assessment of surrounding regions confirms the presence of clonal cell populations that are not yet fully transformed. Given time, these lesions then arise as other preinvasive or invasive lesions in the same patient. In fact, investigators have been able to establish clonality between second lung or esophageal tumors and the original squamous cell carcinoma of the head and neck.

Answer 13.17. **The answer is D.**

It appears that a subgroup of squamous cell carcinomas of the head and neck (up to 25%) are associated with prior HPV infection, specifically HPV 16. Indeed, these patients do share common characteristics, including male sex, younger age at presentation, palatine and lingual tonsil and base of tongue primary tumors, but without the typical risk factors associated with squamous cell carcinoma of the head and neck in general. Molecularly, they are less likely to harbor p53 mutations, which may be related to the ability of the HPV E6 gene to inactivate p53.

CHAPTER **14**

Cancer of the Lung

JANESSA J. LASKIN AND ALAN B. SANDLER

Directions Each of the numbered items below is followed by lettered answers. Select the ONE lettered answer that is BEST in each case unless instructed otherwise.

QUESTIONS

Question 14.1. **A 53-year-old man, ex-smoker, is seen for an increased cough that has not responded to antibiotic therapy. Chest radiograph reveals a new right upper lobe (RUL) mass. Further workup includes a chest and upper abdominal computed tomographic (CT) scan that identify a speculated 4.5-cm RUL mass but no lymphadenopathy or distant metastasis. He is otherwise well, without weight loss or a significant past medical history. The pathology from his right upper lobectomy reveals a 5-cm squamous cell carcinoma that does not invade the visceral pleura. Four hilar nodes, but no mediastinal nodes, were positive. What is the most appropriate therapy for this man?**

A. Adjuvant radiation therapy to the hilum and ipsilateral mediastinum.
B. Adjuvant platinum-based chemotherapy, followed by local radiation.
C. Adjuvant platinum-based chemotherapy alone.
D. The positive hilar nodes mandate a reresection and full pneumonectomy.
E. No further treatment is recommended.

Question 14.2. **A 62-year-old woman is seen by a thoracic surgeon after a left upper lobe (LUL) mass is detected on her chest x-ray. The biopsy from bronchoscopy reveals an adenocarcinoma. Pulmonary function testing is within normal limits for this previously healthy, nonsmoking woman. A CT scan of the chest and upper abdomen identifies a 3.5-cm mass in the LUL, a bulky left hilum, and multiple 2- to 3-cm nodes in the mediastinum. The LUL mass, hilar, and mediastinal nodes are all "positive" on positron emission tomography (PET) scan, and a mediastinoscopy identifies adenocarcinoma in the contralateral subcarinal lymph nodes. Which of the following interventions is most appropriate?**

A. Left pneumonectomy and full bilateral mediastinal lymph node dissection.
B. Left upper lobectomy and bilateral mediastinal lymph node dissection.
C. Induction chemotherapy followed by left pneumonectomy.
D. Palliative chemotherapy alone.
E. Concurrent chemotherapy and radiation.

Corresponding Chapters in *Cancer: Principles & Practice of Oncology*, Seventh Edition: 27 (Cancer of the Lung).

Question 14.3. **A 58-year-old man with chronic obstructive pulmonary disease (COPD) is seen for a new mass in his right supraclavicular fossa and pain in his left thigh. Although he continues to work, he has been feeling more fatigued for 3 months and has lost 10 pounds (from a baseline of 170). Workup includes a CT scan of the chest and abdomen, which identifies an 8-cm mass in the right lower lung, multiple enlarged hilar and mediastinal lymph nodes, 4 discrete liver metastases (the largest measuring 3 cm), and a 3-cm mass on the right adrenal gland. A core biopsy of the right supraclavicular mass reveals adenocarcinoma consistent with a primary lung cancer. A bone scan identifies bone metastases in his left midfemur and several ribs. Serum chemistry, including liver and renal function, is normal. What is the most appropriate course of therapy?**

A. Palliative local radiation to his left femur followed by 4 to 6 cycles of a platinum-based doublet chemotherapy regimen.
B. Administer 4 to 6 cycles of a platinum-based doublet chemotherapy regimen.
C. Administer continuous platinum-based chemotherapy until progressive disease.
D. Hyperfractionated radiation therapy to the lung lesion and local nodes, left femur, and ribs, and concurrent chemoembolization of the liver metastases.
E. Supportive care including pain and symptom management.

Question 14.4. **The man in Question 14.3 receives radiation followed by 4 cycles of cisplatin-gemcitabine chemotherapy. He attains a partial response on CT scan and is able to return to work. Unfortunately, 6 months after his last chemotherapy he presents with increasing shortness of breath (SOB) and a new moderate-sized right-sided pleural effusion. Restaging also shows progressive liver metastases. His effusion is drained and his SOB improves. What is the next course of action?**

A. Repeat administration of 4 to 6 cycles of cisplatin-gemcitabine chemotherapy.
B. Talc pleurodesis and a follow-up CT scan in 3 months.
C. Given his rapid recurrence of disease, he should be treated with best supportive care including pain and symptom management.
D. Consideration of a phase I clinical trial.
E. Second-line chemotherapy with either docetaxel or pemetrexed.

Question 14.5. **A physically fit 76-year-old man presents with a new cough and progressive shortness of breath. His workup includes a CT scan of his chest and abdomen, which reveals a 6-cm mass adjacent to the left hilum, a second 3-cm mass in the right lower lobe, enlarged mediastinal lymphadenopathy, and a suspicious liver nodule. The brushings from bronchoscopy reveal**

a poorly differentiated adenocarcinoma that is thyroid transcription factor-1 (TTF-1) positive (consistent with a primary lung cancer). He is on medications for dyslipidemia and mild chronic asthma. His serum chemistry including liver and renal function is normal. What is the most appropriate course of action?

A. Given his age and comorbidities, he should be treated with the best supportive care including pain and symptom management.
B. After a thorough discussion of the risks and benefits, he should be offered systemic chemotherapy.
C. Administer an oral tyrosine kinase inhibitor of the epidermal growth factor receptor (such as gefitinib or erlotinib) concurrently with 4 to 6 cycles of a platinum-based doublet chemotherapy regimen.
D. Palliative radiation therapy to his lung lesions and mediastinal nodes.

Question 14.6. **Which of the following statements is NOT true about bronchioloalveolar carcinoma (BAC)?**

A. The mucinous subtype is commonly characterized by pools of mucus in the alveoli.
B. BAC may be one subtype of NSCLC that is more responsive to inhibitors of the epidermal growth factor receptor (EGFR).
C. The definition of BAC includes the cases in which there is an invasive focus of carcinoma so long as it is less than 10% of the tumor.
D. The cancerous cells of BAC tend to spread in a monolayer throughout the alveolar walls, interfering in gas exchange and causing a right-to-left pulmonary shunt.

Question 14.7. **A 58-year-old woman presents to the emergency department complaining of increased shortness of breath, a nonproductive cough, and fatigue. She was well and working as an office clerk up until 6 months ago, but in the last 3 months her performance status has significantly deteriorated. She has lost 30 pounds (from a baseline of 130), and in the last 2 weeks she has been unable to get off bed or dress herself without assistance. On examination she is cachectic, she has a moderate-sized left pleural effusion, she has a 5-cm left supraclavicular mass, and her liver edge is palpable 5 cm below the costal margin and extends to the midline of her abdomen. Cytology from her pleural effusion reveals adenocarcinoma consistent with a primary lung cancer. What is the most appropriate course of therapy for this patient?**

A. Best supportive care including pain and symptom management.
B. Administer 4 to 6 cycles of a platinum-based doublet chemotherapy regimen.
C. Concurrent platinum-based chemotherapy with thoracic radiation to include the supraclavicular fossa.
D. Pleurodesis followed by a surgical consultation for consideration of a primary resection.

Question 14.8. **A 53-year-old man is found to have a new left upper lobe mass on chest x-ray. Further workup including a CT scan of his chest and abdomen details a 4-cm LUL mass with an associated hilar nodal mass measuring 2 cm and a 2-cm mass in the subcarinal region. A biopsy specimen from his bronchoscopy reveals a squamous cell cancer. His PET scan is positive in the region of the LUL mass but not in the hilum or mediastinum. What is the most appropriate next step?**

A. Despite the PET scan findings, he requires a preoperative mediastinoscopy.
B. Given the negative PET findings in the mediastinum, he should proceed directly to surgery.
C. He has locally advanced disease and should receive concurrent platinum-based chemotherapy with thoracic radiation.
D. Initial PET scans are frequently inaccurate and the scan should be repeated.

Question 14.9. **A 62-year-old man received combined chemoradiotherapy for his locally advanced (stage IIIB) lung cancer 2 months ago. He had a good response to therapy with a 35% shrinkage in his tumor volume. The shortness of breath and chest discomfort he had prior to diagnosis improved with treatment of the cancer, and he has regained the weight he lost during the course of his therapy. Unfortunately, at his 2-month follow-up visit he complains that in the last week he has developed a nonproductive irritating cough and more shortness of breath going up stairs. He denies any fevers, pain, or other systemic complaints. His chest x-ray shows a diffuse interstitial infiltrate, more pronounced on the side of his initial cancer. What is the most likely diagnosis?**

A. Community-acquired pneumonia.
B. Radiation-induced pneumonitis.
C. Lymphangitic carcinomatosis.
D. Cisplatin-induced pulmonary toxicity.

Question 14.10. **Given that the survival of patients with lung cancer is fundamentally predicated on stage, early detection or screening strategies have been tested in clinical trials. Which of the following statements is true?**

A. Randomized trials of routine chest x-rays and sputum cytology compared to usual care have demonstrated that this screening technique can identify more cases of lung cancer, and this detection makes a significant impact on disease-specific mortality.
B. Screening with CT scans detect more cancers than screening with chest x-rays and thus has a more significant impact on disease-specific mortality.
C. Screening for lung cancer is still an active area of study, and there is no current standard of care for screening.
D. Sputum cytology alone can detect the vast majority of preclinical lung cancers.

Question 14.11. **A 58-year old woman presents with an irritating cough, progressive shortness of breath over 3 weeks, and central chest discomfort. A chest x-ray done 4 months ago when the cough started was normal, but x-rays now reveal a large central lung mass extending into both hila. A CT scan shows a 7-cm mass in the right lung abutting the hilum and extending into the mediastinum but no other masses. A CT-guided biopsy identifies a small cell lung cancer (SCLC). Blood work including a complete blood cell (CBC) and serum chemistry are normal except for hyponatremia (sodium of 128). Bone scan and CT of the head are both normal. What is the most appropriate treatment for this woman?**

A. Admission to hospital for immediate treatment with hypertonic saline for the hyponatremia and further staging investigations, including bone marrow biopsy.
B. As her mass is greater than 6 cm, she has extensive stage disease and should be treated with chemotherapy alone.
C. Referral to a thoracic surgeon for consideration of a resection of her lung cancer.
D. Concurrent cisplatin-etoposide chemotherapy with thoracic radiation.
E. Thoracic radiation therapy alone.

Question 14.12. **The woman in Question 14.11 achieves a complete response to her therapy. She asks about the role of prophylactic cranial radiation (PCI). Which statement is true?**

A. Since her initial CT did not show central nervous system (CNS) metastasis and because she had a complete response to treatment, her chance of getting CNS metastasis is very small and not worth the potential toxicity.
B. Her chance of developing CNS metastasis is at least 25%; PCI can decrease this risk and has been shown to improve overall survival.
C. Her chance of developing CNS metastasis is at least 25%, and while PCI can decrease this risk, it has not been shown to improve overall survival.
D. PCI is associated with significant neurocognitive side effects and is generally not recommended.

Question 14.13. **A 57-year-old man presents to his pulmonologist with a 2-week history of cough with minimal hemoptysis and a hoarse voice. He is fatigued, anorexic, and has lost 20 pounds (from a baseline of 150) in 2 months. Workup includes a CT scan of the chest and abdomen that reveals a 9-cm LUL mass with associated hilar lymphadenopathy, enlarged bilateral supraclavicular nodes, a small left pleural effusion, and a 5-cm right adrenal mass. Serum chemistry, bone scan, and CT of the head are normal. CT-guided biopsy of the lung mass reveals small cell lung cancer. What is the appropriate management?**

A. Palliative chemotherapy with 4 to 6 cycles of platinum-etoposide.
B. Palliative chemotherapy with 4 to 6 cycles of an anthracycline-based regimen.
C. Weekly dose-dense platinum-based chemotherapy with G-CSF (granulocyte colony stimulating factor) support.
D. A or B.
E. A or C.

Question 14.14. **A 43-year-old man presents to his primary care physician complaining of right-sided shoulder pain and a tingling sensation in the medial aspect of his right hand. Chest x-ray identifies a right apical mass which is confirmed on chest CT. The mass measures 5 cm in maximum diameter and appears to be invading the superior chest wall. There is no obvious hilar or mediastinal adenopathy, or distant disease. Bronchial washings identify a moderately differentiated adenocarcinoma. Which treatment is associated with the highest chance of local control?**

A. Neoadjuvant platinum-based chemotherapy with concurrent local radiation therapy followed by surgical resection.
B. Platinum-based chemotherapy with concurrent local radiation therapy.
C. If the PET scan does not suggest mediastinal disease, proceed to immediate surgical resection.
D. High-dose local radiation therapy.

Question 14.15. **Which of the following statements is NOT true?**

A. The p53 gene is the most frequently mutated tumor suppressor gene in human cancers.
B. The fundamental role of p53 is to maintain the genomic integrity after DNA damage causes stress on the cell.
C. It has been proven that cigarette smoking causes alterations in p53 that lead to lung cancer.
D. Mutations in p53 are more common in small cell lung cancer (~90%) than non-small cell lung cancer (~50%).

Question 14.16. **Which of the following statements is NOT true about asbestos exposure as it relates to lung cancer?**

A. Lung cancers typically develop within 5 years of the exposure.
B. Cigarette smoking potentiates the malignant potential of asbestos exposure and other environmental carcinogens.
C. Studies have suggested a 7- to 10-fold increase in the lung cancer risk in individuals who were exposed to asbestos dust in mills or from insulation.
D. Analysis of the risk of lung cancer following secondhand residential exposure has been variable.

ANSWERS

Answer 14.1. **The answer is C.**

This man has a stage IIB non-small cell lung cancer (T2N1). The role for adjuvant radiation therapy has been controversial; although it has been shown to decrease the rate of local recurrence, it does not improve survival and may even be detrimental in some cases. Adjuvant radiation can be considered if patients have a positive resection margin, but otherwise it is not the standard of care. Until recently, there was minimal evidence to suggest a survival benefit for adjuvant chemotherapy. However, recent randomized phase III studies including the International Adjuvant Lung Trial, CALGB 9633, and the NCI-Canada (JBR10), have clearly demonstrated a significant survival benefit associated with a course of platinum-based doublet chemotherapy for patients deemed fit enough to receive this treatment. He has had a complete resection; positive hilar nodes do not warrant any further resection.

Answer 14.2. **The answer is E.**

This woman has a locally advanced cancer, stage IIIB (T2N3). In general, patients with stage IIIB disease are technically inoperable. Combined modality therapy with platinum-based doublet chemotherapy given concurrently with radiation therapy is most appropriate for patients who have good pulmonary function, a good performance status, and disease which is encompassable within a reasonable radiation field. Clinical trials have demonstrated a survival benefit associated with a concurrent chemoradiotherapy approach compared to sequential radiation followed by chemotherapy or conventional radiation therapy alone. It should be noted, however, that the concurrent regimen is also associated with more toxicity, particularly esophagitis, and patients must be carefully selected by a multidisciplinary team of oncologists and surgeons. Although the chance of cure is relatively small, palliative chemotherapy is not a sufficiently aggressive approach in this otherwise well woman.

Answer 14.3. **The answer is A.**

In patients with advanced NSCLC with a good performance status, chemotherapy has been definitively shown to prolong survival and improve a patient's quality of life over best supportive care alone; it is also more cost effective. The current standard of care is treatment with 4 to 6 cycles of a platinum-based doublet regimen. Randomized phase III clinical trials have been unable to clearly discriminate a clinically significant difference between a variety of combinations of cisplatin or carboplatin with either gemcitabine, vinorelbine, docetaxel, or paclitaxel; thus any of these regimens is generally acceptable and allows a clinician to choose based on toxicities, convenience, and cost.

Although chemotherapy will also provide pain relief, palliative radiation therapy can be given prior to chemotherapy to areas of localized pain. In this case, the femur is a weight-bearing bone that carries a high risk of fracture; radiation therapy can help reduce this risk. There is no proven benefit to extend the duration of chemotherapy beyond 4 to 6 cycles.

Answer 14.4. **The answer is E.**

Given he has recurrent disease, it is unlikely he would achieve a meaningful response to the repeat administration of cisplatin-gemcitabine. It has been demonstrated that single-agent docetaxel chemotherapy is superior to best support care in terms of quality of life and median survival. In a randomized trial of pemetrexed, a multitargeted antifolate, versus docetaxel, pemetrexed appeared to have a similar efficacy but with less systemic toxicity, fewer episodes of febrile neutropenia, and fewer hospitalizations. In the second-line setting, there is no evidence that multiagent chemotherapy is more beneficial than a single agent. Phase II studies testing the efficacy of new agents or combinations of agents are frequently considered as options for second-line therapy; however, a phase I trial assessing drug toxicity may not be appropriate when chemotherapies such as docetaxel have clearly demonstrated a survival benefit.

Answer 14.5. **The answer is B.**

Advanced age (over 70 years) alone should not preclude the administration of systemic chemotherapy. Randomized trials restricted to elderly patients with advanced NSCLC have shown that single-agent vinorelbine or gemcitabine therapy is well tolerated and associated with a survival benefit over best supportive care alone. Subgroup analyses from other randomized trials suggest that elderly patients tolerate standard doublet platinum-based chemotherapy regimens and obtain the same benefit as their younger counterparts. Although the single-agent activity of erlotinib and gefitinib is promising, combining such agents with chemotherapy did not improve response or survival rates in large randomized phase III trials.

Answer 14.6. **The answer is C.**

The most recent (1999) World Health Organization definition of BAC specifies that no areas of invasive carcinoma should be identified. If present, as is often the case when BAC is noted at the periphery of an adenocarcinoma, then it should be considered to be a mixed BAC adenocarcinoma.

Answer 14.7. **The answer is A.**

There are several accepted methods of "scoring" performance status including the Karnofsky, ECOG (Eastern Cooperative Oncology Group), or Zubrod scales. In NSCLC, these scales correlate closely with survival and help differentiate subgroups of patients more or less likely to benefit from aggressive treatment. Patients such as this woman, who are unable to care for themselves and/or spend more than 50% of their waking time in bed, are not thought to benefit from chemotherapy. Thus, given her advanced disease state, weight loss, and poor performance status, she should be treated with best supportive palliative care. Although randomized studies have confirmed the benefit of delivering systemic chemotherapy to relatively fit patients with metastatic lung cancer, none of this benefit is achievable in a patient with such a poor performance status.

Answer 14.8. **The answer is A.**

The routine use of mediastinoscopy for patients with early stage disease (clinical stage I) is controversial and likely can be omitted in those patients who have had a CT and/or PET scan that does not identify mediastinal adenopathy. Any patient, like the man in this question, with suspicious disease and/or a clinical stage II or III cancer should undergo mediastinoscopy to rule out the possibility of N3 disease and to identify patients with N2 disease who might benefit from neoadjuvant therapy. Although the PET scan was negative, it could well be false, particularly in the presence of 2- to 3-cm nodes.

Answer 14.9. **The answer is B.**

Although it is generally a diagnosis of exclusion, the clinical features of radiation-induced pneumonitis are cough, dyspnea, fever, and an abnormal chest x-ray. It usually occurs 1 to 3 months after the completion of radiation therapy. Chest x-rays and CT scans typically show an infiltrate in the radiation field, and frequently one can observe a straight line representing the edge of this field. Although this is usually a self-limiting process, radiation pneumonitis can become quite severe and debilitating. Once other causes, such as bacterial pneumonia, are ruled out, the standard therapy is oral corticosteroids with a taper over 10 to 14 days depending on the response.

Answer 14.10. **The answer is C.**

Randomized and nonrandomized trials of screening chest-x-rays with or without paired sputum cytology do demonstrate a higher rate of lung cancer detected in the screened population, but this has had no demonstrable effect on lung cancer specific mortality. Numerous studies show that CT scans are superior to chest x-rays in terms of cancer detection; however, no CT studies have yet demonstrated a significant impact on lung cancer specific mortality. One issue with CT screening is the relatively high rate of false-positive findings that require further investigation, which can be costly and invasive. One aspect of the ongoing studies is an attempt to define the high risk populations that are most likely to develop invasive cancers and, thus, are the most likely to benefit from early detection and intervention.

Answer 14.11. **The answer is D.**

This woman has limited stage SCLC and thus is a candidate for combined modality therapy with curative intent. The majority of randomized trials have suggested that thoracic radiation therapy with the early administration of concurrent cisplatin-etoposide chemotherapy is associated with a better overall survival than sequential treatment. Hyponatremia is commonly noted in patients with SCLC and does not generally require aggressive therapy beyond treating the cancer itself. Though 15% to 30% of patients have bone marrow involvement at presentation, it is rarely the only site of metastatic disease; thus, routine bone marrow biopsies are not recommended. Surgery has a limited role to play in SCLC.

Answer 14.12. **The answer is B.**

Her chance of developing CNS metastasis is approximately 25% and will increase the longer she lives, with estimates of up to 50% to 80% for those patients who survive 2 years. Studies of PCI versus observation have demonstrated a significant reduction in the incidence of clinically detectable brain metastases from 24% to 6% with PCI. In addition, meta-analyses have shown a significant improvement in overall survival associated with PCI (3-year survival of 15% versus 21% for those receiving PCI). Notably, studies focused on assessing the neurotoxic effects of PCI (at standard doses) did not identify sufficient data to demonstrate any more abnormalities in patients receiving PCI than those who did not.

Answer 14.13. **The answer is D.**

This is a classic presentation of extensive stage SCLC. Despite the dismal long-term survival rates, the response to first-line combination chemotherapy is typically 60% to 80% and occurs within 1 to 2 cycles of treatment. Compared to supportive care alone, 4 to 6 cycles of chemotherapy offer substantial quality of life benefits and are associated with median survival time of 7 to 12 months. In extensive stage disease, in which concurrent radiation therapy is not typically administered, cisplatin-etoposide has not demonstrated superiority over anthracycline-based regimens such as CAV (cyclophosphamide, doxorubicin, vincristine). Studies of dose-intensification strategies and growth factor support have served only to increase toxicity but not improve overall survival.

Answer 14.14. **The answer is A.**

Chest wall involvement is a common occurrence in patients with apical or peripheral lung cancers. This patient has a classic presentation of a Pancoast tumor, typically defined as those apical tumors that involve the brachial plexus and/or invade the first rib. These cancers require a multidisciplinary approach and mandate aggressive local control to preserve neurologic function. Although the studies of superior sulcus tumors are not large, there is sufficient evidence to demonstrate the benefit of neoadjuvant combined chemotherapy given concurrently with radiation, followed by surgery in terms of local control and probably long-term survival.

Answer 14.15. **The answer is C.**

Although it is postulated that cigarette smoking is related to p53 mutations, it has not been clearly demonstrated in humans. It is interesting to note that carriers of Li-Fraumeni syndrome (an inherited susceptibility to cancer due to a germline mutation of p53) have an even higher risk of developing lung cancers if they smoke.

Answer 14.16. **The answer is A.**

Lung cancers, including malignant mesothelioma, typically develop 30 to 35 years following asbestos exposure.

CHAPTER **15**

Neoplasms of the Mediastinum

NASSER HANNA

Directions Each of the numbered items below is followed by lettered answers. Select the ONE lettered answer that is BEST in each case unless instructed otherwise.

QUESTIONS

Question 15.1. **A 28-year-old man with a history of Klinefelter syndrome presents to his local physician with complaints of cough and hoarseness of 3 months' duration. A chest x-ray reveals an enlarged mediastinum. A chest CT confirms the presence of an 8-cm anterior mediastinal mass. Serum alpha fetoprotein (AFP) is elevated at 1,500 ng per mL, and b-human chorionic gonadotropin (HCG) is also elevated at 20,000 IU per L. A presumptive diagnosis of nonseminomatous germ cell tumor of mediastinal origin is made. Which of the following is the most appropriate initial management?**

A. Surgical resection of the mass.
B. Four courses of a 3-drug platinum based regimen such as bleomycin + etoposide + cisplatin (BEP) or etoposide + ifosfamide + cisplatin (VIP).
C. Radiation therapy to the mass.
D. Testicular ultrasound.
E. Biopsy of the mass to confirm the diagnosis.

Question 15.2. **A 61-year-old woman with no prior significant medical history reports a 6-month history of diplopia, dysphagia, and fatigue. She is eventually diagnosed as having myasthenia gravis and is treated with an anticholinesterase-mimetic agent without improvement in her symptoms. A CT of the chest reveals a 7-cm anterior mediastinal mass, which appears well encapsulated. A core biopsy is diagnostic for thymoma. The mass is resected and the surgical margins are negative. The final diagnosis was stage I thymoma. Her diplopia, dysphagia, and fatigue significantly improve. What is the next best course of action?**

A. Observation.
B. Adjuvant radiation therapy.
C. Adjuvant chemotherapy.
D. Prednisone.

Corresponding Chapters in *Cancer: Principles & Practice of Oncology*, Seventh Edition: 28 (Neoplasms of the Mediastinum).

Question 15.3. **A 67-year-old man is noted to have an asymptomatic anterior mediastinal mass on a routine preoperative chest x-ray for hip replacement surgery. AFP and b-HCG are normal. A biopsy is consistent with thymoma. Which of the following is least likely associated with this diagnosis?**

A. Pure red cell aplasia.
B. Hypogammaglobulinemia.
C. Myasthenia gravis.
D. Polymyositis.
E. Acute megakaryocytic leukemia.

Question 15.4. **A 33-year-old man presents to his physician with a 3-month history of fatigue, weight loss, and breast tenderness. He is discovered to have a 10-cm anterior mediastinal mass on chest CT. AFP is 1,200 ng per mL and b-HCG is 146,000 IU per L. The patient is diagnosed as having a primary mediastinal nonseminomatous germ cell tumor and is treated with 4 cycles of VIP chemotherapy. Upon completion of his 4 cycles, his tumor markers are declining, but remain slightly elevated. A chest CT demonstrates a significant reduction in the original mass, but a 3-cm mass remains. What is the best next step in management of this disease?**

A. PET imaging and, if negative, observation.
B. Surgical resection of the residual mass.
C. Radiation therapy to the residual mass.
D. Salvage chemotherapy with another platinum-based triplet regimen.
E. High dose chemotherapy with stem cell rescue.

Question 15.5. **Tumors involving the mediastinum**

A. most commonly arise from thymic, neurogenic, lymphatic, germinal, and mesenchymal tissues
B. are less commonly metastases from other sites
C. are common in all age groups
D. are more frequently in the posterior compartment in adults
E. are more frequently in the middle compartment in children

Question 15.6. **Thymomas**

A. occur in the posterior mediastinum most frequently
B. have more malignant features than their thymic carcinoma counterparts
C. more frequently metastasize to the liver compared with the pleura or lung
D. are commonly associated with myasthenia gravis
E. are chemotherapy- and radiation-insensitive tumors

Question 15.7. **Regarding thymic carcinomas, which of the following statement(s) is/are true?**

A. Are rare, aggressive thymic neoplasms.
B. Have a worse prognosis when compared with thymomas.
C. Are rarely associated with myasthenia gravis and other thymoma-associated syndromes.
D. Are surgically resected, when feasible.
E. All of the above.

Question 15.8. **Which of the following is true regarding mediastinal germ cell tumors?**

A. The mediastinum is the most common primary site for extragonadal germ cell tumors.
B. Primary mediastinal seminomas carry a poor prognosis.
C. Teratomas are very chemotherapy-sensitive tumors.
D. Mediastinal germ cell tumors are most commonly diagnosed in the sixth decade of life.
E. Mediastinal seminomas are radiation-resistant tumors.

Question 15.9. **Neurogenic tumors**

A. occur most commonly in the posterior mediastinum
B. are more frequently found in children or young adults
C. may cause significant morbidity depending on their size and location
D. are primarily treated with surgical resection
E. all of the above

ANSWERS

Answer 15.1. **The answer is B.**

The appropriate initial management for patients with primary mediastinal nonseminomatous germ cell tumors is four courses of either BEP or VIP chemotherapy. Germ cell tumor is the most common malignancy in men aged 15 to 35. While the gonads are by far the most common site of origin of germ cell cancers, the mediastinum is the most common site of extragonadal germ cell tumors. A diagnosis of germ cell tumor can be made based upon the clinical presentation associated with the elevated tumor markers in a man this age. A confirmatory biopsy is, therefore, unnecessary. Germ cell cancers found in the anterior mediastinum are almost always the primary site of origin, whereas germ cell cancers in the posterior mediastinum usually arise from a testicular or retroperitoneal primary. In those instances, a testicular ultrasound is mandatory. Radiation therapy plays no role in the management of nonseminomatous germ cell tumors. Surgical resection is only undertaken following chemotherapy.

Answer 15.2. **The answer is A.**

Five-year survival rates for Masaoka stage I tumors is approximately 96%. Complete surgical resection is the mainstay of therapy. Extended total thymectomy, including all tissue anterior to the pericardium from the diaphragm to the neck and laterally from phrenic nerve to phrenic nerve, is recommended in all cases. Three-year recurrence rates for patients with myasthenia gravis and thymoma are reportedly approximately 4.8%. Adjuvant radiation therapy in stage I thymoma has not been shown to improve upon the excellent results of surgery alone. Adjuvant chemotherapy with or without steroids is not standard for stage I thymomas that are completely resected. Adjuvant radiation therapy is frequently given for resected stage II and III tumors resulting in improved local control rates. When tumors are unresectable at presentation, neoadjuvant chemoradiation is frequently administered to improve the chances of complete resection. Single modality treatment with chemotherapy is usually reserved for locally advanced unresectable disease (stage III) or metastatic disease.

Answer 15.3. **The answer is E.**

Answers A, B, C, and D are all associated with thymoma, while answer E is most frequently associated with primary mediastinal germ cell tumors. In addition to those listed in the question, a variety of autoimmune disorders, such as lupus, Sjögren syndrome, ulcerative colitis, thyroiditis, rheumatoid arthritis, sarcoidosis, and scleroderma are associated with thymoma. A variety of blood disorders such as T-cell deficiency, erythrocytosis, and pernicious anemia are also associated with thymomas as are neuromuscular syndromes such as myasthenia gravis, myotonic dystrophy, and Eaton-Lambert syndrome. Mediastinal germ cell tumors are more commonly associated with Klinefelter syndrome and acute leukemias, in particular acute megakaryocytic leukemia.

Answer 15.4. **The answer is B.**

Patients with primary mediastinal nonseminomatous germ cell tumors, by definition, have poor risk disease as defined by the International Germ Cell Consensus Classification. Four cycles of a platinum-based three-drug regimen, such as BEP or VIP, is recommended as initial management. All patients with germ cell tumor would be expected to have an initial response to chemotherapy; however, the majority of patients with a large mass at diagnosis would be expected to have a residual radiographic abnormality following 4 cycles of chemotherapy. The proper management in this patient would be a surgical resection of the residual mass. PET imaging would not be considered standard and is not sensitive enough to detect microscopic disease or teratoma; therefore, it would not be recommended in this instance. Radiation therapy plays little role in the management of nonseminomatous disease. Salvage chemotherapy at standard doses or at high doses with stem cell rescue is rarely curative in the salvage setting for primary mediastinal nonseminomatous germ cell tumors. In the absence of other distant metastatic disease, surgical resection is the recommended therapy, even in the salvage setting.

Answer 15.5. **The answer is A.**

Tumors in the mediastinum are more commonly metastases from other primary sites, are uncommon in all age groups (but are most common in the third to fifth decades of life), and are most frequently in the anterior compartment in both adults and children (although posterior compartment tumors are more frequent in children than in adults).

Answer 15.6. **The answer is D.**

While thymomas are associated with a variety of paraneoplastic syndromes, myasthenia gravis occurs in 30% to 50% of patients with thymomas. Thymomas most frequently occur in the anterior mediastinum, have more bland features when compared with thymic carcinomas, most frequently metastasize to the pleura or lung and rarely to extrathoracic sites, and are very radiation- and chemotherapy-sensitive tumors.

Answer 15.7. **The answer is E.**

All the above statements regarding thymic carcinomas are correct.

Answer 15.8. **The answer is A.**

While mediastinal germ cell tumors comprise only 2% to 5% of all germinal tumors, they constitute 50% to 70% of all extragonadal germ cell tumors and most frequently occur in the third decade of life. Primary mediastinal seminomas are highly curable tumors, carrying a good prognosis. Definitive therapy for primary mediastinal seminomas can be radiation therapy alone or 3 cycles of BEP chemotherapy. Residual radiographic abnormalities can be safely observed following chemotherapy. Teratomas are chemotherapy and radiation therapy insensitive tumors; do not secrete either AFP or b-HCG; are comprised of elements of ectodermal, endodermal, and mesodermal origin; and frequently degenerate into other non-germ cell malignancies, such as sarcoma or primitive neuroectodermal tumors.

Answer 15.9. **The answer is E.**

All of the above statements regarding neurogenic tumors are correct. Neurogenic tumors may occur in the anterior mediastinum but most commonly occur in the posterior mediastinum. They comprise 19% to 39% of all mediastinal tumors, including 75% of posterior mediastinal tumors. They are more frequently discovered in children and young adults, occur without gender predilection, and are often asymptomatic and solitary. They may cause spinal cord compression, pain, Horner syndrome, and muscle atrophy depending on the size and location. They are always treated with surgical resection, when feasible.

CHAPTER **16**

Cancers of the Gastrointestinal Tract

DAVID H. ILSON, SHARLENE GILL, AND RICHARD M. GOLDBERG

Directions Each of the numbered items below is followed by lettered answers. Select the ONE lettered answer that is BEST in each case unless instructed otherwise.

QUESTIONS

Question 16.1. **A 40-year-old man with a 10-year history of reflux disease and Barrett esophagus is found on surveillance endoscopy to have a distal esophageal ulcer, with a biopsy revealing invasive adenocarcinoma. A computed tomographic (CT) scan of the chest and abdomen is normal, and endoscopic ultrasound reveals a T1N0 lesion. The appropriate management for this patient is**

A. photodynamic therapy
B. endoscopic mucosal resection
C. surgical resection
D. preoperative chemotherapy followed by surgical resection

Question 16.2. **A 65-year-old man presents with solid food dysphagia and weight loss. Endoscopy reveals a mass at 28 cm from the incisors, and a biopsy reveals squamous cell carcinoma. A CT scan of the chest and abdomen reveals a midthoracic esophageal mass, and bronchoscopy shows no evidence of invasion of the airway. Endoscopic ultrasound reveals a T3N1 lesion. The best initial therapy for this patient is**

A. brachytherapy
B. radiation therapy
C. chemotherapy followed by radiation therapy
D. combined concurrent chemotherapy and radiotherapy
E. photodynamic therapy

Corresponding Chapters in *Cancer: Principles & Practice of Oncology*, Seventh Edition: 29 (Cancers of the Gastrointestinal Tract).

Question 16.3.

A 45-year-old man presents with solid food dysphagia. Endoscopy reveals a gastroesophageal junction mass, and a CT scan of the chest and abdomen reveals thickening of the distal esophagus. A positron emission tomographic (PET) scan reveals positive uptake in the gastroesophageal junction with no evidence of metastatic disease, and an endoscopic ultrasound reveals a T3N0 lesion. The patient undergoes a thoracoabdominal resection, and surgical pathology reveals a T3 lesion with 5 of 25 lymph nodes involved with metastatic adenocarcinoma, and all surgical margins are clear. Recent studies support the benefit of which of the following postoperative treatments.

A. No study has shown a benefit for postoperative therapy in gastroesophageal (GE) junction cancers.
B. Adjuvant chemotherapy after surgery improves survival compared to surgery alone.
C. Adjuvant radiation therapy after surgery improves survival compared to surgery alone.
D. Combined chemotherapy and radiotherapy reduces local recurrence and improves disease-free and overall survival compared to surgery alone.

Question 16.4.

A 75-year-old patient presents with dysphagia to solid foods and a 15 pound weight loss. He is able to swallow solid foods and is ambulatory. Endoscopy reveals a midthoracic squamous cancer, and a CT scan of the chest and abdomen reveals multiple 1- to 2- cm hepatic metastases, bilateral pulmonary nodules, and retroperitoneal adenopathy measuring up to 3 cm. A PET scan indicates uptake in the primary tumor, lung, liver, and retroperitoneum. Palliative approaches to the patient include all of the following EXCEPT

A. esophageal stent placement
B. external beam radiotherapy
C. single agent or combination chemotherapy
D. esophagectomy and gastric pull up
E. brachytherapy

Question 16.5.

A patient presents with progressive solid food dysphagia, fevers, weight loss, and persistent cough when swallowing. A barium swallow reveals a constricting mass in the midthoracic esophagus, with evidence of a tracheoesophageal fistula. Endoscopy and biopsy reveal a squamous cancer of the midthoracic esophagus, and a bronchoscopy confirms tumor invasion of the trachea. A CT scan reveals bilateral pulmonary nodules and multiple hepatic metastases. The most appropriate first course of action is

A. 5-fluorouracil (5FU), cisplatin, and concurrent radiotherapy
B. combination chemotherapy
C. esophagectomy
D. esophageal stent placement

Question 16.6. **Which of the following statements about chemoradiotherapy in esophageal cancer is true?**

A. Pathologic complete responses are achieved with chemoradiotherapy in 20% to 40% of patients.
B. Chemoradiotherapy may downstage the primary tumor and potentially increase the rate of resection.
C. Surgery after combined chemoradiotherapy may result in a reduction in local recurrence of the cancer compared with chemoradiotherapy alone.
D. Chemoradiotherapy prior to surgery has not been consistently shown to improve survival in randomized trials compared with surgery alone.
E. All of the above.

Question 16.7. **Molecular pathways that may be involved in esophageal adenocarcinoma and squamous carcinoma include**

A. overexpression of cyclin D1
B. mutation of the retinoblastoma gene
C. mutation of p53
D. loss of heterozygosity or promoter hypermethylation of p16
E. all of the above

Question 16.8. **A 50-year-old man presents with episodes of severe nocturnal heartburn occurring 1 to 2 times weekly for nearly 3 years. He is referred for an upper endoscopy, which reveals a short segment of Barrett esophagus in the distal esophagus. Four quadrant biopsies reveal no evidence of dysplasia or carcinoma. Follow-up in this patient should include**

A. antacid therapy, but no follow-up endoscopy is needed given the absence of dysplasia
B. follow-up endoscopy at 6 months
C. follow-up endoscopy at 1 to 2 years
D. photodynamic therapy

Question 16.9. **The most common presentation of esophageal cancer is**

A. anemia
B. abdominal pain
C. dysphagia and weight loss
D. hemoptysis

Question 16.10. **In the staging of a thoracic esophageal cancer, which of the following statements is correct?**

A. For a proximal esophageal cancer, supraclavicular lymph nodes represent stage III disease.
B. For a distal esophageal adenocarcinoma, celiac lymph nodes represent stage III disease.
C. Retroperitoneal lymph nodes for a distal esophageal adenocarcinoma represent M1A (Stage IVA) disease.
D. For stage III esophageal squamous cancers, lymph nodes must not extend outside of the thorax.

Question 16.11. **The T and N stage of an esophageal cancer are best assessed by which modality?**

A. Endoscopic ultrasound.
B. Barium esophagram.
C. CT scan of the chest and abdomen.
D. Magnetic resonance imaging (MRI) scan of the chest and abdomen.
E. PET scan.

Question 16.12. **In the surgical management of a clinically staged T2N1 (stage II) adenocarcinoma of the distal esophagus, which of the following statements is true?**

A. Thoracoabdominal resection is superior to transhiatal resection.
B. Transhiatal resection is superior to thoracoabdominal resection.
C. A three-field lymph node dissection (neck, chest, and abdomen) is performed routinely.
D. The outcome, including postoperative mortality, is generally superior in centers performing a high number of esophageal resections.

Question 16.13. **For stage III esophageal squamous cancer, which of the following statements is true?**

A. Surgery results in superior survival compared to combined chemoradiotherapy.
B. Chemoradiotherapy results in superior survival compared to surgery.
C. Survivals for primary chemoradiotherapy and for surgery are comparable.

Question 16.14. **Which of the following statements is true about combined chemoradiation in esophageal cancer?**

A. Adding brachytherapy after combined chemoradiotherapy improves treatment outcome.
B. High-dose radiotherapy of 64.8 Gy is superior to 50.5 Gy of radiotherapy in combination with 5FU and cisplatin.
C. There is no evidence that radiotherapy administered above a dose of 50.4 Gy in 1.8 Gy daily fractions improves treatment outcome in combined chemoradiotherapy.

Question 16.15. **Which of the following statements is true about combined chemoradiotherapy in esophageal cancer?**

1. **5FU and cisplatin combined with radiation achieves a pathologic complete response in 20–30% of patients.**
2. **Paclitaxel- or irinotecan–based chemotherapy in combination with radiation therapy are superior to 5FU and cisplatin in antitumor response and patient survival.**
3. **Paclitaxel or irinotecan in combination with radiation therapy may reduce rates of gastrointestinal toxicity when combined with radiation therapy.**
4. **All patients require enteral feeding tubes prior to treatment with combined chemoradiotherapy.**

A. All of the above.
B. Statements 2 and 3.
C. Statements 1 and 4.
D. Statements 1 and 3.

Question 16.16. **Which of the following statements is true regarding the recurrence of esophageal adenocarcinoma after surgery?**

A. Local recurrence after surgery is the primary pattern of disease recurrence.
B. Distant metastatic disease is the most common site of recurrence after surgery.
C. Adjuvant chemotherapy results in a significant reduction in distant recurrence of disease after surgery.

Question 16.17. **The most common complication of primary chemoradiotherapy in esophageal cancer is**

A. treatment-related death due to therapy toxicity
B. esophageal stricture
C. radiation pneumonitis
D. tracheoesophageal fistula

Question 16.18. **The most common complication after esophageal cancer surgery is**

A. postoperative death
B. wound dehiscence
C. pulmonary embolism
D. respiratory complications

Question 16.19. **Esophageal squamous cancer and esophageal adenocarcinoma are characterized by which of the following statements.**

1. **Esophageal squamous cancer has a better prognosis for survival than adenocarcinoma.**
2. **Esophageal squamous cancer is more common in African-American males than white males.**
3. **Adenocarcinoma of the esophagus is increasing in incidence in the United States and now exceeds the incidence of squamous cancer in white males.**
4. **Worldwide adenocarcinoma of the esophagus is more common than squamous cancer.**

A. All of the above.
B. Statements 1, 2, and 3.
C. Statements 2 and 3.
D. Statement 4.

Question 16.20. **Which of the following statements is correct about cigarette smoking and the risk of esophageal cancer?**

1. **Smoking increases the risk of both esophageal squamous cancer and adenocarcinoma.**
2. **Smoking plays no role in the risk of developing adenocarcinoma.**
3. **Alcohol and tobacco together increase the risk of adenocarcinoma.**
4. **Ninety percent of squamous cancers of the esophagus in the United States are attributable to cigarette smoking.**

A. Statements 1 and 2.
B. Statements 3 and 4.
C. Statements 1 and 4.
D. Statements 2 and 4.

Question 16.21. **A 73-year-old man presents with iron deficiency anemia. Physical exam is unremarkable except for guaiac positive stool. Colonoscopy is normal, but upper endoscopy reveals a mass in the gastric antrum, with a biopsy revealing adenocarcinoma. Chest x-ray is clear. The patient is taken to surgery and undergoes exploratory laparotomy. At surgery he is found to have miliary deposits of tumor throughout the peritoneum which are millimeter in size, and a biopsy reveals metastatic adenocarcinoma. Open laparotomy most likely would have been avoided if what procedure was done prior to surgery?**

A. Contrast CT scan of the abdomen and pelvis.
B. Ultrasound of the abdomen.
C. PET scan.
D. Endoscopy with ultrasound.
E. Laparoscopy.

Question 16.22. **The Siewert classification recognizes which of the following categories of gastric cancer.**

A. Staging by the number of lymph nodes involved with metastatic cancer.
B. Classification of intestinal versus diffuse histology.
C. Stratification of tumors involving the gastroesophageal junction as involving primarily the distal esophagus, the GE junction, or the gastric cardia.
D. Classification of gastric cancer based on the sites of metastatic disease.

Question 16.23. **A 50-year-old woman presents with anemia, and workup includes an upper endoscopy that reveals a shallow ulcer in the gastric cardia, with a biopsy revealing adenocarcinoma. CT scan of the abdomen and pelvis is unremarkable. The patient is taken to surgery and has gastrectomy, with pathology revealing a T1N0 lesion with 0 of 28 lymph nodes involved with cancer. The most appropriate course of action is**

A. observation alone
B. adjuvant chemotherapy with cisplatin and 5FU
C. combined chemotherapy and radiation therapy with 5FU
D. whole abdominal radiotherapy

Question 16.24. **A 50-year-old man presents with solid food dysphagia and weight loss. Upper endoscopy reveals a mass in the gastroesophageal junction. Endoscopic ultrasound reveals a T3N0 lesion, and a CT scan of the chest, abdomen, and pelvis shows only thickening of the GE junction. Which of the following statements is correct?**

A. Transhiatal esophagectomy results in superior survival compared to transthoracic esophagectomy.
B. Transthoracic esophagectomy results in superior survival compared to transhiatal esophagectomy.
C. Preoperative chemotherapy and radiation therapy is mandatory prior to resection.
D. Choice of the surgical procedure is dependent on the training and experience of the treating thoracic surgeon.

Question 16.25. **A 55-year-old woman presents with abdominal pain after eating and is found to have iron deficiency anemia. Upper endoscopy reveals an ulcer in the gastric fundus, and a biopsy reveals adenocarcinoma. A CT scan of the abdomen and pelvis only shows gastric thickening with no evidence of metastatic disease. The patient undergoes a partial gastrectomy and is found to have a pathologic T3 tumor with 8 of 25 lymph nodes involved with metastatic adenocarcinoma (T3N2). What is the most appropriate course of postoperative therapy?**

A. Observation alone.
B. Postoperative chemotherapy for 6 months with 5FU and leucovorin.
C. Postoperative chemotherapy for 6 months with combination 5FU and cisplatin chemotherapy.
D. Postoperative combined chemotherapy and radiotherapy with 5FU and leucovorin.
E. Radiation of the gastric surgical bed to reduce local recurrence.

Question 16.26. **A 65-year-old man presents with increasing abdominal girth, early satiety, and abdominal pain. He has ascites and hepatomegaly on physical examination. A CT scan of the abdomen and pelvis reveals a mass in the gastric cardia, ascites, and hepatic metastases. Upper endoscopy reveals a mass in the gastric cardia with a biopsy revealing poorly differentiated adenocarcinoma. He undergoes a large volume paracentesis, with cytology revealing signet ring adenocarcinoma, and his symptoms of pain and early satiety resolve. The most appropriate next step in the patient's care is**

A. palliative gastrectomy to prevent obstruction of the GE junction
B. palliative radiation therapy to the primary tumor to prevent obstruction of the GE junction
C. observation and follow-up in 2 to 3 months' time
D. initiation of palliative systemic chemotherapy

Question 16.27. **In evaluating phase III trials of chemotherapy in metastatic gastric cancer, which of the following statements is NOT true?**

A. In a phase III comparison in metastatic disease, there was no difference in response rate or survival for the regimens etoposide/leucovorin/fluorouracil (ELF), fluorouracil/doxorubicin/methotrexate (FAMTX), and cisplatin/fluorouracil (CF).
B. A phase III comparison of FAMTX in comparison to epirubicin/cisplatin/fluorouracil (ECF) indicated a higher response rate and superior survival for ECF.
C. The regimen of fluorouracil, doxorubicin, and mitomycin is superior to single agent fluorouracil in metastatic disease.
D. The addition of docetaxel to cisplatin and fluorouracil may result in higher response rates and survival in metastatic gastric cancer.

Question 16.28. **Which of the following is correct about the definition of resection type after gastrectomy?**

A. An R2 resection indicates a more extensive soft tissue and nodal resection compared with R0 and R1 resections.
B. An R1 resection, in which all disease has been removed but in which microscopic surgical margins are positive, indicates a curative resection.
C. An R2 resection is a palliative resection in which gross disease is left behind; an R1 resection is a complete resection with involved surgical margins; and an R0 resection is a complete, negative-margin resection.

Question 16.29. **Which of the following is true about the surgical management of gastric cancer?**

A. A D1 resection of gastric cancer, gastrectomy with greater and lesser curvature lymph nodes, results in inferior survival compared with a D2 resection, which is an additional resection of gastrohepatic, splenic, and celiac lymph nodes.
B. The most common surgery performed for gastric cancer in the United States is an extended D2 resection.
C. The number of lymph nodes sampled during surgery has no effect on patient survival.
D. More extended D2 resection and more limited D1 resection result in comparable survival in gastric cancer.

Question 16.30. **Which of the following is true about adjuvant chemotherapy in gastric cancer?**

A. Trials of adjuvant chemotherapy in gastric cancer show a consistent survival benefit compared to surgery alone.
B. Cisplatin combination regimens of chemotherapy are more effective than non-cisplatin-based regimens in the adjuvant setting.
C. Preoperative chemotherapy is superior to postoperative chemotherapy in the adjuvant setting.
D. Randomized trials of chemotherapy after resection in gastric cancer have failed to show a consistent benefit for adjuvant chemotherapy alone.

Question 16.31. **After gastrectomy of a T3N1 cancer of the gastric antrum, which of the following is true about pattern of disease recurrence?**

A. Distant metastatic disease is the predominant pattern of disease recurrence.
B. Bone and lung metastasis are the most common sites of distant tumor recurrence.
C. Intraabdominal recurrence, including the surgical bed, peritoneum, and liver, is the most common pattern or disease recurrence.
D. Lymph node recurrence in the abdomen is the most common site of recurrence.

Question 16.32. **Molecular pathways that appear to be implicated in gastric cancer tumorigenesis include all of the following EXCEPT**

A. alteration of p53
B. mutation of E-cadherin
C. mutation of p16
D. allelic loss of chromosome 3p

Question 16.33. **Which of the following is true about the worldwide incidence of gastric cancer?**

A. Gastric cancer is a rare form of cancer worldwide.
B. Gastric cancer is more common in Western Europe than Eastern Europe.
C. Gastric cancer is the second leading cause of cancer-related death worldwide after lung cancer.
D. Proximal cancers of the GE junction and gastric cardia continue to decrease in incidence in the United States.

Question 16.34. **Which of the following statements about gastric cancer is true?**

A. Infection with *Helicobacter pylori* increases the risk of GE junction and gastric cardia cancer.
B. Infection with *H. pylori* leading to atrophic gastritis and intestinal metaplasia in the stomach appears to be significantly associated with the development of gastric cancer.
C. Obesity, smoking, and esophageal reflux significantly increase the risk of cancers of the gastric body and antrum.
D. An increase in antacid consumption may have led to an increase in GE junction cancer in Western countries.

Question 16.35. **Which of the following is true about familial risk of gastric cancer?**

A. There are no familial syndromes associated with gastric cancer.
B. BRCA 1 and 2 carriers have an increased risk of developing gastric cancer.
C. Families with hereditary nonpolyposis colorectal cancer may have an increased risk of developing gastric cancer.

Question 16.36. **Which of the following statements is true regarding outcome differences for Japanese and Western patients with gastric cancer?**

A. Stage for stage, Japanese patients have survival superior to Western patients undergoing gastric cancer surgery.
B. More radical surgical resections in Japanese patients may more accurately stage patients in Japan compared to Western patients, resulting in potential stage migration and superior survival.
C. Proximal cancers of the GE junction and gastric cardia predominate in the West and have an overall worse prognosis than the more distal gastric cancers more commonly seen in Japan.
D. All of the above.
E. None of the above.

Question 16.37. **A 65-year-old man presents with painless jaundice. An abdominal ultrasound reveals biliary obstruction and a fullness in the head of the pancreas, and there is no evidence of gallstones or gallbladder pathology. Which of the following statements about subsequent evaluation and treatment of the patient is correct?**

A. Endoscopic retrograde cholangiopancreatography (ERCP) remains the standard of care for staging and diagnosis of obstructive pancreatic masses.
B. CT scan or MRI of the abdomen is required for staging prior to surgical exploration.
C. A needle biopsy of the mass should be performed prior to any planned surgical intervention.
D. Percutaneous biliary drainage should be performed as the first therapeutic intervention.
E. All of the above.

Question 16.38. **A 70-year-old man presents with back pain and jaundice. A CT scan of the abdomen reveals a 2-cm mass in the head of the pancreas and no evidence of metastatic disease. The patient undergoes a Whipple procedure without complication and surgical pathology reveals a 3.5 cm adenocarcinoma in the head of the pancreas, with clear surgical margins, and 0 of 20 lymph nodes are involved. Which of the following statements about adjuvant therapy is correct?**

A. Gemcitabine plus radiotherapy is better tolerated than 5FU plus radiotherapy as adjuvant treatment.
B. Gemcitabine plus radiotherapy results in superior survival compared to 5FU plus radiotherapy as adjuvant treatment.
C. The recent Radiation Therapy Oncology Group (RTOG) Trial R97-04 administered 5FU plus radiotherapy after pancreatic resection and then compared gemcitabine versus 5FU as additional systemic therapy.
D. All of the above.

Question 16.39. **A 65-year-old woman presents with painless jaundice. A CT scan of the abdomen shows a mass confined to the head of the pancreas with evidence of bile duct obstruction, and there is no evidence of metastatic disease. She undergoes pancreaticoduodenectomy without complication. Surgical pathology reveals a well-differentiated adenocarcinoma with the tumor 2 cm in size, with 5 of 20 lymph nodes involved with metastatic adenocarcinoma, and all surgical margins clear. Which of the following statement(s) about postoperative therapy is/are correct?**

A. Observation alone is an option for this patient.
B. Postoperative 5FU and radiotherapy is a treatment option for this patient.
C. Postoperative chemotherapy with gemcitabine is a treatment option for this patient.
D. All of the above.
E. A and B.

Question 16.40. **A 50-year-old woman presents with weight loss, anorexia, and back pain. A CT scan of the abdomen reveals a 5-cm mass in the head of the pancreas, retroperitoneal lymphadenopathy, and multiple bulky hepatic metastases. A liver biopsy reveals metastatic adenocarcinoma consistent with a pancreatic primary tumor. The patient is referred for medical oncology evaluation and is noted to be deeply jaundiced with significant complaint of pruritus. Which of the following statements is correct?**

A. The patient should be referred for surgical biliary and gastric bypass.
B. Endoscopic biliary stent placement is the preferred intervention.
C. Percutaneous biliary drainage is preferred over endoscopic biliary drainage.
D. Chemotherapy should be instituted as the primary intervention for biliary obstruction.

Question 16.41. **A 45-year-old patient presents with back pain, weight loss, and anorexia. A CT scan of the abdomen reveals a mass in the head of the pancreas with soft tissue encasement of the superior mesenteric and celiac arteries, with no evidence of distant metastatic disease. A biopsy reveals adenocarcinoma consistent with a pancreatic primary tumor. Which of the following treatment approaches is acceptable?**

A. Chemotherapy with weekly gemcitabine.
B. Combined chemotherapy with 5FU and concurrent radiation.
C. Surgical exploration with gastric and biliary bypass.
D. All of the above.
E. A and B.

Question 16.42. **For patients undergoing potentially curative pancreaticoduodenectomy for adenocarcinoma of the pancreas, which of the following statements is correct?**

A. Five-year survival after surgical resection for all patients is generally less than 15% to 20%.
B. Local regional recurrence occurs in 50% or more of patients.
C. Local recurrence of the cancer is uncommon, whereas metastasis to the peritoneum and liver predominate.
D. A and C.
E. A and B.

Question 16.43. **Which of the following is correct about the staging of pancreatic cancer?**

A. Lymph node involvement defines stage III disease for T1–T3 tumors.
B. T1N1 tumors represent stage II disease.
C. T2 tumors represent stage II disease.
D. All of the above.

Question 16.44. **Which of the following statements about the surgical management of pancreatic cancer is true?**

A. The operative mortality for a Whipple procedure at cancer specialty referral centers is generally less than 5%.
B. Laparoscopy is generally recommended prior to full surgical exploration for left sided pancreatic tumors due to the higher incidence of metastatic disease at presentation.
C. Total pancreatectomy is recommended for right-sided pancreatic tumors.
D. All of the above.
E. A and B.

Question 16.45. **Which of the following statements is true regarding chemotherapy for metastatic pancreatic cancer?**

A. In a phase III trial, gemcitabine resulted in superior median and 1-year survival and superior symptom palliation compared with bolus 5FU.
B. Combination chemotherapy has been shown to be consistently superior to single-agent chemotherapy in metastatic pancreatic cancer.
C. Gemcitabine in combination with 5FU is superior to gemcitabine alone in metastatic pancreatic cancer.
D. All of the above.

Question 16.46. **Surgical palliation for adenocarcinoma of the pancreas is usually performed for which of the following reasons.**

A. To relieve biliary obstruction.
B. To relieve gastric outlet obstruction.
C. To debulk disease to enhance response to chemotherapy.
D. All of the above.
E. A and B.

Question 16.47. **Tumors of the exocrine pancreas include all of the following EXCEPT**

A. infiltrating ductal adenocarcinoma
B. acinar cell carcinoma
C. colloid carcinoma
D. adenosquamous carcinoma
E. islet cell carcinoma

Question 16.48. **Which of the following statements is true about cystic neoplasms of the pancreas?**

A. Mucinous cystic neoplasms of the pancreas, which are large cystic lesions with tenacious mucus, are rarely cured with surgery.
B. Serous cystic neoplasms of the pancreas are usually benign.
C. Intraductal papillary mucinous neoplasms with associated invasive carcinoma have an inferior survival to infiltrating ductal adenocarcinoma.

Question 16.49. **Which of the following statements is true about pancreatic cancer?**

A. Given its relative rarity, pancreatic cancer is an uncommon cause of cancer-related death in the United States.
B. The majority of patients with pancreatic cancer present with localized disease amenable to surgical resection.
C. Tobacco abuse plays a significant role in the development of pancreatic cancer.
D. Occupational exposures, including exposure to chlorinated hydrocarbons, nickel and chromium compounds, polycyclic amines, organochloride insecticides, and silica dust, represent the most important patient exposure risk for developing pancreatic cancer.

Question 16.50. **Which of the following statements about pancreatic cancer is NOT true?**

A. The oncogene K-ras is frequently mutated in pancreatic cancer.
B. Mutation of p53 and p16 occur in the majority of pancreatic cancers.
C. Hereditary pancreatic cancer may account for 10% to 20% of cases.
D. Mutation of DNA mismatch repair genes leading to microsatellite instability is common in pancreatic cancer.

Question 16.51. **Which of the following statements about screening and prevention in pancreatic cancer is NOT true?**

A. Tobacco abuse is the leading preventable cause of pancreatic cancer.
B. A combination of endoscopic ultrasound and CT scan plus CA19-9 determination with subsequent ERCP as clinically indicated is undergoing evaluation as a screening approach in high-risk families with pancreatic cancer.
C. Biomarkers under evaluation in pancreatic cancer include cancer-specific DNA alterations, mRNA based markers in pancreatic juice, and protein-based markers evaluated by mass spectrometry by serum proteomics.
D. CA19-9 measurement in the general population may increase pancreatic cancer detection.

Question 16.52. **A 55-year-old Asian woman with a history of chronic hepatitis B and known cirrhosis presents with a rising alpha fetoprotein (AFP) and abnormal liver function tests. Liver ultrasound revealed a 3-cm lesion in the left hepatic lobe. Serum bilirubin is 2.1 mg per dL, serum albumin is 2.7 g per dL, and the prothrombin time (PT) is minimally prolonged, consistent with Child's B cirrhosis. A needle biopsy reveals hepatocellular carcinoma. Which of the following statements about this patient is are correct?**

A. Primary hepatic resection should be considered in this patient with a stage I tumor.
B. Ethanol injection is a reasonable first treatment option for this patient.
C. Primary multiagent chemotherapy should be used initially given the history of severe cirrhosis.
D. Liver transplantation should be considered in this patient early on in management.
E. B and D.

Question 16.53. **A 40-year-old man is found to have abnormal liver function and an elevated serum AFP. Hepatitis serologies are normal. An ultrasound reveals a 4-cm lesion in the left hepatic lobe, and a CT scan reveals no evidence of metastatic disease or vascular involvement. A needle biopsy reveals hepatocellular carcinoma. The patient undergoes successful partial hepatectomy, surgical margins are clear, and the patient recovers from surgery. Which of the following approaches should be followed?**

A. Adjuvant chemotherapy with a multiagent regimen.
B. Intraarterial adjuvant chemotherapy.
C. Whole abdominal radiotherapy.
D. None of the above.

Question 16.54. **Guidelines for selection of patients appropriate for liver transplantation include**

A. patients with solitary tumors 5 cm or less in size
B. patients with multifocal disease with 3 or fewer tumor nodules each 3 cm or less in size
C. patients with Child's B or C cirrhosis
D. patients who are not candidates for primary liver resection
E. tumors with no evidence of macrovascular invasion
F. all of the above

Question 16.55. **All of the following statements about American Joint Committee on Cancer (AJCC) staging of hepatocellular cancers are true EXCEPT**

A. stage I disease identifies a T1 tumor, a solitary lesion without vascular invasion, with no evidence of lymph node involvement or distant metastases
B. for Stage III disease, patients must have lymph node involvement
C. T2 tumors involve a solitary lesion with vascular invasion or multiple tumors that are all less than or equal to 5 cm in size
D. T3 tumors include multiple lesions more than 5 cm in size or a tumor involving a branch of the hepatic or portal vein

Question 16.56. **In the evaluation of patients with hepatocellular cancer, which of the following statements is true?**

A. The presence of vascular invasion, macroscopic or microscopic, is an adverse prognostic factor.
B. AFP elevation is universally found in patients with hepatocellular carcinoma.
C. Ultrasonography is the best imaging modality to assist in the diagnosis of hepatocellular carcinoma.
D. The majority of patients diagnosed with hepatocellular cancer have no presenting symptoms.

Question 16.57. **For ablation of a solitary hepatocellular carcinoma, which of the following statements is correct?**

A. Radiofrequency ablation is appropriate for tumors 5 cm or less in size.
B. Ethanol injection is appropriate for tumors 3 cm or less in size.
C. Radiofrequency ablation can be performed under ultrasound guidance or during laparoscopy.
D. All of the above.

Question 16.58. **Approaches that may potentially improve the outcome for primary surgical management of hepatocellular cancer include**

A. preoperative portal vein occlusion to cause atrophy of the involved lobe of the liver and compensatory hypertrophy of the noninvolved liver
B. inflow occlusion (the Pringle maneuver) during liver resection to decrease blood flow and improve perioperative morbidity
C. reserving hepatic resection for patients with Child's A cirrhosis and stage I–II hepatocellular carcinoma
D. all of the above
E. none of the above

Question 16.59. **Which of the following statements is true about liver transplantation for early stage hepatocellular carcinoma?**

A. In patients with normal liver function and a stage I hepatocellular cancer, liver transplantation is the optimal initial therapy.
B. In patients with Child's B cirrhosis and a stage I hepatocellular cancer, because of the liver disease, the patient may not tolerate a liver transplant and attempted surgical resection may be the preferred initial therapy.
C. In patients with cirrhosis and early stage hepatocellular carcinoma, the most important principle in initial treatment is to utilize the treatment approach that allows for maximal sparing of the hepatic parenchyma.
D. Invasion of the portal vein does not preclude attempted liver transplantation in most patients.

Question 16.60. **Treatment options for early stage hepatocellular carcinoma include**

A. surgical resection
B. liver transplantation
C. ethanol injection
D. radiofrequency ablation
E. hepatic artery embolization
F. all of the above

Question 16.61. **Which of the following statements about chemotherapy in hepatocellular cancer is true?**

A. Combination chemotherapy appears to improve patient survival compared to single agents.
B. Single agents such as doxorubicin, fluorinated pyrimidines, and cisplatin have response rates ranging from 0% to 25%.
C. Tamoxifen is one of the most active single agents in the treatment of hepatocellular cancer.
D. All of the above.

Question 16.62. **Which of the following statements about intraarterial chemotherapy is true?**

A. Response rates to intraarterial chemotherapy appear to be higher than for systemic chemotherapy administration.
B. Survival in patients treated with intraarterial chemotherapy is superior to treatment with systemic chemotherapy.
C. Chemotherapy added to hepatic arterial embolization procedures results in superior response rates and survival compared to arterial embolization alone.
D. All of the above.

Question 16.63. **Radiation-based palliative options for hepatocellular carcinoma include**

A. external beam and conformal external beam radiotherapy
B. ^{90}Y attached to microspheres
C. radiolabeled ^{121}I anti-ferritin antibodies
D. all of the above
E. A and B

Question 16.64. **Paraneoplastic syndromes associated with hepatocellular cancer include**

A. hypercalcemia
B. hypoglycemia
C. erythrocytosis
D. all of the above
E. none of the above

Question 16.65. **Which of the following statements about hepatocellular cancer is correct?**

A. Although uncommon in the United States, hepatocellular cancer is a leading cause of cancer worldwide.
B. Hepatocellular cancer is most common in parts of China and sub-Saharan Africa.
C. Endemic causes of hepatocellular cancer include hepatitis B and mycotoxin exposure.
D. All of the above.

Question 16.66. **In the United States, hepatocellular cancer has been associated with which of the following.**

A. Infection with hepatitis B or C virus.
B. Alcoholism.
C. Estrogen use.
D. All of the above.
E. A and B.

Question 16.67. **Regarding the incidence of hepatocellular carcinoma in the United States, which of the following statements is correct?**

A. Hepatocellular carcinoma is decreasing in incidence due to hepatitis B vaccination programs.
B. The incidence of hepatocellular carcinoma is increasing in incidence due to hepatitis C infection.
C. Aflatoxin exposure in the United States is a significant cause of hepatocellular carcinoma.

Question 16.68. **An increased risk of developing hepatocellular carcinoma is associated with all of the following EXCEPT**

A. Wilson disease
B. hemochromatosis
C. alpha1-antitrypsin deficiency
D. primary biliary cirrhosis

Question 16.69. **Which of the following statements about screening and prevention is true?**

A. The advent of vaccination for hepatitis B has the potential to reduce hepatocellular carcinoma in endemic areas.
B. A combination of AFP and ultrasound screening is employed in high-risk populations.
C. Aggressive screening programs for hepatocellular carcinoma have been shown to improve survival.
D. None of the above.
E. A and C.
F. A and B.

Question 16.70. **A 58-year-old epidemiologist has a screening colonoscopy that notes two hyperplastic polyps and an adenomatous polyp measuring 12 mm in largest diameter with a high degree of dysplasia observed on microscopic evaluation. All three polyps are pedunculated and completely removed at colonoscopy. The patient comes to you for recommendations regarding the best interval for repeating his colonoscopy and wants to know if there are any lifestyle changes or medications that could decrease his risk for future premalignant lesions. You recommend**

A. annual colonoscopy
B. daily use of two scoops of Metamucil or Citracil
C. 500 mg of calcium daily
D. two Tylenol daily
E. two aspirin daily
F. no relevant intervention has proven useful

Question 16.71. **A 47-year-old woman with a single episode of dark red rectal bleeding is operated on after colonoscopy. Pathology reveals a poorly differentiated adenocarcinoma that is not obstructing the lumen of the colon. The tumor is located just proximal to the hepatic flexure. There is vascular and lymphatic involvement noted with tumor invasion to the serosa but not beyond. Surgical margins are clear and five lymph nodes are noted to be negative for metastatic disease. Because of a history of colon cancer in a sibling who was diagnosed at the age of 49, the tumor is evaluated by immunohistochemistry for microsatellite instability and is noted to lack expression of MSH2. In order to confirm a diagnosis of HNPCC (hereditary nonpolyposis colon cancer), a blood sample is obtained and germ-line DNA testing is performed that confirms that she does lack expression of MSH2 in peripheral lymphocytes. She has three other siblings and two preteen children. This patient should be managed with**

A. 5FU + leucovorin for 6 months
B. FOLFOX for 6 months
C. reassurance that she has a high likelihood of cure and referred back to her internist for follow-up at her discretion
D. referral to a cancer geneticist

Question 16.72. **A 59-year-old man who underwent a screening colonoscopy was noted to have a right-sided colon mass that proves on biopsy to be moderately differentiated adenocarcinoma. At laparotomy, a right hemicolectomy is done and the pathology reveals a transmural (T3) tumor involving 5 of 22 lymph nodes (N2). No residual disease is noted on careful abdominal exploration, and a CT scan is negative for lung, liver, or abdominal residual disease. The patient brings Internet printouts with him to the appointment and asks about getting cetuximab, bevacizumab, edrecolomab, and/or interferon in addition to chemotherapy. You would recommend**

A. no treatment
B. 5FU plus leucovorin (5FU/LV)
C. irinotecan plus 5FU and leucovorin (IFL or FOLFIRI)
D. oxaliplatin plus 5FU and leucovorin (FOLFOX)

Question 16.73. **A 68-year-old man in good general health moves to your town 3 years after having completed adjuvant therapy with 5FU/LV for a T3N1 M0 stage III colon cancer. At your recommendation, he has a repeat colonoscopy including a biopsy of the anastomotic site, which is negative. A physical examination is negative but the carcino embryonic antigen (CEA) is 76. He has a CT of the chest, abdomen, and pelvis that notes a low density, 3-cm lesion in segment 6 of the liver. CT scans are not available from his prior follow-up, but a report of a scan done 18 months ago indicates that this lesion was previously present and thought to be a hemangioma. You recommend**

A. FOLFIRI chemotherapy
B. needle biopsy followed by radiofrequency ablation (RFA)
C. a PET scan
D. repeat CEA in 6 weeks
E. repeat CT in 6 weeks

Question 16.74. **A 64-year-old woman with rectal bleeding has a sigmoid colon lesion noted during colonoscopy. An abdominal CT scan shows 9 low density liver lesions consistent with metastases, the largest of which is 6 cm in longest diameter. After resection of a T3N2 tumor with 7/11 positive nodes, she is referred for treatment of unresectable metastatic disease. There is no disease identified outside of the liver either intraoperatively or on CT scan. The bilirubin is 2.2 with a normal aspartate amino transfers (AST) and elevated alkaline phosphatase of twice normal. The reasonable options include**

A. 5FU and leucovorin
B. irinotecan, 5FU, and leucovorin, with the 5FU given as bolus (IFL)
C. irinotecan, 5FU, and leucovorin, with the 5FU given as infusion therapy (FOLFIRI)
D. oxaliplatin plus 5FU and leucovorin (FOLFOX)
E. capecitabine
F. A or D

Question 16.75. **A 64-year-old woman with metastatic colon cancer to the liver and lungs was initially treated with FOLFOX but now has manifestations of disease progression after 11 months of treatment and a significant partial remission. Her liver function studies are normal and her performance score is 1 based upon modest peripheral neuropathy related to the oxaliplatin. She has no tumor related symptoms. You would choose**

A. capecitabine
B. irinotecan
C. irinotecan plus cetuximab
D. best supportive care without chemotherapy
E. enrollment in a clinical trial
F. B or C

Question 16.76. **A 62-year-old accountant presents with a 3-month history of hematochezia. On rectal exam, a friable, circumferential, nonfixed mass is palpated 4 to 6 cm from the anal verge. Physical examination is otherwise unremarkable. Colonoscopy and biopsy confirm a moderately differentiated adenocarcinoma. The remainder of the colon is unremarkable. What staging investigations should be performed at this time?**

A. Complete blood count (CBC), liver, and renal function tests.
B. Chest x-ray (CXR) and CT scan of the abdomen and pelvis.
C. Endorectal ultrasound (EUS).
D. MRI pelvis.
E. PET scan.
F. A, B, and C.
G. All of the above.

Question 16.77. **The patient in Question 16.76 is clinically staged with T3N1 M0 rectal cancer. He is otherwise well with no significant comorbidities. He has been assessed by a surgeon and an abdominal perineal resection (APR) with a total mesorectal excision (TME) has been recommended. He is dismayed at the prospect of a permanent colostomy and returns to you for further discussion. You recommend that he**

A. proceed to primary surgery and return for planned postoperative chemotherapy and radiation (assuming his surgical pathology confirms T3 and/or N+ disease)
B. proceed to primary surgery and return for planned postoperative chemotherapy (assuming his surgical pathology confirms T3 and/or N+ disease); you note that he does not require adjuvant radiotherapy as his resection will include a TME
C. proceed to short-course (25 Gy/5 fractions) preoperative radiotherapy followed by immediate surgery, then postoperative chemotherapy
D. proceed to prolonged-course (50 Gy/25–28 fractions) preoperative radiotherapy with continuous-infusion 5FU followed by surgery and postoperative chemotherapy

Question 16.78. **The patient in Question 16.77 completes preoperative prolonged-course chemoradiation and is able to undergo a sphincter-preserving anterior resection with TME. Pathology reveals a moderately differentiated adenocarcinoma limited to the muscularis mucosa. Sixteen lymph nodes are negative for metastatic disease and all margins are negative. He presents for consideration of postoperative chemotherapy. You recommend**

A. 5FU plus leucovorin (Mayo or Roswell Park, or a biweekly infusional regimen)
B. FOLFOX
C. capecitabine
D. no chemotherapy; he now has stage I disease

Question 16.79. **A 52-year-old lawyer is diagnosed with a clinical stage T1N0 M0 moderately differentiated adenocarcinoma of the rectum, as determined by EUS and CT. The distal margin of the 3-cm tumor is at 6 cm from the anal verge, occupying one third of the luminal circumference. Following transanal excision, there is no pathologic evidence of vascular or lymphatic invasion. All margins are negative. At this time, you recommend**

A. no further therapy
B. low anterior resection
C. adjuvant pelvic chemoradiation
D. none of the above

Question 16.80. **A 45-year-old married nurse presents with hematochezia and altered bowel habits. On examination, a mass is identified at the anorectal junction with biopsy positive for an infiltrating moderately differentiated squamous cell carcinoma. She has a history of cervical carcinoma *in situ* and genital herpes. She denies prior anal intercourse and has no history of anal fissures or condylomata. She is otherwise well, on no medications, and is a lifelong nonsmoker. Which of the following statements about risk factors for anal cancer is/are true?**

A. Human papilloma virus (HPV) is implicated in the development of anal intraepithelial neoplasia (AIN).
B. *Herpes simplex* virus is a risk factor for squamous anal cancers.
C. Anal cancer is an acquired immunodeficiency syndrome (AIDS)-defining neoplasm.
D. Anal fissures are associated with an increased risk of anal cancer.
E. All of the above.

Question 16.81. **Remarkable findings on examination of the patient in Question 16.80 include a firm lesion with central ulceration palpated in the anterior and superior aspect of the anal canal. A 1.5-cm mobile right inguinal node is also noted, which on fine needle aspirate is confirmed to be metastatic squamous cell carcinoma. She proceeds to a CXR and CT scan of the abdomen and pelvis, which are negative for extrapelvic metastases. Transanal ultrasound identifies a 5.5-cm primary lesion with invasion into muscularis propria and associated with a 1.3-cm perirectal lymph node. You recommend**

A. abdominoperineal resection (APR) with nodal dissection
B. radiation
C. chemoradiation with 5FU and mitomycin
D. cisplatin and 5FU chemotherapy alone

Question 16.82. **A previously well 54-year-old woman presents with abdominal discomfort, nausea, early satiety, and weight loss. Esophagogastroduodenoscopy identifies a large smooth, nonulcerated mass in the greater curvature of the stomach. On CT, a 6- X 4-cm heterogeneous soft tissue mass is seen involving the gastric wall and associated with multiple small intraabdominal and hepatic metastases. Biopsy confirms a malignant gastrointestinal stromal tumor with immunostains positive for CD117 (c-kit) and CD34. Numerous mitoses are seen. You recommend imatinib 400 mg po daily. With respect to predicting response to imatinib therapy, which of the following statements is true?**

A. KIT mutations in exon 9 are associated with a higher rate of response.
B. KIT mutations in exon 11 are associated with a higher rate of response.
C. Increased 18FDG uptake on PET scanning performed within days of starting imatinib therapy is an early predictor of objective CT response.
D. Gastrointestinal stromal tumors (GISTs) arising from a genetic syndrome are more likely to respond to imatinib therapy.
E. A high mitotic index is predictive of response to imatinib therapy.
F. None of the above.

ANSWERS

Answer 16.1. **The answer is C.**

In a patient with a T1N0 clinically staged esophageal cancer who can medically tolerate surgery, surgical resection remains the standard of care. Ablative strategies such as photodynamic therapy or endoscopic mucosal resection remain investigational. Preoperative chemotherapy also remains an investigational approach, and such an approach would not be considered in a patient with a clinical stage I tumor that appears surgically resectable.

Answer 16.2. **The answer is D.**

The standard of care in the radiation-based management of locally advanced esophageal squamous cancer treated with radiation therapy is concurrent chemotherapy and radiation therapy, established by the Radiation Therapy Oncology Group Trial 85-01. Radiation therapy alone is inferior in survival outcome and local control. Brachytherapy and photodynamic therapy have been primarily used in the palliative disease setting to relieve dysphagia, and there has been no comparison of brachytherapy to radiation therapy or combined chemoradiotherapy. The use of sequential chemotherapy followed by radiotherapy has not been compared to concurrent chemoradiotherapy, but the demonstrated inferiority of radiation therapy alone to concurrent chemoradiotherapy argues against the use of radiation therapy alone in locally advanced disease.

Answer 16.3. **The answer is D.**

The recent gastric Intergroup Trial 116 evaluated the use post of postoperative 5FU and radiation therapy after surgery compared to surgery alone. Twenty percent of the patients on this trial had GE junction cancers, and postoperative chemoradiotherapy improved survival compared to surgery alone. Chemotherapy alone or radiotherapy alone after surgery has not been consistently shown to improve survival compared to surgery alone.

Answer 16.4. **The answer is D.**

Esophagectomy in the palliation of metastatic esophageal cancer is generally limited to patients with actively bleeding or completely obstructing cancers, and the morbidity and potential mortality of esophagectomy should limit its use as palliation. Stent placement, external beam radiation or brachytherapy, and chemotherapy are all acceptable palliative treatment approaches.

Answer 16.5. **The answer is D.**

Esophageal stenting should be performed in an attempt to seal off a tracheoesophageal fistula. Combined chemoradiotherapy may actually exacerbate a fistula and should also not be used in the face of distant metastatic disease. The presence of a tracheoesophageal fistula is a contraindication to esophagectomy and also should not be considered in the face of distant metastatic disease. Palliative chemotherapy could be considered once an esophageal stent is in place.

Answer 16.6. **The answer is E.**

Chemoradiotherapy achieves pathologic complete responses in a significant proportion of patients. Chemoradiotherapy appears to downstage the primary tumor, and surgery may enhance local control after chemoradiotherapy compared to chemoradiotherapy alone. Despite the activity of combined chemoradiotherapy, it is still unclear whether or not the addition of preoperative chemoradiotherapy to surgery improves survival compared to surgery alone, with trials failing to show a consistent benefit for preoperative therapy.

Answer 16.7. **The answer is E.**

All of these pathways have been implicated as potentially important in the tumorigenesis of both esophageal adenocarcinoma and squamous cell carcinoma.

Answer 16.8. **The answer is C.**

Patients with Barrett esophagus are at increased risk of developing adenocarcinoma, although the risk over 10 years is only 2% to 3%, so that periodic follow-up endoscopy at 1 to 2 years should be considered. Antacid therapy alone provides only symptom relief and will not revert Barrett changes. Follow-up at a 6 month interval is recommended in patients with low grade dysplasia. Photodynamic therapy remains an investigational technique, although it has recently been approved for the attempted ablation of Barrett esophagus with high-grade dysplasia in patients who are medically not surgical candidates.

Answer 16.9. **The answer is C.**

Dysphagia and weight loss are the most common presenting complaints with esophageal cancer. Odynophagia may also be present in some patients.

Answer 16.10. **The answer is D.**

Supraclavicular nodes for a proximal esophageal cancer, or celiac nodes for a distal esophageal cancer, represent stage IV disease but are staged as stage IVA or M1A as these nodal sites are proximal to the primary tumor site. Retroperitoneal lymph nodes are stage IVB or M1B and represent true distant metastatic disease. For esophageal squamous cancers, stage III lymph nodes must be confined to the thorax.

Answer 16.11. **The answer is A.**

Endoscopic ultrasound has the highest accuracy for determining T and N stage. Conventional radiography with esophagram, CT scan, or MRI has a lesser ability to determine T stage and N stage. PET scan has its greatest utility to detect occult metastatic disease.

Answer 16.12. **The answer is D.**

There is a significant association with outcome in esophageal cancer surgery and the volume of esophageal cancer surgery performed at an institution. The optimal surgical approach for esophageal resection remains controversial, with some surgeons advocating transhiatal resection to reduce perioperative complications and thoracoabdominal resection to improve the exploration of mediastinal contents. The benefit of a more radical three-field nodal resection remains to be established.

Answer 16.13. **The answer is C.**

For stage III esophageal squamous cancer, randomized national trials employing surgery alone as a treatment, or combined chemoradiotherapy as a primary treatment, indicate comparable 5-year survival for the two treatment approaches. Trimodality therapy combining chemoradiotherapy followed by surgery remains the subject of active investigation.

Answer 16.14. **The answer is C.**

A radiation dose of 50.4 Gy is the standard dose to combine with chemotherapy. Adding brachytherapy has not been shown to improve treatment outcome, and escalating the radiation dose to 64.8 Gy in Intergroup Trial 0123 also did not improve treatment outcome.

Answer 16.15. **The answer is D.**

Chemoradiation with 5FU and cisplatin achieves a pathologic complete response in roughly 25% of patients, and regimens using irinotecan or paclitaxel may have lesser degrees of gastrointestinal toxicity than 5FU based regimens but are not necessarily more effective. Fifty percent or fewer of patients require enteral feeding tubes during combined chemoradiotherapy so that all patients may not require such an intervention prior to therapy.

Answer 16.16. **The answer is B.**

Occult metastatic disease is likely present at diagnosis in the majority of patients with esophageal adenocarcinoma who have clinically localized disease at presentation, and distant metastatic disease develops in the majority of patients treated with surgical resection. Local recurrence of disease is common as well after surgery, but the development of distant metastatic disease is the predominant pattern of disease recurrence. Adjuvant chemotherapy alone has not yet been clearly demonstrated to reduce distant recurrence of disease compared to surgery alone.

Answer 16.17. **The answer is B.**

Fatality from combined chemoradiotherapy is uncommon and less than 5% at most centers. Radiation pneumonitis is also uncommon. Tracheoesophageal fistula occurs when tumors invade the airway, and irradiating patients with tumor involvement of the airway may exacerbate or precipitate a fistula, but in the absence of tumor invasion into the airway tracheoesophageal (TE) fistula is uncommon.

Answer 16.18. **The answer is D.**

Wound dehiscence and pulmonary embolism occur but are uncommon, and postoperative mortality occurs in 5% or fewer patients after esophagectomy.

Answer 16.19. **The answer is C.**

Esophageal squamous cell and adenocarcinoma have equally poor prognoses despite different epidemiologic and risk factors. Worldwide esophageal squamous cancer is the most common histology, despite recent increases in adenocarcinoma in Western countries. Esophageal squamous cancer is more common in African American males than in white males, but adenocarcinoma of the esophagus is increasing in incidence and is now the predominant histology in white males in the United States.

Answer 16.20. **The answer is C.**

Smoking has been implicated in the development of both adenocarcinoma and squamous carcinoma, and the most important risk factor for the development of squamous cancer in the United States is smoking. Alcohol and tobacco abuse combined increase the risk of squamous cancers.

Answer 16.21. **The answer is E.**

Unexpected peritoneal carcinomatosis is found in 20% to 30% or more of patients undergoing exploratory laparotomy for gastric cancer. A laparoscopy prior to commitment to open surgery is the optimal way to detect small-volume peritoneal disease. Peritoneal deposits are often too small to be imaged on CT, PET scan, or ultrasound, and routine PET scan imaging does not yet have an established role in the staging of gastric cancer. Endoscopic ultrasound may give a clearer indication of T stage at diagnosis but will likely not be able to detect small peritoneal deposits.

Answer 16.22. **The answer is C.**

The Siewert classification identifies three sub-sites of tumor involvement of the GE junction, which may have implication in differing patterns of lymphatic drainage and choice of optimal surgical procedure for each sub-site.

Answer 16.23. **The answer is A.**

Stage I, T1N0 gastric cancers are generally excluded from adjuvant therapy protocols because of the good prognosis with surgical management alone.

Answer 16.24. **The answer is D.**

Outcomes with transhiatal and transthoracic esophagectomy appear to be comparable in most series. The use of preoperative chemotherapy and radiation therapy, although commonly used in the United States, has not been clearly shown to be beneficial in stage II disease compared to surgery alone. Postoperative chemotherapy and radiation therapy, however, based on the positive results of Intergroup Trial 116, may be a consideration as 20% of the patients on this trial had GE junction tumors.

Answer 16.25. **The answer is D.**

The standard of care in the United States, established by Intergroup Trial 116, is postoperative chemotherapy and radiation with 5FU and leucovorin. The majority of patients on this trial had either T3 or node positive disease. Chemotherapy or radiotherapy alone has not consistently shown to improve outcome compared to surgery alone.

Answer 16.26. **The answer is D.**

Palliative gastrectomy should be reserved for an actively bleeding tumor, or for complete GE junction or gastric outlet obstruction. Palliative radiotherapy has similar application and would not be the first choice of palliation in the face of metastatic disease. Untreated metastatic gastric cancer has a median survival of less than 3 to 4 months so that deferring chemotherapy may result in rapid clinical deterioration and the future inability to treat. Palliative chemotherapy is the most appropriate initial therapy of metastatic gastric cancer.

Answer 16.27. **The answer is C.**

The FAM regimen is not superior to single-agent chemotherapy. Randomized comparisons have indicated equivalence for ELF, FAMTX, and CF. ECF was superior to FAMTX in a randomized trial from the United Kingdom. Preliminary analysis of a recent phase III trial indicates potential benefit for the addition of docetaxel to CF compared to CF alone.

Answer 16.28. **The answer is C.**

Both R2 and R1 resections are palliative, with gross disease left behind in an R2 resection. An R1 resection is also palliative given the presence of positive surgical margins. Only an R0 resection defines a curative resection.

Answer 16.29. **The answer is D.**

Recent studies indicate that a D1 resection results in similar patient survival compared with the more extensive D2 resection. In the United States, in a review of surgeries performed, it was found that many patients had only limited lymph node sampling during surgery performed, and many of these samplings did not even reach the recommended minimum of a D1 resection. Studies indicate that a minimum number of lymph nodes should be sampled at surgery, both for prognostic and therapeutic reasons.

Answer 16.30. **The answer is D.**

Chemotherapy alone, either pre- or postoperatively, has yet to be validated as an effective adjuvant treatment in the surgical management of gastric cancer. For high-risk resected gastric cancer, postoperative chemotherapy and radiotherapy as shown on Intergroup Trial 116 improved overall and disease-free survival, with the greatest benefit being in the reduction of local tumor recurrence.

Answer 16.31. **The answer is C.**

Intraabdominal recurrence of gastric cancer is the most common pattern of recurrence, with distant metastatic disease less common. Recurrence is typically in the surgical bed, liver, and peritoneum and is not restricted to lymph nodes.

Answer 16.32. **The answer is C.**

Hypermethylation of the promoter of p16 has been implicated in gastric cancer tumorigenesis, but mutation of p16 has not been consistently demonstrated.

Answer 16.33. **The answer is C.**

Gastric cancer is most common in Japan, South America, and Eastern Europe and remains the second leading cause of cancer-related death worldwide. Although cancers of the body and antrum are declining in the United States and Western Europe, cancer of the GE junction and cardia are increasing in incidence for unclear reasons.

Answer 16.34. **The answer is B.**

H. pylori infection has no relation to GE junction and cardia cancer but is an important risk factor for distal gastric cancer. Obesity and reflux have been implicated in the development of proximal and GE junction cancers, not distal gastric cancer, and there is a lesser association of smoking and the risk of developing distal gastric cancer; smoking, however, has been implicated with an increased risk of GE junction and cardia cancer. Although antacid use has increased in Western countries, there has been no association between the increase in GE junction cancer and antacid use.

Answer 16.35. **The answer is C.**

There are reports of familial gastric cancer in the literature. HNPCC families have an increased risk of uterine, gastric, pancreatic, and renal pelvis cancers. There has been no association between gastric cancer and BRCA.

Answer 16.36. **The answer is D.**

Answer 16.37. **The answer is B.**

ERCP has lost favor as a diagnostic and staging modality for tumors of the pancreas, the vast majority of which are adenocarcinomas. Either CT scan or MRI is an important staging study done prior to surgery to assess for metastatic disease or local unresectability due to vascular encasement prior to commitment to surgery. A tissue diagnosis is usually not mandated prior to surgical exploration if there is clinical suspicion for adenocarcinoma of the pancreas, given the predominance of adenocarcinoma histology. Percutaneous or other biliary decompression may be accomplished at the time of surgery and is not always required in patients presenting with pancreatic cancer.

Answer 16.38. **The answer is C.**

Although gemcitabine appears to be active in combination with radiotherapy in unresectable pancreatic cancer, or given as preoperative therapy prior to surgery in research trials, recent studies suggest greater toxicity for gemcitabine in combination with radiation compared to 5FU and radiation. Although gemcitabine results in superior survival in metastatic pancreatic cancer compared to 5FU, there has not yet been a head-to-head comparison of gemcitabine versus 5FU in combination with radiotherapy either in unresectable disease or as adjuvant treatment. The recent RTOG trial administered 5FU and radiation as adjuvant therapy after resection, and the comparison on this trial was the additional months of systemic chemotherapy with either 5FU or gemcitabine.

Answer 16.39. **The answer is E.**

Phase III trials comparing surgery alone with surgery followed by combined radiotherapy with concurrent 5FU have come to mixed conclusions. The Gastrointestinal Tumor Study Group (GITSG) trial indicated a survival benefit for postoperative therapy, but the European Organization for the Research and Treatment for Cancer (EORTC) trial failed to confirm a benefit for postoperative chemoradiotherapy. Given the conflicting results of phase III trials, either observation alone or postoperative 5FU and radiation therapy are considered standard therapy options after pancreaticoduodenectomy. Gemcitabine is reserved for the palliation of inoperable or metastatic pancreatic adenocarcinoma. Chemotherapy alone as an adjuvant treatment was recently evaluated in the European Study Group for Pancreatic Cancer (ESPAC) trial, which indicated a potential benefit for adjuvant treatment with 5FU and leucovorin alone without radiotherapy, but this trial has a number of methodologic concerns and it has not been subject to a confirmatory trial.

Answer 16.40. **The answer is B.**

Patients presenting with metastatic pancreatic cancer with biliary obstruction, without clinical evidence of gastric outlet obstruction, are best served with endoscopic biliary drainage, with reservation for percutaneous drainage if endoscopic drainage is not technically feasible. Surgical bypass is more invasive and should be considered for patients with clinical evidence of gastric outlet obstruction to relieve both biliary and gastric obstruction with one procedure. Given the limited activity of chemotherapy in pancreatic cancer, it is unlikely that chemotherapy will result in relief of biliary obstruction in the short term.

Answer 16.41. **The answer is E.**

Either chemotherapy alone with gemcitabine or combined chemoradiotherapy is an acceptable option for a locally unresectable pancreatic cancer. Vascular encasement, which is one criterion for inoperability, would argue against surgical exploration, and bypass would not be mandated in a patient without clinical evidence of either biliary or gastric outlet obstruction.

Answer 16.42. **The answer is E.**

Five-year survival after pancreatic resection is generally poor. Local regional recurrence is common after pancreatic resection and occurs in more than 50% of patients. Although metastatic disease is also common, local recurrence of disease is also a predominant problem.

Answer 16.43. **The answer is A.**

Stage I disease includes tumors limited to the pancreas that are T1 (2 cm or less in size) or T2 (>2 cm in size) which are N0 and M0. Stage II disease includes T3 tumors (tumor extension into the duodenum, bile duct, or peripancreatic tissue) that are N0 and M0. Stage III disease includes T1–T3 tumors that are node positive.

Answer 16.44. **The answer is E.**

At high-volume surgical centers, the surgical mortality for pancreaticoduodenectomy is less than 5%. Because left-sided pancreatic tumors are clinically silent, metastatic disease at presentation is more frequent and laparoscopic assessment prior to surgical exploration is recommended. Total pancreatectomy is rarely performed for pancreatic tumors due to the greater morbidity and complication rate.

Answer 16.45. **The answer is A.**

Gemcitabine is the standard of care in the treatment of metastatic pancreatic cancer based on a pivotal phase III trial indicating superiority over bolus 5FU. Phase III trials have failed to show a consistent benefit from combination chemotherapy over single-agent chemotherapy, including some recent trials of gemcitabine combinations. A phase III trial conducted by ECOG failed to show a survival benefit for the combination of bolus 5FU plus gemcitabine compared with gemcitabine alone.

Answer 16.46. **The answer is E.**

Gastric and biliary bypass can offer effective surgical palliation of gastric and biliary obstruction, particularly when the primary tumor is found to be unresectable at the time of attempted surgery. Surgical debulking plays no role in the treatment of metastatic pancreatic cancer.

Answer 16.47. **The answer is E.**

Islet cell tumors arise from the endocrine pancreas.

Answer 16.48. **The answer is B.**

Serous cystic neoplasms are a benign entity. Mucinous or serous tumors of the pancreas have a superior survival in comparison to ductal adenocarcinomas of the pancreas. Mucinous cystic neoplasms represent lower grade malignancies than infiltrating ductal adenocarcinoma, and in tumors with a component of invasive carcinoma, the 5-year survival with surgery is 50%; without an invasive component, the 5-year survival with surgery approaches 100%. Intraductal papillary mucinous neoplasms have a superior survival in comparison with ductal adenocarcinoma, with a 5-year survival rate of 40% with surgical management.

Answer 16.49. **The answer is C.**

Tobacco is the most significant risk factor for pancreatic cancer identified in recent epidemiologic studies, with occupational exposures a less likely common causative factor. Although pancreatic cancer is a relatively uncommon malignancy, because the case fatality rate nearly equals its incidence, death from pancreatic cancer is common and is the fifth leading causing of U.S. cancer deaths. Only a minority of patients (20%) have potentially resectable pancreatic cancer, and the majority either have metastatic disease or inoperable disease at presentation.

Answer 16.50. **The answer is D.**

K-ras, p53, and p16 mutations are common in pancreatic cancer, but microsatellite instability is uncommon. Hereditary pancreatic cancer, although rare, occurs in 10% to 20% of cases and may also be associated with BRCA2 carriers, families with HNPCC, familial atypical multiple mole melanoma syndrome, hereditary pancreatitis, ataxia telangiectasia, and Peutz-Jeghers syndrome.

Answer 16.51. **The answer is D.**

CA19-9 elevation is not specific for pancreatic cancer and may occur in benign biliary or pancreatic conditions. CA19-9 levels may be normal when the cancers are small and asymptomatic and may not be secreted in 10% to 15% of individuals as a function of their Lewis antigen status. Screening of high-risk families for pancreatic cancer using imaging and endoscopic modalities is the subject of ongoing trials, and DNA, RNA, and protein-based biomarkers are also under active investigation.

Answer 16.52. **The answer is E.**

Primary resection of an early stage hepatocellular carcinoma (HCC) should be reserved for patients with Child's A cirrhosis as patients with significant cirrhosis may not tolerate loss of a significant degree of hepatic parenchyma. Chemotherapy, which has marginal activity in HCC, should be reserved for the palliation of metastatic disease or treatment of inoperable tumors. Liver transplantation should be considered in patients with Child's B and C cirrhosis with early-stage primary tumors, an intervention that treats both the cirrhosis and the cancer. While awaiting transplantation, ethanol injection of a small HCC may lead to some local control of the tumor.

Answer 16.53. **The answer is D.**

There is no clearly proven adjuvant strategy after hepatic resection for HCC, although a recent meta-analysis indicated a potential survival benefit for postoperative intraarterial chemotherapy.

Answer 16.54. **The answer is F.**

Answer 16.55. **The answer is B.**

Stage III includes T3 (IIIA) and T4 (IIIB) tumors without lymph node involvement, and N1 lesions are stage IIIC.

Answer 16.56. **The answer is A.**

AFP is elevated in only 50% of patients in the United States and Europe and in 70% of Asian patients with newly diagnosed HCC. Triple phase helical CT scan is the current imaging standard for HCC. Only 25% of patients diagnosed with HCC have no symptoms at diagnosis, with common presenting symptoms including abdominal pain, abdominal swelling, weight loss, and anorexia.

Answer 16.57. **The answer is D.**

Answer 16.58. **The answer is D.**

Answer 16.59. **The answer is C.**

Patients with significant liver dysfunction, even with an early stage hepatocellular cancer, may not tolerate a large loss of hepatic parenchyma, and initial therapies (which may be required while awaiting availability of a liver transplant) should be geared to sparing hepatic parenchyma in anticipation of future transplantation. Surgical resection, not transplant, would be the optimal initial approach for a patient with normal liver function and an early stage hepatocellular cancer. Liver transplantation is the optimal therapy for patients with liver dysfunction and cirrhosis who have an early stage hepatocellular cancer. Vascular invasion portends an extremely poor prognosis and identifies a far less optimal patient for consideration for management with either surgery or liver transplantation.

Answer 16.60. **The answer is F.**

All of the above are options to treat an early stage hepatocellular cancer, depending on the clinical status of the patient and the availability of surgical expertise.

Answer 16.61. **The answer is B.**

There is no evidence from randomized trials that combination chemotherapy is superior to single-agent chemotherapy, with all agents having marginal activity of less than 25%. Tamoxifen has been evaluated in randomized trials in HCC and is an inactive agent.

Answer 16.62. **The answer is A.**

Although response rates to intraarterial chemotherapy appear to be higher than for systemic chemotherapy, a survival benefit has yet to be demonstrated for this treatment approach. Hepatic arterial embolization is an accepted regional therapy for HCC, but it is unclear whether or not adding chemotherapy to hepatic artery embolization (HAE) improves response rates or survival.

Answer 16.63. **The answer is E.**

Phase III trials of antiferritin antibodies have failed to demonstrate a survival benefit, and this agent is no longer in clinic use.

Answer 16.64. **The answer is D.**

Answer 16.65. **The answer is D.**

Answer 16.66. **The answer is E.**

Estrogen use has never been linked to the development of hepatocellular carcinoma, although benign adenomas may be associated with estrogen use.

Answer 16.67. **The answer is B.**

Despite the advent of hepatitis B vaccination programs, the incidence of hepatocellular carcinoma is increasing in the United States, and the increase is thought to be due to hepatitis C infection. Aflatoxin exposure in agricultural products is thought to account for a significant number of cases of hepatocellular cancer in China and Africa.

Answer 16.68. **The answer is D.**

Primary biliary cirrhosis is associated with an increased risk of cholangiocarcinoma.

Answer 16.69. **The answer is F.**

Although screening programs are in place in endemic areas of HCC and in high-risk populations, it is unclear whether or not screening identifies earlier stage patients or improves patient survival.

Answer 16.70. **The answer is E.**

The National Polyp Study has shown that in patients such as this with premalignant polyps, a screening interval for repeat colonoscopy of 3 years is as good as annual colonoscopy. Because of the cost, potential risk for colonic perforation, and need to optimize the use of scarce resources, a 3-year interval is recommended. Data from this group also indicate that optical colonoscopy is better than double contrast barium enema in detecting polyps, especially as this procedure also permits both diagnosis and removal. The use of CT colonography remains problematic because of the need for excellent radiology interpretation and limited availability of this test.

Data from several large randomized trials have shown no benefit to the use of fiber supplements in preventing or decreasing the incidence of premalignant polyps. COX-2 inhibitors have been shown to be of benefit in reducing the incidence of polyps. In patients with familial adenomatous polyposis (FAP), celecoxib led to a dramatic reduction in polyps and appeared to decrease new polyp formation, leading to its Food and Drug Administration (FDA) approval for that indication. Large screening trials in patients with premalignant polyps that do not have FAP are in progress. Several large randomized trials have shown that the incidence of polyps is decreased by aspirin use at a dose of either 325 or 650 mg daily. Aspirin is a nonspecific inhibitor of both COX-1 and COX-2. Calcium supplementation has been associated with a decrease in the incidence of polyps, but doses of at least 1,000 mg daily appear to be optimal.

Answer 16.71. **The answer is D.**

Approximately 10% of patients with colon cancer will have tumors that have a defect in the mechanism known as mismatch repair that results in correction of errors in the matching of the components of DNA that can occur during DNA replication. These tumors can result from an inherited defect known as hereditary nonpolyposis colon cancer (HNPCC) or, especially in older patients, from hypermethylation of the promoter regions that results in the silencing of the genes that control the mismatch repair machinery. HNPCC commonly affects younger patients, causes right-sided colon cancer, and exhibits a poorly differentiated histologic appearance under the microscope, so this patient seems likely to have HNPCC particularly since she has a first-degree relative, her sister, who also had the disease. Testing of germline DNA will confirm whether the defective mismatch repair is inherited or acquired. In this patient the findings indicate that it is hereditary. The syndrome of HNPCC is associated with other malignancies including duodenal cancer and cancers of the urothelium, uterus, biliary tract, and brain. Because of the very high incidence of these cancers, screening is recommended and the patient's siblings and children should be offered germline DNA testing for a mismatch repair defect with screening recommendations based upon these results after counseling. Follow-up for her colon cancer including screening for additional polyps, possible consideration for total colectomy, and screening for other HNPCC-associated malignancies should be a part of her future care.

Whether or not to recommend chemotherapy in this case is controversial. The patient has factors. the lymphatic and vascular invasion, that suggest that she may fit into a group with a higher recurrence risk. Ideally 12 to 14 lymph nodes should be examined in order to be confident that this is a stage II tumor. Asking the pathologist to search for additional lymph nodes is recommended in this case. Seven additional negative nodes were identified with careful repeat sectioning of the surgical specimen leading to a conclusive staging determination. In average risk patients with colon cancer, the 5-year overall survival is approximately 80% and adjuvant chemotherapy appears to confer a 2% to 4% overall survival benefit in multiple pooled analyses and in several clinical trials. None of these individual studies was adequately powered to show a survival advantage. Therefore, recommendations for treatment are still done on a case-by-case basis in stage II disease. There are two other relevant findings in the literature in patients with HNPCC. On a stage-by-stage basis, patients with HNPCC have a better prognosis than other colon cancer cases with identical stage. Also, there are data that 5FU based adjuvant chemotherapy may not be as beneficial in cases of HNPCC-associated colon cancer as in other cases. For these reasons, referral to a geneticist is the recommended intervention and adjuvant chemotherapy, while still a matter of personal patient/physician choice, seems unwarranted in this individual.

Answer 16.72. **The answer is D.**

This patient is potentially curable but at high risk of recurrence due to positive lymph nodes. With no further therapy, the likelihood of cure is approximately 35%, and a large meta-analysis shows that 6 months of adjuvant chemotherapy with 5FU/LV or FOLFOX will increase the cure rate respectively to 51% and 60%. There are no data to suggest that irinotecan-based regimens are of benefit in this setting, and data specifically show that IFL is more toxic and no more effective than 5FU/LV. Data comparing 5FU/LV to FOLFIRI are pending. There are currently no data in the adjuvant setting to indicate that bevacizumab or cetuximab add to adjuvant chemotherapy, although trials are underway to investigate this issue. There are negative studies indicating that interferon adds toxicity but no efficacy to 5FU/LV and that edrecolomab is not useful in this setting. The recommended therapy for this patient is FOLFOX based on the activity and toxicity profile of this regimen and this patient's high risk for recurrence.

Answer 16.73. **The answer is C.**

American Society of Clinical Oncology (ASCO) guidelines recommend colonoscopy every 3 years, CEA screening, and physical examination periodically after a diagnosis of colon cancer. If the CEA is elevated, screening for recurrence should be done with chest, abdominal, and pelvic CT scans as was done in this case. With an abnormality that is of an equivocal nature in this setting, a PET scan is recommended. Two things can be gained from the scan: a determination of whether the lesion is hypermetabolic and thus likely to be malignant, and identification of any extrahepatic disease. In this case the PET scan revealed increased uptake in the solitary lesion in the liver with no evident disease identified elsewhere. In this circumstance, referral to a surgeon experienced in hepatic resection is a good alternative as the liver disease appears to be indolent in that the lesion has not apparently changed much in 18 months. In addition, it is a single lesion and the CEA is only modestly elevated. Retrospective data would suggest this patient has a better than 30% likelihood of cure with resection. While a single randomized study suggests that intraarterial chemotherapy after resection may be of benefit in this setting, the acceptance of this therapeutic approach has been limited. It is also unclear if postoperative intravenous chemotherapy is of additional benefit in this circumstance.

Answer 16.74. **The answer is F.**

This patient has liver-limited disease that it is judged not to be amenable to surgical removal. Chemotherapy is therefore the primary modality and, should she have a good response, the potential for hepatic resection needs to be reconsidered during ongoing care. To discern the reason for the bilirubin elevation, the CT scan needs to be reviewed to be sure that there is no dilatation of the biliary tree indicating obstruction. Assuming on rereview that no dilation is seen, the bilirubin should be fractionated. In this case the indirect bilirubin is found to be elevated at 1.7 mg per dL. This indicates that the patient likely has Gilbert syndrome, which is characterized by an inherited polymorphism leading to decreased efficacy of the enzyme that catalyzes the conjugation of bilirubin known as glucuronidase. This is relevant because irinotecan is a prodrug that is transformed to an active metabolite, SN-38, which then is detoxified by glucuronidase. Toxicity with irinotecan is augmented in patients with Gilbert syndrome. The early death rate observed in the IFL arm of the NCCTG N9741 trial comparing FOLFOX to IFL to IROX and the CALGB adjuvant study comparing IFL to 5FU plus leucovorin may be linked in part to patients with decreased ability to detoxify SN-38, that is, those with Gilbert syndrome.

While data from the Tournigand trial of FOLFOX versus FOLFIRI suggests equivalent first-line outcomes among patients randomized to either regimen with comparable toxicity, FOLFOX would be a better choice in a patient with Gilbert syndrome. Another reason to consider using the FOLFOX regimen relates to the potential for future hepatic resection that is more commonly associated with oxaliplatin regimens in preliminary data. Whether or not to add bevacizumab in this case is uncertain at this time. The data from the 800 patient comparison of IFL to bevacizumab + IFL (B-IFL) indicates an advantage to B-IFL. When the FDA approved bevacizumab, it specifically permitted the drug to be given with any regimen containing intravenously administered 5FU. Since this patient is not an optimal candidate for irinotecan, the potential to use bevacizumab with either FOLFOX or 5FU plus leucovorin should be explored. At this time there are no phase III data on the efficacy of FOLFOX plus bevacizumab although the combination has been shown to be safe. There is data on over 100 patients that shows B-FL to be better than IFL from the Hurwitz trial. Based upon available data, one could choose FOLFOX or 5FU plus leucovorin with or without bevacizumab in this case.

Answer 16.75. **The answer is F.**

With best supportive care alone, this patient's estimated median survival is limited to approximately 6 months. With irinotecan alone, the median survival expectation approaches 10 months. Cetuximab alone or coupled with irinotecan has been tested mainly in irinotecan refractory patients. The response rate to cetuximab alone in irinotecan refractory patients is approximately 10%, while that with cetuximab plus irinotecan is 23%. However, the FDA has approved cetuximab only for use in irinotecan refractory patients whose tumors are shown by immunohistochemistry to overexpress the epidermal growth factor receptor (EGFR). No data currently exist that would support the addition of bevacizumab to chemotherapy in this setting nor would that strategy be consistent with the FDA approval of bevacizumab as it is indicated in combination with an intravenously administered, 5FU-based therapy in patients who have not been previously treated for metastatic disease. Additionally, a phase II trial of capecitabine after progression on IFL showed no responses in that treatment setting.

The best option for this patient is to either consider enrollment in a clinical trial or to use an irinotecan based therapy as standard therapy. It is not known whether patients are benefited more with single agent irinotecan or through adding 5FU plus leucovorin to the irinotecan as those two strategies have never been compared in this setting. However, in the Tournigand study, the response rate in patients treated with FOLFIRI after FOLFOX was a modest 4%, suggesting that single-agent therapy may be a reasonable alternative based on the comparative toxicities of single versus combination therapy. Testing of the tumor for EGFR overexpression would be useful for consideration of third-line therapy in the future.

Answer 16.76. **The answer is F.**

Appropriate clinical staging for rectal cancer is critical both for prognosis and management as it is the basis for the decision to offer neoadjuvant chemoradiation. While a complete blood count (CBC), liver, and renal function tests are routinely performed to assess organ function, these tests have poor sensitivity for metastatic disease. CXR and CT scan of the abdomen and pelvis are useful for detecting metastatic disease. Conventional CT, however, lacks sufficient accuracy for staging of the primary tumor site. In experienced hands, EUS has an overall accuracy of 75% to 95% for T-stage and 62% to 83% for N-stage. Understaging of nodal metastases is often due to the fact that involved nodes from rectal cancer are typically small and not easily detectable. Primary use of MRI or PET is not standard: they are typically used to clarify abnormalities. Endorectal MR offers similar performance to EUS but may not be routinely available.

Answer 16.77. **The answer is D.**

This patient has a low-lying rectal cancer (<6 cm from the anal verge). Issues that need to be addressed in conjunction with resection of the primary tumor include the risk of recurrence, the desire for sphincter preservation, and the toxicities of treatment.

With surgical therapy alone, the risk of local failure for patients with T3–4 and/or N+ disease is historically in the range of 25% to 50%. This risk is lower with the use of TME. In the Dutch trial of TME alone versus short course preoperative radiation followed by TME, the local failure rate after TME was 15% in N+ patients at 2 years. While it has been suggested that adjuvant radiation may not be required following an adequate TME, pelvic radiotherapy remains the standard for any T3 or greater rectal cancers. Defining the optimal strategy of radiotherapy (e.g., preoperative versus postoperative) has been an area of much investigation. From two large meta-analyses, the risk of local recurrence is reduced by approximately 50% with preoperative radiation and 40% with postoperative radiation. Postoperative radiation has not been shown to impact overall survival. A single Swedish study of short-course preoperative radiation compared to surgery alone showed a long-term survival advantage (58% vs 48% at 5 years); however, these results have not been reproduced. For the purposes of sphincter preservation, short-course preoperative radiation (25 Gy for 5 fractions) is not enough to yield sufficient downstaging. A preoperative or neoadjuvant chemoradiation approach has been shown to increase the chance for sphincter preservation for patients with low-lying tumors. Continuous infusion 5FU is the preferred regimen for concurrent administration. In addition, prolonged-course preoperative chemoradiation is recommended for locally advanced disease (T4 tumors with invasion into adjacent structures) to allow for a potentially curative resection.

In terms of toxicity, radiotherapy delivered preoperatively may be better tolerated as much of the irradiated bowel is subsequently removed at surgery and, in contrast to postoperative therapy, preoperative radiation circumvents the risk of radiation injury to a postsurgical perineum and to any normal bowel that has been relocated into the pelvis following resection. The early results of the recently completed randomized German Rectal Cancer Study of preoperative versus postoperative chemoradiation confirms advantages to a preoperative approach with improved local control, improved sphincter preservation, and less acute and long-term toxicity. The final results of this trial are awaited with interest. The preferred recommendation for this patient would be prolonged-course (50 Gy/25–28 fractions) preoperative radiotherapy with continuous-infusion 5FU followed by surgery and postoperative chemotherapy.

Answer 16.78. **The answer is A.**

Based upon his preoperative clinical staging, the risk of micrometastatic disease in this patient is estimated to be greater than 50%. Trials of adjuvant therapy for stage II and III rectal cancer have established the use of 5FU plus leucovorin for postoperative chemotherapy. For resected high-risk colon cancer, the FOLFOX regimen has demonstrated superior 3-year disease-free survival (MOSAIC trial), and capecitabine has demonstrated less toxicity and equivalent efficacy to 5FU plus leucovorin (X-act trial). However, data for these regimens in rectal cancer are lacking. Nonetheless, their use is gaining popularity. For this patient, preoperative therapy resulted in a good tumor response with downstaging to pT1N0. However, the risk of micrometastatic disease and, consequently, the plan for postoperative chemotherapy is determined by the pretreatment clinical staging. Based on available evidence, the appropriate recommendation is 5FU plus leucovorin.

Answer 16.79. **The answer is A.**

For T1 lesions with no evidence of nodal involvement, transanal excision provides adequate resection of the primary tumor. Staging should include endorectal ultrasound to accurately assess the T-stage. While local excision may be offered for selected T2 lesions (located within 8 to 10 cm of the anal verge, encompassing <40% of the bowel circumference, well or moderate differentiation, and no lymphovascular invasion on biopsy), this should be undertaken with caution as a review of the National Cancer Database suggests inferior outcomes for T2 lesions following local excision. Post-local excision adjuvant pelvic chemoradiation should be considered for T2 tumors and for T1 tumors with adverse prognostic features including lymphovascular invasion, poor differentiation, and close margins. This patient has a T1N0 tumor with no adverse features.

Answer 16.80. **The answer is A.**

As with squamous cancers of the lower female genital tract, sexually transmissible HPV, particularly subtype 16, is highly associated with squamous cell anal cancer and its precursor lesion, AIN. There is no definitive evidence that Herpes Simplex Virus (HSV) plays an etiologic role. Immunosuppression including iatrogenic and HIV exposure are associated with an increased risk of anal cancer. However, anal cancer is not presently an AIDS-defining neoplasm. The impact of human immunodeficiency virus (HIV) independent of sexual practices and behavior is unclear. Benign anal conditions such as fistulae, fissures, and hemorrhoids do not increase the risk for anal cancer.

Answer 16.81. **The answer is C.**

This patient has clinical T3N2 M0, stage IIIB disease. APR was previously considered the treatment of choice; however, three randomized trials (UKCCCR, EORTC, RTOG-ECOG) have established primary combined modality therapy, using radiation with 5FU and mitomycin as the standard of therapy for stage I, II, and III disease with 5-year colostomy-free survival rates of 60% (range 55% to 100%) and overall survival rates of 65% to 75% (range 45% to 80%). Compared to radiation alone, chemoradiation is associated with better locoregional control and colostomy-free survival. Control rates for inguinal and pelvic node metastases can also approach

80% with primary chemoradiation. APR and/or nodal dissection is reserved for surgical salvage of residual or recurrent disease after radiation-based treatment. It is important to recognize that residual masses after chemoradiation may take several weeks to months to regress fully. Suspected residual cancer should be confirmed by biopsy. Salvage surgery offers a 40% to 50% potential for long-term control and survival. The rate of distant metastases following chemoradiation is approximately 20%. There is no proven benefit to adjuvant chemotherapy following initial chemoradiation. Primary treatment with chemotherapy alone with cisplatin and 5FU is not a curative-intent option. This combination is used extensively for the treatment of metastatic squamous cell carcinoma of the anal canal. The appropriate recommendation for this patient is chemoradiation with 5FU and mitomycin.

Answer 16.82. **The answer is B.**

Mutations in the KIT protooncogene result in constitutive activation of the KIT receptor tyrosine kinase and are characteristic of the overwhelming majority of malignant GISTs. These activating mutations are most commonly identified in exon 11 (the intracellular juxtamembrane domain) of KIT and have also been described in exons 9, 17, and 18. Imatinib mesylate was initially identified as an inhibitor of the tyrosine kinase function of the BCR-ABL oncoprotein, implicated in the pathogenesis of chronic myeloid leukemia. It was also shown to be a potent inhibitor of the tyrosine kinase function of both KIT and platelet-derived growth factor receptor (PDGFR). In the US-Finland trial of advanced GIST, objective responses and/or disease control were observed in over 80% of patients with 400 or 600 mg of imatinib daily. No additional benefits were seen with the higher dose. In this trial, patients whose GIST harbored KIT mutations in exon 11 had higher rates of objective response when compared to patients whose disease had exon 9 KIT mutations.

The prognostic impact of KIT genotyping is unclear. Known adverse prognostic features for GIST are age, tumor size, and mitotic index—none of these factors are predictive of response. Functional PET imaging can be an early predictor of treatment response. Decreased uptake of 18FDG can be detected soon after the first dose of imatinib and is a reliable early predictor of beneficial response to therapy. Familial syndromes of GIST or in association with GIST, such as Carney's triad (GIST, pulmonary chondromas, and extraadrenal paraganglioma), or with neurofibromatosis Type 1 have been identified. It is unknown whether the response to imatinib therapy differs in this setting compared to sporadic GIST.

CHAPTER **17**

Genitourinary Cancer

WALTER M. STADLER

Directions Each of the numbered items below is followed by lettered answers. Select the ONE lettered answer that is BEST in each case unless instructed otherwise.

QUESTIONS

Questions 17.1–17.6.

A 63-year-old white male smoker presents to his physician with a 2-month history of urinary frequency, urgency, and dysuria without hesitancy or decreased stream. He denies hematuria, fever, chills, or abdominal pain. He has normal erections and is sexually active. Past medical history is significant for hypertension, well controlled on a beta blocker and diuretic, hypercholesterolemia controlled on an 3-hydroxy-3-methylglutaryl coenzyme A (HMG coA) reductase inhibitor, and diet-controlled type 2 diabetes. General physical exam is significant for some scattered expiratory wheezes, normal cardiac exam, and normal abdominal exam. Rectal exam reveals a mildly enlarged prostate that is nontender.

Question 17.1. **The appropriate initial workup should include which of the following?**

A. Urinalysis.
B. Urine culture.
C. Contrast-enhanced computed tomography (CT) scan of the abdomen and pelvis.
D. A and B.
E. All of the above.

Corresponding Chapters in *Cancer: Principles & Practice of Oncology*, Seventh Edition: 30 (Cancers of the Genitourinary System).

Question 17.2. **Urine dipstick reveals no protein or ketones, but there is 1+ blood. Microscopic analysis reveals 10 to 15 red blood cells (RBCs), 2 to 3 white blood cells (WBCs), 0 to 1 squamous epithelial cells, and no bacterial cells per high power field. Urine culture is negative. Prostate specific antigen (PSA) is 2.5, complete blood count (CBC) is unremarkable, and general chemistries reveal normal electrolytes, normal liver function tests, and a creatinine of 1.2 mg per dL. The next appropriate diagnostic step is**

A. intravenous pyelogram (IVP)
B. contrast-enhanced CT scan of the abdomen and pelvis
C. abdominal ultrasound
D. cystoscopy

Question 17.3. **Flexible cystoscopy in the urology office reveals a papillary tumor in the dome of the bladder approximately 3 cm in size, as well as diffuse erythema of the remainder of the bladder wall. The patient is subsequently taken to the operating room where an exam under general anesthesia reveals a mobile bladder. Resection of the papillary lesion reveals grade III papillary carcinoma, and multiple biopsies of the erythematous areas of the bladder all reveal diffuse carcinoma *in situ*. Muscle is present in the pathologic specimens and there is no evidence for invasive tumor. The appropriate therapy is**

A. intravesicle Bacillus Calmette–Guérin (BCG) vaccine
B. intravesicle cyclosphosphamide
C. radiation
D. cystectomy

Question 17.4. **The patient is treated with intravesicle BCG weekly for 6 weeks, as well as with a follow-up maintenance program; however, 4 months after initiating the maintenance BCG program, the urologist notes multiple recurrent papillary lesions. Repeat biopsy reveals transitional cell cancer invasive into muscle. CT scan of the chest, abdomen, and pelvis is unremarkable. Appropriate therapy at this point is**

A. reinduction with intravesicle BCG
B. intravesicle chemotherapy with mitomycin-C
C. partial cystectomy
D. radical cystectomy

Question 17.5. **After consultation with an oncologist regarding the risks and benefits of neoadjuvant chemotherapy, the patient elects to proceed with a cystectomy and orthotopic neobladder. Pathologic specimen reveals a diffuse carcinoma *in situ* with an invasive tumor at the dome. The tumor invades into but not through the muscular layer, and evaluation of 15 lymph nodes shows no metastatic cancer. After additional discussion with the oncologist, the patient decides not to have adjuvant chemotherapy and opts only for routine follow-up. By 6 months, he has only mild stress incontinence, is impotent, feels well, but routine serum chemistries reveal a creatinine of 4.1 mg per dL. The most likely diagnosis is**

A. acute glomerulonephritis
B. calcium oxalate stone nephropathy
C. obstructive nephropathy
D. renal tubular acidosis

Question 17.6. **The patient is found to have obstruction at the urethral anastomosis, which is surgically corrected, but the creatinine remains abnormal at 2.5 mg per dL. Six months later, a routine follow-up non-contrast enhanced CT scan reveals two 3-cm lung nodules. Biopsy of one is consistent with metastatic transitional cell cancer. Appropriate therapy at this time includes**

A. surgical resection of all visible metastatic disease
B. palliative care
C. cisplatin-based multiagent chemotherapy
D. interferon-based immunotherapy

Question 17.7. **A 63-year-old uncircumcised man without any significant past medical history presents to his physician with an inability to retract the foreskin. Examination reveals phimosis, with an underlying painless ulcerated mass 1 × 2 cm in size. A 2.5-cm hard node is palpated in the left inguinal region. Biopsy of the penile lesion reveals squamous cell cancer. In addition to wide surgical resection of the primary lesion, other appropriate therapeutic and/or diagnostic maneuvers at this time include**

A. a 4-week course of a broad-spectrum antibiotic
B. left inguinal lymph node dissection
C. bilateral lymphangiography
D. bilateral inguinal radiotherapy
E. taxane-based chemotherapy

Questions 17.8–17.12.

A 71-year-old white gentleman with a history of hypertension, hyperlipidemia, coronary artery disease, and prior angioplasty with stent placement, but no prior myocardial infarction, is noted to have a rise in his PSA from 3.0 to 4.1 ng per mL over 1 year. He is a semiretired accountant, swims actively 3 times per week, and helps care for his mildly demented 95-year-old father. General physical exam is unremarkable; a rectal exam reveals a mildly enlarged prostate gland without any palpable nodules.

Question 17.8. **The most correct statement about this case is**

A. biopsy should be discussed because the PSA rise is greater than 0.75 ng/mL/yr
B. biopsy should not be discussed because PSA is normal for his age
C. biopsy should not be discussed because his expected survival makes treatment not worthwhile, even if prostate cancer is discovered
D. biopsy should be discussed because the PSA is greater than 4 ng per mL
E. the free to total PSA ratio will determine the need for biopsy

Question 17.9. **Biopsy reveals Gleason 8 prostate cancer in 6/6 cores. CT scan of the abdomen and pelvis and bone scan are unremarkable. The most appropriate therapy is**

A. radical retropubic prostatectomy
B. 3-D conformal radiotherapy with concomitant androgen ablation
C. interstitial radiotherapy with ^{125}I
D. all of the above

Question 17.10. **After discussion with a radiation oncologist and a urologist, the patient elects to undergo combined androgen ablation and external beam radiation therapy. The androgen ablation is administered prior to the radiation therapy and continued for 3 months thereafter. Radiotherapy is complicated only by a mild diarrhea that resolves once the radiation therapy is complete. The PSA nadirs at 1.2 ng per mL; however, 9 months after his last dose of the luteinizing hormone-releasing hormone (LH-RH) agonist, the PSA rises to 2.4 ng per mL and then to 3.6 ng per mL 1 month later. The most appropriate next therapeutic and/or diagnostic maneuver is**

A. an MRI of the pelvis to assess for local recurrence
B. reinitiate androgen ablation
C. refer the patient to a urologist for salvage prostatectomy
D. initiate a docetaxel-based chemotherapy

Question 17.11. **The patient elects to undergo androgen ablation with an LH-RH agonist along with the antiandrogen Casodex. PSA declines to 0.8 ng per mL, but after 10 months, the PSA begins to slowly rise to a value of 3.7. He continues to feel well, has minimal urinary symptoms, no bone pain, and no weight loss. The most appropriate therapy at this point is**

A. docetaxel-based chemotherapy
B. discontinuing the antiandrogen Casodex
C. hospice care
D. radionuclide therapy with strontium-98 (Metastron)

Question 17.12. **The patient does not have a PSA response to antiandrogen withdrawal and in fact develops bone pain and documented bone metastases on bone scan. Appetite, weight, functional status, and organ function as assessed by routine chemistries remain normal. In addition to initiating docetaxel-based chemotherapy, other therapeutic maneuvers to be considered include**

A. megestrol acetate
B. local radiotherapy
C. opiate pain control
D. bisphosphonates
E. B, C, and D
F. all of the above

Questions 17.13–17.14.

A 51-year-old black male executive with no prior medical history undergoes a routine PSA screening evaluation and is found to have a PSA of 5.5 ng per mL. Biopsy reveals a Gleason 3 + 3 prostate cancer in 2/6 biopsy cores. After discussion with a radiation oncologist and urologist, he elects to receive treatment with a radical retropubic prostatectomy. Surgical pathology confirms a Gleason score 6 tumor in both lobes of the prostate. There is focal capsular penetration in the right posterolateral region, but surgical margins are negative. There is no evidence of seminal vesicle or lymph node invasion. His postoperative PSA is undetectable. No additional therapy is administered and the patient does well until 3 years postsurgery when the PSA rises to 0.1 ng per mL. Continued observation reveals a persistent elevated PSA, but no value greater than 0.3 ng per mL within the next 12 months. His urinary function is normal. He is impotent but not concerned about his lack of sexual activity, and he has developed mild hypertension in the interim.

Question 17.13. **The appropriate next step is**

A. repeat surgical exploration with possible reexcision of the prostatic bed
B. CT scan
C. watchful waiting
D. local radiotherapy
E. C and D

Question 17.14. **The patient responds to salvage radiotherapy with an undetectable PSA nadir, but 8 years later, now at the age of 63, recurrent biochemical disease is noted. After appropriate discussion, androgen ablation with an LH-RH agonist alone is initiated, and the PSA once again becomes undetectable. The patient maintains an undetectable PSA while on androgen ablation for 3 years when he develops sudden midback pain after lifting his grandson. There are no associated neurologic signs or symptoms. Bone scan shows marked uptake at the T8 vertebra, and PSA remains undetectable. The most appropriate therapeutic or diagnostic maneuver is**

A. immediate radiotherapy to T8
B. therapy with ketoconazole, 400 mg 3 times daily with hydrocortisone replacement
C. spinal MRI to rule out cord compression
D. bone densitometry to assess for osteoporosis
E. docetaxel-based chemotherapy

Questions 17.15–17.17.

A 56-year-old moderately obese woman with a past medical history of chronic hypertension well controlled on a thiazide diuretic comes to the Emergency Department with a 1-day history of abdominal pain, diarrhea, nausea, and fever. General physical exam is significant only for some mild abdominal tenderness; negative stool guaiac; a white blood cell (WBC) count of 14.2 per μL; hemoglobin of 14.5 d per dL; a normal platelet count; normal electrolytes, amylase, lipase, and transaminases; and a creatinine of 0.9 mg per dL. Workup includes an abdominal CT scan, which was remarkable only for a 3.5-cm left renal mass in the left lower pole that is enhancing and interpreted by the radiologist as a "probable renal cell carcinoma." The patient's abdominal symptoms resolve without sequelae.

Question 17.15. **The appropriate next step(s) is/are**

A. CT scan of the chest
B. open radical nephrectomy
C. open partial nephrectomy
D. laparoscopic nephrectomy
E. all of the above

Question 17.16. **The patient undergoes a laparoscopic nephrectomy; there are no postoperative complications, and she is back to work 3 weeks later. Postoperative creatinine is 1.3 and pathology reveals a 4.5-cm renal cell carcinoma, granular cell type with invasion into the renal vein, but confined to the renal parenchyma. No lymph nodes were recovered. The next appropriate step is**

A. open retroperitoneal lymph node dissection
B. high-dose interleukin-2 (IL-2)
C. adjuvant local radiotherapy
D. submission of pathology specimen for second review

Question 17.17. **Review of the pathologic specimen by an experienced genitourinary pathologist reveals clear cell carcinoma of the kidney, Fuhrman grade III. Invasion into the renal vein is confirmed. The patient does well for 8 years, at which time she develops a pathologic intratrochanteric fracture of her left hip. CT scanning of the chest, abdomen, pelvis, and brain and bone scan reveal no other sites of disease. The most appropriate next step is**

A. radiation alone
B. high-dose IL-2 alone
C. orthopedic resection of the tumor with reconstruction followed by radiation
D. multiagent cytotoxic chemotherapy
E. hospice care

ANSWERS

Answer 17.1. **The answer is D.**

The differential diagnosis for dysuria, frequency, and urgency include cystitis, prostatitis, and obstructive uropathy, most commonly due to benign prostatic hyperplasia in men. Notably, significant dysuria without hesitancy or decreased stream is unusual with obstruction due to benign prostatic hyperplasia. It is also notable that prostate cancer, although occasionally presenting with local urinary obstructive symptoms, rarely presents with this constellation of findings unless there is obvious extensive local disease on rectal exam. This is due to the fact that prostate cancer more typically arises in the peripheral zone of the prostate, and thus causes obstructive symptoms only when the tumor is more locally advanced. The appropriate workup thus includes urinalysis and urine culture to assess for infection; the assessment of renal function and PSA is also appropriate.

Answer 17.2. **The answer is D.**

Dysuria, hematuria, and a lack of demonstrable lower urinary tract infection raise the possibility of a bladder cancer. The sensitivity of CT scan, ultrasound, and IVP are all extremely low for the detection of bladder cancer. Cystoscopic evaluation is indicated.

Answer 17.3. **The answer is A.**

Indications for intravesicle therapy are multiple recurrent Ta lesions, especially if they are high grade, or carcinoma *in situ*. It is critical that the pathologic specimen in patients diagnosed with superficial bladder cancer contains muscle in order to determine whether there is an invasive component. Most, but not all, studies have suggested that intravesicle BCG is more effective than intravesicle chemotherapy. Although other chemotherapy agents are being investigated, cyclophosphamide needs to be activated to 4-hydroxy-cyclosphosphamide in the liver in order to act as an alkylating agent, and thus bladder instillation of the parent compound is not expected to be effective. Radiation and/or cystectomy, although potentially useful for invasive carcinoma and/or refractory bladder cancer, are not appropriate as initial therapy.

Answer 17.4. **The answer is D.**

Patients with muscle-invasive bladder cancer require definitive local therapy. Additional intravesicle therapy is inappropriate. Partial cystectomies are only rarely indicated and should be performed in only a very highly select group of patients, which does not include patients with a history of carcinoma *in situ* or patients with multiple tumors. The standard definitive therapy for bladder cancer is cystectomy. Combined chemotherapy and radiation therapy is reasonable but does lead to the need for salvage cystectomy in approximately 20% to 30% of patients and is accompanied by a relatively high risk of recurrent superficial disease. Recent data suggest that neoadjuvant chemotherapy for patients with invasive bladder cancer has a modest effect on survival.

Answer 17.5. **The answer is C.**

Complications of orthotopic neobladders include metabolic acidosis, renal calculi, and obstructive nephropathy, and, of these, only obstruction commonly causes renal failure. Acute glomerulonephritis is not a recognized complication in the absence of other underlying medical history. Obstructive nephropathy can occur at the level of ureteral implantation or at the urethral sphincter anastomosis.

Answer 17.6. **The answer is B.**

Metastatic urothelial cancer, even when only a limited number of metastatic deposits are visible on radiologic scanning, is almost always widely disseminated, and surgical resection alone has little role. Cisplatin-based multiagent chemotherapy is appropriate in patients with good performance status and normal organ function. The combination of methotrexate, vinblastin, doxorubicin (adriamycin), and cisplatin (MVAC) has been shown to improve survival over other multiagent and single-agent chemotherapies, and gemcitabine/cisplatin has been shown to have similar outcomes to MVAC. However, less than 5% of patients have long-term survival with multiagent chemotherapy, and cisplatin is inappropriate for patients with abnormal renal function. Taxanes, which can be administered in patients with renal failure, do have anticancer activity in this disease, but whether they provide any long-term benefit in patients such as this is unclear. Immunotherapy, although effective in superficial bladder cancer when applied intravesically, is not effective in patients with systemic disease. Palliative care is thus the most appropriate option.

Answer 17.7. **The answer is A.**

Penile carcinoma is a rare malignancy that presents most commonly with phimosis in an uncircumcised patient. Metastatic spread of penile carcinoma is via superficial inguinal lymphatics, followed by deep inguinal lymphatics, and then to the pelvic lymphatics. Systemic metastatic disease almost never develops in the absence of pelvic lymphadenopathy. Therefore, surgery and occasionally radiotherapy form a cornerstone of treatment of lymph node positive patients. Importantly, however, half of the patients with clinically palpable nodes will have inflammatory lesions only. Thus, a course of antibiotics prior to any further therapy is indicated.

If the nodes persist after a course of antibiotics, biopsy and surgical dissection are indicated. Management of clinical N0 patients is more controversial, with some authors recommending immediate lymph node dissection and others recommending a watchful waiting approach. Pathologic risk factors as assessed in the primary lesion may assist in decision making. Lymphangiography prior to a course of antibiotics is generally not considered helpful.

Answer 17.8. **The answer is A.**

The decision to screen for and diagnose prostate cancer always needs to be a discussion between the physician and the patient regarding risks and benefits of screening. To this end it should be recognized that the median survival of an average 70-year-old man without significant comorbidities is over 10 years, and, thus, he could benefit from treatment of localized disease. Nonetheless, there is a risk of treating disease that will never become clinically significant within the patient's lifetime. It also needs to be recalled that the sensitivity and specificity of all PSA-based screening methods are limited, and there are no absolute "normal" criteria. Therefore no single test can determine the absolute need for a biopsy. Predictors of cancer on biopsy include PSA greater than 4.0 ng per mL, PSA greater than age-adjusted PSA norms (based on normal increasing PSA with age), free-to-total PSA ratio, and PSA velocity. Of these, and in this case, the rapid rise in the PSA is most predictive and is also predictive of aggressive disease.

Answer 17.9. **The answer is D.**

Based on the high Gleason score, the aforementioned rapid PSA doubling time, and tumor in all cores, this patient is at a high risk for locally advanced disease and systemic recurrence. As such, staging CT scan and bone scan are reasonable, although not generally necessary in patients with lower risk disease. Because of the high-risk nature of the disease and the general good health of the patient, watchful waiting is probably not an appropriate option. Radiotherapy, with external beam radiotherapy or interstitial brachytherapy, or surgical prostatectomy is equally appropriate for patients with clinically localized disease. The choice is dependent on a discussion of expected risks and benefits.

Answer 17.10. **The answer is B.**

Patients with rapidly rising PSA prior to diagnosis, a high Gleason score, a PSA nadir of greater than 1.0 following radiotherapy, a short interval between definitive local therapy and biochemical recurrence, and rapid PSA rise once recurrence is identified have a poor prognosis. Clinical probability of locally recurrent disease alone is extremely low, and there is not much value to pelvic MRI for assessing local recurrence. Despite the poor prognosis, the role of chemotherapy in patients whose testosterone axis is intact is controversial. Although timing of androgen ablation is controversial, some retrospective data suggests that "early" ablation in high-risk patients such as this provides a long-term survival advantage over "later" ablation.

Answer 17.11. **The answer is B.**

Approximately 10% to 15% of patients on treatment with an antiandrogen will experience an antiandrogen withdrawal response. Although the majority of these responses are of brief duration, it is obviously the easiest therapeutic maneuver. Although docetaxel-based chemotherapy leads to improved survival in hormone refractory prostate cancer, the "hormone refractory" state is generally defined as a progressive disease following androgen ablation, an antiandrogen, and antiandrogen withdrawal. Radioactive nuclides are occasionally useful for treatment of diffuse bone pain but by themselves have not been shown to have an impact on survival.

Answer 17.12. **The answer is E.**

Docetaxel-based chemotherapy is appropriate and has been shown to improve survival of patients with hormone-refractory prostate cancer. Nevertheless, local radiotherapy to painful bony lesions remains an important component of palliative care, as does the use of opiate and nonopiate pain medication. Megestrol acetate can occasionally cause a "flair" response and should not be used to prevent cachexia. Randomized phase III data suggest that the use of bisphosphonates in hormone refractory prostate metastatic cancer decreases the incidence of bone complications, including the need for radiotherapy, and fractures.

Answer 17.13. **The answer is E.**

Following radical retropubic prostatectomy, prognostic factors for recurrent disease include the diagnostic PSA value, Gleason score, the presence of capsular invasion, margin positivity, and the presence of lymph or seminal vesicle invasion. Additional molecular markers are being developed. A number of nomograms are available for predicting recurrence risks. For this patient, following prostatectomy, the expected risk of biochemical recurrence within 5 years and based on the pathologic variables is approximately 10%. For patients in whom cancer recurs, one major question is whether the recurrence is local only or whether the patient has additional microscopic systemic disease. For patients with local only recurrence, additional radiotherapy may be effective. CT scans have not been useful for assessing the presence of systemic disease because their sensitivity is limited. Some studies suggest that a ProstaScint exam may have a good specificity and be helpful in this scenario. Most useful are, however, the clinical parameters. Predictors for good response and outcome in patients treated for recurrent biochemical disease following prostatectomy include PSA of less than 1.0 at time of treatment, Gleason score less than 8 on initial diagnosis, absence of lymph node or seminal vesicle invasion at surgery, interval of greater than 12 months between surgery and recurrent disease, and PSA doubling time of greater than 10 to 12 months. The patient meets all of these criteria and is thus a good candidate for salvage radiotherapy. Toxicities of salvage radiotherapy are the same as a primary radiotherapy for prostate cancer with perhaps a somewhat higher incidence of urinary and sexual symptoms. Thus, whether to proceed with salvage radiotherapy or simply watchful waiting is based on the patient's perception of the risks and benefits. Androgen ablation for recurrent biochemical disease is not unreasonable in this patient, but long-term benefit is unclear, especially in light of systemic toxicity and the long expected interval from biochemical recurrence to bone scan positivity and/or death.

Answer 17.14. **The answer is D.**

Patients on long-term androgen ablation are at high risk for development of osteoporosis and its complications, and an osteoporotic fracture must be considered in this patient prior to initiating any therapy for progressive metastatic disease. If progressive disease were to be diagnosed, ketoconazole is not an unreasonable second-line hormonal therapy, but, in this patient, addition of an antiandrogen would likely be more appropriate. Chemotherapy would generally require failure of both androgen ablation as well as an antiandrogen. In the absence of neurologic signs or symptoms, an MRI is not necessary.

Answer 17.15. **The answer is E.**

Although flank pain, and/or hematuria, and/or an abdominal mass have traditionally been considered the presenting symptoms for renal cancer, one of the most common manners in which this disease is currently diagnosed is during a CT scan performed for an unrelated reason. Contrast-enhanced CT scan has a high specificity for renal cancer, and biopsy prior to definitive surgical removal is usually not necessary. Assessment for the presence of metastatic disease with a chest CT is reasonable. Traditionally, open radical nephrectomy has been the operation of choice for an abnormal enhancing lesion. However, most urologists are beginning to prefer laparoscopic and partial nephrectomies, the latter of which has the advantage of preserving maximal renal function.

Answer 17.16. **The answer is D.**

Renal cell cancer is currently divided into clear cell and non-clear cell subtypes. The non-clear cell subtypes have been further divided into papillary, chromophobe, and collecting duct tumors. A number of renal cancers cannot be accurately subtyped, often due to poor histologic differentiation such that the originating subtype cannot be easily recognized. Such tumors are often classified as "sarcomatoid." Granular cell carcinoma has been used in the past but is not currently an accepted pathologic classification, and thus a second opinion and pathologic review should be requested. The presence of renal vein invasion is an adverse prognostic feature, but if this is the only adverse prognostic feature, the recurrence risk is only 20% to 30%. High dose IL-2 has not been shown to be effective adjuvant therapy. Patients who do recur following radical nephrectomy almost always recur systemically and thus additional local radiotherapy is not indicated. Likewise, the role of extensive lymph node dissection is highly controversial and generally not recommended. In any case, formal retroperitoneal lymph node dissection as is carried out in testes cancer would certainly not be standard in patients with localized renal cell carcinoma.

Answer 17.17. **The answer is C.**

Patients with renal cancer can develop recurrent disease more than 5 years after initial definitive therapy. Development of a single metastatic site is not unusual. Patients with a single site of metastatic disease and a long interval between initial diagnosis and recurrent metastatic disease typically have a good prognosis. Thus, aggressive surgical resection including orthopedic stabilization is indicated. Because orthopedic surgery such as this often leaves microscopic tumors behind in the surgical field, additional radiotherapy to the site is appropriate. Radiation alone, however, is insufficient to completely eradicate metastatic renal cancer and does not repair the underlying structural bony abnormality. Cytotoxic chemotherapy is not standard for metastatic renal cancer. High-dose IL-2 is approved for metastatic renal cancer but is less effective than aggressive local surgery for complete eradication of disease when possible. Because patients with a single site of metastatic renal cancer have a 5-year survival of approximately 30%, hospice is not appropriate.

CHAPTER **18**

Cancer of the Testis

DANIEL MORGENSZTERN AND BENJAMIN R. TAN

Directions Each of the numbered items below is followed by lettered answers. Select the ONE lettered answer that is BEST in each case unless instructed otherwise.

QUESTIONS

Question 18.1. **A 26-year-old man presented with cough and a left testicular mass. Workup revealed multiple retroperitoneal lymph nodes and several lung nodules. Serum (β-HCG) human chorionic gonadotropin was 80 mIU per mL and alpha-fetoprotein (AFP) was normal. Pathologic diagnosis was pure seminoma. What is the best treatment?**

A. Two cycles of bleomycin, etoposide, and cisplatin (BEP).
B. Three cycles of BEP.
C. Four cycles of BEP.
D. Three cycles of etoposide and cisplatin (EP).

Question 18.2. **A 22-year-old man presents with an enlarging testicular mass. A computed tomography (CT) scan of the abdomen and pelvis reveals no enlarged lymph nodes and a horseshoe kidney. Chest x-ray and serum lactate dehydrogenase (LDH), AFP, and β-HCG are normal. An orchiectomy is performed and the pathology shows pure seminoma. What subsequent therapy should be recommended?**

A. Observation.
B. Radiation therapy.
C. Adjuvant chemotherapy with 2 cycles of BEP.
D. Retroperitoneal lymph node dissection.
E. Retroperitoneal lymph node dissection followed by 2 cycles of BEP.

Question 18.3. **A 25-year-old man presented with a painless enlargement of the right testicle, and visual symptoms including blurred vision and photophobia. CT of the abdomen showed no enlarged lymph nodes but chest x-ray revealed bilateral hilar lymphadenopathy. Serum markers were normal and orchiectomy led to the diagnosis of pure seminoma. Biopsy of the hilar lymph nodes is likely to be consistent with**

A. metastases from the seminoma
B. lymphoma
C. tuberculosis
D. sarcoidosis
E. histoplasmosis

Corresponding Chapters in *Cancer: Principles & Practice of Oncology*, Seventh Edition: 31 (Cancer of the Testis).

Question 18.4. **A 29-year-old man presented with nonseminomatous germ cell tumor involving the retroperitoneal lymph nodes and lungs. Serum markers were elevated with AFP of 1,000 ng per mL and β-HCG of 500 mIU per mL. Serum markers normalized after the third cycle of chemotherapy with BEP, and most of the enlarged retroperitoneal lymph nodes and all lung lesions had disappeared. One of the retroperitoneal lymph nodes, however, continued to grow and began to cause severe discomfort. What is the most likely diagnosis?**

A. Refractory disease.
B. Lymphoma.
C. Teratoma.
D. Infection.
E. Lymph node necrosis.

Question 18.5. **What would be your treatment recommendation for the patient in Question 18.4?**

A. Observation.
B. Surgery.
C. Radiation therapy.
D. Continue chemotherapy with 2 additional cycles of BEP.
E. Change chemotherapy to vindesine-ifosfamide-platinum (VIP).

Question 18.6. **A 25-year-old man with good risk stage III seminoma was treated with 3 cycles of BEP. At the end of the therapy, there was a solitary 3.5-cm residual retroperitoneal mass. What is the best next step in the management of his disease?**

A. Observation.
B. Positron emission tomography (PET) scan.
C. Retroperitoneal lymph node dissection.
D. Two additional cycles of BEP.
E. Change chemotherapy to VIP.

Question 18.7. **Which of the following is a risk factor for the development of germ cell tumors?**

A. Exposure to diethylstilbestrol.
B. Vasectomy.
C. Intratubular germ cell neoplasia (carcinoma *in situ*).
D. Mumps.
E. Trauma.

Question 18.8. **A 32-year-old man presented with a testicular mass and a 6- X 4-cm retroperitoneal mass. Orchiectomy revealed pure seminoma. Serum markers are within normal limits. What is the next therapeutic intervention?**

A. Observation.
B. Radiation therapy.
C. Retroperitoneal lymph node dissection.
D. Two cycles of BEP.
E. Three cycles of BEP.

Question 18.9. **What is the expected 5-year overall survival for a patient with nonseminomatous germ cell tumor metatastatic to the brain?**

A. 85%.
B. 65%.
C. 45%.
D. 25%.
E. 10%.

Question 18.10. **Which metastatic site from patients with germ cell tumors is associated with the best overall survival?**

A. Bone.
B. Brain.
C. Liver.
D. Lung.

Question 18.11. **What is the most frequent primary testicular neoplasm in men over the age of 50?**

A. Seminoma.
B. Nonseminomatous germ cell tumor.
C. Lymphoma.
D. Sertoli cell tumor.
E. Leydig cell tumor.

Question 18.12. **Which chromosomal marker is present in virtually all patients with germ cell tumors?**

A. 47, XXY karyotype.
B. t(11;22).
C. t(8;21).
D. i(12p).
E. t(8;14).

Question 18.13. **A 28-year-old man presents with a painless testicular mass and dyspnea. CT scan of the abdomen and pelvis showed multiple retroperitoneal lymph nodes and liver metastases. CT of the chest showed several lung nodules. Serum AFP is 16,000 ng per mL and β-HCG is 200 mIU per mL. At the beginning of the third cycle of BEP, dyspnea has resolved and serum markers are as follows: AFP 200 ng per mL, β-HCG undetectable. What is the next step in the management?**

A. Continue current therapy for a total of 4 cycles.
B. Change chemotherapy to VIP.
C. Repeat CT of the chest and abdomen for restaging.
D. PET scan.
E. Autologous stem cell transplant.

Question 18.14. **A 22-year-old man presented with diffuse testicular pain. Symptoms did not improve with a trial of antibiotic therapy, and a testicular ultrasound showed a discrete hypoechoic intratesticular mass. Serum markers including AFP, β-HCG, and LDH are within normal limits. What is the next diagnostic step?**

A. Fine-needle aspiration.
B. Transscrotal biopsy.
C. Scrotal orchiectomy.
D. Radical inguinal orchiectomy.

Question 18.15. **A 25-year-old man presented with a testicular mass and two small ipsilateral retroperitoneal lymph nodes. Orchiectomy revealed nonseminomatous germ cell tumor (NSGCT) and serum markers were normal. Retroperitoneal lymph node dissection showed metastatic disease in four lymph nodes measuring 1.2 to 1.8 cm in greatest dimension. Patient was very compliant to previous appointments. What is the best subsequent management?**

A. Observation.
B. Radiation therapy.
C. Two cycles of BEP.
D. Three cycles of EP.
E. Three cycles of BEP.

Question 18.16. **A 32-year-old man presented with pancytopenia and immature white blood cells in the peripheral blood smear. Bone marrow studies led to the diagnosis of acute myeloid leukemia. He has a history of testicular seminoma treated 3 years ago with 4 cycles of BEP. What is the most likely chromosomal abnormality expected in this patient?**

A. 47, XXY.
B. t(9;22).
C. t(11;14).
D. Translocation involving 11q23.
E. 13q deletion.

Question 18.17. **What is the most likely diagnosis in a 10-year-old boy with virilization and a testicular mass?**

A. Seminoma.
B. Embryonal carcinoma.
C. Yolk sac tumor.
D. Leydig cell tumor.
E. Lymphoma.

Question 18.18. **A 22-year-old man presented with nonseminomatous germ cell tumor metastatic to retroperitoneal lymph nodes and lung. AFP was 8,000 ng per mL and β-HCG was 5 mIU per mL. What is the best treatment?**

A. Two cycles of BEP.
B. Three cycles of BEP.
C. Four cycles of BEP.
D. Three cycles of EP.
E. Four cycles of EP.

Question 18.19. **What is the treatment of choice for a 32-year-old man with seminoma and metastases to two retroperitoneal lymph nodes measuring 3.5 cm and 5.5 cm in greatest dimension?**

A. Radiation therapy.
B. Retroperitoneal lymph node dissection.
C. Retroperitoneal lymph node dissection followed by 2 cycles of BEP.
D. Two cycles of BEP.
E. Three cycles of BEP.

Question 18.20. **Which of the following patients has a poor-prognosis germ cell tumor?**

A. A 55-year-old man with seminoma, lung metastases, and a β-HCG of 120 mIU per mL.
B. A 22-year-old man with seminoma, lung and brain metastases, and a β-HCG of 300 mIU per mL.
C. A 25-year-old man with nonseminoma, lung metastases, and an AFP of 15,000 ng per mL.
D. A 33-year-old man with nonseminoma, lung metastases, an AFP of 8000 ng per mL, and a β-HCG of 4000 mIU per mL.
E. Both B and C.

Question 18.21. **A 25-year-old man with poor-prognosis nonseminoma and increased AFP is treated with 4 cycles of BEP. At the end of the therapy, AFP is normalized but there are 5 residual lesions in the lung measuring between 2.0 and 4.2 cm in greatest dimension. What is the best appropriate therapy?**

A. Observation.
B. Radiation therapy.
C. Surgery.
D. Two additional cycles of BEP.
E. Change chemotherapy to VIP.

Question 18.22. **What is the best therapy for a 32-year-old patient with nonseminomatous germ cell tumor of the mediastinum and multiple lung nodules who had incomplete response to BEP?**

A. Chemotherapy with vinblastin, ifosfamide, and etoposide.
B. Chemotherapy with etoposide, ifosfamide, and etoposide.
C. Chemotherapy with taxol, ifosfamide, and etoposide.
D. Radiation therapy.
E. High-dose chemotherapy followed by autologous peripheral stem cell transplant.

Question 18.23. **What is the percentage of viable tumor in residual retroperitoneal masses after salvage chemotherapy in germ cell tumors?**

A. 90%.
B. 70%.
C. 50%.
D. 30%.
E. 15%.

Question 18.24. **A 28-year-old man presented with a painless testicular mass, bulky retroperitoneal adenopathy, and an AFP of 700 ng per mL. Orchiectomy was performed and showed a nonseminomatous germ cell tumor. Patient was subsequently treated with 3 cycles of BEP. At the completion of therapy, AFP was normalized but a residual mass persisted in the retroperitoneum. Pathologic specimen from retroperitoneal lymph node dissection revealed immature teratoma. What is the best therapeutic approach?**

A. Observation.
B. Radiation therapy.
C. Two cycles of BEP.
D. Three cycles of BEP.
E. Four cycles of BEP.

Question 18.25. **What would be the management if the above patient had more than 10% viable tumor in the specimen?**

A. Observation.
B. Radiation therapy.
C. Two cycles of BEP.
D. Three cycles of BEP.
E. Two cycles of EP.

Question 18.26. **High-dose chemotherapy in preparation for stem cell transplant in germ cell tumors utilizes the following agents EXCEPT**

A. carboplatin
B. cisplatin
C. etoposide
D. ifosfamide
E. cyclophosphamide

Question 18.27. **What is the dose-limiting toxicity of bleomycin?**

A. Myelosuppression.
B. Mucositis.
C. Arthritis.
D. Pulmonary fibrosis.
E. Skin toxicity.

Question 18.28. **Which surgical finding characterizes a pathologic stage T3 testicular germ cell tumor?**

A. Invasion of the spermatic cord.
B. Invasion of the tunica albuginea.
C. Involvement of the tunica vaginalis.
D. Lymphovascular invasion.
E. Involvement of the scrotum.

Question 18.29. **In patients with good-prognosis germ cell tumors, which of the following statements is true?**

A. Four cycles of BEP is superior to 3 cycles of BEP.
B. Three cycles of BEP is equivalent to 3 cycles of EP.
C. Three cycles of BEP is equivalent to 4 cycles of EP.
D. Four cycles of EP is equivalent to 4 cycles of EC (etoposide and cyclophosphamide).
E. Four cycles of BEP is superior to 4 cycles of EP.

Question 18.30. **Which of the following immunohistochemical markers is present in the majority of patients with seminoma?**

A. Blood group antigen A.
B. Low–molecular weight keratins.
C. Placental alkaline phosphatase (PLAP).
D. Vimentin.
E. CD30.

ANSWERS

Answer 18.1. **The answer is B.**

According to the International Germ Cell Consensus Classification, this patient has good-risk seminoma due to the absence of nonpulmonary visceral metastases. Standard therapy includes either 3 cycles of BEP or 4 cycles of EP. In a randomized study, 3 cycles of BEP has been shown to be equivalent to 4 cycles of therapy for patients with good prognosis. Treatment with 2 cycles of BEP or 3 cycles of EP is suboptimal.

Answer 18.2. **The answer is A.**

Although radiation therapy remains the treatment of choice for patients with clinical stage I seminoma, it is contraindicated in patients with horseshoe kidney due to the high likelihood of radiation-induced renal failure. Retroperitoneal lymph node dissection is usually not indicated for seminomas, and 2 cycles of BEP are probably not necessary in this population with a very high probability of cure.

Answer 18.3. **The answer is D.**

Sarcoidosis appears to be more frequent in patients with seminoma. The presence of bilateral hilar and paratracheal adenopathy without involvement of retroperitoneal lymph nodes in patients with seminoma should suggest the possibility of sarcoidosis. Visual symptoms in this case are attributed to uveitis. Of course, every attempt should be made to obtain tissue diagnosis.

Answer 18.4. **The answer is C.**

The presence of a growing mass despite disappearance of most lesions and normalization of serum markers during or after therapy for nonseminomatous germ cell tumors constitutes the growing teratoma syndrome. Lymphoma, infection, and lymph node necrosis are unlikely causes for the growing mass in this patient. Refractory disease is less likely in the presence of normalized serum markers and complete resolution of most lesions.

Answer 18.5. **The answer is B.**

Growing teratomas are usually refractory to chemotherapy and radiation therapy but can be cured with surgery alone. Observation is not a reasonable option for this patient with a symptomatic enlarging mass.

Answer 18.6. **The answer is B.**

Observation is a valid option for tumors smaller than 3 cm. Retroperitoneal lymph node dissection following chemotherapy is usually difficult due to the severe desmoplastic reaction and obliteration of tissue planes. A recent study has shown that PET is useful in the detection of residual viable seminoma in patients with masses larger than 3 cm in diameter after chemotherapy. In patients with NSGCT, PET has not been consistently able to identify residual viable malignant GCT and/or teratoma.

Answer 18.7. **The answer is C.**

Carcinoma *in situ* (CIS) precedes invasive testicular cancer in virtually all cases of germ cell tumors. The median time to progression from CIS to invasive carcinoma is 5 years. Epidemiologic studies have failed to identify an association between testicular germ cell tumors and diethylstilbestrol, vasectomy, trauma, or mumps.

Answer 18.8. **The answer is E.**

This patient has a bulky retroperitoneal lymph node (N3) and should be treated as good-prognosis germ cell tumors with 3 cycles of BEP. Relapse rates are high with observation or radiation therapy alone, retroperitoneal lymph node dissection is not indicated in this case, and 2 cycles of BEP are probably insufficient.

Answer 18.9. **The answer is C.**

The expected 5-year overall survival for patients with poor-prognosis nonseminomatous germ cell tumors is approximately 45%.

Answer 18.10. **The answer is D.**

The presence of any nonpulmonary visceral metastasis is associated with worsened prognosis. Whereas seminomas with nonpulmonary visceral metastases are classified as intermediate risk, nonseminomas are classified as high risk.

Answer 18.11. **The answer is C.**

Germ cell tumors are most common between the ages of 25 and 40. Sertoli and Leydig cell tumors are rare tumors. Therefore, the development of a painless testicular mass in patients over the age of 50, particularly if associated with systemic B symptoms such as fever and weight loss, is likely to be caused by a non-Hodgkin lymphoma.

Answer 18.12. **The answer is D.**

Klinefelter syndrome, characterized by the 47, XXY karyotype, is associated with increased incidence of mediastinal germ cell tumors. Answers B, C, and E are associated with Ewing sarcoma, acute myeloid leukemia, and Burkitt lymphoma respectively. Virtually all germ cell tumors have increased copies of 12p. The fact that even testicular carcinomas *in situ* have this chromosomal abnormality suggests that it may be one of the earliest genetic changes associated with these tumors.

Answer 18.13. **The answer is A.**

This patient has poor-prognosis nonseminoma and should be treated with 4 cycles of BEP. The serum half-life of AFP is 5 to 7 days, and after 6 weeks of therapy, serum levels are expected to be between 62 and 250 ng per mL. Due to the shorter serum half-life of β-HCG, levels are expected to be within the normal range after 2 cycles of therapy. In the absence of clinically refractory or progressive disease, imaging studies should be performed at the completion of the therapy. There are no indications in this case for changing chemotherapy or performing autologous stem cell transplant.

Answer 18.14. **The answer is D.**

Radical inguinal orchiectomy minimizes local tumor recurrence and aberrant lymphatic spread, representing the only acceptable diagnostic and therapeutic procedure. Answers A, B, and C are associated with scrotal violation and are, therefore, contraindicated.

Answer 18.15. **The answer is A.**

This patient has pathologic stage IIa (any pT, pN1, M0) NSGCT. Treatment of choice in compliant patients is surveillance. This approach is associated with a 20% risk of relapse. Indications for chemotherapy with 2 cycles of BEP include lack of compliance, geographic location, and psychological factors.

Answer 18.16. **The answer is D.**

This patient likely developed secondary leukemia due to etoposide. The characteristic chromosomal abnormality is located at the 11q23. The 47, XXY genotype is characteristic of Klinefelter syndrome, which is associated with mediastinal germ cell tumors. The translocation t(9;22) is more commonly associated with chronic myeloid leukemia or acute lymphoblastic leukemia and rarely seen in acute myeloid leukemia, whereas the translocation t(11;14) is associated with acute lymphoblastic leukemia and mantle cell lymphoma. The 13q deletion represents the most common genetic aberration in patients with chronic lymphocytic leukemia (CLL).

Answer 18.17. **The answer is D.**

Leydig cell carcinoma represents approximately 2% of the testicular tumors. Although most commonly seen in adults, approximately 25% occur in children, where it may be associated with pubic hair and enlarged genitalia. Virilization is not a common feature of classic germ cell tumors or lymphoma.

Answer 18.18. **The answer is C.**

This patient has intermediate risk nonseminoma due to the absence of nonpulmonary metastases and increased levels of AFP between 1,000 and 10,000 ng per mL. The treatment of choice is 4 cycles of BEP.

Answer 18.19. **The answer is E.**

The presence of a retroperitoneal lymph node larger than 5 cm in greatest dimension places the patient at stage IIIc (any T, N3, M0). These patients should be treated with standard therapy for good-prognosis stage III seminoma, which includes 3 cycles of BEP or 4 cycles of EP. Radiation therapy is associated with increased relapse rate, and 2 cycles of BEP would be appropriate in cases with nonbulky stage II. Retroperitoneal lymph node dissection is not indicated in this patient with advanced stage seminoma.

Answer 18.20. **The answer is C.**

Patients are diagnosed as having poor-prognosis germ cell tumors if they have nonseminoma with nonpulmonary visceral metastases, mediastinal primary site, an AFP greater than or equal to 10,000 ng per mL, a β-HCG greater than or equal to 50,000 mIU per mL, or LDH greater than or equal to 10 times the upper limit of normal.

Answer 18.21. **The answer is C.**

The treatment of choice for patients with nonseminoma with resectable residual masses at the end of the therapy and normalization of serum markers is surgical removal of all residual masses. Radiation therapy and observation are not indicated. The requirements for additional therapy will be guided by the pathologic surgical findings.

Answer 18.22. **The answer is E.**

This patient has two unfavorable prognostic features for poor response to additional conventional chemotherapy including extratesticular primary site and incomplete response. In this subset of cisplatin-refractory patients, the 3-year survival is less than 10% with conventional cisplatin-based chemotherapy. The best alternative appears to be the use of high-dose chemotherapy followed by peripheral stem cell transplant. With this approach, 30% to 57% of the patients are expected to achieve complete remission and 15% to 48% will be cured.

Answer 18.23. **The answer is C.**

Unlike residual masses after primary chemotherapy for germ cell tumors where the percentage of viable tumor after resection is 10% to 15%, approximately 50% of residual masses after salvage chemotherapy contain viable tumor.

Answer 18.24. **The answer is A.**

Due to the low risk of relapse in patients with fibrosis, necrosis, or teratoma, further therapy is not necessary after complete resection of the lesion.

Answer 18.25. **The answer is E.**

The prognosis for patients with viable tumor in the resected specimen is very poor in the absence of additional chemotherapy. Due to the cumulative toxicity of bleomycin, the additional chemotherapy may include 2 cycles of EP; vinblastine, ifosfamide, and cisplatin (VeIP); or taxol, ifosfamide, and cisplatin (TIP).

Answer 18.26. **The answer is B.**

Most preparative regimens for autologous stem cell transplant in germ cell tumors include a combination of carboplatin, etoposide, and either cyclophosphamide or ifosfamide. Although cisplatin is the backbone of conventional chemotherapy for germ cell tumors, this agent is not used in high-dose therapy due to its toxicity profile including cumulative peripheral neuropathy, ototoxicity, and nephropathy.

Answer 18.27. **The answer is D.**

Skin toxicities including hyperpigmentation and hyperkeratosis occur commonly in patients treated with bleomycin. Acute arthritis and mucositis are also frequently seen. Myelosuppression is not a prominent side effect. Pulmonary fibrosis, however, occurs in 10% of the patients and is the dose-limiting toxicity of bleomycin. It occurs more commonly in patients treated with more than 400 units and in those with a history of chest radiotherapy.

Answer 18.28. **The answer is A.**

Invasion of the tunica albuginea and vaginalis constitute pT1 and pT2 respectively, whereas involvement of the scrotum characterizes pT4. Vascular invasion may be present in pT2 to pT4. Pathologic stage T3 occurs in the presence of spermatic cord invasion, with or without lymphovascular invasion.

Answer 18.29. **The answer is C.**

Three cycles of BEP and 4 cycles of EP are equivalent and represent the standard of care for patients with good-prognosis germ cell tumors. Four cycles of BEP have not shown advantage over 3 cycles of BEP and, although they produced better complete response rates than 4 cycles of

EP, they did not translate into a significant improvement in survival. Three cycles of EP are inferior to 3 cycles of BEP. The use of cyclophosphamide instead of cisplatin resulted in similar complete response rates but inferior survival.

Answer 18.30. **The answer is C.**

Seminomatous tumors are almost always positive for PLAP by immunohistochemistry. Markers of somatic differentiation such as blood group antigens, low-molecular-weight keratins, and vimentin are typically absent in seminoma. The CD30 antigen, which is characteristic of Hodgkin disease and anaplastic large cell lymphoma, may also be expressed in embryonal carcinoma.

CHAPTER **19**

Gynecologic Cancers

GINI F. FLEMING AND DAVID G. MUTCH

Directions Each of the numbered items below is followed by lettered answers. Select the ONE lettered answer that is BEST in each case unless instructed otherwise.

QUESTIONS

Question 19.1. **A 35-year-old premenopausal woman of Ashkenazi Jewish ancestry presents to you because her 60-year-old paternal aunt was recently diagnosed with ovarian cancer, and she is concerned about her own risk for ovarian cancer. She has no siblings and there is no other family history of cancer. She has two living children, is in good health, and her pelvic exam is unremarkable. You should advise her that**

A. ovarian cancer cannot be inherited through the paternal side, and she does not need any particular screening
B. a single second-degree relative with cancer at age over 50 does not confer a significantly increased risk for her
C. she should visit a genetic counselor
D. annual transvaginal ultrasound and CA-125 screening can reduce her risk of mortality
E. she should have a prophylactic total abdominal hysterectomy/bilateral salpingo-oopherectomy (TAH/BSO) if/when she does not wish to have any more children

Question 19.2. **A 35-year-old woman presents to you for recommendations regarding therapy of her newly diagnosed mucinous ovarian cancer. This was a 5-cm, grade 1, left-sided mass that was incidentally found at the time of surgery for endometriosis as part of an infertility workup. The ovary was removed, and the operative note states that there was no evidence of tumor on the external surface of the ovary or elsewhere in the abdomen, but full surgical staging was not performed. A postoperative computed tomographic (CT) scan of the abdomen and pelvis is unremarkable and CA-125 is within normal limits. Pelvic exam is unremarkable.**

Corresponding Chapters in *Cancer: Principles & Practice of Oncology*, Seventh Edition: 32 (Gynecologic Cancers).

The patient would like to have children but does not want to compromise her survival. You should advise her that

A. she is unlikely to have any residual cancer or a recurrence, and further surgery or chemotherapy is not needed
B. she should have a positron emission tomographic (PET) scan, and if there is no uptake, she does not need further surgery or chemotherapy
C. since her CT and CA-125 are normal, she is unlikely to have any residual disease, and further surgery is not needed; however, because the mucinous subtype of ovarian cancer has a very poor prognosis, she will require 3 to 6 cycles of carboplatin/paclitaxel chemotherapy
D. she should have complete surgical staging, if possible, via laparoscopy, with the option of preserving her uterus and contralateral ovary if no further evidence of tumor is found; if no further tumor is found, she would have a greater than 90% chance of 5-year survival, and chemotherapy would not be required
E. she should have complete surgical staging, including TAH/BSO; if no further disease is found, she will need only 3 cycles of carboplatin/paclitaxel chemotherapy, but if there is disease outside the ovary, she will need 6 cycles

Question 19.3. **A 55-year-old woman who has just achieved a complete clinical remission (normal CT scan, pelvic exam, and CA-125) after 6 cycles of chemotherapy for stage IIIC optimally debulked serous ovarian cancer presents to you for a second opinion regarding her prognosis and treatment options at this point. She is in excellent general health and tolerated chemotherapy well except for some numbness in her fingers and toes, which caused her treating oncologist to switch her from paclitaxel/carboplatin to docetaxel/carboplatin after cycle 3. You should advise her that**

A. the risk of eventual relapse for an optimally debulked patient with a complete clinical remission is about 30%; no therapy is proven to be of any further survival benefit at this point
B. she should have second-look surgery; if residual disease is found, she should have 4 to 6 cycles of intraperitoneal platinum-based therapy as this can improve survival in patients with platinum-sensitive, minimal residual disease
C. she should have a PET scan; if residual disease is found, she should have 4 to 6 cycles of a noncross resistant drug, such as topotecan
D. her risk of eventual relapse is about 70%; she should be offered consolidation therapy with paclitaxel 175 mg per m^2 every 3 weeks for 12 months with the expectation of a 30% improvement in survival
E. her risk of relapse is about 70%; no therapy is proven to be of any survival benefit at this point

Question 19.4. **Which of the following statements is true about low malignant potential (borderline) tumors of the ovary?**

A. They occur more often in younger women.
B. They are usually stage III/IV.
C. Survival of patients with stage I disease is excellent, but they tend to relapse late, particularly if the tumor is large.
D. Survival of patients with stage III/IV disease is poor, and they should receive chemotherapy.
E. They are always of serous histology.

Question 19.5. **Which of the following statement(s) is/are true about granulosa cell tumors of the ovary?**

A. They usually occur in premenopausal women.
B. They are usually stage III/IV.
C. Survival of patients with stage I disease is generally good, but they may relapse late.
D. Survival of patients with stage III/IV disease is poor, and they should consider chemotherapy.
E. They may be associated with endometrial cancer.
F. C, D, and E.

Question 19.6. **Which of the following statements is true about germ cell tumors of the ovary?**

A. They occur more often in younger women.
B. They are usually stage III/IV.
C. Appropriate therapy includes TAH/BSO/full surgical staging and chemotherapy regimens similar to those used in male testicular cancer.
D. Survival of patients with stage III/IV disease is poor.
E. The chemotherapy will usually result in infertility.

Question 19.7. **A 51-year-old woman presents to you for recommendations regarding the treatment of her recurrent ovarian cancer. She was optimally debulked for stage IIIC serous ovarian carcinoma and completed 6 cycles of carboplatin/paclitaxel 36 months ago with a clinical complete remission. She now has recurrent ascites, which is histologically positive for tumor compatible with her original primary. CT scan shows peritoneal carcinomatosis and a pelvic mass. You should advise her that**

A. prognosis of recurrent ovarian cancer is poor; she may get short-term benefit from chemotherapy, but hospice is a reasonable option
B. tamoxifen has a 40% chance of shrinking her disease
C. she has a very high likelihood of disease shrinkage and symptom palliation with further platinum-based chemotherapy
D. she has a chance of cure with autologous stem cell transplant
E. liver metastases and liver failure will probably be her ultimate cause of death

Question 19.8. **Cervical cancer is the leading cause of death in many medically underserved countries. There is a relationship between human papillomavirus (HPV) and preinvasive and invasive cancer such that**

A. 95% of cervical cancers are associated with HPV
B. 80% of cervical cancers are associated with HPV
C. 50% of cervical cancers are associated with HPV
D. 25% of cervical cancers are associated with HPV

Question 19.9. **When HPV is associated with cervical cancer it is thought that**

A. p53 is inactivated by E7
B. p53 is inactivated by E6
C. E2 inactivates transcription of E6 and E7
D. the E6 proteins of high-risk types of HPV have a greater affinity for p53 than other E6 proteins

Question 19.10. **More than 100 subtypes of HPV have been isolated. Some HPV subtypes show a significant predilection for geographic regions such that**

A. HPV-45 is found in Western Africa
B. HPV-59 is found in the United States
C. HPV-70 is found in Eastern Europe
D. HPV-16 is found in South America

Question 19.11. **HPV infection is necessary for cervical cancer to develop. It is probably not sufficient to cause cancer without other factors to encourage persistent infection. These include all of the following EXCEPT**

A. smoking
B. DNA integration
C. oral contraceptives
D. multiple sexual partners

Question 19.12. **International incidences of cervical cancer tend to reflect cultural differences that are reflected in all of the following EXCEPT**

A. attitudes toward sexual promiscuity
B. penetration of mass screening programs
C. incidence of smoking
D. cultural differences within society

Question 19.13. **The incidence of adenocarcinoma is increasing (29% from 1973 to 1996) despite a significant decrease in the incidence of squamous cell carcinoma (42%) during the same period. This may reflect all of the following EXCEPT**

A. increased recognition of cases with glandular elements
B. decreased effectiveness of cytologic screening in detecting premalignant conditions of adenocarcinomas more than squamous lesions
C. a decrease in "other categories of cervical malignancy"
D. a change in the type of HPV-causing adenocarcinoma

Question 19.14. **All of the following statements are true of cervical cancer EXCEPT**

A. in 1993 the Centers for Disease Control added cervical cancer to the list of acquired immunodeficiency syndrome (AIDS) defining neoplasms
B. data strongly suggests that human immunodeficiency virus (HIV)-related immunosuppression is correlated with an increased risk of cervical HPV infection
C. HIV infection seems to correlate with a higher prevalence and infection rate of high-risk HPV types
D. HIV infection appears to be associated with a faster rate of progression to high grade cervical intraepithelial neoplasia (CIN)

Question 19.15. **An 18-year-old intravenous (IV) drug abuser is seen in your office. She complains of frequent apparent viral infections and decreased energy. You test her for HIV and it returns positive. You inform her. Your recommendations for her gynecologic care include all of the following EXCEPT**

A. condom use if she chooses to be sexually active
B. pelvic examination with Pap smear
C. routine colposcopic evaluation of the cervix
D. colposcopic evaluation of the cervix if the Pap smear is abnormal

Question 19.16. **Dysplasia is said to progress to cancer when**

A. lymph node metastases are observed
B. lung metastases are observed
C. local spread is observed
D. the basement membrane is breached

Question 19.17. **Despite large tumor size, fewer than 5% of invasive cervical cancers have**

A. bladder involvement
B. vaginal involvement
C. pelvic sidewall involvement
D. paraaortic nodal involvement

Questions 19.18–19.19.

A 23-year-old woman is seen for a routine Pap smear. She has a normal physical examination and leaves the office. Two weeks later the she is notified that her Pap smear returned showing atypical cells of undetermined significance.

Question 19.18. **The most appropriate next step is to**

A. perform HPV typing
B. perform colposcopy
C. repeat the Pap smear in 4 months
D. none of the above

Question 19.19. **The patient returns for colposcopic evaluation and is found to have a low-grade intraepithelial lesion on biopsy. There is no endocervical involvement. The recommendation would be**

A. judicious observation
B. frequent colposcopy and biopsy
C. loop electrosurgical excision procedure (LEEP)
D. cold knife cone biopsy

Question 19.20. **The most common cytologic abnormality diagnosed in United States cytologic laboratories is**

A. low grade squamous intraepithelial lesion (SIL)
B. high grade SIL
C. normal
D. atypical squamous cells of undermined significance (ASCUS)

Question 19.21. **Cone biopsy margins are unreliable for adenocarcinoma *in situ* because**

A. the lesion is often multifocal
B. a high fraction of adenocarcinomas are associated with squamous carcinoma *in situ*
C. glandular cells often penetrate deeply into the cervical stroma
D. adenocarcinoma *in situ* is often associated with invasive cancer

Question 19.22. **Treatment of microinvasive carcinoma of the cervix includes all of the following EXCEPT**

A. cold knife cone biopsy
B. simple hysterectomy
C. radical hysterectomy with nodes
D. observation

Question 19.23. **Verrucous carcinoma of the cervix is often confused with**

A. small cell carcinoma
B. condyloma
C. papillary carcinoma
D. sarcomatoid variant of carcinoma

Question 19.24. **All of the following make cervical cancer an ideal candidate for general screening EXCEPT**

A. long preinvasive component
B. relatively high prevalence in the unscreened population
C. high specificity of the cytologic test
D. high sensitivity of the cytologic screening test

Question 19.25. **All of the following are screening recommendations developed by the American Cancer Society (ACS) in 2001 EXCEPT**

A. screening should begin 3 years after first intercourse
B. Pap smears can be done every 2 years with liquid-based Pap cytology
C. Pap smear screening can stop after age 70
D. after age 30, if the patient has had normal smears for 3 years, the screening interval can increase

Question 19.26. **The rate of false-negative Pap smears in patients with high grade CIN is**

A. less than 5%
B. 5% to 10%
C. 10% to 15%
D. 20% to 30%

Question 19.27. **Once an abnormal Pap smear is reported, which of the following is the next step in the evaluation of the abnormality?**

A. Repeat Pap smear immediately; if normal, then repeat every 3 months. Once normal for 3 consecutive times, regular screening intervals may be re-instituted.
B. Refer for immediate colposcopy.
C. Repeat Pap smear and test for high-risk HPV.
D. Perform cervical biopsies with repeat Pap smear.

Question 19.28. **Which of the following features is indicative of invasive cancer on colposcopy?**

A. Mosaic pattern.
B. Atypical vessels.
C. Punctation.
D. White epithelium.

Question 19.29. **Indications for excisional procedures (cold knife cone or LEEP cone) include all of the following EXCEPT**

A. Pap smear demonstrates high-grade lesion but biopsy shows only mild dysplasia
B. Pap smear demonstrates invasive cancer
C. biopsy shows invasive cancer with an identified lesion on Pap
D. adequate colposcopy demonstrates CIN 3

Question 19.30. **A 32-year-old woman presents with vaginal bleeding and lower back pain. You perform a general examination and then a pelvic examination. You see an exophytic lesion which you biopsy, and bimanual with rectal vaginal examination reveals a lesion in the parametrium. Your colleague examines the patient and feels that the lesion extends to the pelvic sidewall. You both agree that the lesion does not extend down to the vagina. According to conventional staging, the patient has what stage of disease?**

A. Stage IIA.
B. Stage IIB.
C. Stage IIIA.
D. Stage IIIB.

Question 19.31. **The most widely accepted staging system is defined by which organization?**

A. FIGO (International Federation of Gynecology and Obstetrics).
B. SGO (Society of Gynecologic Oncology).
C. ACS (American Cancer Society).
D. TNM (Tumor size, Nodal metastasis, Metastasis).

Question 19.32. **In the United States, the most accepted definition of microinvasive carcinoma of the cervix is**

A. FIGOs
B. SGOs
C. ACSs
D. TNMs

Question 19.33. **Surgical staging is a procedure adopted by some physicians to improve treatment by identifying patients with lymph node involvement. Which of the following carries the highest published complication rate when combined with radiation therapy?**

A. Transabdominal.
B. Extraperitoneal.
C. Laparoscopic.
D. Postradiation therapy nodal evaluation.

Question 19.34. **All of the following are associated with poorer prognosis EXCEPT**

A. lymphovascular space involvement
B. deep stromal invasion
C. uterine body involvement
D. a strong inflammatory response to tumor invasion

Question 19.35. **Lymph node metastases are prognostic of survival. If a patient with a IB carcinoma of the cervix has positive lymph nodes, this patient's survival is reduced by**

A. 10%
B. 25%
C. 50%
D. 70%

Question 19.36. **All of the following are acceptable management plans for a patient with stage IA1 cancer of the cervix EXCEPT**

A. radical hysterectomy
B. cold knife conization
C. simple hysterectomy
D. radiation therapy

Question 19.37. **A 45-year-old woman was diagnosed 2 years ago with a IB carcinoma of the cervix. This was treated with a radical hysterectomy and pelvic and para-aortic lymph node dissection. All nodes were negative and the margins were free. There was some lymphovascular space involvement, but with no positive nodes and free margins no further therapy was recommended. The patient presented to your office for routine follow-up. You notice a nodule at the vaginal apex and biopsy it. It returns showing recurrent squamous cell cancer. Which of the following treatments would you recommend?**

A. Pelvic exenteration.
B. Radical excision.
C. Radiation therapy.
D. Radiation therapy with concurrent chemotherapy.

Question 19.38. **Patients with noninvasive lesions can be treated with ablative therapy if invasion has been completely ruled out. Which of the following treatments is generally preferred at this time?**

A. Cryotherapy double freeze technique.
B. Laser vaporization.
C. Loop diathermy excision.
D. Cold knife conization.

Question 19.39. **For patients with IA2 lesions, the risk of lymph node metastases is approximately**

A. 1% to 2%
B. 5%
C. 10%
D. 15%

Question 19.40. **The chances of adjuvant radiation therapy in the case of a large IB tumor where the patient undergoes radiation therapy first is**

A. 10%
B. 20%
C. 50%
D. 80%

Question 19.41. **A 50-year-old woman presents with a 6-cm cervical lesion. Metastatic workup is negative. The most appropriate therapy for this patient is**

A. radiation therapy with weekly cisplatin chemotherapy
B. radiation therapy followed by completion hysterectomy
C. simple hysterectomy followed by radiation therapy
D. radiation therapy alone

Question 19.42. **The standard surgical treatment for stage IB cervical cancer is**

A. type I radical hysterectomy
B. type II radical hysterectomy
C. type III radical hysterectomy
D. type IV radical hysterectomy

Question 19.43. **The most common complication from radical hysterectomy is**

A. pulmonary embolism
B. ureterovaginal fistula
C. small bowel obstruction
D. bladder dysfunction

Question 19.44. **Eligibility criteria for inclusion in the Gynecologic Oncology Group (GOG) trial of intermediate risk factors included all of the following EXCEPT**

A. positive pelvic nodes
B. lymph vascular space involvement
C. tumor diameter of greater than 4 cm
D. greater than one-third stromal invasion

Question 19.45. **Radiation therapy alone can achieve cure rates of what percent in patients with IB carcinoma of the cervix?**

A. 67%.
B. 75%.
C. 82%.
D. 90%.

Question 19.46. **Brachytherapy is a critical element in the treatment of patients with cervical cancer and allows delivery of large radiation doses to the cervix and surrounding tissues. The dose typically delivered to point A, a point 2 cm lateral to and 2 cm above the cervical os, using this technique is**

A. 50 to 60 Gy
B. 70 to 75 Gy
C. 80 to 85 Gy
D. 90 to 95 Gy

Question 19.47. **The cure rates for patients with large volume IIIB disease treated with radiation is reported to be**

A. 10% to 15%
B. 35% to 50%
C. 50% to 65%
D. greater than 75%

Question 19.48. **A complication of low-energy radiation (4 to 6 MeV photons) that is NOT as common with high-energy radiation (15 to 18 MeV) is**

A. superficial tissue damage
B. bowel injury
C. bladder injury
D. microvascular damage

Question 19.49. **What percentage of patients with gross paraaortic disease exhibit a long-term survival with proper radiation therapy?**

A. 10% to 15%.
B. 15% to 20%.
C. 25% to 30%.
D. 35% to 40%.

Question 19.50. **Fletcher described three features that must be met for successful cervical brachytherapy. These include all of the following EXCEPT**

A. the geometry of the radioactive sources must prevent underdosed regions on and around the cervix
B. an adequate dose must be delivered to the paracervical areas
C. tolerable doses to the paravaginal areas should not be exceeded
D. mucosal tolerance should be respected

Question 19.51. **Ideal placement of the uterine tandem and vaginal ovoids produces a distribution shaped like**

A. a box
B. a sphere
C. a pear
D. an ellipse

Question 19.52. **Brachytherapy's low dose rate is useful because it does all of the following EXCEPT**

A. permits repair of sublethal cellular injury
B. preferentially spares normal tissues
C. optimizes the therapeutic ratio
D. decreases the damage to normal tissue

Question 19.53. **Recently, technology has made it possible for brachytherapy to be delivered at higher dose rates. One of the isotopes used to deliver the higher rate is**

A. ^{32}P
B. ^{60}Co
C. ^{137}Cs
D. ^{131}I

Question 19.54. **Most long-term complications from radiation therapy occur in the first**

A. year
B. 3 years
C. 5 years
D. 10 years

Question 19.55. **The treatment of choice for central recurrence in a patient treated with prior radiation therapy is**

A. additional radiation therapy
B. chemotherapy
C. pelvic exenteration
D. radical hysterectomy

Question 19.56. **Conization in the first trimester of pregnancy is associated with an abortion rate of**

A. 10%
B. 25%
C. 50%
D. 75%

ANSWERS

Answer 19.1. **The answer is C.**

This woman should be referred for genetic counseling and possible genetic testing. Forty percent to 60% of epithelial ovarian cancer patients of Jewish descent carry one of three founder BRCA-1 or BRCA-2 mutations (irrespective of family history). These, like other BRCA mutations, are inherited in an autosomal dominant manner, through either the paternal or maternal side. If this woman carries a BRCA-1 mutation, her lifetime risk of ovarian cancer is 20% to 60%, and her risk of breast cancer is even higher. While transvaginal ultrasound and CA-125 screening are generally recommended for mutation carriers who have their ovaries in place, there is no good evidence that such screening will decrease mortality. Oral contraceptives have been suggested to decrease the risk of ovarian cancer by up to 50%. Removal of the ovaries likely confers the best method for reducing the risk of ovarian cancer; it remains controversial whether the uterus should be removed as well.

Answer 19.2. **The answer is D.**

Understaging is common, particularly when the preoperative diagnosis is that of a benign process. Earlier laparoscopic surgical staging series suggested that up to 30% to 40% of patients thought to have FIGO stage I or II disease actually had disease in the upper abdomen. The incidence of extraovarian spread will be lower with a grade 1 tumor. Nonetheless, complete surgical staging, if possible, is advised in this case, since the recommendation for a stage IA grade 1 mucinous tumor is no chemotherapy. While there have been some data to suggest that advanced stage mucinous tumors may respond less well to chemotherapy than serous tumors, a low-grade early stage mucinous tumor does not have a poor prognosis. However, chemotherapy would be recommended in the case of any extraovarian spread. In the hands of an experienced surgeon, laparoscopic staging, including omentectomy and paraaortic lymph node examination, is an option. Preservation of the uterus and contralateral ovary is reasonable if no further disease is found at the time of staging. CA-125 is frequently normal in women with mucinous ovarian tumors, even when of advanced stage. A PET scan will not detect microscopic disease, may not be positive in low-grade malignancies, and is not likely to be helpful.

Answer 19.3. **The answer is E.**

While the majority (almost 80%) of patients with advanced stage (III–IV) ovarian cancer will achieve a clinically complete remission with taxane/platinum combination therapy, about 70% will ultimately relapse from a clinical complete remission. Even patients with a surgically confirmed complete remission (negative second look) have an eventual relapse rate of about 50%. Although patients with optimally debulked stage III disease are a relatively favorable subgroup, those optimally debulked patients who have a larger presurgical tumor burden (IIIC) fare worse that those with a lesser presurgical tumor burden (IIIA). One randomized trial has demonstrated that maintenance paclitaxel improved progression-free survival of women with a clinical complete response (66% with optimal stage III disease) from 21 to 28 months in a randomized trial, and this option should be discussed with this patient. However, no survival benefit was observed at the time the trial was ended and the randomization code was broken, and there is a significant incidence of neuropathy. No data exist on PET scans in this situation, and consolidation topotecan has shown no benefit in two randomized trials. While intraperitoneal therapy is a theoretically attractive option, cisplatin, the most widely used drug, carries a significant risk of neurotoxicity, and there are no data showing any survival benefit to its use in the setting of minimal residual disease.

Answer 19.4. **The answer is A.**

Low malignant potential tumors are uncommon, but not rare, comprising about 15% of all ovarian epithelial carcinomas (4% to 14% of all ovarian malignancies). The majority are stage I. They occur much more frequently in younger women and have an excellent prognosis, with a long-term survival rate of over 95%. They tend to be quite large, and while careful sampling is required to rule out foci of invasive disease, the size does not affect survival. They may be of serous or mucinous histology. Those with stage III disease still have excellent survival (88% 10-year relative survival), and there is no evidence to suggest that they benefit from front-line chemotherapy, although it is often considered for the subset of patients with invasive implants who have a somewhat poorer prognosis.

Answer 19.5. **The answer is F.**

Sex cord-stromal tumors (of which granulosa cell tumors are the most common subtype) comprise only about 5% of all ovarian neoplasms. The peak incidence is in women over 50, although a significant proportion occurs in premenopausal women. Granulosa cell tumors may secrete estrogen and be associated with endometrial hyperplasia and endometrial carcinoma. A large majority are diagnosed in stage I, and these patients have 10-year survivals of 75% to 95%. However, late relapses may be observed. Patients with advanced stage disease fare much more poorly. Although the rarity of the tumor precludes randomized trial data, most such patients will be offered chemotherapy, traditionally with bleomycin, etoposide, cisplatin (BEP) or other regimens used in germ cell tumors.

Answer 19.6. **The answer is A.**

Germ cell tumors almost always occur in young women, with a peak incidence in the early 20s. Sixty percent to 70% are stage I at diagnosis. With the use of platinum-based chemotherapy regimens similar to those employed for males with testicular cancer, even advanced stage patients have a good prognosis. Because most of these tumors occur in young women, often before they have had children, and because the type of chemotherapy used will not cause infertility in most young female patients, the surgical approach is critical; in many patients, the contralateral ovary and uterus can and should be spared.

Answer 19.7. **The answer is C.**

Recurrent ovarian cancer is not generally curable with transplant or any other modality, but patients whose disease recurs with a disease-free interval of over 1 year have over a 50% chance of responding to platinum-based combination therapy and should usually be offered chemotherapy. Secondary debulking surgery may also be of benefit. Hormonal therapy in ovarian cancer generally produces response rates of only 10% to 15% and is usually reserved for patients who cannot tolerate other therapy. It has also been recommended as the initial salvage therapy in patients who have a rising CA-125 as their only manifestation of recurrent disease.

Answer 19.8. **The answer is A.**

Carcinoma of the cervix is one of the leading causes of cancer death in women throughout the world. This is probably because most underdeveloped countries do not have an organized screening system for this cancer. Countries that have established screening systems tend to have an increase in the incidence of dysplasia and a concomitant decrease in the incidence of cervical cancers. Though death from this disease is relatively uncommon in the United States, infection with HPV and associated dysplasia is very common. Infection with HPV leads to a premalignant condition called cervical intraepithelial neoplasia (CIN) or dysplasia that is detected through cervical cytologic screening. The premalignant condition that leads to cancer is caused by the integration of HPV DNA into the human genomic DNA. Once this has occurred, expression of E6 protein leads to inactivation of p53 that in turn leads to progressive malignant transformation.

Answer 19.9. **The answer is D.**

The E6 proteins of high-risk types of HPV have a greater affinity for p53 than other E6 proteins.

Answer 19.10. **The answer is A.**

There are many HPV types. Over 100 subtypes have been identified to date. Certain subtypes are associated with an increased likelihood of progression to high-grade dysplasias and cervical cancers (16, 18, 31, 33, 45). These subtypes are often isolated in various regions of the world. For instance, HPV-45 is most common in Western Africa, and HPV-39 and HPV-59 most common in Central and South America. Most HPV infections are transient and do not lead to cancer. Persistent infection is needed to develop dysplasia and subsequent cervical cancer. Therefore, other factors are necessary to allow persistent infection and progression to dysplasia.

Answer 19.11. **The answer is D.**

Although multiple sexual partners are a risk factor for exposure to HPV and therefore development of cervical cancer, it is not a factor that promotes persistent infection.

Answer 19.12. **The answer is C.**

Whereas smoking may increase the likelihood that a patient will develop cervical cancer, there have been no studies that demonstrate an increase in the incidence of this disease by country or cultural origin.

Answer 19.13. **The answer is D.**

The first three options are cited by Smith et al. in their paper utilizing the Surveillance, Epidemiology, and End Results (SEER) database to at least partially explain the increased incidence of adenocarcinoma of the cervix. Although adenocarcinoma of the cervix is associated with HPV, there has been little change in the HPV types associated with this disease.

Answer 19.14. **The answer is C.**

There is no evidence that HIV infection changes the type of HPV infecting the cervix, only that HIV infected individuals are more susceptible to infection and that they progress at a more rapid rate.

Answer 19.15. **The answer is C.**

Some advocate colposcopic evaluation immediately upon diagnosis because of the high risk of dysplasia. Few advocate routine colposcopic screening.

Answer 19.16. **The answer is D.**

Cervical cancers usually arise at the squamocolumnar junction on the cervix. This area is the most metabolically active region of the cervix and therefore carries the greatest risk of neoplastic change. The mean age of CIN is about 15 years younger than women with invasive cancer. This fact represents part of the data that strongly supports a prolonged premalignant condition. The rate of progression of cervical dysplasia to cancer varies from study to study, but it seems clear that a substantial number of patients infected with HPV regress spontaneously and only a minority actually progress to cancer. Cancer is diagnosed once it displays the ability to invade the basement membrane. The most common means of spread once dysplasia becomes a cancer is by direct extension or via lymphatics. Lymph node involvement is directly correlated with tumor stage and overall volume of tumor. On the average, stage I tumors have a 15% to 20% chance of having pelvic lymph node involvement and about a 1% to 5% chance of having paraaortic nodal metastasis. Cervical cancer generally follows an orderly progression of metastatic spread. This is usually to primary-echelon nodes in the pelvis, then to paraaortic nodes, and finally to distant sites. Hematogenous spread is somewhat rare.

Answer 19.17. **The answer is A.**

Despite its close proximity to the cervix, the bladder itself is uncommonly involved by direct extension of tumor.

Answer 19.18. **The answer is A.**

The most appropriate next step is to perform HPV typing on the cervical cytology. If there is detectable high-risk HPV, then the patient should undergo colposcopy, though all three treatment regimens are reasonable. Regarding HPV, typing with triage to colposcopy if positive is the most cost-effective method of follow-up. This was demonstrated by the ASCUS/LSIL Triage Study (ALTS) trial.

Answer 19.19. **The answer is A.**

Since most low-grade lesions will resolve spontaneously and few will progress, careful observation is the best course of action.

Answer 19.20. **The answer is D.**

ASCUS is the most common abnormal Pap smear. There have been several systems that have been developed to describe abnormal cervical cytology and abnormal cervical histology. Richart proposed the term *cervical intraepithelial neoplasia* (CIN). This term is now preferred over dysplasia. The Bethesda system was designed to standardize cervical cytology.

Squamous intraepithelial lesion (SIL) is used to describe all squamous alterations induced by HPV. SILs are divided into two different groups: low grade LSIL and high grade HSIL. LSIL tends to be associated with low-risk HPV and HSIL tends to be associated with high-risk HPV types. The Bethesda system also introduced a new term: *atypical squamous cells of undetermined significance* (ASCUS). This ASCUS smear is the most common abnormal diagnosis in cytology laboratories in the United States. Management of ASCUS smears can follow three paths: (a) repeat in 3 to 4 months, (b) colposcopy, and (c) reflex HPV testing followed by colposcopy if positive. The most cost-effective treatment is reflex HPV testing followed by colposcopy if positive for high-risk HPV type and was determined by the ALTS.

There are several diagnostic dilemmas in the diagnosis of cervical abnormalities. One of these is adenocarcinoma. This is because cytology is often unreliable as these cells are difficult to distinguish and the rate of pickup is markedly less than that for squamous cell abnormalities. When adenocarcinoma *in situ* is suspected, a diagnostic excisional procedure is usually required. Microinvasive carcinoma of the cervix must be diagnosed with an excisional biopsy such as a cone biopsy or LEEP. These procedures offer both complete excision of the lesion in question as well as exact measurement of its dimensions.

Answer 19.21. **The answer is A.**

Because the lesion is often multifocal, negative margins are often meaningless.

Answer 19.22. **The answer is D.**

The only unacceptable treatment of a lesion that demonstrates less than 5 mm of invasion is observation. There are seldom lymph node metastases when invasion is less than 3 mm, and most in the United States feel that a simple hysterectomy or even a cone biopsy, if the patient desires future childbearing, is acceptable. If invasion is greater than 3 mm but less than 5 mm, most in the United States would perform a radical hysterectomy with lymph node dissection.

Answer 19.23. **The answer is B.**

Verrucous carcinoma of the cervix is often so well differentiated that it is mistaken for condyloma. Often complete excision is required to make the diagnosis and even then it can be difficult.

Answer 19.24. **The answer is C.**

The Pap smear is quite sensitive but not very specific. There are many reasons for false-positive tests and false-negative tests. The Pap smear is a good screening test because it is sensitive. The specificity is less of an issue because the prevalence of the premalignant lesion is quite high in the general population.

Answer 19.25. **The answer is C.**

Screening can stop at 70 only if the patient has had normal Pap smears for 10 years. In 2001 the American Cancer Society (ACS) developed a series of guidelines for screening. These include all of the following:

1. Screening should begin at age 21 or 3 years after first intercourse.
2. Screening should be performed at 1-year intervals if conventional Pap smears are used or every 2 years if liquid based cytology is used.
3. Starting at age 30, the screening interval can increase if all Pap smears have been normal for 3 years.
4. Women over the age of 70 can discontinue screening if all Pap smears have been normal for 10 years.

These recommendations are not endorsed by all for several reasons. First, the prevalence of HPV is so high in our society that patients can express the HPV virus at any point. Also, because of screening, younger women have a lower incidence of cervical cancer than in the past; now the most common age of diagnosis for cervical cancer is in the 70s. However, these recommendations can be used as excellent guidelines for screening. The clinical situation of the patient must always be considered, such as new sexual partners.

Answer 19.26. **The answer is D.**

Even in patients with invasive cancer, the false-negative rate is as high as 15%. This false-negative rate is the reason that yearly Paps are recommended. The sensitivity increases significantly with regular routine screening. The technique of obtaining the Pap smear is also important. For instance, obtaining the specimen with a cytobrush increases the sensitivity significantly as well as being better at picking up high endocervical lesions.

Answer 19.27. **The answer is B.**

Colposcopy is always the next step in the evaluation of a patient with an abnormal Pap smear. Colposcopy is performed by staining the cervix with 3% acetic acid; the cervix is then examined under 10- to 15-fold magnification. Abnormal areas are biopsied. Endocervical curettage should always be performed to evaluate unseen areas in the endocervix. Ablative or excisional treatment should be performed based on the pathology of the biopsies.

Answer 19.28. **The answer is B.**

All of the above patterns are abnormal. Mosaicism, punctation, and white epithelium are generally signs of dysplasia. Only atypical vessels are a sign of invasive cancer until proven otherwise. Atypical vessels are identified by winding or corkscrew patterns. They also often change caliber along their course.

Answer 19.29. **The answer is B.**

If there is an identified lesion so that a non-microinvasive cervical cancer is diagnosed, no further workup is indicated. The patient must be treated definitively for her cancer either with radiation or surgery. The other cases represent situations where an invasive cancer cannot be ruled out. In these cases, a larger excision of the cervix must be performed to completely exclude the possibility of an invasive cancer as well as excise the abnormal area. Indications for a cone biopsy or LEEP cone include: (a) the squamocolumnar junction is not completely visualized and a high-grade lesion is suspected, (b) a high-grade lesion extends into the endocervical canal and is not completely visualized, (c) a microinvasive carcinoma is found on directed biopsy, (d) the cytologic findings are worrisome for adenocarcinoma *in situ*, (e) the endocervical curettage is positive, and (f) sometimes when the biopsy shows a high-grade dysplasia and the colposcopist feels that there could be a worse lesion.

Answer 19.30. **The answer is B.**

According to FIGO rules, if two experienced examiners disagree, the correct stage is designated as that which is the lower of the two. Since the disease does not extend down the vagina but involves the parametrium, the correct stage is IIB. The other examiner felt that the disease extended to the sidewall. If both examiners had agreed on this, the correct stage would have been IIIB. Once a stage has been established, it cannot be changed.

Answer 19.31. **The answer is A.**

FIGO established a general staging system in 1994. This staging system is based on a clinical evaluation and imaging of the kidneys as well as a chest x-ray. The reason that high technology imaging is not included in the staging is that most cervical cancers occur in countries or regions where CT or MRI may not be available.

Answer 19.32. **The answer is B.**

Most gynecologic oncologists accept 3 mm of invasion as the cutoff for microinvasion. This defines the cutoff where a radical hysterectomy is necessary if the invasion is greater than 3 mm. If the invasion is less, then a simple hysterectomy is adequate. This is because the incidence of lymph node metastasis is almost zero when there is less than 3 mm of invasion.

Answer 19.33. **The answer is A.**

Transabdominal staging of the lymph node metastases has the highest complication rate when combined with radiation therapy. The complication rate over the long term can be as high as 30%. This is presumably because of the adhesions formed as a result of the surgery that fixes the small bowel to other abdominal structures. This procedure is controversial because, even though the exact location of nodal metastases is identified and can therefore be more accurately treated, there has never been a study that clearly documents a survival advantage. The extraperitoneal approach has a very low complication rate (<5%), and the laparoscopic approach has not been adequately evaluated to determine its efficacy.

Answer 19.34. **The answer is D.**

A strong inflammatory response is associated with a better prognosis. This is presumably because an immune response can be mounted.

Answer 19.35. **The answer is C.**

The survival in patients with a IB carcinoma of the cervix is 85% to 95%. If positive lymph nodes are detected, the survival falls to 45% to 55%. Lymph node metastases are clearly a poor prognostic feature. Unfortunately, there is no good way of detecting lymph node metastases. CT scan will detect only about one third of positive nodes; a PET scan may be slightly more sensitive but at this time empiric treatment of the nodes appears to be the best solution to this dilemma.

Answer 19.36. **The answer is A.**

Radical hysterectomy is excessive treatment for this limited lesion with little or no chance of lymph node metastases. A cone biopsy is adequate therapy in a patient who desires future childbearing. These patients must have invasion of less than 3 mm and no lymph vascular space involvement. A simple hysterectomy is adequate for patients who do not wish future childbearing. Radiation therapy is an acceptable treatment modality for those patients who may not be good surgical candidates.

Answer 19.37. **The answer is D.**

Pelvic exenteration is not needed but would be the treatment of choice if the patient had already received radiation therapy. Radical excision is never appropriate therapy in this setting. Radiation therapy would have been appropriate therapy before 1999. Now most people would treat this patient with concurrent radiation therapy and chemotherapy.

Answer 19.38. **The answer is C.**

All of the above therapies are acceptable treatment options. Cryotherapy is cheap and easily performed in the office. The cervix must be frozen twice to ensure adequate ablation. Some authors feel that this technique has a higher failure rate especially with extensive high-grade lesions involving multiple quadrants. Laser is also acceptable but is expensive and requires anesthesia with the attendant risks. Loop diathermy is cheap and can be performed in the office. It has the advantage of having a pathology specimen for evaluation. Some authors have published reports indicating that invasive cancer can be found in some of these specimens. This leads one to wonder how many cancers have been missed by ablative techniques. Cold knife conization requires an anesthetic as well and is associated with increased infertility.

Answer 19.39. **The answer is B.**

The risk is approximately 5%. For this reason, nodal evaluation must be undertaken to ensure adequate therapy in all but the most superficial cervical cancers.

Answer 19.40. **The answer is D.**

Overall survival rates for patients with stage IB cervical cancer treated with surgery or radiation is said to be 80% to 90%. This suggests that the two treatment options are equivalent. However, biases introduced by patient selection and variable indications for postoperative radiation therapy confound comparisons of these two treatment modalities. In the only randomized comparative trial, the use of radiation therapy in the surgery arm was quite high. In this trial, 54% of patients with lesions less than 4 cm received radiation therapy, and a staggering 84% of patients with lesions of this size were advised to get adjuvant radiation therapy. The survival rates were similar in both arms but combined treatment led to significantly increased morbidity.

Answer 19.41. **The answer is A.**

Some surgeons advocate the use of radical hysterectomy as initial treatment for patients with IB2 tumors. However, patients with tumors measuring more than 4 cm in diameter usually have poor prognostic features, and, therefore, postoperative radiation therapy is usually recommended. Consequently, many recommend radiation therapy as the primary modality for treatment of IB2 lesions. Two recent prospective randomized trials indicate that patients with bulky central tumors benefit from concomitant cisplatin-containing chemotherapy.

Answer 19.42. **The answer is C.**

Type I hysterectomy is a simple hysterectomy and clearly has no role in this situation. Type II radical hysterectomy is a modified radical hysterectomy and does not take all of the parametrium or the uterosacral ligaments. Type III radical hysterectomy has become the surgical standard for treatment of stage IB cervical cancers. This procedure consists of en bloc removal of the uterus, cervix, and parametrial, paracervical, and paravaginal tissues. The uterine vessels are ligated at their origin, and the proximal third of the vagina and the paracolpium are resected. The type IV radical hysterectomy requires resection of the same structures as a Type III as well as additional structures such as the bladder or ureter. The complication rate is too high with a Type IV procedure and thus it is seldom performed.

Answer 19.43. **The answer is D.**

Complications of radical hysterectomy include pulmonary embolism (1% to 2%), bowel obstruction (1% to 2%), and postoperative fever (25% to 30%). Most patients have transient bladder dysfunction, and about 3% to 5% have long-term clinically significant bladder dysfunction.

Answer 19.44. **The answer is A.**

In 1999, the Gynecologic Oncology Group (GOG) reported on a prospective trial of adjuvant pelvic radiotherapy in patients with an intermediate risk of recurrence after radical hysterectomy for stage IB carcinoma. Patients were eligible if they had at least two of the following risk factors: greater than one third stromal invasion, lymph vascular space involvement, or clinical tumor diameter of at least 4 cm. Patients with involvement of the pelvic lymph nodes, parametria, or surgical margins were excluded. After surgery, 277 patients were randomly assigned whole pelvic radiotherapy (46 to 50 Gy). Overall there was a 47% reduction in the recurrence rate in patients treated with adjuvant radiotherapy.

Answer 19.45. **The answer is D.**

Eifel reported a 5-year survival of 90% in 701 patients with IB carcinoma of the cervix treated with radiation alone. The central pelvic control rates were 99%. The disease-specific survival in patients with large tumors greater than 5 cm was 67%. Recent data have emerged suggesting that survival in patients with large IB tumors can be improved with combination radiation therapy and platinum-based chemotherapy.

Answer 19.46. **The answer is C.**

As with radical surgery, the goal of radiotherapy is to sterilize disease in the cervix, paracervical tissues, and regional lymph nodes. Patients are usually treated with a combination of external beam therapy and internal brachytherapy. Brachytherapy allows radiation to be delivered directly to the affected tissue. This significantly improves the local control rate and hence the cure rate. Doses of around 80 to 85 Gy can be delivered to the affected area using the combination therapy.

Answer 19.47. **The answer is B.**

Radiotherapy is the primary treatment modality for most patients with locally advanced cervical cancer (patients with IIB or greater). The success of therapy depends on a careful balance between external-beam therapy and brachytherapy that optimizes the dose to tumor and normal tissues. Five-year survival rates of 65% to 75%, 35% to 50%, and 15% to 20% are reported for patients treated with radiotherapy alone for stage IIB, IIIB, and IV tumors respectively. With appropriate radiotherapy, even patients with massive locoregional disease have a significant chance of cure. These survival rates can be improved even more with the addition of concurrent chemotherapy to the treatment regimen.

Answer 19.48. **The answer is A.**

High energy photons (15 to 18 MeV) are usually preferred for pelvic treatment because they spare superficial tissues that are unlikely to be involved with the tumor. At these energies, the pelvis can be treated either with four-field technique or with anterior/posterior fields alone. When high-energy beams are not available, four fields are usually used because less-penetrating 4- to 6-MeV photons often deliver an unacceptably high dose to superficial tissues when two fields are used. However, lateral fields must be designed with great care because estimation of tumor location from the lateral position is often inaccurate.

Answer 19.49. **The answer is A.**

Numerous small series of patients with documented paraaortic node involvement demonstrate that 25% to 50% of these patients enjoy long-term survival. Patients with microscopic disease have a better survival than do those with gross lymphadenopathy, but even 10% to 15% of patients with gross lymphadenopathy appear to be curable with aggressive management.

Answer 19.50. **The answer is C.**

Geometry and appropriate dosing to surrounding areas is important. The mucosal tolerance rule applies to the appropriate dose to the surrounding tissues as well as the principle of the inverse square law. The larger the volume of the implant, the less surface dose.

Answer 19.51. **The answer is C.**

Treatment dose has been specified in a number of ways, making it difficult to compare experiences. Paracentral doses are most frequently expressed at a single point usually designated as point A. This reference point is calculated in a number of ways.

Answer 19.52. **The answer is D.**

Brachytherapy does not decrease damage to normal tissue more than teletherapy.

Answer 19.53. **The answer is B.**

During the past two decades, computer technology has made it possible to deliver brachytherapy at a much higher rate. The sources used are high activity ^{60}Co or ^{192}Ir. Also, the technology of remote afterloading allows the sources to be loaded into the patient safely without exposing health care providers to radiation. Clinicians have found high-dose radiation attractive because it does not require patient hospitalization. However, unless it is heavily fractionated high-dose radiation, brachytherapy loses the radiobiologic advantage of conventional low-dose therapy.

Answer 19.54. **The answer is B.**

Estimates of the risk of late complications of radical radiotherapy vary according to the grading system, duration of follow-up, method of calculation, treatment method, and prevalence of risk factors in the study population. However, most reports quote an overall risk of major complications of 5% to 15%. In a report from the Patterns of Care Study, Lanciano et al. reported an actuarial risk of 8% at 3 years. In a study of 1,784 patients with stage IB disease, Eifel et al. reported an actuarial risk of 7.7% at 5 years. The actuarial risk was greatest at 3 years with continuing risk to patients at 0.3% per year.

Answer 19.55. **The answer is C.**

Generally, central pelvic recurrences after definitive radiation therapy are treated with pelvic exenteration. Tumor involvement of the pelvic sidewall is a contraindication for exenteration, but this may be difficult to assess because of pelvic radiation fibrosis. The triad of unilateral leg edema, sciatic pain, and ureteral obstruction almost always indicates unresectable disease. The cure rate of pelvic exenteration is usually quoted around 50% if the lesion can be resected. Mathews and colleagues reported a 5-year survival rate of 46% and an operative mortality of 11% in patients over 65 undergoing pelvic exenteration compared with a survival rate of 45% and an operative mortality rate of 8.5% for patients who were younger.

Answer 19.56. **The answer is B.**

Conization in pregnancy should be avoided. Blood loss is quoted at an average of 500 cc per procedure. Abortion rate is said to be around 25%, and, therefore, conization should be performed in the second trimester.

CHAPTER **20**

Cancer of the Breast

LEANNE S. BUDDE AND KATHY D. MILLER

Directions Each of the numbered items below is followed by lettered answers. Select the ONE lettered answer that is BEST in each case unless instructed otherwise.

QUESTIONS

Question 20.1. **Mechanisms of DNA alteration in oncogenes or tumor suppressor genes implicated in breast cancer include all of the following EXCEPT**

A. gene amplification (Her-2/neu)
B. point mutation (p53)
C. gene methylation (E-cadherin)
D. loss of heterozygosity at a single locus
E. loss of heterozygosity at multiple loci

Question 20.2. **Which of the following statements about hormone receptors is FALSE?**

A. The estrogen-positive epithelial and proliferative cell populations in breast cancer function independently of one another.
B. The progesterone receptor is dependent on the estrogen receptor.
C. Estrogen α-receptor activation and nuclear localization are regulated by phosphorylation.
D. The estrogen receptor may regulate lobular cells as well as ductal cells.
E. The estrogen receptor may interact with cyclin D1 to promote transcriptional activity.

Question 20.3. **With regard to epithelial growth factor family of receptors (EGFR), which of the following is true?**

A. Five subtypes of EGFR have been identified.
B. The complex dimeric pattern of EGFR probably governs its multiple responses.
C. Trastuzumab acts through a series of steps to upregulate cyclin D1, thereby slowing cell cycle progression.
D. Her-2/neu overexpression is typically associated with EGFR gene amplification.

Corresponding Chapters in *Cancer: Principles & Practice of Oncology*, Seventh Edition: 33 (Cancer of the Breast).

Question 20.4. **Which of the following about tamoxifen is NOT true?**

A. Its half-life is 2 to 3 days.
B. It binds to the estrogen receptor, leading to dimerization of the receptor and, ultimately, inhibition of transcriptional processes.
C. It is extensively metabolized by the liver cytochrome p450 enzymes.
D. It is best not given to patients with a history of deep vein thrombosis (DVT), pulmonary embolism (PE), or cerebrovascular disease.
E. It can inhibit metabolism of warfarin, leading to increased anticoagulation.

Question 20.5. **With regard to trastuzumab, which of the following is NOT true?**

A. It acts against a receptor that is present in 25% to 30% of breast cancers.
B. It acts against the type-2 epithelial growth factor receptor (EGFR).
C. It downregulates the expression of Her-2/neu receptors.
D. It stimulates Her-2/neu intracellular signaling pathways.

Question 20.6. **Which of the following regarding autologous tissue breast reconstruction is NOT true?**

A. A transrectus abdominal muscle (TRAM) flap allows the surgeon the most versatility in autologous tissue breast reconstruction.
B. A single TRAM flap results in only 25% loss of abdominal strength.
C. The risk of total flap loss is approximately 2%.
D. There is no difference in the rate of breast cancer recurrence after a skin-sparing mastectomy.
E. Patients undergoing autologous tissue reconstruction may still require a complementary prosthetic implant to achieve a satisfactory cosmetic result.

Question 20.7. **All of the following statements about prosthetic breast reconstruction are true EXCEPT**

A. a tissue expander can be placed at the time of mastectomy or in a separate operation
B. approximately 2% of patients will require removal of the tissue expander due to wound complication or persistent or recurrent disease
C. adjuvant chemotherapy can be given during the tissue expansion period
D. the prosthetic implant cannot be placed during adjuvant chemotherapy
E. a contralateral symmetry procedure may be needed at the time the prosthetic implant is placed

Question 20.8. **Which of the following regarding immediate breast reconstruction is true?**

A. There is still an equal likelihood (compared to delayed reconstruction) that a symmetry procedure on the contralateral breast will be required to achieve an acceptable cosmetic result.
B. Previous radiation treatment excludes a patient from consideration for a skin-sparing mastectomy with immediate reconstruction.
C. Only the integrity of the breast skin envelope is crucial for optimizing breast form and symmetry.
D. Only the integrity of the inframammary fold is crucial for optimizing breast form and symmetry.
E. The integrity of both the breast skin envelope and the inframammary fold is important for optimizing breast form and symmetry.

Question 20.9. **The following statements about autologous breast reconstruction after breast irradiation are true EXCEPT**

A. blood supply is decreased
B. the infection rate is increased
C. the rate of flap survival is lower
D. reconstruction necessitates the use of autologous tissue
E. skin elasticity is decreased

Question 20.10. **With regard to the Breast Imaging Reporting and Data System (BI-RADS) for categorizing mammography findings, which of the following is true?**

A. A BI-RADS score of zero means the mammogram is normal.
B. A BI-RADS score of one means the mammogram is normal.
C. A BI-RADS score of three represents a benign finding.
D. A BI-RADS score of four represents malignancy.
E. Possible BI-RADS scores range from one to five (i.e., a possible score of zero does not exist).

Question 20.11. **With regard to breast biopsies, which of the following is true?**

A. Approximately 10% of breast biopsies showing atypical hyperplasia are associated with underlying ductal carcinoma *in situ* (DCIS).
B. Biopsies showing proliferation but no atypia are not associated with an increased risk of breast cancer.
C. If a woman has a nonexcisional biopsy for an abnormal finding on mammography, and the biopsy reveals lobular carcinoma *in situ* (LCIS), an excisional biopsy must be done.
D. The false-positive rate for fine needle aspiration (FNA) is about 5%.

Question 20.12. **Concerning breast cancer staging, which of the following is true?**

A. The number of axillary lymph nodes involved does not impact disease-free or overall survival in early breast cancer.
B. The greatest decrement in 5-year survival rates is seen between women without axillary lymph node involvement and those with 1 to 3 positive lymph nodes.
C. Within stage I breast cancer, T-stage impacts disease-free survival rates.
D. Downstaging axillary lymph nodes with neoadjuvant chemotherapy does not affect 5-year survival.
E. T-stage has a greater impact on survival for women with locally advanced breast cancer than N-stage.

Question 20.13. **A 55-year-old African American woman with a remote history of ER-positive, Her-2/neu-positive stage I breast cancer comes to you for follow-up. A lumbar x-ray obtained by her primary care physician to evaluate severe low back pain revealed a lytic lesion. Chest, abdominal, and pelvic computed tomography (CT) and a bone scan are normal, but her primary care physician is concerned she has recurrent breast cancer. Appropriate steps to consider include the following EXCEPT**

A. magnetic resonance imaging (MRI) to exclude cord compression
B. serum and urine protein electrophoresis
C. implementation of paclitaxel and trastuzumab
D. CT-guided biopsy of the lesion
E. prescription of narcotic pain medication

Question 20.14. **For which of the following patients is a full staging evaluation NOT mandatory?**

A. A patient with an 8-cm tumor with movable ipsilateral axillary lymph nodes.
B. A patient with peau d'orange and 2 positive axillary lymph nodes.
C. A patient with a 4-cm tumor with matted ipsilateral axillary lymph nodes.
D. A patient with a 6-cm tumor with clinically apparent internal mammary lymph nodes.
E. A patient with skin ulceration and matted axillary lymph nodes.

Question 20.15. **A number of changes were made in 2002 to the American Joint Committee on Cancer (AJCC) staging system for breast cancer. These changes have been shown to affect stage-specific survival. Of the following, which of the statements about the changes is NOT correct?**

A. Changes were made based on the number of involved axillary lymph nodes.
B. Additional N-stage categories were introduced to discriminate between micrometastases and isolated tumor cells.
C. The new system reclassifies metastases to internal mammary nodes.
D. The new system introduced identifiers to highlight the use of special diagnostic procedures.
E. Supraclavicular lymph node metastases are now categorized as M1 disease.

Question 20.16. **Concerning DCIS, the following are true EXCEPT**

A. DCIS is classified based on architectural grade and/or subtype
B. $^2/_3$ of cases with comedonecrosis are high grade
C. the association of an underlying mass with DCIS indicates the need for mastectomy
D. the risk of local recurrence with radiotherapy after lumpectomy is reduced by 50%
E. postoperative radiotherapy does not increase survival

Question 20.17. **The benefits of neoadjuvant chemotherapy in breast cancer include all of the following EXCEPT**

A. the possibility of downgrading the necessity of a mastectomy to breast-conserving surgery
B. the opportunity to test the chemosensitivity of the tumor
C. an increase in survival compared to administering chemotherapy in the adjuvant setting
D. the opportunity to downgrade the extent of the patient's lymph node involvement, thereby lowering the risk of recurrence

Question 20.18. **A 74-year-old woman presents after mastectomy for a 1-cm breast cancer found on routine mammography. The pathology report notes that the tumor is ER-negative, PR-negative, and Her-2/neu-negative. As an appropriate next step, you**

A. tell the patient she has a high chance of cure and there is no need for chemoprevention with hormonal therapy
B. ask the pathologist to retest the specimen for estrogen-receptor positivity
C. tell the patient she should take tamoxifen; despite her tumor being ER-negative, tamoxifen will lower the chance of development of breast cancer in the contralateral breast
D. tell the patient she should take tamoxifen; despite her tumor being ER-negative, tamoxifen will lower the chance of recurrence of her breast cancer
E. order staging exams to ensure there is no metastatic disease

Question 20.19. **With regard to the risks and benefits of chemotherapy, which of the following is NOT true?**

A. Deaths due to chemotherapy are most often due to neutropenic sepsis or thromboembolic events.
B. Chemotherapy confers an increased benefit with each advancing decade of patient age.
C. Lethal toxicities are estimated to occur in approximately 1 of every 200 to 500 women.
D. Deaths from chemotherapy are more common in postmenopausal patients.
E. Deaths from chemotherapy are more common in patients receiving concomitant tamoxifen therapy.

Question 20.20. **All of the following are important factors when considering adjuvant chemotherapy for stage I breast cancers less than 1cm in size EXCEPT**

A. recurrence-free survival is influenced by the size of the tumor and its histologic classification
B. prognostic factors associated with a higher risk of relapse include tumor size, poor histologic grade, poor nuclear grade, and lymphatic vessel invasion
C. the absolute reduction in relapse and death will be the same regardless of a patient's risk for recurrence
D. studies have shown that physicians tend to overestimate a patient's risk for recurrence and overestimate the benefit of adjuvant chemotherapy

Question 20.21. **Regarding the use of taxanes in addition to doxorubicin and cyclophosphamide in the neoadjuvant treatment of early breast cancer, which of the following is true?**

A. Taxanes are more effective if used concurrently rather than sequentially.
B. Paclitaxel is more effective than docetaxel.
C. The addition of paclitaxel in the neoadjuvant setting increases disease-free survival.
D. The addition of docetaxel has no effect on pathologic complete response.
E. Adjuvant taxanes augment toxicity minimally.

Question 20.22. **Of the following, which does NOT exclude a woman for consideration of breast conservation therapy (BCT) (e.g., lumpectomy)?**

A. Residual invasive ductal carcinoma after neoadjuvant chemotherapy.
B. Progression or no response to chemotherapy.
C. Extensive microcalcifications associated with an extensive intraductal component.
D. A T4 lesion.
E. Islands of tumor throughout the specimen after induction chemotherapy.

Question 20.23. **According to the American Society of Clinical Oncology (ASCO) guidelines for postmastectomy radiotherapy (PMRT) for patients with localized breast cancer, which of the following is true?**

A. PMRT is indicated for women with T1/2 tumors with one to three positive axillary lymph nodes.
B. PMRT is not needed for patients with T3 tumors as long as they have no axillary lymph node involvement.
C. Supraclavicular lymph node irradiation is necessary for women with one to three positive axillary lymph nodes.
D. Full axillary radiotherapy is still necessary for women who have undergone a level I/II axillary lymph node dissection.
E. Axillary radiotherapy is required for women with BRCA-1-positive tumors regardless of their axillary lymph node status.

Question 20.24. **The following statements characterize Paget disease EXCEPT**

A. it is associated with *in situ* or invasive breast cancer in 97% of cases
B. wedge or punch biopsy of the nipple is the preferred diagnostic procedure
C. about half the cases of Paget disease are hormone-receptor positive
D. it tends to be associated with underlying high-grade disease
E. underlying breast cancers are almost always located within 2 cm of the nipple

Question 20.25. **Regarding Paget disease, which of the following is true?**

A. It should be treated according to the type of any underlying disease.
B. 75% of cases are associated with an underlying mass.
C. 80% of cases are associated with a mammographic abnormality.
D. 5% of cases are seen with mammography only.
E. 10% of cases do not have any associated underlying neoplasm.

Question 20.26. **According to the ASCO guidelines for PMRT for women with locally advanced breast cancer, which of the following is NOT true?**

A. PMRT is recommended for women with four or more positive axillary lymph nodes.
B. Internal mammary radiation is recommended as part of PMRT for women with positive supraclavicular lymph nodes.
C. PMRT is recommended for patients with operable stage III tumors.
D. A supraclavicular field should be used in patients with four or more positive axillary lymph nodes.
E. In patients given PMRT, treatment of the chest wall is mandatory.

Question 20.27. **Which of the following regarding locally advanced breast cancer is true?**

A. Chemotherapy given in the adjuvant setting obviates the need for postmastectomy radiation.
B. Hormonal therapy does not improve outcome.
C. There is no difference in outcome regardless of whether chemotherapy is given in the neoadjuvant or the adjuvant setting.
D. Surgery should be done first to debulk disease and achieve local control.
E. Women with locally advanced breast cancer represent a relatively homogeneous population.

Question 20.28. **Which of the following regarding locally advanced breast cancer is NOT true?**

A. NSABP-B18 failed to demonstrate that T3 tumors can sometimes be converted from requiring a mastectomy to being eligible for breast conservation surgery.
B. NSABP-B18 showed that a significant number of patients who received neoadjuvant chemotherapy had fewer positive lymph nodes than women who did not receive neoadjuvant treatment.
C. NSABP-B18 showed that fewer women who received neoadjuvant chemotherapy had four or more positive lymph nodes.
D. For women with inoperable locally advanced tumors, surgery may still be considered if neoadjuvant chemotherapy is able to convert the tumor into operable disease.

Question 20.29. **Which of the following does NOT accurately characterize inflammatory breast cancer (IBC)?**

A. Almost all women with IBC have lymph node involvement.
B. The 10-year survival rate exceeds 30%.
C. IBC is staged as T4d, stage IIIC.
D. Dermal lymphatic invasion must be seen on biopsy to confirm IBC.
E. Fever and leukocytosis should be excluded.

Question 20.30. **The following statements regarding clinical features that predict responsiveness to endocrine therapy in the metastatic setting are true EXCEPT**

A. isolated bone or soft tissue involvement predicts response to endocrine therapy
B. a prior response to endocrine therapy predicts response to endocrine therapy
C. a long relapse-free survival (after initial treatment) predicts response to endocrine therapy
D. tumors that express the estrogen receptor (but not the progesterone receptor) are likely to respond to endocrine therapy
E. tumors that express the progesterone receptor (but not the estrogen receptor) are unlikely to respond to endocrine therapy

Question 20.31. **A 39-year-old woman with a history of ER-negative, Her-2/neu-positive stage II breast cancer (history of treatment with doxorubicin, cyclophosphamide, and paclitaxel; surgery and adjuvant radiation 5 years ago) is evaluated by abdominal CT scan for intermittent right upper quadrant pain. In addition to gallstones, she is found to have multiple liver lesions, the largest of which is 3 cm. This is biopsied and confirmed to be metastatic breast cancer. You start her on trastuzumab. Three months later, repeat CT scan reveals enlargement of the liver lesions. Appropriate treatment alternatives include the following EXCEPT**

A. treatment with capecitabine; discontinue trastuzumab because it will not add any benefit
B. treatment with liposomal doxorubicin
C. treatment with docetaxel
D. treatment with gemcitabine
E. enrollment in a clinical trial

Question 20.32. **The benefit of combination chemotherapy will likely be the greatest for which of the following patients with breast cancer metastatic to the liver?**

A. ER-positive disease recently found to have several asymptomatic hepatic lesions but elevated transaminases.
B. Her-2/neu-negative disease found to have liver metastases 3 months ago and started on single-agent chemotherapy, now with replacement of her liver parenchyma by tumor.
C. ER-positive disease and several asymptomatic hepatic lesions, increasing in size despite treatment with hormonal therapy.
D. Her-2/neu-positive disease, recently found to have several liver metastases.
E. Her-2/neu negative disease found to have liver metastases 3 months ago and started on single-agent chemotherapy, asymptomatic, but now with an increase in the hepatic lesions and transaminases.

Question 20.33. **A 60-year-old woman with a remote history of stage II ER-positive, Her-2/neu-negative breast cancer is found to have elevated hepatic transaminases. An abdominal CT scan reveals numerous lesions throughout both hepatic lobes. One of the lesions is biopsied and found to be consistent with metastatic breast cancer. Additional tests do not reveal any additional sites of disease. She is asymptomatic. Which of the following would you recommend?**

A. Start chemotherapy.
B. Start hormonal therapy.
C. Consider starting therapy once she develops symptoms.
D. Consider chemoembolization.
E. Consider metastatectomy.

Question 20.34. **The ASCO recommendations regarding the use of bisphosphonates in metastatic breast cancer include which of the following.**

A. Zoledronic acid is more efficacious than pamidronate.
B. Starting bisphosphonates in women with an abnormal bone scan, but additional imaging evidence of bone destruction, is still considered reasonable.
C. Starting bisphosphonates in women who have demonstrated bone destruction by imaging studies, but normal plain radiographs, is considered reasonable.
D. Bisphosphonates should not be started unless a patient has bone pain.

Question 20.35. **Which of the following statements about male breast cancer is NOT true?**

A. The BRCA-2 gene has been implicated in male breast cancer, but its prevalence in male breast cancer is low.
B. As with breast cancer in females, male breast cancer appears to be associated with increased exposure to estrogen.
C. Regions with the highest incidence of male breast cancer coincide with areas of increased incidence of liver disease.
D. About 1,500 cases of male breast cancer occur in the United States each year.
E. As compared to female breast cancer, family history of breast cancer is not as much a risk factor in male breast cancer.

Question 20.36. **With regard to the clinical and pathologic characteristics of male breast cancer, which of the following is NOT true?**

A. Male breast cancer is found, more often than in female breast cancer, to be estrogen-receptor positive, and the older a male with breast cancer, the more likely it is to be estrogen-receptor positive.
B. Both lobular carcinoma *in situ* and invasive lobular carcinoma have been reported in male patients.
C. The most common presenting symptom is a painless, firm subareolar mass, seen in more than 75% of patients.
D. In addition to a palpable mass, common physical exam findings include changes in the areola with nipple retraction, inversion or fixation, or eczematous skin changes.
E. On mammography, an uncalcified mass is most commonly seen, and microcalcifications are less frequent.

Question 20.37. **Concerning the staging and treatment of male breast cancer, which of the following is NOT true?**

A. The same TNM staging system is used to stage male breast cancer.
B. Stage and axillary node status are the more important prognostic indicators in male breast cancer.
C. In cases of DCIS in men, simple mastectomy with axillary node dissection is the treatment of choice.
D. For localized disease, a simple mastectomy, or modified radical mastectomy, with local radiation treatment are effective therapies; there are no data to suggest that more extensive surgical resection improves survival.
E. For metastatic disease, hormonal therapy is the mainstay of treatment.

Question 20.38. **In pregnant patients, which of the following regarding breast masses and cancer is NOT true?**

A. Most breast cancers in pregnant women present as palpable masses.
B. Mammography is safe but less sensitive during pregnancy.
C. A single unilateral MLO (medial lateral oblique) mammographic view may be sufficient and minimize x-ray exposure.
D. Serum alkaline phosphatase levels are decreased in pregnancy.

Question 20.39. **In staging pregnant breast cancer patients, which of the following is true?**

A. Neither CT nor MRI is safe in pregnancy.
B. Radiation exposure to the fetus is estimated to be low using radioisotope labeling in a sentinel lymph node procedure.
C. Sentinel lymph node biopsy is an important procedure because a high number of pregnant women with breast cancer will be found to have positive axillary lymph nodes.
D. Breast cancer during pregnancy is usually detected at the same stage as in nonpregnant patients.
E. Breast cancer in pregnancy is associated with the same survival as in nonpregnant patients.

Question 20.40. **Which of the following regarding treatment of breast cancer in the pregnant patient is NOT true?**

A. Breast irradiation is contraindicated in the pregnant patient.
B. Mastectomy has no place in the treatment of pregnant patients who have tumors amenable to breast conservation.
C. Adjuvant chemotherapy should be avoided in the first trimester because almost all chemotherapeutic agents cross the placenta and are associated with a 15% to 20% risk of fetal malformation.
D. Chemotherapy can generally be administered safely during the second and third trimesters of pregnancy; the risk of fetal malformation is 1% to 3% during this time, similar to the risk of fetal malformation in healthy women.
E. Breast surgery can be performed safely during pregnancy and is not associated with an increased risk of fetal abnormalities.

Question 20.41. **A 60-year-old female presents to a dermatologist for evaluation of a hyperkeratotic nodule on her neck that has become ulcerated. Biopsy is consistent with breast cancer, metastatic to the skin, ER-positive, Her-2/neu-negative. She is referred to you for treatment recommendations. Clinical breast exam reveals a 3-cm upper outer quadrant mass in the right breast with associated fixed, matted axillary lymph nodes. Staging exams do not reveal any additional sites of disease. You immediately start her on tamoxifen. Two weeks later, she calls to say that new nodules are beginning to appear. You explain to her that**

A. her breast cancer is resistant to tamoxifen and she should start a different hormonal therapy
B. her breast cancer is resistant to tamoxifen and she should start chemotherapy
C. her breast cancer is resistant to tamoxifen; despite being Her-2/neu-negative, there is still a possibility that she will respond to trastuzumab (Herceptin)
D. her breast cancer may be responding to tamoxifen and she should keep her follow-up appointment with you in 1 month
E. she should return to the dermatologist for a repeat biopsy

Question 20.42. **A 64-year-old female is diagnosed with ER-positive breast cancer diffusely metastatic to bone and is started on anastrozole and zolendroic acid. One week later, her daughter calls to say the patient is lethargic. You instruct the daughter to bring her mother in for immediate medical evaluation because you are concerned that the patient most likely has**

A. a pulmonary embolus
B. a cerebrovascular accident
C. hypercalcemia
D. an infection
E. overdosed on her narcotic medication

Question 20.43. **Which of the following statements regarding chemotherapy-induced cardiac toxicity is NOT true?**

A. Without medication, cardiac toxicity related to both adriamycin and trastuzumab is irreversible.
B. Heart failure occurs in less than 2% of patients who receive anthracyclines for breast cancer.
C. As a general rule, the total dose of doxorubicin should be restricted to less than 360 mg per m^2, and the total dose of epirubicin should be restricted to less than 720 mg per m^2.
D. When used as a single agent, the rate of cardiac events related to trastuzumab is approximately 5%.
E. When trastuzumab and anthracyclines are used in combination, the rate of cardiac events can be as high as 25%.

Question 20.44. **Which of the following statements regarding chemotherapy-related premature ovarian failure (POF) is NOT true?**

A. Development of POF appears to correlate with patient age.
B. The probability for developing POF varies by which chemotherapeutic regimen a patient receives.
C. Development of POF is a function of the total dose of drugs given.
D. The time of onset and intensity of symptoms related to POF are similar to natural menopause.
E. Chemotherapy destroys ovarian follicles, leading to lower estrogen levels, higher follicle-stimulating hormone (FSH) and luteinizing hormone (LH) levels, and menopausal symptoms.

Question 20.45. **Arm and hand precautions to avoid impairment of lymphatic drainage in women at increased risk for lymphedema include all of the following EXCEPT**

A. regular exercise
B. avoid skin puncture
C. avoid hot baths
D. wear loose clothes
E. practice careful nail care

Question 20.46. **With regard to lymphedema,**

A. overall incidence is estimated at 10%
B. breast irradiation has no effect on its development
C. lymphedema may result from a sentinel node biopsy
D. it affects the skin, subcutaneous tissue, and underlying muscle
E. it typically occurs within 1 year of treatment

Question 20.47. **With regard to the risk of development of hematologic malignancies after chemotherapy for breast cancer, which of the following statements is true?**

A. The incidence of leukemia is approximately 5% at 10 years.
B. The risk of leukemia has increased by the introduction of taxanes.
C. The latency of myelodysplastic syndrome (MDS) or leukemia is the same regardless of whether a patient receives anthracyclines or alkylating agents.
D. The risk for developing MDS or leukemia ranges from 0.1% to 1.5% depending on the regimen the patient receives and the length of the follow-up period.

Question 20.48. **Indications for kyphoplasty, in which cement is injected percutaneously to reexpand a pathologic vertebral compression fracture, include the following EXCEPT**

A. no neurologic compromise
B. no pain relief with noninvasive measures
C. poor prognosis to withstand recovery from aggressive neurosurgical intervention
D. no chance of cure from en bloc resection
E. involvement of the posterior vertebral elements

Question 20.49. **Factors influencing the appropriate use of intravenous radionuclides, such as samarium, for the treatment of painful skeletal metastases include all of the following EXCEPT**

A. painful osteoblastic metastases
B. diffuse skeletal involvement
C. hormone-insensitive tumor
D. inadequate pain control with analgesics, or analgesic intolerance
E. further consideration of cytotoxic chemotherapy

Question 20.50. **Considerations for referring a patient with a long bone metastasis to an orthopedic surgeon for internal fixation include all of the following EXCEPT**

A. 50% cortical involvement
B. blastic bone lesion
C. 4-cm lesion
D. no response to radiotherapy
E. functional pain

Question 20.51. **A 45-year-old woman with ER-negative, Her-2/neu-positive stage III breast cancer presents with diplopia. Physical exam is most notable for lateral deviation of the left eye but no other focal neurologic deficits. Steroid medication is begun. A brain MRI with and without contrast is obtained, which fails to demonstrate any evidence of metastatic disease. The most appropriate next step is to**

A. order whole-brain radiotherapy
B. consult a neurologist
C. order an MRI of her orbits
D. do a lumbar puncture
E. consult an ophthalmologist

Question 20.52. **A woman with a history of stage II ER-negative, Her-2/neu-positive breast cancer presents to your office complaining of progressively worsening low-back pain. She denies incontinence of bowel or bladder. She has no focal neurologic complaints. Physical exam reveals lumbar spinal tenderness but no focal neurologic findings; sensation and strength are intact. As the single most important next step, you**

A. order a lumbar x-ray
B. order a bone scan
C. order a lumbar MRI
D. prescribe nonsteroidal antiinflammatory medication
E. prescribe narcotic pain medication

Question 20.53. **The tumor of a woman with newly diagnosed breast cancer is found, according to the Scarff-Bloom-Richardson (SBR) histologic grading system (Contesso modification), to have a tubule formation score of 2, a nuclear pleomorphism score of 2, and a mitotic index of 2. Based on the SBR grading system, her tumor score**

A. is 6 and represents a well-differentiated tumor
B. is 6 and represents a moderately well-differentiated tumor
C. is 6 and represents a poorly differentiated tumor
D. is 8 and represents a moderately well-differentiated tumor
E. is 8 and represents a poorly differentiated tumor

Question 20.54. **With regard to persistent lymph node involvement after neoadjuvant chemotherapy in patients with operable breast cancer, which of the following is NOT true?**

A. The increase in the number of positive nodes is almost linearly correlated with a decline in survival and the potential to achieve cure.
B. Tumor grade is an independent prognostic factor for survival.
C. Hormonal receptor status is an independent prognostic factor for survival.
D. Clinical response to neoadjuvant chemotherapy does not contribute prognostic information regarding survival.

Question 20.55. **Which of the following regarding the "Adjuvant!" program for projecting breast cancer prognosis is true?**

A. It does not provide additional data with regard to prognosis if no further therapy is given.
B. It provides 5-year survival projections.
C. It provides 10-year survival projections.
D. It will only consider the effect of a chemotherapy regimen on survival.
E. It will only consider the effect of a hormonal therapy regimen on survival.

Question 20.56. **With regard to surveillance for patients with early stage breast cancer, all of the following are true EXCEPT**

A. screening mammography and breast ultrasound are the only imaging studies recommended for routine surveillance
B. there is no role for intense surveillance because early detection of relapse has not been shown to improve overall survival or other meaningful clinical endpoints
C. survival data from surveillance strategies to detect early recurrence of disease may be affected by lead-time bias
D. survival data from surveillance strategies to detect early recurrence of disease may be affected by length bias
E. there is a role for routine surveillance because early detection of in-breast recurrence has been shown to improve survival for women who have undergone breast conservation

Question 20.57. **With regard to breast cancer surveillance, all of the following are NOT true EXCEPT**

A. approximately 30% of all patients with stage I and stage II breast cancer will eventually experience a relapse of their disease
B. the hazard risk of recurrence of disease is constant for each year of follow-up
C. patients who are disease-free for over 5 years have miniscule risk for recurrence and, therefore, are not suitable for clinical trials of risk reduction agents
D. in high-risk patients, CA 27.29 can be followed to detect early recurrence of disease
E. tumors that lack the estrogen receptor are less likely to relapse in visceral organs than those that do not lack the receptor

Question 20.58. **Which of the following statements about newly discovered metastases is true?**

A. Bony metastases tend to be associated with recurrent disease in other sites.
B. Liver metastases tend to be associated with recurrent disease in other sites.
C. Pulmonary metastases tend to be isolated (i.e., not associated with recurrent disease in other sites).
D. Central nervous system (CNS) metastases tend to be isolated.

Question 20.59. **Accepted alternatives to surveillance of lobular carcinoma *in situ* (LCIS) include all of the following EXCEPT**

A. risk reduction bilateral mastectomy
B. risk reduction bilateral salpingo-oophorectomy, regardless of BRCA mutation status
C. risk reduction bilateral salpingo-oophorectomy for patients with known or strongly suspected BRCA-1 or BRCA-2 mutations
D. tamoxifen
E. enrollment on a clinical trial

Question 20.60. **Which of the following patients should be offered genetic counseling to determine if she or her family members are at increased risk for breast cancer?**

A. A woman whose 40-year-old sister has been diagnosed with breast cancer.
B. A woman whose 50-year-old brother has been diagnosed with breast cancer.
C. A woman who has been diagnosed with bilateral breast cancer but has no family history of breast cancer.
D. A and B.
E. A, B, and C.

Question 20.61. **All of the following are factored into a patient's Gail model risk for breast cancer EXCEPT**

A. age
B. age at menarche
C. age at menopause
D. number of children
E. number of first-degree relatives with breast cancer

Question 20.62. **Accurate statements about the Gail model for breast cancer include all of the following EXCEPT**

A. it underestimates hereditary influences on the risk of breast cancer
B. it does not take family cases of male breast cancer into account
C. it does not take family cases of ovarian cancer into account
D. it calculates the 5-year and lifetime risk of breast cancer
E. it explicitly asks whether the patient is pre- or postmenopausal

Question 20.63. **Established criteria for high-risk status for breast cancer include all of the following EXCEPT**

A. family history of early age at diagnosis of breast cancer
B. family history of colon cancer
C. family history of ovarian cancer
D. family history of bilateral breast cancer
E. family history of male breast cancer

Question 20.64. **A woman considering prophylactic mastectomy should understand that all of the following statements are true EXCEPT**

A. it does not remove all breast tissue
B. bilateral subcutaneous mastectomies are as effective as bilateral total (simple) mastectomies
C. it has been shown to reduce risk of breast cancer in women with BRCA mutations by 90%
D. she may further reduce her risk of breast cancer by having prophylactic oophorectomy as well
E. she may further reduce her risk of breast cancer by taking chemoprevention as well

Question 20.65. **Conclusions of the ASCO Technology Assessment on breast cancer risk reduction include which of the following.**

A. The greatest clinical benefit of tamoxifen with fewest side effects is derived by premenopausal women.
B. The greatest clinical benefit of tamoxifen with fewest side effects is derived by women with a uterus.
C. The higher a woman's risk for breast cancer, the lower the absolute benefit she will derive from tamoxifen.
D. Raloxifene is an acceptable substitute for tamoxifen in preventing breast cancer.
E. Aromatase inhibitors are acceptable substitutes for tamoxifen in preventing breast cancer.

Question 20.66. **All breast cancer patients should be screened for risk of developing osteoporosis. Which of the following does not place a woman in the high risk category for osteoporosis?**

A. Age older than 65.
B. Age 60 to 64 and a family history of osteoporosis.
C. Age 60 to 64 and body weight less than 70 kg.
D. Age 60 to 64 and history of a nontraumatic fracture.
E. Poor calcium intake.

Question 20.67. **With regard to screening breast cancer patients who are on tamoxifen for osteoporosis, which of the following is NOT true?**

A. Women at low risk should receive lifestyle advice about preventing osteoporosis, but bone mineral density (BMD) scanning is not necessary.
B. All women at high risk should undergo BMD density screening of the vertebral spine and hip.
C. Acceptable therapies for osteoporosis include alendronate, risedronate, zoledronic acid, and raloxifene.
D. The screening interval for BMD in women with osteoporosis is 1 year.
E. The screening interval for BMD in high-risk women regardless of their baseline BMD is 1 year.

ANSWERS

Answer 20.1. **The answer is D.**

Amplification of oncogenes as well as loss of heterozygosity at multiple loci of tumor suppressor genes is implicated in tumorigenesis. Point mutation and gene methylation may lead to inactivation of the nondominant allele of a tumor suppressor gene, prior to loss of heterozygosity of the other dominant, normal allele due to changes in DNA at multiple loci.

Answer 20.2. **The answer is A.**

In the normal breast gland, estrogen receptor–positive epithelial and proliferative cells function independently of one another, whereas in cancer there is aberrant coupling of the epithelial cells which promote an estrogen-driven proliferative response.

Answer 20.3. **The answer is B.**

Four subtypes of EGFR have been identified: EGFR-1, c-erbB2, c-erbB3, and c-erbB4. The four subtypes form homo- and heterodimers, likely governing the multiple responses of the EGFR receptor family. Trastuzumab acts through a series of steps to downregulate cyclin D1, thereby slowing cell cycle progression. Her-2/neu overexpression is associated with Her-2/neu gene amplification.

Answer 20.4. **The answer is A.**

The half-life of tamoxifen is 7 days. Thus it may take up to 1 month before tumor response may be evaluated under the full effect of tamoxifen.

Answer 20.5. **The answer is D.**

Trastuzumab inhibits Her-2/neu intracellular signaling pathways.

Answer 20.6. **The answer is B.**

A single TRAM flap results in 10% loss of abdominal strength.

Answer 20.7. **The answer is D.**

Both tissue expansion and prosthetic implantation may be accomplished concurrently with the administration of adjuvant chemotherapy.

Answer 20.8. **The answer is E.**

In immediate reconstruction, the inframammary fold, which is preserved or reconstructed, and the breast skin envelope, which is preserved, are critical landmarks for optimizing breast form and symmetry. The other statements are false.

Answer 20.9. **The answer is C.**

Despite a decreased blood supply, increased infection rate, and fat necrosis, there is no significant difference in the rate of flap survival for autologous breast reconstruction before or after radiation treatment.

Answer 20.10. **The answer is B.**

BI-RADS scores range from zero to five. A score of zero represents a mammogram on which there is a finding for which additional imaging is requested by the radiologist. A score of one represents a normal mammogram. A score of two represents a benign finding, whereas a score of three represents a probable benign finding for which follow-up imaging in 6 months is typically recommended. A score of four is indicative of a suspicious abnormality and should prompt biopsy, and a score of five is highly suggestive of malignancy.

Answer 20.11. **The answer is C.**

Depending on the size of the core needle used, greater than 20%, and as many as 50%, of breast biopsies showing atypical hyperplasia may be associated with underlying DCIS. Biopsies showing proliferation but no atypia are associated with a two-fold increased risk of breast cancer. LCIS is usually mammographically occult. Therefore, if a woman has a nonexcisional biopsy for an abnormal finding on mammography, and the biopsy reveals LCIS, an excisional biopsy must be done because there is a high chance that DCIS or invasive disease may have been missed. The false-positive rate for FNA is less than or equal to 1%, although differentiating between DCIS and invasive disease may be difficult.

Answer 20.12. **The answer is C.**

Even within stage I disease, disease-free and overall survival rates are higher for patients with tumors measuring less than 1 cm than for patients with tumors measuring 1 to 2 cm. The number of axillary lymph nodes involved impacts survival in early breast cancer. The greatest decrement in 5-year survival rates is seen between women with 1 to 3 positive lymph nodes and those with 4 to 10 positive lymph nodes. Downstaging of axillary lymph nodes by neoadjuvant chemotherapy has been shown to affect 5-year survival. The number of involved axillary lymph nodes has a greater impact on survival than T-stage for women with locally advanced breast cancer.

Answer 20.13. **The answer is C.**

Confirmation of metastatic disease, particularly in women with a history of early stage disease or who present with solitary lesions, is of utmost importance. For example, this woman could have multiple myeloma; serum and urine protein electrophoresis would help exclude this possibility. Back pain is often the first symptom preceding cord compression, regardless of whether the patient has neurologic findings on physical exam. CT-guided biopsy could help confirm the etiology of the lesion, and narcotic pain medication would provide great relief to the patient.

Answer 20.14. **The answer is A.**

The first patient has T3N1 disease; the second patient has T4N1 disease; the third patient has T2N2 disease; the fourth patient has T3N2 disease; and the fifth patient has T4N2 disease. Staging data for over 400 patients have been reviewed to ascertain which patients are more likely to have metastatic disease and, therefore, for whom a complete staging workup is more likely to yield useful information Three different risk groups were defined. Groups I (T1N0-1) and II (T2N0-1) were found to be at relatively low risk for having metastatic disease; the detection rate for metastatic disease was less than 3%. Group III (T4N1, or patients with N2 disease) had substantially higher risk. The yield for an evaluation for metastatic disease was closer to 15%.

Answer 20.15. **The answer is E.**

Supraclavicular lymph node metastases are now categorized as N3 disease. In the absence of other M1 disease, women with breast cancer with supraclavicular lymph node involvement have disease that behaves more consistently with stage III rather than metastatic disease.

Answer 20.16. **The answer is C.**

There are several contraindications to breast-conserving surgery, such as diffuse microcalcifications, gross multicentric disease, prior radiotherapy, and active collagen vascular disease, but an associated underlying mass in and of itself is not a contraindication to breast conserving surgery.

Answer 20.17. **The answer is C.**

While administering chemotherapy in the neoadjuvant setting does not confer a survival benefit, it may result in breast conservation. However, if a breast tumor progresses during neoadjuvant chemotherapy, chemotherapy should be aborted and the tumor should be surgically removed. The lower the number of lymph nodes involved by cancer after neoadjuvant chemotherapy, the lower the risk a patient will develop recurrent disease.

Answer 20.18. **The answer is B.**

Because 95% to 98% of grade I breast cancers in postmenopausal women are ER-positive, the specimen should be retested to ensure it is truly ER-negative. If it is found to be ER-positive, the patient should be started on hormonal therapy.

Answer 20.19. **The answer is B.**

A review by the Early Breast Cancer Trialists' Collaborative Group (EBCTCG) found a decrement in benefit with adjuvant chemotherapy with each advancing decade of patient age.

Answer 20.20. **The answer is C.**

Adjuvant chemotherapy confers the same reduction in the risk of recurrent disease to all groups of patients. In other words, the *relative* risk reduction is the same. However, since some patients are at higher risk of having disease relapse, their *absolute* benefit will be greater. Thus, the absolute reduction in relapse and death will be greatest in high-risk patients and smallest in low-risk patients.

Answer 20.21. **The answer is C.**

The optimal way to incorporate taxanes into the neoadjuvant treatment of early breast cancer is not clear. Paclitaxel and docetaxel are both effective agents, but there has been no head-to-head comparison of them in the neoadjuvant setting to know whether one is better than the other. There are also no data to know whether they are more effective if used concurrently or sequentially. The use of taxanes increases pathologic complete response. Despite the increase in disease-free survival conferred by taxanes, toxicity is augmented.

Answer 20.22. **The answer is A.**

As long as any residual intraductal carcinoma does not extend beyond the quadrant in which a woman's tumor was located, small-volume residual intraductal carcinoma is not a contraindication for BCT.

Answer 20.23. **The answer is B.**

Insufficient evidence exists to recommend the routine use of PMRT in patients with T1/2 tumors with one to three positive axillary lymph nodes. Sufficient evidence also fails to exist to support the use of a supraclavicular field in patients with one to three axillary lymph nodes. Full axillary radiotherapy is not needed if a woman has undergone a level I/II axillary lymph node dissection. There is insufficient evidence to suggest that the ASCO radiotherapy guidelines should be applied differently to special subgroups of patients.

Answer 20.24. **The answer is E.**

It is not uncommon for an underlying tumor to be several centimeters away from the nipple. A wedge or punch biopsy of the nipple, particularly in cases without a palpable breast mass, is the preferred procedure to make the diagnosis and, importantly, exclude melanoma. Half of cases are hormone-receptor negative, consistent with the higher rate of underlying high-grade tumors.

Answer 20.25. **The answer is A.**

Fifty percent of cases of Paget disease are associated with a palpable mass. Twenty percent of cases present without a palpable mass but abnormal findings are seen on mammogram. Twenty-five percent of cases present with neither a mass nor a mammographic abnormality. In 5% of cases, no underlying neoplasm is found.

Answer 20.26. **The answer is B.**

There is insufficient evidence to know whether internal mammary nodal irradiation should be used in any patient subgroup.

Answer 20.27. **The answer is C.**

Neoadjuvant chemotherapy plays a multifaceted role in the treatment of locally advanced breast cancer. It may downsize a tumor, making it more amenable to breast-conserving treatment or helping to achieve a more acceptable cosmetic result. It may downstage the patient's disease by decreasing the number of positive axillary lymph nodes, thereby improving survival. Giving neoadjuvant chemotherapy allows the oncologist to gauge the chemosensitivity of the tumor. Regardless of whether chemotherapy is given in the neoadjuvant or adjuvant setting, post-surgical radiation is still required, and outcome is the same. Hormonal therapy improves outcome and should be given after any additional adjuvant treatment. Locally advanced breast cancers include patients with chest wall disease, inflammatory breast cancer, aggressive histologic subtypes, and supraclavicular involvement, and therefore represent a heterogeneous population.

Answer 20.28. **The answer is A.**

NSABP-B18 demonstrated that 14% of patients who initially required mastectomy were able to have breast-conserving treatment after receiving neoadjuvant chemotherapy.

Answer 20.29. **The answer is D.**

IBC is a clinical diagnosis. Dermal lymphatic invasion on full-thickness skin biopsy is often seen but not required for diagnosis. Fever and leukocytosis should be excluded to ensure the absence of cellulitis or granulytic sarcoma. Most women will have lymph node involvement. In the absence of distant metastases, IBC is staged as T4d, stage IIIC disease.

Answer 20.30. **The answer is E.**

Tumors that express both the estrogen and progesterone receptors are associated with a 70% chance of response to endocrine therapy. Those that express either the estrogen receptor or the progesterone receptor (but not the other) are associated with a 40% chance of response to endocrine therapy. However, those that express neither are associated with a less than 10% chance of response to endocrine therapy.

Answer 20.31. **The answer is A.**

Despite her disease progressing on trastuzumab, the patient may benefit from combination chemotherapy with capecitabine and trastuzumab. Studies have shown synergy between these drugs.

Answer 20.32. **The answer is B.**

Combination chemotherapy has demonstrated increased response rates but no definite improvement in overall survival. Although some studies have suggested an improvement in survival, these trials have been limited by lack of adequate crossover to ensure a survival advantage even when patients on what appears to be the inferior arm receive alternative treatment. Combination chemotherapy comes at the cost of additional toxicity and is best reserved for patients with severely symptomatic or rapidly progressive disease to maximize the chance of response and remission of disease. As long as a patient does not have severe symptoms or clinical findings concerning the patient's imminent demise, hormonal or single-agent chemotherapy may be implemented, based on the patient's receptor status.

Answer 20.33. **The answer is B.**

Hormonal therapy is the appropriate consideration for this patient. Visceral disease does not mandate chemotherapy. If the patient develops rapidly progressive disease, then chemotherapy could be considered as positive effects may be realized more rapidly than for hormonal therapy. Treatment should be initiated immediately, before the patient's performance status declines. Neither chemoembolization nor metastatectomy are appropriate considerations for this patient with diffuse hepatic disease.

Answer 20.34. **The answer is C.**

There is insufficient data to support the efficacy of one bisphosphonate over another. In the absence of bone destruction on imaging exams, bisphosphonates are not indicated. The presence or absence of bone pain should not affect the decision to initiate treatment with bisphosphonates.

Answer 20.35. **The answer is E.**

In addition to the other risk factors mentioned, family history is a key risk factor for development of male breast cancer.

Answer 20.36. **The answer is A.**

Approximately 80% of cases of male breast cancer are estrogen-receptor positive, presumably since men are effectively postmenopausal. There does not appear to be a difference in the chances a tumor will be estrogen-receptor positive depending on the age of a male patient with breast cancer.

Answer 20.37. **The answer is C.**

As in women, DCIS is primarily a local disease with excellent prognosis, and axillary node dissection is not necessary.

Answer 20.38. **The answer is D.**

Serum alkaline phosphatase levels are increased in pregnancy and should be interpreted in conjunction with clinical findings in assessing patients for liver or bone metastases.

Answer 20.39. **The answer is B.**

Breast cancer during pregnancy is usually detected at a later stage and is generally associated with a poorer survival than breast cancer detected in nonpregnant patients. The fetus may incur significant radiation exposure with CT scanning; therefore CT should be avoided. MRI, however, is safe and poses no harm to the fetus. Pregnant patients may undergo a sentinel lymph node procedure with little risk to the fetus; however, as many as 60% of pregnant patients with breast cancer will be found to have positive axillary nodes, and so a full axillary dissection remains the preferred procedure for most patients.

Answer 20.40. **The answer is B.**

Since breast irradiation is contraindicated in the pregnant patient, mastectomy may prove to be a more appropriate management approach even in patients with tumors amenable to breast conservation, particular in women early in pregnancy.

Answer 20.41. **The answer is D.**

As with bone metastases, patients with metastatic skin changes from breast cancer who are on tamoxifen or antiestrogen medications may experience a "flare reaction" in which new nodules may appear or skin erythema worsens. Tamoxifen has a half-life of 7 days. Tumor flare reactions may occur as early as 2 days and as late as 3 weeks. Treatment response is best assessed at 4 to 6 weeks. In the meantime, patients should be treated symptomatically. If there is no improvement in their skin changes or bone pain by after 6 weeks on tamoxifen, alternative treatment should be considered.

Answer 20.42. **The answer is C.**

Though more commonly seen in patients on tamoxifen or antiestrogen medications, aromatase inhibitors may also cause a tumor flare response. Five percent of patients with tumor flare will also develop hypercalcemia.

Answer 20.43. **The answer is A.**

Without cardiac medication, toxicity related to adriamycin is generally irreversible, whereas heart failure related to trastuzumab generally improves with discontinuation of the drug.

Answer 20.44. **The answer is D.**

Symptoms related to chemotherapy-related premature ovarian failure are often more rapid in onset and severe in intensity than in natural menopause.

Answer 20.45. **The answer is A.**

Two main principles of lymphedema prevention are to avoid increased lymph production or blood flow and to avoid blockage of lymph transport. Patients should be advised to avoid strenuous exertion, but, if they choose to exercise, a compression arm garment should be worn.

Answer 20.46. **The answer is C.**

The long-term incidence of lymphedema is fully 25% to 30%. Breast irradiation is estimated to double the incidence of lymphedema. The risk of lymphedema is decreased for a sentinel node biopsy as opposed to lymph node dissection, but is still a risk, particularly if a lymph node bridge is destroyed or the node is close to the lymph trunk. Lymphedema spares effect on underlying muscle but has dreaded effects on the skin and subcutaneous tissue. Lymphedema can occur several years after treatment.

Answer 20.47. **The answer is D.**

The incidence of leukemia is approximately 1% at 10 years. Data with short-term follow-up suggest that taxanes do not increase the risk of hematologic malignancy. The latency period for hematologic malignancies after treatment with anthracyclines ranges from 6 months to 5 years, whereas the latency period for developing disease after treatment with an alkylating agent, such as cyclophosphamide, is longer—often 5 to 7 years and preceded by MDS.

Answer 20.48. **The answer is E.**

Patients with neurologic compromise from a vertebral compression fracture require neurosurgical intervention, particularly if their life expectancy is estimated to be greater than the length of time to recover from the surgery. Patients who may be cured from en bloc resection should also be referred for neurosurgical intervention. Patients whose pain is mild to moderate and controllable with analgesics may not require an invasive procedure like kyphoplasty, but a patient whose pain is severe or acute will likely benefit from the procedure. Patients with involvement of the posterior vertebral elements are more likely to have spinal instability and should be referred for neurosurgical intervention.

Answer 20.49. **The answer is E.**

Patients with skeletal metastases are most likely to benefit from radionuclide treatment if their tumor is osteoblastic because the radionuclide will localize to blastic lesions. Radionuclides are used for patients with severe pain in multiple locations. Patients with severe pain in only one or two locations or pain uncontrolled by analgesics should be referred for radiation for external beam palliation of pain. Patients who have not yet exhausted cytotoxic chemotherapy treatment options, or who have hormone-sensitive tumors and have not exhausted antihormonal treatment options, receive these treatments. Radionuclides used to treat diffuse skeletal metastases cause significant, prolonged myelosuppression. It should be noted that patients included in the samarium study by Serafini were not heavily pretreated with cytotoxic chemotherapy. Patients who are heavily pretreated will likely have more prolonged recovery from cytopenias than did patients in the study whose median recovery from thrombocytopenia was 2 months.

Answer 20.50. **The answer is B.**

The classic criteria for internal fixation include 50% cortical involvement, a 2.5-cm lesion, and no response to radiotherapy. Lytic bone lesions require orthopedic prosthetic support due to the weak nature of lytic bone matrix. Functional pain is especially debilitating to patients and requires aggressive intervention.

Answer 20.51. **The answer is C.**

Even in the absence of grossly metastatic CNS disease, breast cancer has a predilection for tracking along the optic nerve and extraocular muscles. An MRI of her orbits would reveal metastatic disease, and a radiation oncology consult to plan for radiotherapy of the orbit would be appropriate.

Answer 20.52. **The answer is C.**

Despite having neither focal neurologic complaints nor findings on physical exam, it is crucial to exclude impending spinal cord compression from metastatic disease. Pain is the first symptom heralding cord compression. Even with a normal lumbar x-ray, the patient could still have impending cord compression. Although a bone scan will identify multifocal bony metastatic disease, it will not exclude cord compression.

Answer 20.53. **The answer is B.**

The three component scores are added to arrive at the global SBR histologic grade. A score of 3 to 5 represents a well-differentiated tumor, a score of 6 to 7 represents a moderately well-differentiated tumor, and a score of 8 to 9 represents a poorly differentiated tumor.

Answer 20.54. **The answer is D.**

In addition to tumor grade, hormonal status, and pathologic node status, clinical response to neoadjuvant chemotherapy is an independent prognostic factor for survival.

Answer 20.55. **The answer is C.**

Studies have shown that oncologists routinely overestimate the potential benefit of adjuvant therapy. Patients overestimate the risk and benefit of such therapy. The "Adjuvant!" program provides 10-year overall and disease-free survival data to give a woman a more precise picture of the potential impact adjuvant therapy may have on her disease. "Adjuvant!" has been clinically validated and provides remarkably accurate projections, although it currently tends to overestimate slightly the benefit of combined chemotherapy and hormonal therapy.

Answer 20.56. **The answer is A.**

Screening mammography is the only imaging study recommended for routine surveillance. A woman should have a mammogram of her conserved breast 6 months after completion of radiotherapy and at least annually thereafter.

Answer 20.57. **The answer is A.**

Approximately 30% of all patients with stage I and stage II breast cancer will eventually experience a relapse of their disease. The hazard risk for recurrence is not constant and peaks within the first 2 years following surgery. Even patients beyond 5 years of follow-up have measurable relapse rates and are candidates for risk reduction trials looking at novel agents. There is no proven role for the use of tumor markers in the surveillance of breast cancer. Tumors that lack the estrogen receptor are more likely to relapse in visceral organs than those that do not lack the receptor.

Answer 20.58. **The answer is B.**

As with lung and liver metastases, CNS metastases tend to be associated with recurrent disease in other sites and, therefore, a full restaging evaluation including CT scans of the chest, abdomen, and pelvis, as well as a bone scan, should be done. Bony metastases tend to be isolated. A full restaging evaluation is not mandatory unless the patient has symptoms or other clinical findings to warrant further evaluation. However, as much as is possible, new disease that appears to be metastatic disease should be confirmed by biopsy to exclude the possibility of a new primary tumor.

Answer 20.59. **The answer is B.**

For women who desire risk-reduction therapy, all of the other options listed are acceptable, but a risk-reduction bilateral salpingo-oophorectomy should only be recommended for patients with known or strongly suspected BRCA-1 or BRCA-2 mutations.

Answer 20.60. **The answer is E.**

Factors associated with hereditary breast cancer include multiple family members with breast cancer, bilateral disease, ovarian cancer, male breast cancer, and young age at diagnosis (less than or equal to age 40).

Answer 20.61. **The answer is D.**

In calculating a woman's Gail model risk for breast cancer, the number of breast biopsies she has had with and without atypia are also taken into account. Age at first live birth is also factored into this calculation of a woman's risk for breast cancer, but total number of children is not.

Answer 20.62. **The answer is E.**

The Gail risk model underestimates hereditary influences on the risk of breast cancer because it considers only how many first-degree relatives have breast cancer. It does not count how many men in the family have had breast cancer, nor does it consider how many family members may have had ovarian cancer. Although it takes a patient's age into consideration, it does not ask whether the patient is pre- or postmenopausal.

Answer 20.63. **The answer is B.**

A family history of ovarian cancer places a patient at higher risk for developing breast cancer than does a family history of colon cancer. A family at high risk has features suggestive of an autosomal dominant predisposition to breast cancer.

Answer 20.64. **The answer is B.**

A prophylactic mastectomy removes most, but not all, of breast tissue. Bilateral total (simple) mastectomies are more effective than bilateral subcutaneous mastectomies. In addition to prophylactic mastectomy, women at high risk for breast cancer should consider prophylactic oophorectomy as well as chemoprevention.

Answer 20.65. **The answer is A.**

The greatest clinical benefit of tamoxifen with fewest side effects is derived by premenopausal women who have a lower risk for thromboembolic events. Women without a uterus who are on tamoxifen are unlikely to develop uterine cancer. The higher a woman's risk for breast cancer, the greater the absolute benefit she will derive. Neither raloxifene nor aromatase inhibitors are currently acceptable alternatives for chemoprevention of breast cancer.

Answer 20.66. **The answer is E.**

While a risk factor, poor calcium intake itself does not place women in the high-risk category for osteoporosis. All breast cancer patients, regardless of their risk for osteoporosis, should be instructed to begin calcium and vitamin D.

Answer 20.67. **The answer is C.**

Because it is structurally similar to tamoxifen, and there is evidence of detriment when tamoxifen has been used for longer than 5 years, caution should be used in considering raloxifene for the treatment of osteoporosis.

CHAPTER 21

Cancer of the Endocrine System

MOUHAMMED AMIR HABRA

Directions Each of the numbered items below is followed by lettered answers. Select the ONE lettered answer that is BEST in each case unless instructed otherwise.

QUESTIONS

Question 21.1. **A 35-year-old woman is found to have a left thyroid mass on routine physical examination. She is healthy otherwise and denies any compressive symptoms. There is no past history of radiation exposure or family history of thyroid cancer. Neck ultrasound reveals a 2-cm hypoechoic left thyroid nodule with microcalcifications and a 0.5-cm hypoechoic nodule in the right thyroid lobe without evidence of cervical lymphadenopathy. Fine needle aspiration shows thyroid follicular cells with nuclear grooves and intranuclear cytoplasmic inclusions suggestive of papillary thyroid carcinoma. The appropriate initial management in this patient is**

A. total thyroidectomy with modified left neck dissection
B. left thyroid lobectomy
C. total thyroidectomy
D. total thyroidectomy with bilateral neck dissection

Question 21.2. **A 30-year-old woman with multinodular goiter elects to have near-total thyroidectomy for cosmetic reasons. Preoperative neck ultrasound does not reveal cervical lymphadenopathy and thyroid functions are normal. She had successful surgery 1 week ago and her pathology specimen showed a 0.3-cm focus of papillary thyroid carcinoma but otherwise confirmed the diagnosis of benign multinodular goiter. The best management of this patient is**

A. start thyroid hormone replacement only
B. radioactive iodine scan followed by radioactive iodine ablation if there is neck uptake
C. resect the remaining thyroid tissue followed by radioactive iodine ablation
D. radioactive iodine ablation followed by thyroid hormone suppression

Corresponding Chapters in *Cancer: Principles & Practice of Oncology*, Seventh Edition: 34 (Cancer of the Endocrine System).

Question 21.3. **A 50-year-old woman is found to have a left thyroid mass on routine physical examination. Thyroid functions are normal and her neck ultrasound reveals a 3-cm hypoechoic nodule in the left lobe only. Fine needle aspiration biopsy yields a cellular aspirate with scant colloid and is read as follicular neoplasm. The appropriate initial management in this patient is**

A. left lobectomy followed by completion thyroidectomy later if malignancy was found
B. total thyroidectomy
C. left lobectomy and intraoperative frozen section biopsy to plan the extent of resection
D. repeat ultrasound-guided biopsy to obtain more tissue

Question 21.4. **A 42-year-old woman has a history of papillary thyroid carcinoma diagnosed 10 years ago. She underwent total thyroidectomy with neck dissection and was found to have multifocal disease (largest focus 2.5 cm) with six positive lymph nodes bilaterally. She initially received 100 mCi ^{131}I with posttreatment scan showing thyroid bed uptake only. Thereafter, she had two negative whole body iodine scans but her serum thyroglobulin remained detectable (5 to 8 ng per mL) while thyroid-stimulating hormone (TSH) was suppressed. The next step in evaluation is**

A. neck ultrasound
B. positron emission tomography (PET) scan
C. continued observation
D. chest x-ray

Question 21.5. **A 20-year-old woman was recently found to have a left thyroid nodule. She is totally asymptomatic except for a 6-month history of diarrhea. Her mother died suddenly at the age of 32 and her maternal grandfather had a history of nephrolithiasis and goiter. Her examination is unremarkable except for a 3-cm thyroid mass with a few palpable cervical lymph nodes bilaterally. Fine needle aspiration biopsy showed neuroendocrine cells with positive calcitonin staining. The next most appropriate steps are**

A. serum calcitonin/thyroglobulin, then proceed with total thyroidectomy
B. measure metanephrines and catecholamines/serum calcium/serum calcitonin/carcinoembryonic antigen (CEA)/*RET* protooncogene
C. measure metanephrines and catecholamines/serum calcium/calcitonin/CEA
D. proceed with emergent surgery, then perform postoperative evaluation

Question 21.6. **A 65-year-old man presents with a 6-month history of right neck mass and a 2-week history of intermittent hoarseness. Neck ultrasound reveals a 5-cm hypoechoic right thyroid mass. Fine needle aspiration biopsy highly suggests papillary thyroid carcinoma. Total thyroidectomy is attempted without complications. The specimen contains a 5-cm papillary thyroid carcinoma in the right lobe only without extrathyroidal extension. None of the resected lymph nodes contains papillary thyroid carcinoma. The next appropriate step is**

A. radioactive iodine ablation
B. radiation therapy
C. chemotherapy
D. combined concurrent chemotherapy and radiotherapy
E. careful observation only

Question 21.7. **A 75-year-old patient had papillary thyroid carcinoma in 1975 and was treated with total thyroidectomy followed by radioactive ablation. Thereafter, he was followed for 15 years and his whole-body iodine scans and chest x-rays were normal. Further follow-up was discontinued. Recently, he presented with dysphagia, mainly to solids. Laboratory workup showed a thyroglobulin level of 120 ng per mL with negative antibodies while the patient is on thyroid hormone suppression therapy. Computed tomography (CT) scan of the neck and chest revealed a 4-cm cervical mass in the tracheoesophageal groove; otherwise CT scan of the chest is normal. A positron emission tomography (PET) scan showed a fluorodeoxyglucose-avid (FDG) lesion corresponding to the mass discovered on CT; otherwise, there was physiologic tracer uptake. The best treatment option at present is**

A. esophageal stent placement
B. external beam radiotherapy
C. chemotherapy
D. radioactive iodine ablation
E. surgical resection to achieve local control followed by external beam radiation therapy

Question 21.8. **A 28-year-old woman was found to have a right thyroid mass. At age 12, she had Hodgkin disease and was treated with combination chemotherapy and radiation therapy involving the neck. Fine needle aspiration therapy was diagnostic for papillary thyroid carcinoma. The expected abnormality in this case is**

A. *RET* protooncogene mutation
B. *APC* gene mutation
C. *BRAF* mutation
D. *RET/PTC* rearrangement

Question 21.9. **Which of the following factors negatively affects survival in papillary thyroid carcinoma in a 35-year-old man?**

A. Age.
B. Cervical lymphadenopathy.
C. Large tumor size.
D. All of the above.

Question 21.10. **A 40-year-old woman with a history of (T1N1a, M0) papillary thyroid carcinoma was treated 2 years ago with total thyroidectomy followed by radioactive iodine ablation for thyroid bed activity. Last year, her thyroglobulin level was 0.5 ng per mL and her neck ultrasound and whole-body iodine scan were both negative. This year she came for follow-up and reported feeling well on thyroid hormone suppression. Her thyroglobulin is 0.4 ng per mL with negative antibodies, while her TSH is 0.1 μ unit per mL. The suggested approach in follow-up is**

A. repeat whole body iodine scan
B. obtain stimulated thyroglobulin value
C. reduce thyroid hormone dose to keep TSH in normal range
D. obtain PET scan

Question 21.11. **In the workup of medullary thyroid carcinoma, which of the following is correct?**

A. Genetic testing is needed even in the absence of family history of medullary thyroid carcinoma.
B. Plasma metanephrines should be assessed within a few weeks after thyroidectomy.
C. PET scan should be part of the initial staging.
D. Calcium stimulation is needed to identify family members at risk.

Question 21.12. **The goal of surgical treatment in patients with anaplastic thyroid carcinoma is**

A. local disease control
B. disease cure
C. facilitate radioactive iodine ablation
D. none of the above

Question 21.13. **Which of the following is needed in the follow-up of patients with medullary thyroid carcinoma and elevated calcitonin?**

A. Contrast CT scan of the chest/abdomen.
B. Ultrasound of the neck.
C. Serum CEA.
D. Bone scan.
E. All of the above.

Question 21.14. **All of the following variants of papillary thyroid carcinoma are associated with worse prognosis EXCEPT**

A. follicular variant
B. columnar variant
C. tall cell variant
D. all of the above
E. none of the above

Question 21.15. **Anaplastic thyroid carcinoma is considered stage IV disease in the presence of**

A. cervical lymphadenopathy
B. lung or bone metastases
C. anaplastic thyroid carcinoma is considered stage IV at presentation
D. none of the above

Question 21.16. **The agent most commonly used chemotherapy agent in metastatic thyroid carcinoma is**

A. doxorubicin (Adriamycin)
B. 5-fluorouracil (5FU)
C. cisplatin
D. methotrexate (MTX)

Question 21.17. **A 55-year-old man presents with a 1-month history of fatigue and polyuria. His past medical history and family history are unremarkable. On laboratory workup, his serum calcium is 15.5 mg per dL, phosphorus 1.9 mg per dL, and intact parathormone (PTH) 450 pg per mL (normal 10 to 65). The patient feels better after treatment with intravenous (IV) hydration, intravenous bisphosphonates, and subcutaneous calcitonin. Parathyroid sestamibi scan reveals an intense tracer uptake in the area of the right inferior parathyroid gland that persists on delayed images. CT of the neck also confirms the presence of a 3-cm mass matching the area of uptake seen on the parathyroid scan. Parathyroid carcinoma is suspected in the presence of severe PTH-mediated hypercalcemia and neck mass. Further imaging studies do not suggest the presence of metastases. The suggested treatment in this case is**

A. total or subtotal parathyroidectomy
B. en bloc resection followed by adjuvant external beam irradiation to the neck
C. external beam irradiation only
D. chemotherapy after confirming the diagnosis

Question 21.18. **A 70-year-old woman with parathyroid carcinoma was referred for recurrent hypercalcemia 6 months after initial surgical resection of her primary tumor. Her initial tumor measured 4 cm and was resected successfully along with the left thyroid lobe and the surrounding soft tissue. Serum calcium and intact PTH were normal for 3 months after surgery, but for the past 3 months, there has been a gradual increase in serum calcium. Currently her serum calcium is 14.4 mg per dL, intact PTH 270 pg per mL, and serum phosphorus is 2.0 mg per dL. Imaging studies reveal multiple nodules in the neck measuring 5 to 8 mm in addition to numerous new pulmonary nodules. Which of the following is indicated to control her hypercalcemia?**

A. Cinacalcet.
B. Mithramycin.
C. Hydration.
D. IV bisphosphonates.
E. All of the above.

Question 21.19. **Which of the following syndromes is associated with parathyroid carcinoma?**

A. Hyperparathyroidism/Jaw tumor syndrome.
B. Familial hypercalciuric hypocalcemia.
C. Multiple endocrine neoplasia-2 (MEN-2).
D. Familial hypocalciuric hypercalcemia.

Question 21.20. **The staging of parathyroid carcinoma is based on**

A. tumor, nodes, metastases (TNM)
B. age, gender, metastases, tumor size
C. no clear staging system

Questions 21.21–21.22.

A 28-year-old man presents with a 12-month history of impotence and loss of libido. He is adopted and no family history could be obtained. He is married and has two healthy children, and his past medical history is otherwise negative except for an episode of nephrolithiasis at 20 years of age. Laboratory workup reveals a prolactin level of 300 ng per mL, serum testosterone of 110 ng per dL (250 to 800), serum calcium of 11 mg per dL, and intact PTH of 150 pg per mL. MRI of the sella reveals a 1.5-cm sellar mass displacing the pituitary stalk to the left but not affecting the optic chiasm.

Question 21.21. **The expected genetic disorder in this case is**

A. *menin* gene mutation
B. *RET* protooncogene mutation
C. inactivating calcium sensing receptor *(CaSR)* mutation
D. *RET/PTC* rearrangement

Question 21.22. **The appropriate treatment of this patient includes**

A. dopamine agonists (bromocriptine or cabergoline) with subtotal parathyroidectomy
B. subtotal parathyroidectomy with prophylactic pancreatectomy
C. transsphenoidal pituitary resection with subtotal parathyroidectomy

Questions 21.23–21.24.

A 25-year-old man presents with a neck mass and cervical lymphadenopathy. Ultrasound-guided fine needle aspiration biopsy suggests the diagnosis of medullary thyroid carcinoma (MTC). Preoperative laboratory workup shows serum calcium of 9.1 mg per dL, intact PTH of 28 pg per mL, serum calcitonin of 2,300 pg per mL (normal 0 to 4), and plasma free metanephrine of 2.2 nmol per L (normal is <0.5). MRI of the abdomen shows a 2-cm right adrenal mass that appears hyperintense on T2-weighted images.

Question 21.23. **The appropriate management of this case is**

A. proceed with total thyroidectomy and central neck dissection followed by right adrenalectomy
B. right adrenalectomy, then proceed with total thyroidectomy and neck dissection
C. right adrenalectomy followed by subtotal parathyroidectomy and total thyroidectomy
D. total thyroidectomy with neck dissection alone

Question 21.24. **The patient reports having chronic pruritic rash on his back and family history of MEN-2. The expected RET protooncogene mutation in this family is**

A. codon 609 mutation
B. codon 634 mutation
C. codon 768 mutation
D. codon 918 mutation

Question 21.25. **The most common MEN-1 related cause of death is**

A. hypercalcemia
B. pituitary insufficiency
C. metastatic pancreatic neuroendocrine tumors (PNETs)
D. gastric carcinoid

Question 21.26. **Which disorder is associated with mutated *RET* protooncogene?**

A. MEN-1.
B. Hirschsprung disease.
C. Sporadic MTC.
D. Familial paraganglioma.

Question 21.27. **A 50-year-old woman is found to have a 4-cm right adrenal mass on CT scan obtained to evaluate left-sided abdominal pain. She is healthy otherwise and is not taking any medications. There is no history of systemic hypertension, hypokalemia, or diabetes mellitus. Her weight is stable [body mass index (BMI): 24 kg per m^2], and she denies palpitations, hirsutism, skin changes, or muscle weakness. Her family history is negative for adrenal masses, thyroid cancer, or hypercalcemia. On physical examination her blood pressure (BP) is 145/89 mm Hg and her pulse is 85 beats per minute. Otherwise her physical examination is normal. The next step in evaluation is**

A. CT-guided fine needle aspiration
B. plasma metanephrines, overnight dexamethasone suppression, plasma rennin activity, and plasma aldosterone concentration
C. MRI of the abdomen
D. laparoscopic adrenalectomy

Question 21.28. **A 40-year-old man presents with a 6-month history of right shoulder pain. His past medical history is significant only for left adrenalectomy for pheochromocytoma at the age of 35. He is otherwise asymptomatic and denies any history suggestive of familial disorder. Further workup suggests the presence of multiple bone metastases and reveals elevated plasma free normetanephrine. Both diagnostic metaiodobenzoguanidine (MIBG) scan and Octreoscan show multiple areas of uptake in the spine, ribs, and shoulders. The suggested treatment in this patient is**

A. local irradiation therapy and systemic chemotherapy (cyclophosphamide, vincristine, and doxorubicin)
B. high-dose MIBG therapy
C. long-acting octreotide
D. interferon therapy
E. B and C
F. A and B

Question 21.29. **A 55-year-old woman presents with a 3-month history of unintentional weight loss, fatigue, and hirsutism. She complains of vague left upper quadrant discomfort and is otherwise asymptomatic. CT of the abdomen shows a heterogeneous 7-cm left adrenal mass. Chemical workup shows a serum testosterone level of 350 ng per dL; other tests are normal. The next step in management is**

A. systemic chemotherapy
B. CT-guided fine needle aspiration
C. laparoscopic adrenalectomy
D. open adrenalectomy

Question 21.30. **CT scan features that suggest adrenal adenoma include**

A. heterogeneous appearance
B. density of less than 10 Hounsfield units on nonenhanced CT
C. washout less than 50% at 15 minutes postcontrast
D. irregular borders

Question 21.31. **Mutations of all of the following genes are associated with extraadrenal pheochromocytoma EXCEPT**

A. *RET* protooncogene
B. *VHL* gene (von Hippel–Lindau gene)
C. *SDHB*
D. *SDHD*

Question 21.32. **The expected side effects of mitotane during the treatment of adrenocortical carcinoma include**

A. neuropathy
B. gastrointestinal (GI) side effects
C. adrenal insufficiency
D. fatigue
E. all of the above

Question 21.33. **A 30-year-old man presents with hematemesis. He reports having a 1-year history of diarrhea and occasional epigastric discomfort. He denies recent use of corticosteroids or nonsteroidal antiinflammatory drugs (NSAIDs). His past medical history is negative otherwise. His mother has a history of nephrolithiasis and was treated successfully with medical therapy only for infertility. His father has diabetes mellitus and hypertension. Laboratory workup shows hemoglobin level of 10 g per dL, blood urea nitrogen (BUN) of 25 mg per dL, creatinine of 1.2 mg per dL, serum calcium of 10.7 mg per dL, and intact parathormone (PTH) of 78 pg per mL. Upper GI endoscopy reveals multiple duodenal ulcers without active bleeding. Serum gastrin is 600 pg per mL with gastric pH of 2 obtained at the time of endoscopy. The most likely diagnosis in this case is**

A. hypergastrinemia in the presence of atrophic gastritis
B. gastrinoma in the presence of MEN-1
C. hypergastrinemia secondary to acid-reducing therapy
D. sporadic gastrinoma

Question 21.34. **A 55-year-old man presents with diarrhea and occasional flushing after alcohol drinking. He is healthy otherwise. The diarrhea is not controlled by over-the-counter medications. He denies other symptoms except for occasional dyspnea and wheezing. The most appropriate test in this case is**

A. serum gastrin
B. serum vasoactive intestinal peptide (VIP)
C. twenty-four hours urinary 5-hydroxy indole acetic acid (5-HIAA)
D. serum glucagon
E. calcitonin

Question 21.35. **The least malignant pancreatic endocrine tumor is**

A. glucagonoma
B. gastrinoma
C. PPoma
D. VIPoma
E. insulinoma

ANSWERS

Answer 21.1. **The answer is C.**

Total thyroidectomy is indicated in this young patient with papillary thyroid carcinoma, especially considering that her preoperative ultrasound raises the possibility of multifocal disease. Neck dissection is not routine in the absence of clinical or ultrasound evidence of cervical lymphadenopathy.

Answer 21.2. **The answer is A.**

This young patient has incidental microscopic papillary thyroid carcinoma. There is no need for further cancer-directed therapy in this case in the absence of multifocal disease or cervical lymphadenopathy. Thyroid hormone replacement should be initiated to maintain TSH in the normal range.

Answer 21.3. **The answer is A.**

Fine needle aspiration biopsy cannot distinguish benign from malignant follicular lesions. Intraoperative frozen section is theoretically useful but has resulted in added expense without adding useful information in the many patients with follicular neoplasms. The distinction between benign and malignant follicular lesions should be made upon finding vascular or capsular invasion.

Answer 21.4. **The answer is A.**

This patient has a low level of thyroglobulin that is most likely secondary to cervical lymphadenopathy. Neck ultrasound is likely to be sufficient to identify the extent of her disease and facilitate ultrasound-guided fine needle aspiration if needed. PET scan is indicated in patients with negative iodine scans and higher levels of thyroglobulin (>10 to 20 ng per mL). Chest x-ray is likely to be normal in this patient with low levels of thyroglobulin.

Answer 21.5. **The answer is B.**

This patient has multiple endocrine neoplasia 2-A. Pheochromocytoma has to be excluded prior to any intervention. Calcitonin and CEA can be used as tumor markers in medullary thyroid carcinoma. Genetic testing (*RET* protooncogene) is important even in cases that initially appear sporadic.

Answer 21.6. **The answer is A.**

This patient has (T3N0, Mx) disease and because of his age (older than 45), he is considered to have stage III disease. Postoperative radioactive iodine ablation is justified using doses 100 to 150 mCi. This will help to eradicate the normal residual thyroid tissue, reveal distant metastases if present, and improve the interpretation of the thyroglobulin level during follow-up. Radiation therapy is unnecessary in the absence of extrathyroidal extension or cervical lymphadenopathy. Chemotherapy is not indicated in the absence of widely metastatic disease with rapid growth.

Answer 21.7. **The answer is E.**

This patient has dedifferentiated papillary thyroid carcinoma as illustrated by the previously negative iodine scans and positive PET scan. He also illustrates the importance of life long-term follow-up and utilizing thyroglobulin monitoring in addition to imaging studies. Considering his age, the best treatment option is to achieve local control and prevent local recurrence.

Answer 21.8. **The answer is D.**

RET/PTC rearrangement is the expected abnormality in patients with papillary thyroid carcinoma and prior history of radiation exposure. *BRAF* mutation is another finding in patients with papillary thyroid carcinoma but it is not associated with radiation exposure. *APC* gene mutation is found in patients with familial adenomatous polyposis, and some of these patients might develop differentiated thyroid carcinoma. *RET* protooncogene mutations are associated with multiple endocrine neoplasia type 2.

Answer 21.9. **The answer is C.**

Large tumor size increases disease-specific mortality in patients with papillary thyroid carcinoma. In contrast, the prognosis is remarkably better for individuals diagnosed between the ages of 20 and 45. Cervical lymphadenopathy increases the recurrence rate but is unlikely to affect long-term survival in this case.

Answer 21.10. **The answer is B.**

This patient is at low risk of long-term complications from papillary thyroid carcinoma. Stimulated thyroglobulin has proven to be more sensitive in detecting disease when compared to iodine scans. PET scan is indicated in the presence of negative whole-body iodine scan and serum thyroglobulin in excess of 10 ng per mL. TSH suppression may still be of value in the first few years after initial diagnosis in a low-risk patient who had positive lymph nodes initially.

Answer 21.11. **The answer is A.**

RET protooncogene testing is indicated even in cases that appear to be sporadic. Genetic testing helps in identifying and screening family members and has replaced the previous stimulation tests. PET scan is not part of the essential screening. Pheochromocytoma needs to be ruled out prior to attempting surgical resection in these cases.

Answer 21.12. **The answer is A.**

Anaplastic thyroid carcinoma carries poor prognosis. Surgery is reserved to selected cases when local disease control is aimed for. These patients usually have distant metastases at the time of presentation, and radioactive iodine has no role in therapy.

Answer 21.13. **The answer is E.**

Medullary thyroid carcinoma can metastasize early to cervical lymph nodes, bone, and liver. It can be hard to distinguish benign hepatic hemangiomas from liver metastases secondary to medullary thyroid carcinoma. CEA is often used in follow-up in parallel to serum calcitonin as some cases show more CEA production compared to calcitonin.

Answer 21.14. **The answer is A.**

The follicular variant of papillary thyroid carcinoma is not associated with worse prognosis in contrast to the other variants.

Answer 21.15. **The answer is C.**

Anaplastic thyroid carcinoma carries poor prognosis and is considered stage IV at presentation.

Answer 21.16. **The answer is A.**

Doxorubicin is the best single chemotherapeutic agent in metastatic differentiated thyroid carcinoma. It is still reserved to selected cases as the partial response rate is close to 30%. Combining cisplatin with doxorubicin is not superior to doxorubicin alone.

Answer 21.17. **The answer is B.**

Parathyroid carcinoma is a rare malignant neoplasm with mortality and morbidity attributed mainly to hypercalcemia. Surgery is the mainstay of therapy, and there is some data to suggest the beneficial role of adjuvant external beam irradiation to achieve local control and reduce recurrence. Resection of other parathyroid glands is not necessary as parathyroid carcinoma originates from one parathyroid gland. Chemotherapy is generally ineffective in these cases.

Answer 21.18. **The answer is E.**

Normalizing serum calcium is among the priorities when treating parathyroid carcinoma. Cinacalcet is a novel agonist of the calcium sensing receptor with FDA approval in the management of hypercalcemia in patients with parathyroid carcinoma. Mithramycin (Plicamycin) is another agent used in the past in patients with metastatic parathyroid carcinoma. Hydration is also essential in managing these patients who often require repeated IV bisphosphonate infusions to reduce hypercalcemia by inhibiting osteoclast activity.

Answer 21.19. **The answer is A.**

Hyperparathyroidism/Jaw tumor syndrome (HPT/JT) is a rare autosomal dominant disorder presenting with recurrent parathyroid adenomas in 90% of cases along with fibro-osseous tumors of the maxilla or mandible in 50% of cases. Other manifestations include renal cysts or tumors as well as parathyroid carcinoma in 5% to 10% of cases. The disease is secondary to mutation in the *HRPT-2* gene (1q25-32) that encodes for a protein of unknown function called parafibromin. There are very few reports of parathyroid carcinoma in patients with MEN-1 but not MEN-2. Familial hypercalciuric hypocalcemia and familial hypocalciuric hypercalcemia are secondary to mutations in the calcium sensing receptor and not associated with parathyroid carcinoma.

Answer 21.20. **The answer is C.**

There is still no staging system for this rare malignancy that infrequently metastasizes to lymph nodes. Disease course is not well correlated with tumor size, age at diagnosis, or gender.

Answer 21.21. **The answer is A.**

This patient meets the diagnostic criteria for MEN-1. Hyperparathyroidism is the most common manifestation in this disorder. The other endocrine disorders include pituitary adenomas, pancreatic neuroendocrine tumors (PNETs), foregut carcinoid tumors, and occasionally adrenocortical adenomas. Other manifestations include lipomas, collagenomas, and angiofibromas. The *menin* gene is a tumor suppressor gene on chromosome 11 (11q13) that encodes for a protein of unclear function celled menin. *RET* protooncogene mutation is associated with MEN-2A (medullary thyroid carcinoma, hyperparathyroidism, and pheochromocytoma) and MEN-2B (medullary thyroid carcinoma, mucosal neuromas, intestinal ganglioneuromas, and pheochromocytoma). Inactivating calcium-sensing receptor *(CaSR)* mutation is responsible for familial hypocalciuric hypercalcemia, whereas *RET/PTC* rearrangements are seen in some cases of papillary thyroid carcinoma.

Answer 21.22. **The answer is A.**

Prolactin-producing pituitary adenomas usually respond well to dopamine agonists, and transsphenoidal resection is a second-line therapy in selected cases. Subtotal parathyroidectomy (or total parathyroidectomy with autotransplantation of a parathyroid tissue in the arm) is the preferred approach in treating hyperparathyroidism in MEN-1 as these patients have multigland parathyroid hyperplasia. Prophylactic thymectomy is occasionally done in these cases to remove supernumerary parathyroid glands and in some cases to prevent malignant thymic carcinoid. Pancreatectomy is not done unless justified by the presence of a resectable pancreatic neuroendocrine tumor.

Answer 21.23. **The answer is B.**

This patient meets the criteria for MEN-2 as he presents with MTC and right-sided pheochromocytoma. Pheochromocytoma should be resected prior to addressing the other disorders to prevent complications related to untreated pheochromocytoma.

Answer 21.24. **The answer is B.**

MEN-2 syndrome is a great example of genotype–phenotype correlation. Knowing the mutation site helps predicting clinical manifestations and behavior in mutation careers. This patient has MEN-2A with cutaneous lichen amyloidosis (CLA). CLA is a rare skin condition associated with MEN-2A in some families. *RET* codon 634 mutations have been described in MEN-2A/CLA families. Codon 609 mutation is found in familial medullary thyroid carcinoma (FMTC) and MEN-2A whereas FMTC is the only manifestation of codon 768 mutation. Mutated codon 918 manifests as MEN-2B.

Answer 21.25. **The answer is C.**

Metastatic PNETs are the most common cause for MEN-1 related deaths.

Answer 21.26. **The answer is B.**

Mutated *RET* protooncogene can cause Hirschsprung disease as well as MEN-2.

Answer 21.27. **The answer is B.**

This patient has right adrenal incidentaloma. There are no features to suggest hormonal overproduction though her blood pressure is mildly elevated. Pheochromocytoma must be ruled out prior to any intervention. Dexamethasone suppression is required to rule out subclinical Cushing syndrome, and obtaining plasma aldosterone/renin activity ratio is justified in the presence of hypertension. Imaging studies can only suggest the etiology of the neoplasm but cannot substitute the chemical workup.

Answer 21.28. **The answer is F.**

This patient has metastatic pheochromocytoma. The most commonly used regimen contains cyclophosphamide, vincristine, and doxorubicin. High-dose MIBG treatment can be of some value in a few patients. External beam irradiation is often used in treating localized bone metastases. Interferon and octreotide are not helpful in these cases.

Answer 21.29. **The answer is D.**

This patient is likely to have adrenocortical carcinoma manifested as a large heterogeneous adrenal mass and hyperandrogenism. Intervention should be postponed until ruling out pheochromocytoma. Fine needle aspiration is indicated mainly in patients with prior history of other malignancy, and it carries the risk of needle tract or peritoneal seeding in cases of adrenocortical carcinoma. In patients with adrenal tumors greater than 6 cm, surgery is indicated regardless of the hormonal production as the risk of malignancy is high in this group. Open adrenalectomy is usually done when adrenocortical carcinoma is suspected to attempt full resection of the tumor without taking the risk of peritoneal seeding.

Answer 21.30. **The answer is B.**

At a threshold of 10 HU, the sensitivity of nonenhanced CT for characterizing adrenal adenomas is 79%, with a specificity of 96%. A washout more than 50% at 10- to 15-minute images is highly suggestive of benign adenoma with 96% sensitivity and 100% specificity. Irregular borders and heterogeneous appearance raise the possibility of malignancy.

Answer 21.31. **The answer is A.**

Mutated *RET* protooncogene causes adrenal pheochromocytoma that can be bilateral, but is not known to cause extraadrenal pheochromocytoma in contrast to the other listed genes.

Answer 21.32. **The answer is E.**

Mitotane is associated with multiple side effects that are dose related. Monitoring serum levels during therapy is recommended to adjust the dose and avoid toxicity. These patients require higher-than-usual doses of corticosteroids as mitotane increases the level of corticosteroid-binding globulin.

Answer 21.33. **The answer is B.**

This patient has the classic presentation of Zollinger–Ellison syndrome (ZES) and also has primary hyperparathyroidism. His family history is also suggestive of MEN-1 as his mother had nephrolithiasis presumably secondary to primary hyperparathyroidism and infertility that could be secondary to prolactin-producing adenoma managed successfully with medical therapy. Gastric pH measurement is very important to distinguish hypergastrinemia secondary to acid-lowering therapy or atrophic gastritis from hypergastrinemia in the presence of ZES. The only other explanation for high gastrin and low gastric pH is retained antrum syndrome after gastric surgery.

Answer 21.34. **The answer is C.**

The presence of flushing, diarrhea, and wheezing is highly suggestive of the carcinoid syndrome, which should be confirmed by measuring 5-HIAA (end product of serotonin metabolism). Elevated serum gastrin or VIP can produce secretory diarrhea but is usually not associated with wheezing or skin changes. Glucagon-producing tumors are associated with a unique skin rash (necrolytic migratory erythema) and not associated with diarrhea or wheezing. Medullary thyroid carcinoma can also manifest with diarrhea secondary to high calcitonin levels.

Answer 21.35. **The answer is E.**

Insulinoma is rarely malignant in contrast to other pancreatic endocrine tumors.

CHAPTER **22**

Sarcomas

WILLIAM L. READ

Directions Each of the numbered items below is followed by lettered answers. Select the ONE lettered answer that is BEST in each case unless instructed otherwise.

QUESTIONS

Question 22.1. **Which of the following syndromes increases the risk for malignant peripheral nerve sheath tumors (MPNST)?**

A. Multiple endocrine neoplasia (MEN) type I.
B. Gardner syndrome.
C. Li–Fraumeni syndrome.
D. Type I neurofibromatosis (NF-1).

Question 22.2. **The translocation t(X;18)(p11.2;q11.2) is characteristic of which neoplasm?**

A. Synovial sarcoma.
B. Malignant fibrous histiocytoma (MFH).
C. Ewing sarcoma.
D. Round cell liposarcoma.

Question 22.3. **A 45-year-old man is referred to you after having a 3-cm leiomyosarcoma resected from his flank. Preoperatively, the surgeon believed this mass to be a benign lipoma, and the pathologic specimen has multiple positive margins. The most appropriate next step is**

A. radiation
B. reresection
C. watchful waiting, with serial exam and computed tomographic (CT) scans of the chest
D. chemotherapy

Corresponding Chapters in *Cancer: Principles & Practice of Oncology*, Seventh Edition: 35 (Sarcomas of the Soft Tissues and Bone).

Question 22.4. **A 36-year-old woman presented with mild arm stiffness and was found to have a desmoid tumor near the clavicle. It was thought to be associated with her cosmetic breast implants. She underwent a complete resection with negative margins. Two years later she again experienced mild arm stiffness, and magnetic resonance imaging (MRI) found her to have locally recurrent disease. Reresection would cause cosmetic deformity and possibly impair the use of her arm. What is the most appropriate next treatment?**

A. Reresection, followed by radiation.
B. Radiation alone.
C. Trial of tamoxifen and sulindac.
D. Trial of methotrexate.
E. Watchful waiting, with opiates for pain.

Question 22.5. **Which of the following would affect the American Joint Committee on Cancer (AJCC) stage of an adult soft tissue sarcoma?**

A. One positive lymph node versus four positive nodes.
B. Young patient (<25 years) versus older patient (more than 26 years).
C. High grade versus low grade.

Question 22.6. **A 45-year-old man undergoes extensive resection for a high-grade leiomyosarcoma arising in the retroperitoneum. Two years later, two new 1-cm pulmonary nodules are seen on chest CT. One is in the right lung and one is in the left lung. What is the most appropriate next treatment?**

A. Ifosfamide and doxorubicin chemotherapy.
B. Resection of both lung metastases.
C. Definitive radiation to lung metastases.
D. Resection, then adjuvant radiation.

Question 22.7. **A 77-year-old man presents with a 1-cm purple nodule on his right temple. Biopsy reveals angiosarcoma. The operating surgeon orders intraoperative frozen sections and must return twice for additional margins, but ultimately the tumor is resected with negative margins. It measures 2 cm on pathologic examination. What is the most appropriate next treatment?**

A. Adjuvant chemotherapy with pegylated liposomal doxorubicin.
B. Adjuvant chemotherapy with paclitaxel.
C. Imaging of neck to look for nodal metastases and adjuvant radiation.
D. Watchful waiting, with close dermatologic follow-up.

Question 22.8. **A 59-year-old man develops jaundice and is found to have several large lesions in the liver. Biopsy finds this to be a high-grade spindle cell neoplasm. What further workup is most important?**

A. Upper and lower endoscopy to find the primary lesion.
B. Immunoperoxidase staining of tumor for CD117.
C. Evaluation for the presence of lung metastases.
D. All of the above.

Question 22.9. **A 50-year-old man presents with a large painless thigh mass. MRI shows it to measure 14 cm, and on biopsy it is found to be a high-grade round cell liposarcoma. CT scans show no evidence of lung metastasis. Appropriate treatment is**

A. preoperative radiotherapy followed by limb sparing resection
B. preoperative chemotherapy followed by limb-sparing resection, followed by radiation
C. limb-sparing resection followed by radiation
D. any of the above

Question 22.10. **A 22-year-old man complains of pain in his right upper arm. MRI reveals a 2-cm destructive mass centered on the humerus, and he is referred to an orthopedic oncologist. Biopsy reveals a nonossifying spindle cell lesion, which is described as a malignant fibrous histiocytoma. CT of the chest and bone scan reveal no other sites of disease. What is the appropriate treatment?**

A. Limb-sparing resection and radiation.
B. Limb-sparing resection with wide margins.
C. Radiation alone.
D. Preoperative chemotherapy, limb-sparing resection, and adjuvant chemotherapy.

Question 22.11. **A 19-year-old woman with osteosarcoma of the knee receives preoperative chemotherapy with high-dose methotrexate alternating with cisplatin and infusional doxorubicin. She undergoes limb-sparing surgery and is found to have an excellent response, with greater that 90% necrosis. She is treated postoperatively with the same regimen. Two years later, surveillance CT scans discover two new lung nodules, each 1 cm. Subsequent CT scan 6 weeks later shows both to have slightly increased in size and the possible appearance of one additional small nodule. The appropriate next treatment is**

A. retreatment with high-dose methotrexate alternating with cisplatin and doxorubicin
B. chemotherapy with high-dose ifosfamide
C. resection of all nodules
D. watchful waiting with consideration of radiation or chemotherapy for symptom management

Question 22.12. **A 17-year-old boy with an osteosarcoma of the distal femur is treated with amputation at the knee and no further treatment. What is his likelihood of surviving 2 years?**

A. 80%.
B. 50%.
C. 35%.
D. 15%.

Question 22.13. **A 60-year-old patient presents with pain on sitting. Evaluation discovers a destructive 4-cm lesion in the proximal femur. Biopsy finds this to be a giant cell tumor (GCT). What is the best treatment?**

A. Resection.
B. Resection and radiation.
C. Resection, radiation, and multiagent chemotherapy.
D. Steroids and bisphosphonates.

Question 22.14. **A 25-year-old woman has pain and swelling in the left lower leg, and imaging finds her to have a destructive lesion in the left popliteal fossa. Ten years previously she had been treated for a Ewing sarcoma in this area, using a combination of radiation and chemotherapy. What is the most likely diagnosis?**

A. Recurrent Ewing sarcoma.
B. GCT of bone.
C. Osteosarcoma.
D. Malignant fibrous histiocytoma.

Question 22.15. **In chondrosarcomas, which of the following is associated with worse prognosis?**

A. Childhood onset.
B. Painlessness.
C. Low histologic grade.
D. Peripheral location.

ANSWERS

Answer 22.1. **The answer is D.**

Approximately 5% of patients with NF-1 will develop a MPNST, often arising from a neurofibroma. These tumors are aggressive and have a poor prognosis. However, most patients diagnosed with MPNST do not have NF-1. Gardner syndrome is a subset of familial adenomatous polyposis. These patients are prone to colon cancer and can also develop abdominal desmoid tumors, which are benign but locally aggressive fibromatoses. Patients with Li-Fraumeni syndrome inherit one defective copy of p53 and are at increased risk for a wide variety of tumors, including sarcomas of soft tissue and bone. Patients with MEN-1 are not at increased risk for sarcomas.

Answer 22.2. **The answer is A.**

Molecular testing for the t(X;18)(p11.2;q11.2) translocation can be helpful in confirming the diagnosis of synovial sarcoma. This diagnosis can be tricky as these sarcomas stain positive for keratin and can be mistaken for epithelial neoplasms, and can calcify and be mistaken for thyroid tumors. Myxoid/round cell liposarcoma typically has a t(12;16)(q13-14;p11) translocation. Ewing sarcoma/primitive neuroectodermal tumors have a t(11;22)(q24;q11.2-12) translocation. Malignant fibrous histiocytoma does not have a characteristic translocation.

Answer 22.3. **The answer is B.**

Positive surgical margins increase the risk for local relapse, and reexcision should be attempted. If repeat surgery is not practicable, radiation should definitely be used in hopes of sterilizing residual disease. If reresection can obtain adequate margins, the chance of recurrence for this small (<5 cm) tumor is only about 10%, making adjuvant radiation unnecessary. Chemotherapy has minimal, if any, benefit in this case.

Answer 22.4. **The answer is C.**

Desmoid tumors are locally aggressive, clonal fibromatoses. They often occur at the site of a prior surgery, such as a cesarean section. Resection is the primary treatment of choice, and even if there are positive margins these tumors sometimes do not recur. On recurrence, as with other benign tumors, reresection should be done if possible. Adjuvant radiation should be considered for recurrent tumors. Primary radiation can be used if surgery would be impossible or unacceptably morbid. Desmoid tumors are unique in that some respond to treatment with NSAIDS, especially sulindac, and tamoxifen. Given the low toxicity of this combination, it is reasonable to give it a try in hopes of avoiding more aggressive treatment. Responses to this regimen may last for years. If this treatment fails, she can go on to surgery and/or radiation.

Answer 22.5. **The answer is C.**

Grade (G) is considered along with the usual T (size), N (nodes), and M (metastases) variables in assigning a stage to a soft tissue sarcoma. Because adult soft tissue sarcomas rarely involve lymph nodes, any positive node (N1) is equivalent to M1, or distant metastatic disease. Young patients develop a different subset of sarcomas than do older patients, but even for the same diagnoses young patients fare better. Age is not considered when assigning stage.

Answer 22.6. **The answer is B.**

The lung is the usual metastatic site for most adult soft tissue sarcomas, including leiomyosarcoma. Resection of lung metastases is the treatment of choice as they might represent the only site of metastatic disease. This is especially true after a disease-free interval of 2 years—the lack of recurrence in the retroperitoneum suggests that his disease there has been cured. Radiation is not commonly used after resection of lung metastases. If comorbid conditions prevent surgery, radiation could be considered as a substitute in a situation analogous to the primary treatment of sarcomas. Chemotherapy might be considered if resection were impossible because of the number or location of metastases. In a series from MD Anderson, chemotherapy did not improve survival over metastasectomy alone.

Answer 22.7. **The answer is C.**

Only a small series comparing surgery plus adjuvant radiation to surgery alone has been reported, but the addition of radiation improved local control in this group. Angiosarcoma of the scalp is a locally aggressive tumor, and recurrence after surgery is common. The addition of radiation to primary surgery is reasonable and certainly should be done after recurrence. Unlike other adult soft tissue sarcomas, angiosarcomas have a relatively high incidence of metastasis to lymph nodes, and evaluation of neck lymph nodes should be part of the treatment of angiosarcoma of the scalp. Angiosarcoma of the scalp is also relatively chemoresponsive, and complete responses have been described to taxanes and pegylated liposomal doxorubicin, as well as older regimens. Unfortunately, rapid recurrence after chemotherapy is the rule. There is no proven benefit to adjuvant chemotherapy.

Answer 22.8. **The answer is B.**

Bulky metastatic sarcoma in the liver has a dismal prognosis, unless the sarcoma is a gastrointestinal stromal tumor (GIST). This subset of sarcomas expresses CD117, or C-KIT, and treatment with the specific C-KIT inhibitor imatinib mesylate can cause partial regression and long periods of disease stabilization. Other workup is unnecessary as these lesions are non-GIST high grade sarcomas, and the disease course will be determined by the liver metastases.

Answer 22.9. **The answer is D.**

Surgical resection is the mainstay of treatment. Large lesions, which would have been treated with amputation in the past, can now often be managed with a limb-sparing operation and adjuvant radiation. There is no clear advantage to presurgical versus postsurgical radiation: presurgical radiation may offer smaller treatment volumes at the expense of delays in wound healing. Both offer comparable survival. Chemotherapy is of questionable benefit for soft tissue sarcomas when taken as a group, with a survival improvement of 4% or less. The survival advantage conferred may be slightly greater in extremity sarcomas. Round cell liposarcoma is among the more chemoresponsive of sarcomas, and treatment preoperatively will allow assessment of response *in vivo,* as well as possibly facilitating subsequent surgery. There is no consensus on the use of chemotherapy in this context, but given that this patient has at least a 50% chance of dying from his disease, aggressive treatment is not unreasonable.

Answer 22.10. **The answer is D.**

MFHs in the soft tissue behave like other soft tissue sarcomas, and adjuvant chemotherapy is of marginal benefit. MFHs of the bone, however, are treated the same as osteosarcomas, with a combination of multiagent chemotherapy and resection. Although the response rate to preoperative chemotherapy is lower for MFH than for osteosarcoma, outcomes are comparable. Radiation is reserved for unresectable disease and palliative treatment.

Answer 22.11. **The answer is C.**

With aggressive resection of all sites of disease, up to 40% of patients may survive 5 years after relapse. Unless there is a contraindication, every attempt should be made to resect lung metastases from osteosarcoma if they represent the only known site of disease. The operating surgeon may find additional smaller nodules on thoracotomy, which should also be resected. Additional chemotherapy with different agents (e.g., ifosfamide) can be considered in patients with early (6 to 12 months postoperative) appearance of metastases, though there is no proven survival benefit. Given the long disease-free interval for this patient, she is best treated with surgery alone.

Answer 22.12. **The answer is D.**

Osteosarcoma is arguably the solid tumor in which adjuvant chemotherapy has the most importance. Before its routine use, the majority of patients died of metastatic disease within 2 years. With multiagent adjuvant chemotherapy, between 60% to 80% of patients can be cured.

Answer 22.13. **The answer is A.**

GCTs of bone are low-grade sarcomas. They infrequently metastasize, though they can be locally destructive. The treatment of choice is resection. Adjuvant radiation can be considered if complete resection is not possible, although malignant transformation of GCTs after radiation was described in older literature. There is no clear role for chemotherapy. There are reports of successful palliative treatment of unresectable/recurrent GCTs with steroids and bisphosphonates. Their role in curative treatment is unclear.

Answer 22.14. **The answer is C.**

After 10 years, she is likely to be cured of her original Ewing sarcoma. Osteosarcomas are the most common radiation-induced sarcoma, with an incidence of about 5%. Radiation-induced sarcomas usually occur 5 or more years after radiation. Soft tissue sarcomas, including MFH, can also occur as a result of prior radiation though less common than osteosarcomas. GCTs of bone are not known to be related to prior radiation.

Answer 22.15. **The answer is A.**

Unlike osteosarcomas, chondrosarcomas are tumors of adults. Those that occur in children have a worse prognosis. Pain is a marker of high-grade and aggressive behavior. Low-grade tumors have a better prognosis than high grade, and peripheral tumors are more likely to be low grade than those that are centrally located.

CHAPTER 23

Cancer of the Skin and Melanoma

GERALD P. LINETTE, LYNN A. CORNELIUS, J. ANDREW CARLSON,
AND J. WILLIAM HARBOUR

Directions Each of the numbered items below is followed by lettered answers. Select the ONE lettered answer that is BEST in each case unless instructed otherwise.

QUESTIONS

Question 23.1. **A 69-year-old man presents with a crusted nodule on his scalp, which had been gradually enlarging over the past 2 months. He has a history of multiple skin malignancies, including basal cell carcinoma, squamous cell carcinoma *in situ*, and invasive squamous cell carcinoma. The tumor was excised. Routine staining with hematoxylin and eosin revealed a dermal nodule composed of small cells with hyperchromatic nuclei arranged in sheets and solid nests and showing numerous mitotic figures. The mortality rate for patients affected by this cancer has been reported to be approximately**

A. 90%
B. 5%
C. 10%
D. 30%
E. 70%

Question 23.2. **At what site(s) does cutaneous squamous cell carcinoma have a high rate of metastasis?**

A. Nose.
B. Ear and lip.
C. Scalp.
D. Extremity.
E. Trunk.

Corresponding Chapters in *Cancer: Principles & Practice of Oncology*, Seventh Edition: 37 (Cancer of the Skin) and 38 (Melanoma).

Question 23.3. **A 17-year-old girl presents with greater than 50 macular to slightly raised, plaquelike 0.4- to 1.8-cm dark brown pigmented lesions on both sun-exposed and nonsun-exposed regions of her body. Her sister has similar skin lesions, and their mother and an uncle have both developed melanoma. Which statement most accurately describes the significance of her pigmented macules?**

A. They both have benign skin lesions with no risk for skin cancer.
B. These two siblings have a high risk for developing melanoma.
C. These lesions are not a reflection of sun exposure.
D. They are markers for internal malignancy.
E. Both siblings have superficial fungal infection.

Question 23.4. **An 80-year-old woman of Celtic ancestry presents for routine physical examination. She mentions a spot on her eyelid that has been bothering her. It is a pink-white, ulcerated papule on her nasal bridge close to the medial canthus. What is the most likely diagnosis?**

A. Basal cell carcinoma, nodular type.
B. Xanthoma.
C. Intradermal melanocytic nevus.
D. Squamous cell carcinoma.
E. Sebaceous hyperplasia.

Question 23.5. **A 58-year-old white woman presents with a lifelong history of a lymphangioma on the right hand. This lesion was surgically debulked when she was 15 years old and subsequently remained stable. Five years before presentation, the hand and digits began to slowly enlarge. Two years ago the patient noticed the onset of dark-colored lesions and hardening of the hand. Although otherwise asymptomatic, progressive loss of function of the hand was noted. What population is most commonly affected by this tumor; what is the most common site of distant metastasis; and what is the 5-year overall survival (OS) rate?**

A. Immunosuppressed individuals; lymph nodes; and 50% OS.
B. Elderly men; lungs; and 12% OS.
C. Adolescents; skin; and 90% OS.
D. Women after mastectomy and lymph node dissection; bone; and 30% OS.
E. Metal workers; brain; and 70% OS.

Question 23.6. **A 49-year-old man presents with a changing mole on the back noticed by his wife who urged him to get checked for skin cancer. The lesion had been there for years but recently started to enlarge and change color. Which statement is INCORRECT?**

A. This melanoma may be undergoing regression.
B. Tenderness and bleeding are the first signs of malignancy.
C. Enlargement and color change are not signs of potential malignancy.
D. Early diagnosis can affect long-term prognosis.
E. Excisional biopsy is the diagnostic method of choice.

Question 23.7. **Which statement is true regarding the expression of melanoma-related antigens?**

A. Melanomas all express the same antigens.
B. They are lost by metastatic melanoma.
C. Serologic levels of these antigens are unrelated to melanoma recurrence or response to treatment.
D. These antigens are the suspected targets for spontaneous and therapy induced regression of melanoma and paraneoplastic vitiligo.
E. The development of paraneoplastic vitiligo following immunotherapy is not a measure of treatment potency.

Question 23.8. **A 36-year-old woman is diagnosed with a 0.76-mm nonulcerated melanoma on her right calf. Her follow-up schedule with clinical exam should be**

A. every 6 months for the first 2 to 3 years and then yearly 2 to 3 years beyond that
B. once a year for 5 years; then as needed
C. every 3 to 6 months for the first 2 to 3 years and every 6 to 12 months for the next 2 to 3 years
D. every 3 to 4 months for the first 2 years and then every 6 months up to year 5 and yearly beyond that
E. a cutaneous exam whenever a new or worrisome lesion is noted

Question 23.9. **A 45-year-old man presents with a changing skin lesion on his back. Punch biopsy revealed a level 4, ulcerated melanoma with a depth of 4.2 mm. In addition, he has an in-transit metastasis. He has no clinical adenopathy. What statement is incorrect regarding his stage and clinical workup?**

A. The American Joint Committee on Cancer (AJCC) clinical stage is IIc (T4bN0, M0).
B. A wide local excision with 2-cm margins should be performed.
C. A lymphatic mapping and sentinel lymph node biopsy is warranted for further staging.
D. Initial and periodic examination of his entire cutaneous surfaces and mucosa should be performed to identify second primary melanoma or other skin cancer.
E. Periodic history and physical exams should be performed.

Question 23.10. **A 79-year-old woman had a 3-month history of a 1-cm, ulcerated nodule on the left helix of the ear. Shave biopsy demonstrated an anaplastic spindle cell tumor. Which one of these statements is INCORRECT?**

A. The clinical differential diagnosis includes basal cell carcinoma, squamous cell carcinoma, metastatic carcinoma, pyogenic granuloma, and chondrodermatitis helicis.
B. The histologic differential diagnosis includes spindle cell variants of squamous cell carcinoma and melanoma, atypical fibroxanthoma (AFX), and leiomyosarcoma.
C. The immunophenotype for the tumor is positive for vimentin, and negative for desmin, actin, keratins, and S100 protein. Therefore, the tumor is an AFX.
D. The histologic diagnosis is AFX, confirmed by immunohistochemistry; therefore, the estimated 5-year survival rate is over 90% with local excision.
E. Superficial malignant fibrous histiocytomas have the same prognosis as deep malignant fibrous histiocytomas.

Question 23.11. **A young boy presents violaceous patches, plaques, and nodules affecting his legs and feet, some of which appear fixed to underlying soft tissue and bone. No lymphadenopathy is found. He complains of fever. His family has recently emigrated from central Africa. Which statement is INCORRECT?**

A. He comes from a region with a high prevalence of human herpesvirus type 8 (HHV-8) infection.
B. Prognostic factors include tumor burden, presence or absence of opportunistic infections, and the presence or absence of systemic symptoms.
C. His clinical stage is IIB.
D. His condition has a 100% fatality rate.
E. Punch biopsy of a plaque revealed the diagnostic changes of a spindle cell proliferation forming slitlike spaces containing erythrocytes.

Question 23.12. **Which of the following statements is correct regarding the current model of melanoma development and progression?**

A. Genes involved in melanocyte development [e.g., *WNT* signaling pathway, microphthalmia-associated transcription factor (*MITF*), *PAX3*, *SOX10*] are implicated in transformation of melanocytes into melanoma.
B. A histologic stepwise pathway exists where melanoma evolves from acquired melanocytic nevi to atypical/dysplastic melanocytic nevi to radial growth phase melanoma to vertical growth phase melanoma to metastatic melanoma.
C. Known susceptibility genes for melanoma include *16INK4A* on 9p21 and *CDK4* on 12q4.
D. A and C.
E. All of the above.

Question 23.13. **Several years after heart transplant, a 49-year-old man develops numerous keratotic papules and plaques over photoexposed sites; some of the larger plaques are ulcerated. Which statement most accurately describes this patient?**

A. After wide local excision, these tumors are associated with a high rate of local recurrence, regional lymph node and visceral metastases, and mortality.
B. Biopsies will show that he has multiple basal cell carcinomas.
C. Many of the smaller lesions will be warts/human papillomavirus infection.
D. A and C.
E. All of the above.

Question 23.14. **Nonmelanoma skin cancer (e.g., basal cell and squamous cell carcinoma) has which attributes.**

A. It has a low mortality rate.
B. It is one of the most costly cancers to care for amongst Medicare patients, ranking amongst lung, prostate, colon, and breast carcinomas.
C. It has incidence that exceeds that for lung, breast, prostate, and colon cancers combined, with one in five Americans expected to develop skin cancer.
D. It is suspected to be a marker of risk for an internal malignancy.
E. All of the above.

Question 23.15. **A 70-year-old man presents to another physician after a year of treatment for monocular cicatricial bullous pemphigoid. He has extensive loss of eyelashes, eyelid induration, and erythema of eyelid and conjunctiva. A punch biopsy reveals an intraepidermal and infiltrative proliferation of atypical basaloid and squamous cells. Which statement is INCORRECT regarding this patient?**

A. Ancillary pathologic tests such as Oil-Red-O on fresh tissue or EMA immunohistochemistry will aid in the confirmation of the diagnosis.
B. Workup examining for an internal, second malignancy is not necessary.
C. Poor prognostic factors include a duration of more than 6 months, multicentric origin, poor differentiation, infiltrative pattern, pagetoid changes, vascular invasion, lymphatic channel involvement, previous radiation, and orbital spread.
D. After treatment, patients affected by this cancer should be followed up for recurrence or progression through regular examination of skin and lymph nodes.
E. Spread of this skin cancer can occur by lymphatic or hematogenous routes or by direct extension with distant metastases reported in up to 20% of cases.

Question 23.16. **A 59-year-old white female with a history of recurrent infiltrating ductal carcinoma of the breast presents status–post-radical mastectomy, and 2 courses of locoregional radiation therapy. Her chief complaint is that of a new lesion of the right chest, presenting 3 years following her last treatment. On examination, there is a 5-mm crusted erythematous papule at the central portion of her mastectomy scar. The differential diagnosis includes all of the following, the least likely being**

A. recurrent carcinoma
B. melanoma
C. angiosarcoma
D. squamous cell carcinoma

Question 23.17. **A 62-year-old white male with a history of renal transplantation and cutaneous squamous cell carcinoma presents with a hypopigmented, firm 7-mm nodule of the back. His medications include cyclosporine, azothioprine, and prednisone. Your differential diagnosis includes scar, morpheaform basal cell carcinoma, and amelanotic melanoma. The patient does not recall previous surgery at the site. You perform an excisional biopsy. Pathology reveals an amelanotic melanoma, nodular type, Breslow depth 1.54 mm. Management of the patient includes**

A. wide local excision with 2-cm margins
B. sentinel lymph node biopsy
C. consultation with the transplant management team regarding his immunosuppressive medications
D. treatment with interferon (IFN) for stage III disease
E. A, B, and C

Question 23.18. **A 19-year-old white male presents with a history of xeroderma pigmentosa. Following his initial diagnosis at age 2, he has been appropriately managed throughout childhood with strict sun avoidance, protective clothing, and sunscreen. Despite these precautions, he has developed several cutaneous malignancies. What is the correct statement regarding this disease?**

A. This is an autosomal recessive disorder, with a defect in DNA nucleotide excision repair (NER).
B. These patients are at increased risk for both melanoma and non-melanoma skin cancers.
C. The most common melanoma subtype these patients develop is nodular.
D. These patients are at increased risk for conjunctival melanoma.
E. A, B, and D are all correct.

Question 23.19. **An elderly white male presents with a history of localized cellulitis of the scalp that is asymptomatic and resistant to oral antibiotic therapy. On physical examination, he has a localized erythematous, indurated 10-cm plaque of the vertex of the scalp, extending to the forehead area. You perform a punch biopsy, and pathology shows irregularly dilated vascular channels lined by flattened endothelial cells that stain positively for CD31. The diagnosis is**

A. desmoplastic melanoma
B. dermatofibrosarcoma protuberans
C. angiosarcoma
D. squamous cell carcinoma

Question 23.20. **A 45-year-old white female presents for a skin exam. She notes no previous history of skin cancer. On examination, she has an 8-mm firm tan-brown plaque with surrounding erythema on her midback that clinically resembles a keloid. She has no history of acne or other trauma to the area and no other hypertrophic scars. The lesion has been present for several years. You perform a punch biopsy, and pathology reveals dermal spindle cells in a storiform pattern, consistent with a dermatofibrosarcoma protuberans (DFSP). Which of the following statements apply to this tumor?**

A. Treatment is surgical and may include Mohs micrographic surgery.
B. These tumors commonly extend beyond the visible margins of the tumor.
C. DFSPs recur locally and rarely metastasize.
D. These tumors occur predominantly on the trunk.
E. All of the above.

Question 23.21. **A 75-year-old white female presents with a history of "intertrigo" that is painful and has not resolved despite repeated treatment with antibiotics and topical antifungal creams. On physical exam, she has an erythematous ulcerated plaque of the vulva. You perform a biopsy. Pathology reveals numerous atypical clear cells in the epidermis. The most likely diagnosis is**

A. squamous cell carcinoma *in situ* (Bowen disease)
B. Lichen sclerosis et atrophicus
C. Extramammary Paget disease
D. Basal cell carcinoma

Question 23.22. **Which of the following statements are INCORRECT?**

A. The rising incidence of melanoma is primarily due to increased diagnosis of disease, as opposed to actual increase in disease occurrence.
B. The use of sunscreen has been unequivocally linked to the development of melanoma.
C. Mortality rates from melanoma are decreasing.
D. Melanoma is the leading cause of death in women aged 25 to 32.
E. A, B, and C are all incorrect.

Question 23.23. **A 48-year-old African American male presents with a 1-year history of a lesion on the plantar surface of his right foot. The clinical diagnosis was plantar verrucae, although the nodule was unresponsive to liquid nitrogen therapy. On exam, he has a 1-cm nonpigmented hyperkeratotic nodule with a superficial erosion, overlying the fourth proximal metatarso-phalangeal joint (MTP). Black puncta, typically seen in verrucae, are notably absent. Due to the location of the lesion, you perform an incisional biopsy. Pathologic diagnosis is amelanotic melanoma, acral lentiginous type, Breslow depth 2.3 mm, ulceration present. Which of the following statements are NOT correct?**

A. The patient should undergo wide local excision (2- to 3-mm margins) and sentinel lymph node biopsy.
B. The patient is clinical stage IIB (T3bN0, M0).
C. According to the most recent (2002) National Comprehensive Cancer Network (NCCN) guidelines, the workup for this patient should include a positron emission tomographic (PET) scan, abdominal and pelvic computed tomography (CT), and a chest x-ray.
D. Due to the location, the patient should receive adjuvant radiation therapy.
E. C and D.

Question 23.24. **According to the most recent NCCN guidelines, follow-up for the above patient should include**

A. physical exam with directed skin and nodal exam every 3 to 6 months for 3 years, then every 4 to 12 months for 2 years, then annually as clinically indicated
B. chest x-ray
C. lactate dehydrogenase (LDH) every 6 to12 months (optional)
D. annual skin exam for life
E. all of the above

Question 23.25. **A 15-year-old white female with many "moles" is referred to you for evaluation and management. She has a family history of melanoma in her mother and her older brother. On physical examination, she has more than 50 nevi, 10 of which are brown to salmon-colored macules greater than 5 mm, some having a papular component and indistinct borders. It has been recommended to her that she have several of her nevi prophylactically excised under general anesthesia. She is seriously considering this option. Which of the following statements is INCORRECT?**

A. Even without her significant family history, she would still have a greater than 10-fold increased risk of melanoma due to the presence of 10 atypical, or "dysplastic," nevi.
B. Her atypical, or "dysplastic," nevi are both markers of risk and potentially precursors to melanoma.
C. She should prophylactically excise all of her atypical nevi as these nevi invariably transform to melanoma.
D. Her lifetime risk to develop melanoma, due to her family history and her atypical nevi, has been estimated to be greater than 50%.
E. Her genetic predisposition to develop nevi is affected by her exposure to ultraviolet (UV) light.

Question 23.26. **After seeing the above patient, you then see a 49-year-old white female with a history of two primary stage I melanomas but no family history of melanoma. Which of the following statements are correct?**

A. It has been estimated that only 1% to 2% of melanoma patients will develop a second primary melanoma.
B. Less than 10% of patients with multiple primary melanomas are found to have germline *CDKN2A* mutations.
C. In the majority of patients with multiple primary melanomas, the melanomas are diagnosed concomitantly.
D. In familial melanoma, the frequency of second primary melanomas is higher than in sporadic melanoma.
E. B and D.

Question 23.27. **All of the following are correct statements regarding patients with melanoma *in situ* (stage 0) EXCEPT**

A. appropriate treatment is wide local excision using 5-mm margins
B. according to the most recent NCCN guidelines, patients should have yearly chest x-ray and LDH
C. follow-up includes periodic skin examinations for life
D. patients have a greater than 95% 10-year survival rate

Question 23.28. **A 20-year-old white man presents with a history of five previous basal cell carcinomas. He does not have significant sun exposure history but does have a positive family history for the early development of basal cell carcinomas. He also gives a history of frequent dental problems and odontoid cysts. On physical examination, he has hypotelorism and well-healed surgical scars of the left preauricular area, back, and scalp. He also has numerous tan-brown, somewhat shiny papules, which on biopsy are confirmed to be basal cell carcinomas. The most likely diagnosis is**

A. xeroderma pigmentosa
B. atypical nevus syndrome
C. basal cell nevus syndrome
D. cockayne syndrome
E. Li-Fraumeni syndrome

Question 23.29. **A 35-year-old white woman with a previous history of stage I melanoma 2 years prior to presentation is referred to you for evaluation and follow-up. There is no family history of melanoma. She has been informed by other physicians that she should not become pregnant due to the risk of disease progression. She asks you specifically about this risk. You can tell her all of the following EXCEPT**

A. there is convincing evidence that there is an increased frequency of melanoma during pregnancy
B. a melanoma that develops during pregnancy has the same prognosis as a melanoma of the same Breslow depth in a similarly matched, nonpregnant female
C. changes in nevi may occur during pregnancy; however, changing nevi during pregnancy that meet the ABCD criteria need to be biopsied
D. studies have supported the need for women with a history of stage I and II melanoma to avoid both the use of oral contraceptives and becoming pregnant
E. A and D

Question 23.30. **A 20-year-old white woman presents with a history of a large (covering 20 cm) congenital nevus that was excised during her first 2 years of life using staged excisions, tissue expanders, and skin grafts. On physical exam, there is extensive scarring covering her back, but no residual primary nevus. She does have numerous light tan, regularly bordered macular nevi, resembling café-au-lait macules. Which of the following statements applies to congenital nevi?**

A. Congenital nevi, of any size, occur in approximately 1% of the population.
B. Small congenital nevi have an increased incidence of melanoma development and should be routinely excised.
C. Giant congenital nevi, also known as bathing suit trunk nevi (covering >20 cm), have a 6% incidence of melanoma development.
D. The greatest risk of melanoma development in a giant congenital nevus is during the teenage years.
E. There is an increased risk of melanoma development in the café-au-lait–like satellite macules.
F. A and C.

Question 23.31. **A 39-year-old woman presents with a 1.4-mm depth, nonulcerated primary cutaneous melanoma diagnosed by excisional biopsy performed by her dermatologist. The primary lesion was found on her left shoulder and the patient is now referred to you for follow-up. On physical examination, no cervical or axillary adenopathy is noted. The appropriate clinical management is**

A. PET scan to complete the staging evaluation
B. wide local excision only
C. sentinal lymph node mapping followed by wide local excision performed during the same procedure
D. wide local excision followed by administration of interferon for 1 year
E. full skin examination performed yearly

Question 23.32. **A 48-year-old woman recently diagnosed with stage IIIB primary cutaneous melanoma (T3bN2a, M0) is referred to you for a second opinion about adjuvant therapy. The 3.1-mm depth primary ulcerated lesion was removed from her right calf. Wide local excision was performed and the sentinel node (right inguinal area) was positive for microscopic disease. Completion lymphadenectomy revealed two additional nodes positive for microscopic disease from 20 nodes removed during the procedure. Her physical examination is unremarkable and she is otherwise healthy. All of the following are true statements EXCEPT**

A. adjuvant high-dose interferon alpha is a treatment option
B. participation in a vaccine clinical trial is a treatment option
C. adjuvant granulocyte-macrophage colony-stimulating factor (GM-CSF) is a treatment option
D. adjuvant radiation therapy has no role as initial treatment
E. surveillance radiologic tests have not been shown to reduce morbidity and mortality

Question 23.33. **A retired 72-year-old farmer presents to your clinic with a chief complaint of a firm, nonpigmented nodule on the scalp that has changed in appearance according to his wife. Excisional biopsy reveals a primary cutaneous nonulcerated melanoma 4.5-mm depth (desmoplastic variant) with perineural invasion. Preoperative CT imaging of the neck and chest x-ray (CXR) are unremarkable for metastatic disease. Sentinal lymph node mapping and wide local excision reveals negative margins with no evidence of metastatic melanoma in the excised occipital node (pathologic stage T4N0, Mx). You meet with the patient and his wife after surgery to discuss clinical management issues. Which of the following statements is NOT true?**

A. Desmoplastic melanoma is an uncommon variant (represents about 1% to 2% of all melanoma) and most often found in the head and neck area.
B. Desmoplastic melanomas often do not express melanoma-lineage antigens such as gp100 (HMB-45) and MART-1 (MELAN-A) and, thus, can sometimes be difficult to diagnose.
C. Desmoplastic variants have a lower rate of regional metastases compared with superficial spreading cutaneous melanoma.
D. Adjuvant high-dose interferon alpha has been shown in randomized controlled clinical trials to increase relapse-free survival in patients with T4N0, M0 (pathologic stage IIB) desmoplastic variants.
E. Adjuvant postoperative radiation therapy with the goal of reducing the rate of local recurrence should be considered for patients with desmoplastic melanoma.

Question 23.34. **Indications for radiation therapy in the treatment of melanoma include**

A. newly diagnosed brain metastases
B. recurrent regional (nodal) disease deemed unresectable
C. adjuvant postoperative therapy for poor prognosis melanoma of the head and neck area
D. palliation for symptomatic subcutaneous, skin, and bone metastases
E. all of the above

Question 23.35. **A 55-year-old man was recently diagnosed with stage IIIC primary cutaneous superficial spreading melanoma. At the time of completion lymphadenectomy, extranodal extension was found within the left axilla, and all detectable tumor was completely resected. CT imaging of the chest, abdomen, and pelvis is unremarkable for distant disease. He is otherwise healthy except for type II diabetes that is well controlled by an oral hypoglycemic agent. You have been asked to consult and advise the patient about his prognosis and treatment options. No protocols are open at your institution. What is the best treatment option for this patient?**

A. Low-dose IFN for 2 years.
B. An abbreviated course of adjuvant radiation therapy to the involved axilla (30 Gy in 5 fractions) followed by high dose IFN for 1 year.
C. Dacarbazine for 6 cycles.
D. Referral to a tertiary center for hematopoietic stem cell transplantation.

Question 23.36. **A 60-year-old woman recently diagnosed with stage III primary cutaneous melanoma is referred to you for discussion of systemic treatment options. She is currently without evidence of disease. She has searched the Internet and inquires about the side effects and toxicities of interferon. Which of the following statements are false?**

A. Leukopenia is a common toxicity.
B. Thyroid dysfunction occurs in some patients receiving interferon.
C. Mild to moderate depression is frequently reported.
D. Greater than 90% of patients receiving high-dose interferon require dose delays and/or reductions.
E. None of the above.

Question 23.37. **A 48-year-old woman previously diagnosed with stage IIB primary cutaneous melanoma is being followed by you with history and physical exam every 3 months and annual CXR. The patient reports new onset headaches for the past week that are only partially relieved by acetaminophen. The patient denies diplopia, nausea, and seizures and has a nonfocal neurologic examination. You order a brain MRI with gadolinium, which reveals a solitary 2.5-cm enhancing lesion in the right parietal lobe with mild edema, but there is no midline shift. You decide to begin dexamethasone and complete the staging evaluation. FDG-PET scan obtained the next day fails to show uptake in the chest, abdomen, and pelvis. The serum LDH is normal. What is the most appropriate next step in the management of this patient?**

A. Begin temozolomide.
B. Whole brain radiation therapy.
C. Begin biochemotherapy.
D. Referral to a neurosurgeon.
E. Change her analgesics and wait for 2 weeks.

Question 23.38. **Investigational therapies for stage IV melanoma include all of the following EXCEPT**

A. IL-2
B. IL-18
C. vaccination with GM-CSF transduced autologous melanoma
D. gene therapy with plasmid DNA encoding HLA-B7
E. *BRAF* inhibitor (small molecule)

Question 23.39. **A 29-year-old man is recently diagnosed with metastatic melanoma and is referred to you for a second opinion. He has searched the Internet and has multiple questions concerning the treatment options. He inquires about high-dose IL-2 and asks if he is a "good candidate" for this treatment. Which of the following statements are true?**

A. Patients with subcutaneous metastases have a higher response rate.
B. Men have a higher response rate.
C. Patients receiving prior adjuvant interferon have a higher response rate.
D. Patients with bone metastases have a lower response rate.
E. All of the above.

Question 23.40. **A close friend informs the patient above that his next door neighbor was "cured" of metastatic melanoma after receiving biochemotherapy several years ago. The patient wants to learn more about biochemotherapy and its track record in treating melanoma. Which of the following statements are true?**

A. Biochemotherapy is Food and Drug Administration (FDA) approved for the treatment of metastatic melanoma.
B. Biochemotherapy regimens containing tamoxifen are superior to regimens without tamoxifen.
C. Patients responding to biochemotherapy often recur with central nervous system (CNS) relapse.
D. Several randomized cooperative group studies show consistent response rates of approximately 50% to 60% with significant improvement in overall survival.
E. Sequential biochemotherapy is clearly superior to other regimens (i.e., concurrent biochemotherapy).

Question 23.41. **All of the following agents have demonstrated single-agent activity (defined as response rates >10%) in melanoma EXCEPT**

A. paclitaxel
B. cisplatin
C. temozolomide
D. imatinib
E. interferon alpha

Question 23.42. **A 37-year-old man with a history of stage II primary cutaneous melanoma of the left lower extremity recurred 3 years after his initial diagnosis with a solitary cutaneous (1.5-cm diameter) regional metastasis. Fine needle aspiration (FNA) confirmed the diagnosis of metastatic melanoma. The lesion was resected with clear surgical margins and no adjuvant therapy was administered. Fifteen months after surgery, the patient recurs now with innumerable (>50) in transit lesions involving the proximal and distal portions of the left lower extremity. Biopsy confirms the presence of melanoma and the patient is sent to you for consultation. After restaging, you determine that the disease is limited to the patient's left lower extremity. What is the most appropriate step in the management of this patient?**

A. Initiation of high-dose interferon.
B. Initiation of temozolomide.
C. Referral for isolated limb perfusion.
D. External beam radiation therapy.
E. Surgical resection followed by adjuvant isolated limb perfusion.

Question 23.43. **A 71-year-old retired construction worker from Arizona presents with a firm, rapidly growing (2.5 cm in diameter) red papule on his right forearm. Excisional biopsy performed last week reveals Merkel cell carcinoma, and he is referred to you for further management. You inform the patient that this is a rare and aggressive skin cancer that is often seen in patients that are immunosuppressed. The patient is active and otherwise healthy but does comment that he has played golf several times a week for the past 15 years. Physical examination reveals a palpable 3-cm node in the right axilla. You recommend wide local excision of the primary site followed by elective lymph node dissection. Surgical margins of the primary site are negative and pathology confirms the presence of tumor in the single (3 cm) node of a total 35 nodes removed from the right axilla. What is the most appropriate recommendation for adjuvant therapy?**

A. No additional treatment is indicated.
B. One year of high-dose interferon.
C. Radiation therapy administered to the primary site and involved nodal basin.
D. Radiation therapy administered to the involved nodal basin only.
E. Radiation therapy administered to the primary site and involved nodal basin followed by 6 cycles of platinum-based chemotherapy.

Question 23.44. **Patients with invasive cutaneous squamous cell carcinoma (SCC) are known to be at risk for developing regional and occasionally distant metastases. Risk factors include locally recurrent SCC, poorly differentiated SCC, and lesions greater than 4 mm in depth. Which of the following statements are true regarding management of patients with invasive SCC?**

A. Total body skin exam and lymph node examination are recommended every 3 months during the first year following initial treatment.
B. Mohs surgery is superior to traditional excisional biopsy based on lower recurrence rates.
C. Solid organ transplant recipients (on standard immunosuppression medications) are at increased risk for SCC.
D. Ten-year survival rates are less than 10% for patients with distant metastases.
E. All of the above.

Question 23.45. **A 45-year-old (non-smoker) woman with a history of recurrent DFSP presents to your office after being told that her employment CXR is abnormal. Her condition has been managed surgically to date with excellent local control despite several recurrences limited to her lower extremity. A follow-up body CT scan confirms the presence of a 4-cm right middle lobe mass as well as a 7-cm mass in the posterior mediastinum. CT-guided biopsy reveals malignancy consistent with metastatic DFSP. She declines surgery and inquires about medical therapy. What treatment recommendation would you offer this patient as initial therapy?**

A. Platinum-based chemotherapy.
B. Imatinib.
C. Gefitinib.
D. Bortezomib.
E. Cetuximab.

Question 23.46. **The most common route of extraocular dissemination for ocular melanoma is**

A. hematogenous spread to the lungs
B. direct extension into the brain via the optic nerve
C. spread to regional lymph nodes in the head and neck
D. hematogenous spread to the liver
E. direct extension through the sclera into the orbit

Question 23.47. **Which of the following conditions is NOT associated with ocular melanoma?**

A. Cutaneous melanoma.
B. Dysplastic nevus syndrome.
C. Oculo (dermal) melanocytosis.
D. Light iris color.
E. Light skin color.

Question 23.48. **Which of the following genetic factors has NOT been linked to ocular melanoma?**

A. Loss of chromosome 3.
B. Gain of chromosome 8.
C. *BRAF* gene mutation.
D. p16INK4a promoter methylation.
E. *c-Myc* gene amplification.

Question 23.49. **Which of the following statements is true regarding the histopathology of ocular melanoma?**

A. Spindle cell melanomas have the worst prognosis.
B. Ocular melanomas exhibit three discrete pathologic stages.
C. Complex extracellular matrix patterns called *networks* and *parallel with cross-linking* show a strong correlation with metastatic disease.
D. No association has been established between extracellular matrix patterns and melanoma cell type.
E. Epithelioid melanomas comprise the vast majority of ocular melanomas and have the most favorable prognosis.

Question 23.50. **Which of the following statements is true regarding the clinical diagnosis of ocular melanoma?**

A. Accurate diagnosis of ocular melanoma cannot be achieved without a biopsy, which should be performed prior to any treatment.
B. Orbital CT is performed routinely to determine tumor location.
C. Orbital MRI is performed routinely to assess tumor size.
D. Retinal angiography using intravenous fluorescein demonstrates a pattern of intratumoral vascularity that is pathognomonic of ocular melanoma.
E. Ocular ultrasonography is the most important ancillary test for diagnosing ocular melanoma.

Question 23.51. **Which of the following statements is true regarding systemic metastasis from ocular melanoma?**

A. Metastatic disease is detected in about half of patients at the time of ocular diagnosis.
B. Systemic workup prior to treatment of ocular melanoma should include PET scan and bone marrow biopsy.
C. Liver function studies are possibly the most important component of the routine metastatic workup.
D. The median survival after diagnosis of metastatic ocular melanoma is about 3 years.
E. Liver function studies are sensitive and specific for ocular melanoma metastasis.

Question 23.52. **Which of the following statements is FALSE regarding treatment of ocular melanoma?**

A. Small melanomas less than 2.5 mm in thickness can be observed for growth prior to treatment.
B. Plaque radiotherapy is appropriate for most patients with medium-sized melanomas between 2.5 and 10 mm in thickness and less than 16 mm in basal diameter.
C. Enucleation is recommended for very large melanomas and those invading the optic nerve.
D. The radiation dose used for plaque radiotherapy of ocular melanoma is similar to that used for lymphoma.
E. Histopathologic diagnosis is not required prior to plaque radiotherapy.

Question 23.53. **A 73-year-old healthy man presents with a complaint of vision loss in his left eye for 2 months. Indirect ophthalmoscopy and ocular ultrasound examination reveal a large (13 mm thickness and 17 mm base) intraocular tumor located anterior to the ocular equator with features highly consistent with ocular melanoma. Which of the following statements is true regarding this patient?**

A. The tumor should be followed for evidence of growth prior to treatment.
B. A fine needle biopsy is needed prior to making a management decision.
C. The patient should be treated by enucleation preceded by external beam radiotherapy to minimize the risk of metastasis in this very large tumor.
D. The statistical likelihood of developing metastatic disease is lower in this patient than in a 36-year-old man with an identical tumor.
E. The statistical likelihood of developing metastatic disease is higher in this patient than in the same patient with an identical tumor located posterior to the ocular equator.

Question 23.54. **A 42-year-old healthy woman presents with 2 weeks of blurred vision in her right eye. On examination, she is found to have a pigmented choroidal tumor measuring 8 mm in basal diameter and 3 mm in thickness. The tumor is located 2 mm temporal to her fovea and is producing subretinal fluid that is tracking into her fovea, causing her visual symptoms. Which of the following statements is true regarding this patient?**

A. The statistical likelihood of developing metastatic disease is lower in this patient than in the same patient with an identical tumor located in the ciliary body.
B. Because of the delicate location of the tumor adjacent to the fovea, the standard of care is to remove the tumor by endoresection using a small vitrectomy instrument.
C. Plaque radiotherapy would be a good treatment choice because of the Bragg peak effect that limits collateral radiation damage to the fovea.
D. Plaque radiotherapy would not be a good treatment choice because the 5-year survival rate is inferior to enucleation.
E. The tumor should not be treated because the presence of subretinal fluid connotes a benign tumor.

Question 23.55. **A 69-year-old woman underwent enucleation of the right eye for a large ocular melanoma. She died 18 months later with widespread metastasis to the liver and lungs. Upon review of the histopathologic specimen from her enucleated eye, which of the following feature(s) would be least consistent with her clinical outcome?**

A. A predominance of spindle melanoma cells.
B. *Networks* and *parallel with cross-linking* extracellular matrix patterns.
C. Involvement of the ciliary body.
D. Tumor cell invasion through the sclera with focal extraocular extension.
E. Numerous mitotic figures.

Question 23.56. **A 54-year-old man is found to have a medium-sized ocular melanoma in his left eye. He says that he wants the treatment that has the strongest scientific support for reducing the risk of metastasis, and he is willing to lose his eye if necessary. Which of the following responses to the patient would be MOST accurate?**

A. Enucleation, charged particle therapy, and plaque radiotherapy have all been investigated extensively, but there is no evidence that any of these modalities provides a survival advantage superior to the other two.
B. Enucleation and plaque radiotherapy are both associated with 5-year survival rates superior to no treatment.
C. There is no statistically significant difference in the survival of patients treated with laser photocoagulation, transpupillary thermotherapy, local tumor resection, plaque radiotherapy, and enucleation.
D. If vision is not a consideration, enucleation is always the best treatment for minimizing the risk of metastasis.
E. Plaque radiotherapy combined with transpupillary thermotherapy provides survival benefit equal to enucleation.

Question 23.57. **The main complications of plaque radiotherapy include all of the following EXCEPT**

A. radiation retinopathy in the ipsilateral eye
B. radiation retinopathy in the contralateral eye
C. ocular inflammation
D. ocular dryness
E. cataract

Question 23.58. **Which of the following is most closely associated with poor visual outcome following plaque or charged particle radiotherapy?**

A. Close tumor proximity to the lens.
B. Decreased tumor thickness.
C. Increase in radiation dose from 50 centigray equivalent (CGE) to 70 CGE.
D. Decreased radiation dose rate.
E. Close tumor proximity to the fovea.

Question 23.59. **Radioisotopes that have been used for plaque radiotherapy of ocular melanoma include all of the following EXCEPT**

A. palladium-103
B. ruthenium-106
C. helium ions
D. iodine-125
E. cobalt-60

Question 23.60. **A 67-year-old man presents with a 6-month history of progressive vision loss in his right eye and is found to have a juxtapapillary ocular melanoma with frank invasion of the optic nerve head. Which of the following statements is MOST correct regarding this patient?**

A. The tumor should be treated with plaque radiotherapy because enucleation may disseminate tumor cells into the orbit.
B. Cranial MRI is indicated because there is a high risk of brain metastasis.
C. The risk of metastasis to the liver is greater than it would be for a similar tumor located 5 mm away from the optic disc.
D. Exenteration (removal of all orbital contents) is required.
E. The juxtapapillary location of this tumor necessitates the use of transpupillary thermotherapy since plaque or charged particle radiotherapy would result in severe vision loss.

ANSWERS

Answer 23.1. **The answer is D.**

Merkel cell carcinoma (MCC) or cutaneous neuroendocrine carcinoma is a rare highly aggressive tumor that commonly recurs locally and metastasizes to both lymph nodes and distal sites. The overall mortality rate is 30% to 35%. MCC is typically found on sun-exposed skin of the elderly. The average age at diagnosis is 69 years, and there is no predilection for either sex. The tumor is most commonly seen in white people with an estimated 470 new cases in the United States each year. Patients present with a solitary, flesh-colored or red, nontender nodule or plaque that has grown rapidly over weeks to months. The average size is less than 2 cm but can reach up to 20 cm. MCC usually occurs on the head and neck (50%), extremities (40%), and the trunk and genitals (10%). Definitive diagnosis is made by histologic examination including immunohistochemical staining where, typically, a collection of uniform small cells with scant cytoplasm and round to oval nuclei is found in the dermis. MCC expresses neuroendocrine markers and low-molecular-weight keratin and cytokeratin (CK) 20, which give a characteristic perinuclear dot pattern. Small cell carcinoma of the lung, the major histologic differential diagnosis, marks with CK7 stain and is negative for CK20.

Answer 23.2. **The answer is B.**

Squamous cell carcinomas (SCC) of the ear and lip are associated with a higher risk of local recurrence and metastasis than SCC at most other anatomic sites. In a meta-analysis of SCC by Rowe et al., the 5-year local recurrence rate for SCC of the ear was 18.7%, and the rate of metastasis was estimated to be 11%. Although these rates may be falsely elevated by the reporting bias inherent in the meta-analysis, recurrence and metastatic rates are clearly elevated for SCCs on the ear in addition to the lip. SCCs of the lip and ear have the highest associated mortality and metastasis rate of approximately 10%. Other factors that influence both local and systemic recurrence are the depth of invasion (deep dermis and subcutis), presence of neural invasion, and poor differentiation. Because 91% of metastases and 93% of recurrences associated with SCC occur within 3 years, clinical follow-up should initially be done within approximately 6 months and should include palpation of the regional lymph nodes to detect metastases. Radiologic and blood tests are not routinely indicated in patients without symptoms. Detection of soft enlarged lymph nodes warrants search for an infectious or inflammatory cause. Hard adenopathy in a regional nodal basin should be investigated either with fine-needle aspiration or nodal biopsy. The finding of metastatic SCC portends a poor prognosis, with a 34% 5-year survival.

Answer 23.3. **The answer is B.**

The number of nevi an individual has appears to be genetically determined, but modifiable by sun exposure. In this scenario, the clinical appearance, family history of melanoma, and occurrence in two siblings implicates a familial melanoma syndrome. The lifetime risk for melanoma for these individuals exceeds 50%. Atypical or dysplastic nevi are suspected by some to be precursors of melanoma, but most authorities consider them to represent markers of risk for melanoma. Most cutaneous melanomas arise *de novo*, not in association with a melanocytic nevus, but in patients with familial melanoma they can arise in association with an atypical or dysplastic nevus.

Answer 23.4. **The answer is A.**

Basal cell carcinoma (BCC) is the most common malignancy amongst white people, particularly those with fair skin, light-colored eyes, and who have early history of recreational sun exposure (intermittent, intense sun exposure resulting in sunburns). BCC accounts for approximately one fourth of all cancers diagnosed in the United States. BCCs rarely metastasize, but because they are locally aggressive and affect anatomic high-risk sites such as the nose, ears, and eyelids, they produce extensive morbidity via local tissue destruction. Sun-exposed areas are most commonly involved with the head and neck in 90% of patients (nose in 30%), but BCC can occur on non-sun-exposed sites such as the genitalia. Men are affected more commonly than women and most patients are over 50 years of age, but younger individuals developing BCC has become more common. The typical presentation is of a slowly enlarging, pearly translucent papule with rolled borders and telangiectases, which with time enlarge and show central ulceration (so-called rodent's ulcer). The diagnosis of basal cell carcinoma is easily confirmed by punch or shave biopsy.

Answer 23.5. **The answer is B.**

Angiosarcomas of soft tissue including skin are uncommon malignancies compromising approximately 2% of all soft tissue sarcomas. Angiosarcomas arise most frequently (60% of reported cases) in skin or superficial soft tissue, although occurrences in the liver, spleen, breast, and bone have been reported. Cutaneous angiosarcoma most commonly occurs on the face and scalp (50%), with a predilection for elderly men. Approximately 10% of cutaneous angiosarcoma cases occur in a setting of chronic lymphedema (i.e., associated with a persistent lymphangioma of the hand in this case). Stewart-Treves syndrome comprises angiosarcoma developing in a lymphedematous upper extremity after a radical mastectomy and axillary lymph node dissection for breast cancer. Angiosarcoma has also been described in areas of lymphedema secondary to a variety of other mechanisms, both primary and acquired. Angiosarcomas are biologically aggressive with a poor prognosis. The reported 5-year survival rate is 12%, with 50% of patients dying within 15 months. Disseminated intravascular coagulopathy can be the ultimate cause of death in patients with local disease. Lesions may metastasize widely; lung, liver, and spleen are the most common sites. Several prognostic factors have been identified, including small tumor size (<5 cm), aggressive mode of treatment (surgical excision with margins plus chemotherapy), low mitotic counts (<10 per 10 high-power fields), and possibly a brisk lymphocytic host response.

Answer 23.6. **The answer is C.**

The ABCD(EF) describe the clinical signs of melanoma and represent asymmetry, border irregularities, color change or variegation, large diameter, enlargement/evolution/elevation, and "funny looking." Loss of pigmentation with a white color change is a clinical sign of melanoma regression, but can also be found in halo melanocytic nevi. Most melanocytic nevi are small, symmetric, and uniform in color. Dysplastic nevi can show many features that overlap with melanoma. A changing or atypical appearing mole should be assumed to be melanoma until proven otherwise. Excisional biopsy is the method of choice. Early diagnosis and treatment can reduce mortality.

Answer 23.7. **The answer is D.**

Patients with melanoma can have spontaneous and therapeutically induced regression of their disseminated disease as well as develop areas of depigmentation (paraneoplastic vitiligo). Immunotherapy-related vitiligo is predictive of tumor response and is a measure of treatment potency. Both antibodies and T cells recognize melanogenesis-related proteins, which include GM2 ganglioside, MART-1 (MELAN-A), gp100, and TRP1/2.

Answer 23.8. **The answer is A.**

For most patients with surgically treated stage I, II, or III disease, recommended follow-up is primarily with periodic history and physical exam. Routine radiologic tests or screening blood tests have not been documented to improve survival. However, periodic chest x-rays are reasonable in an effort to identify lung metastases prior to the onset of symptoms as early detection may increase the therapeutic options available to the patient. Although routine performance of CT scans is not indicated, directed CT scans can be very useful in evaluating patients with suspicious symptoms, physical findings, laboratory abnormalities (anemia, or elevated LDH), or an abnormal chest x-ray. The follow-up schedule for patients who have surgically resected disease is based on the depth of the primary lesion and the presence or absence of nodal disease. For patients with a thin primary melanoma and negative nodes, a follow-up is with clinical exam for evidence of occurrence every 6 months for the first 2 to 3 years and then yearly for 2 to 3 years beyond that. For patients with intermediate or thick melanomas and negative regional nodes, follow-up should be every 3 to 6 months for the first 2 to 3 years and every 6 to 12 months for the next 2 to 3 years. For patients with resected regional disease, their follow-up should be every 3 to 4 months for the first 2 years and then every 6 months up to year 5 and yearly beyond that. All patients must understand that they need routine lifelong dermatologic screening.

Answer 23.9. **The answer is B.**

The correct AJCC stage is IIIB (T4bN2c, M0); he has "in transit" or satellite metastases, which makes his nodal stage N2c. These deposits represent intralymphatic metastases and portend a very poor prognosis. In melanomas greater than 4 mm in thickness, wide local excision with at least 2-cm margins is recommended. In transit metastases occur in about 3% to 4% of stage I and II patients and increase to about 10% to 15% in patients with stage III disease. When present, in transit metastases are usually multiple and evolve over time. Although previous staging systems distinguished between satellitosis (within 2.0 cm of the primary tumor) and in transit metastases (more than 2.0 cm from the primary tumor), pathophysiologically these two events represent different points on a continuum of the same biologic process, lymphatic dissemination of metastases. At the time when an in transit metastasis is surgically removed, it is generally recommended that lymphatic mapping and sentinel node excision be performed in all patients with clinically negative regional lymph nodes, since the probability of occult nodal metastases is as high as 50%. For most patients with surgically treated stage I, II, or III disease, recommended follow-up is primarily with periodic history and physical exam; the schedule is dependent on the thickness of the melanoma and presence or absence of regional disease. All patients must understand that they need routine lifelong dermatalogic screening. Patients who have had one melanoma remain at higher than average risk of a second primary melanoma and also are at risk of basal cell and squamous cell carcinomas.

Answer 23.10. **The answer is E.**

A typical fibroxanthoma (AFX) is an intermediate-grade dermal fibrohistiocytic neoplasm that typically arises on sun-exposed skin in the elderly patient with a mean age of onset at 70 years. Clinically, AFX is a solitary, often ulcerated nodule, usually measuring less than 2 cm. The clinical differential diagnosis of AFX includes basal cell carcinoma, squamous cell carcinoma, metastatic carcinoma, pyogenic granuloma, and ulcerated chondrodermatitis helicis. AFX may be a superficial variant of malignant fibrous histiocytoma (MFH) with a significantly lower metastatic potential. Unlike the cytologically indistinguishable MFH, AFX arises within the dermis and usually does not invade deep subcutaneous tissue, fascia, or muscle. AFX is characterized histologically by an expansile dermal spindle-cell neoplasm, often with a Grenz or clear zone separating it from the epidermis (spindle cell variants of melanoma and squamous cell carcinoma are often contiguous with an *in situ* component). The neoplasm consists of pleomorphic cells with irregular cytology, nuclear atypia, multiple mitoses, and bizarre multinucleation. The histologic differential diagnosis includes desmoplastic melanoma, spindle-cell squamous cell carcinoma, malignant fibrous histiocytoma, metastatic carcinoma, and malignant neural and muscular tumors. AFX reacts with stains for vimentin, CD68 (macrophage marker), antichymotrypsin, and antitrypsin, but not for S-100 protein, cytokeratin, and desmin. Unlike the highly lethal, deeper MFH, AFX carries an excellent prognosis; local recurrence occurs in only 7% of cases and metastasizes rarely.

Answer 23.11. **The answer is D.**

Kaposi sarcoma (KS) can be divided into four epidemiologic variants, all of which are associated with HHV-8 infection. The four variants include classic KS, African endemic KS, iatrogenic KS, and epidemic, acquired immunodeficiency syndrome–associated (AIDS-associated) KS. African endemic KS can be further subdivided into three forms: indolent nodular, locally aggressive (florid and infiltrative), and disseminated aggressive. Nodular African endemic KS presents clinically and behaves similarly to classic KS. The more aggressive forms predominantly affect young black Africans, with the fulminant lymphadenopathic disease with visceral organ involvement usually without cutaneous manifestations. The prognosis is very poor, with a 100% fatality rate within 3 years. A classification system, inclusive of all clinical variants, divides KS into four stages: stage I: locally indolent cutaneous lesions, stage II: locally invasive lesions, stages III and IV: disseminated and systemic KS with generalized lymphadenopathy. Each stage is further subdivided as A or B according to the absence or presence of systemic symptoms such as fever or weight loss greater than 10%. Three distinct prognostic factors exist: (a) the extent of the disease (tumor burden), (b) the presence or absence of systemic symptoms, and (c) the presence of opportunistic infections. Punch biopsy of any of his cutaneous lesions would be diagnostic, but the pathologic findings would vary depending on whether a patch, plaque, or nodule is biopsied. All would show a spindle cell proliferation forming vascular spaces.

Answer 23.12. **The answer is E.**

Clinical and histologic studies have resulted in defining five major steps of melanoma development and progression: (a) common acquired and congenital nevi with structurally normal melanocytes; (b) dysplastic nevi with structural and architectural atypia; (c) radial growth phase (RGP), nontumorigenic primary melanomas without metastatic competence; (d) vertical growth phase (VGP), tumorigenic primary melanomas with competence for metastasis; and (e) metastatic melanoma. Although not proven, genes involved in melanocyte development are suspected to play a crucial role in melanoma development, such as those genes from the *WNT* signaling pathway, microphthalmia-associated transcription factor (*MITF*), *PAX3*, and *SOX10*. Growth factor receptor genes such as *c-KIT* or endothelin receptor-B (*EDNRB*) can also have a potential role in melanocyte transformation. Cytogenetic studies have identified the 9p21 locus, which is frequently affected in familial melanoma and encodes two distinct proteins, p16INK4A and *p14ARF*. Both of these genes exhibit tumor suppressor activity in genetically distinct anticancer pathways (i.e., the "Rb pathway" for p16INK4A and the "p53 pathway" for *p14ARF*). To date, the p16INK4A and *CDK4* (located on chromosome 12q4) genes have been found to be mutated in some familial melanoma families.

Answer 23.13. **The answer is D.**

Immunosuppressed patients with lymphoma or leukemia, patients with AIDS, and organ transplant patients have a higher risk for nonmelanoma skin cancers (NMSC) such as infiltrative basal cell carcinoma and squamous cell carcinoma (SCC). Ultraviolet light radiation is the primary pathogenic factor for the development of NMSC, but degree and duration of immunosuppression are also factors. Although organ transplant recipients have an increased incidence of viral warts, the role of HPV in skin cancer is not clearly defined. For organ transplant recipients, up to a 65 times increased risk for SCC exists compared to the general population. SCCs in this setting occur at a younger age and are more aggressive with an increased risk of local recurrence, regional and distant metastasis, and mortality. Metastasis from skin cancer in organ transplant recipients is mostly due to SCC. The 3-year overall and disease-specific survival was 48% and 56%, respectively, for patients who developed metastatic SCC. Preventive, early, and aggressive therapeutic interventions are required to minimize this serious complication of transplant-associated immunosuppression due to large tumor burden and aggressive nature of these tumors.

Answer 23.14. **The answer is E.**

One in five Americans will develop skin cancer during their lives, and more than 97% of these will be nonmelanoma skin cancer (NMSC). The rising incidence of NMSC is probably due to a combination of increased sun exposure, more frequent outdoor activities, changes in clothing style, increased longevity, and ozone depletion. Although NMSC has a low mortality and morbidity, it is more common than all other cancers and has a higher incidence than lung cancer, breast cancer, prostate cancer, and colon cancer combined. If cancers are classified according to cost of care in addition to number of cases and number of deaths, the financial impact of treatment can also be used to prioritize importance of different malignancies. Utilizing such a scheme ranks NMSC far higher than would death statistics as the five most costly cancers to Medicare are lung, prostate, colorectal, breast, and NMSC. Some epidemiologic studies suggest that development of NMSC, including basal cell carcinoma (BCC) and squamous cell carcinoma (SCC), may indicate increased risk for internal malignancy.

Answer 23.15. **The answer is B.**

Sebaceous carcinoma (SC) mostly frequently affects the eye, with the upper eyelids the most frequent site of involvement, and less than 25% of all SC present at extraocular sites such as the head and neck, trunk, salivary glands, and external genitalia. Approximately 50% of SCs are initially incorrectly diagnosed histologically or, in some series, initially misdiagnosed clinically. SC may present as chronic diffuse blepharoconjunctivitis or keratoconjunctivitis, particularly when pagetoid or intraepithelial spread of tumor onto the conjunctival epithelium occurs. Histologically, SC exhibits varying basaloid, squamoid cells and sebaceous differentiation with nuclear pleomorphism, hyperchromatism, and local infiltration of surrounding tissues. Special stains, including lipid stains such as Oil-Red-O or Sudan IV for fresh tissue, and immunohistochemical stains, such as EMA or LeuM1, are helpful for the its diagnosis. SC is associated with sebaceous adenomas, radiation exposure, Bowen disease, and Muir-Torre syndrome. In Muir-Torre syndrome, an autosomal dominant heritable condition, SC, and, more commonly, sebaceous adenoma (or sebaceous epithelioma) are associated with a second internal malignancy, usually a carcinoma of the colon or urogenital tract, and occasionally keratoacanthomas. Therefore, patients with SC should have routine screening for internal malignancy (stool for occult blood, analysis of urine, colonoscopy), and a family history for internal malignancy should be sought and family members screened, if indicated. Poor prognostic indicators in SC include a duration of more than 6 months, multicentric origin, poor differentiation, infiltrative pattern, pagetoid changes, vascular invasion, lymphatic channel involvement, previous radiation, and orbital spread. After treatment for SC, patients should be followed for recurrence or progression through regular examination of skin and lymph nodes. A mortality rate of 20% to 22% has been reported in ocular and extraocular SC. SC can spread by lymphatic or hematogenous routes or by direct extension with distant metastases in up to 20% of cases involving the lungs, liver, brain, bones, and/or lymph nodes.

Answer 23.16. **The answer is B.**

Both squamous cell carcinoma (SCC) and angiosarcoma (AS) are known to occur in areas of previous radiation therapy. AS is also seen in the context of chronic lymphedema (Stewart-Treves syndrome) and SCC in areas of burn scars, chronic inflammatory dermatosis, and ulceration. Although ultraviolet radiation in the form of frequent sunburns has been implicated in the pathogenesis of melanoma, ionizing radiation, of the type used in radiation therapy, has not. Finally, the range for local recurrence of breast carcinoma (median follow-up of approximately 80 months) following surgery alone has been reported in the range of 18% to 35% and for surgery plus radiation 2% to 13%. The typical clinical presentation is one or more asymptomatic skin or subcutaneous chest wall nodules within, or in the vicinity of, the surgical scar. Cutaneous metastasis at distant sites may also occur in other types of cancer, including colon and melanoma in women and lung, colon, and melanoma in men. By far, the most common malignancy that metastasizes to the skin in women is breast.

Answer 23.17. **The answer is E.**

This patient has stage II (T2N0, M0) melanoma. Appropriate care includes wide local excision at the time of sentinel lymph node biopsy. He has a history of nonmelanoma skin cancer and now melanoma. As the patient is immunocompromised due to his transplant status, further management of his disease poses important questions, such as the specific immunosuppressive agents used and their dosages.

The chronic use of immunosuppressive agents in transplant patients increases their long-term risk of malignancy—approximately 100 times that of the general population. Nonmelanoma skin cancer (NMSC) is the most common type of malignancy in the transplant patient. The increased incidence of SCCs is greater than or equal to 65 times, BCC 10 times, and melanoma 3 times over the general population, most likely due to a combination of decreased immune surveillance and a direct carcinogenic effect of cyclosporine and/or azothioprine. Studies suggest there is a dose-response relationship between the type and level of immunosuppression and the development of malignancies. Carcinomas most frequently arise on sun-exposed sites and in patients who have a history of high sun exposure both prior to, and following, transplantation. In addition, these carcinomas are often associated with cutaneous HPV infections. Most importantly, however, SCCs presenting in these patients have a high metastatic risk. It is unclear whether risk of metastasis for melanoma is increased in this patient population. Interestingly, rapamycin may be an agent of choice in the management of graft rejection in these patients as transplant patients on this agent have been noted to have fewer incidences of cutaneous malignancies.

IFN, due to its immunostimulatory properties, is contraindicated in the treatment of stage III disease in the transplant population.

Answer 23.18. **The answer is E.**

Xeroderma pigmentosa (XP) is an autosomal recessive disorder resulting in either a defect in DNA excision repair or in the capacity to replicate damaged DNA. Affected patients are predisposed to UV-induced DNA damage and ultimately develop both nonmelanoma and melanoma skin cancers. The skin is normal at birth but progressively develops dyspigmentation and atrophy in areas of sun exposure and, ultimately, cutaneous malignancies. Mean age of onset of symptoms, in both the skin and the eyes, is 2 years, and skin cancer onset is usually by 10 years of age. The majority of melanomas that occur in these patients are on sun-exposed areas (face, head, and neck) and are of the lentigo maligna subtype, one commonly associated with chronic sun exposure. These patients are at increased risk for UV-induced ocular neoplasms of the lid and conjunctiva and may suffer from neurologic abnormalities as well.

Seven XP complementation groups (*XP-A* through *XP-G*) have been identified, based upon cell fusion experiments and complementation of repair synthesis, each of which carry a separate genetic mutation necessary for NER *in vitro* (except for *XP-E*). The clinical phenotype (skin cancer severity and associated abnormalities) is determined by the complementation group.

Answer 23.19. **The answer is C.**

Angiosarcoma is an aggressive, often fatal vascular neoplasm. Four variants are recognized: AS of the scalp and face (as in this patient), AS in the setting of chronic lymphedema (Stewart-Treves syndrome), radiation-induced AS, and epitheliod AS. AS of the head and scalp usually affects the elderly, most commonly men. The clinical presentation (an erythematous ill-defined plaque) is similar in all types, as is the aggressive biologic behavior and poor prognosis. Some patients present as unexplained facial edema. Induration and ulceration may occur as the lesions progress, and metastasis to the lymph nodes, lung, and brain are common. Local recurrence rates are high: greater than 80% in certain series. Five-year survival as low as 34% has been reported.

Microscopic examination reveals anastomosing dilated vascular channels lined by atypical endothelial cells that stain positively for several endothelial markers: *Ulex europeas* I lectin, factor VIII-related antigen, CD34, and CD31.

Answer 23.20. **The answer is E.**

Dermatofibrosarcoma protuberans (DFSP) is a low-grade cutaneous sarcoma having aggressive local behavior but low metastatic potential. The tumor typically presents as a plaque on the trunk in young to middle-aged adults and clinically resembles a dermatofibroma or keloid. Microscopic exam reveals monomorphous spindle cells in a storiform pattern that surrounds adipocytes or extends eccentrically in stratified horizontal plates. Immunostaining of DFSP is positive for CD34 and negative for factor XIIIa, while dermatofibromas are diffusely positive for factor XIIIa and negative for CD34.

Due to their eccentric and extensive local infiltration, these tumors are treated by wide local excision using wide (2- to 3-cm) margins. Recurrence rates are related to the adequacy of surgical margins and have been reported as high as 33% to 60% when conservative margins are taken. Overall, recurrence rates of 50% have been reported. Mohs micrographic surgery (MMS) using frozen sections with confirmation by paraffin-embedded sections has also been advocated in the treatment of these tumors, particularly tumors of the head and neck, where tissue conservation is of utmost importance.

Answer 23.21. **The answer is C.**

Primary extramammary Paget disease is a cutaneous neoplasm of apocrine gland origin, most commonly affecting the anogenital area and axilla. Some feel that it represents an epidermotropic apocrine adenocarcinoma with its origin in the epidermis or epidermal appendages. On microscopic exam, characteristic cytologically atypical clear cells ("Paget cells") are seen within the epidermis.

The vulva is the most common presenting site. Intraepithelial vulvar Paget disease rarely progresses to frank invasive carcinoma, although microscopic foci of dermal invasion by "Paget cells" may be present. Treatment is primarily local excision. In contrast, perianal extramammary Paget disease may be associated with regional local rectal or anal carcinoma internally, and may, in fact, represent pagetoid spread of these extracutaneous malignancies (secondary Paget disease). Immunohistochemical staining for cytokeratins may aid in distinguishing primary from secondary Paget disease.

Bowen disease, or squamous cell carcinoma *in situ*, commonly occurs in the genital area, and may present as an erythematous plaque with scale. Histology reveals full thickness keratinocyte atypia. Bowenoid papulosis, associated with infection with HPV subtypes 16 and 18, presents as a verrucous papule of the genital area.

Answer 23.22. **The answer is E.**

Melanoma incidence has risen continuously in the United States, and it is estimated that over 55,000 cases of invasive melanoma will be diagnosed in the year 2004. The increase in melanoma incidence is felt to be real and not solely the result of increased diagnosis, because the absolute number of patients dying from melanoma in the United States continues to rise even though the overall survival rate has improved. In addition, deaths from melanoma have risen consistently over the last several decades.

The controversy regarding the use of sunscreen contributing to the development of melanoma is an interesting one that has received much media attention. Published series to date, including several meta-analyses, do not support a causal relationship between sunscreen use and melanoma development. Nonetheless, it has been suggested that educational campaigns advocate the use of sunscreen in conjunction with other methods of sun protection (protective clothing) and sun avoidance during peak hours of UV intensity as effective methods for skin cancer prevention.

Answer 23.23. **The answer is E.**

This patient has an acral lentiginous melanoma, stage IIB (T3bN0, M0). This melanoma subtype comprises approximately 10% of all melanomas and may occur on the palms, soles, and subungual regions of white people, as well as in persons of color: African, Hispanic, and Asian individuals. The pathogenesis of this tumor is most likely distinct from that of the other melanoma subtypes and is not related to UV exposure.

Matched for Breslow depth, these tumors do not behave more aggressively than other melanoma types; however, they do tend to be diagnosed at a more advanced stage due to their location. Workup of stage II disease, according to NCCN guidelines, specify the optional performance of chest x-ray and LDH and do not include PET or CT examination. Similarly, the same treatment guidelines apply to all melanoma subtypes and are based upon Breslow depth. Adjuvant radiation therapy is not recommended, and as outlined in the text, radiation as a treatment modality in melanoma is advocated judiciously, and only in certain clinical situations.

Answer 23.24. **The answer is E.**

Workup of stage II disease, according to NCCN guidelines, specify the optional performance of chest x-ray and LDH. The same treatment guidelines apply to all melanoma subtypes and are based upon Breslow depth.

Answer 23.25. **The answer is C.**

This patient has a significant positive family history of melanoma in the setting of clinically atypical nevi: similar families have previously been associated with an increased risk of melanoma development due to a genetic abnormality in the *CDKN2A* gene located on chromosome 9p21. Although the phenotype of atypical nevi in the setting of a positive family history of melanoma does not necessarily translate into *CDKN2A* mutation status, approximately 50% of such patients may carry the mutation, according to findings in one study.

Although her atypical nevi are both markers of risk and, potentially, precursors to melanoma, there is no evidence to suggest that prophylactic excision of all of her atypical nevi is indicated. As for all patients, nevi that demonstrate change in size, color, border irregularity, or bleeding should be excised for histopathologic evaluation. In sporadic melanoma, most tumors arise *de novo.* In familial melanoma, these tumors may arise more frequently in a precursor lesion (i.e. atypical nevus), although not all dermatopathologists subscribe to the high numbers often reported (70%).

Answer 23.26. **The answer is E.**

It is estimated that approximately 5% to 10% of melanoma patients will develop a second primary melanoma over their lifetime, the frequency being higher in patients with familial melanoma. In patients with sporadic (nonfamilial) melanoma having multiple primaries, 8% are found to have *CDKN2A* germline mutations. Two-thirds of these tumors occur subsequent to the initial melanoma diagnosis. Interestingly, a significant number (approximately 50% in one study) of melanomas are found by patients themselves or close family members. In addition, patients performing skin self-examination have been reported to detect their melanomas at an earlier stage. These findings emphasize the importance of patient education and self-examination in addition to routine skin examinations performed by a physician.

Answer 23.27. **The answer is B.**

According to NCCN Practice Guidelines for Melanoma, patients with melanoma *in situ* (stage 0 disease) do not require staging workup. These patients should have a total body skin examination and periodic skin examination for life.

Answer 23.28. **The answer is C.**

Basal cell nevus syndrome, or Gorlin syndrome, is an autosomal dominant disorder clinically characterized by multiple basal cell carcinomas that occur early in life and other developmental defects, including odontoid keratocysts, skeletal abnormalities, plantar or palmar pits, and predisposition to other cancers. Germline mutations in the tumor suppressor gene *PTC*, or *patched*, have been identified in the pathogenesis of this disease. Interestingly, somatic mutations in *patched* have also been identified in sporadic tumors.

Answer 23.29. **The answer is E.**

There is no convincing evidence to support a causal link between pregnancy or the use of estrogens and melanoma. Particularly in early stage disease (stage I and II), melanomas diagnosed during pregnancy do not appear to have a worsened prognosis: studies have found no decrease in 10-year disease-free or overall survival. Prognosis remains dependent on tumor thickness and the presence of ulceration. The issue of pregnancy *following* the diagnosis of melanoma may be somewhat less straightforward, and recommendations are usually based upon risk of recurrence and patient age. Some physicians advise waiting from 0 to 5 years following initial diagnosis based upon tumor thickness and stage. There is presently no evidence to demonstrate increased risk of melanoma or melanoma recurrence with the use of oral contraceptives or hormone replacement therapy.

Answer 23.30. **The answer is F.**

Congenital nevi, by definition, are nevi that are present at birth or that may become apparent during infancy. The classic microscopic findings include nevus cells that are present in the deeper dermis, reticular dermis, or subcutis. Congenital nevi are characteristically divided according to their diameter into small (<1.5 cm), medium (1.5 to 20 cm) and large (≥20 cm). The most significant risk for the development of melanoma exists in large congenital nevi; lifetime risk of melanoma development has been estimated to be between 5% to 20%, with approximately 60% of these occurring in the first few years of life. Interestingly, the majority of melanomas that develop in these large nevi do not have an epidermal component, and characteristic changes associated with melanoma may not be clinically apparent. Taken together, it is therefore recommended that these large lesions be prophylactically excised, typically in a staged fashion. In contrast, the risk of melanoma development in small and intermediate congenital nevi is low, and prophylactic excision is not routinely recommended. In small and intermediate congenital nevi that have regular pigmentation, symmetry, and borders, it is generally agreed upon that clinical observation is an appropriate management strategy.

Answer 23.31. **The answer is C.**

Initial management of early stage (intermediate thickness) melanoma is straightforward. It is essential that dermatologists, general practitioners, and internists as well as medical oncologists have a firm understanding of the guidelines in order to expedite referral to the appropriate surgical specialist for wide local excision and sentinel lymph node (SLN) mapping. Excisional biopsy is the most appropriate method for diagnosis and permits the accurate measurement of primary depth (Breslow thickness). Intraoperative lymphatic mapping with sentinel node lymphadenectomy has emerged as the standard practice as a method to accurately stage patients with primary cutaneous melanoma. At most academic centers, SLN mapping is performed for primary lesions greater than or equal to 1 mm depth; in selected thin (<1.0 mm) lesions with features of regression or ulceration, SLN mapping is advised. Recommendations for surgical margins are based on data from randomized clinical trials and in this case, a surgical margin of 2 cm was obtained. Several reports conclude that PET-FDG imaging is not sensitive for the detection of micrometastasis in nodal tissue and should not replace intraoperative techniques. There is no proven benefit for adjuvant interferon in patients with T2aN0, Mx (stage I) melanoma.

Answer 23.32. **The answer is C.**

Treatment options for patients diagnosed with stage III (surgically resected) melanoma include adjuvant high-dose interferon α-2b, participation in a clinical trial, or observation. The risk of recurrence in this patient with stage IIIB disease is significant (expected 5-year survival is 49%), so adjuvant systemic therapy is a reasonable choice for this woman. High-dose interferon α-2b approved by the FDA in 1995 is the only adjuvant therapy that has proven benefit to prolong relapse-free survival or overall survival in melanoma and is best tolerated in patients under the age of 60 with no other comorbidities. Adjuvant GM-CSF has been reported in a single arm (uncontrolled) study to increase the disease-free survival in patients with resected stage III or stage IV melanoma; this observation awaits confirmation in a larger controlled trial and should not be considered as first-line treatment. In patients with measurable (metastatic) melanoma, GM-CSF alone or in combination with dacarbazine has little to no clinical activity based on no objective responses seen in a group of 32 patients.

Answer 23.33. **The answer is D.**

Desmoplastic variants of cutaneous melanoma tend to be neurotropic and locally aggressive. A recent report suggests that radiation therapy can reduce the risk of local recurrence and thus, this modality might play an important role in the management of patients with desmoplastic melanoma (in contrast to the more common histologic types); however, controlled studies are needed to address this question. There are no published data that suggest adjuvant interferon has efficacy in desmoplastic melanoma.

Answer 23.34. **The answer is E.**

Although the role for radiation therapy in the management of advanced melanoma is limited, there are several indications advocated for patients with regional and metastatic disease. For regional disease, the most common indications include the use of adjuvant radiotherapy for primary head and neck melanoma, desmoplastic (or neurotropic variants) melanoma, after salvage lymphadenectomy for recurrent disease, and palliation of unresectable nodal disease. For metastatic disease, the most common indications include the symptomatic palliation for skin, subcutaneous, bone, and brain metastases. Radiotherapy can successfully palliate smaller (<5 cm diameter) subcutaneous lesions in approximately 60% to 80% of cases. Whole brain radiotherapy (30 Gy in 10 fractions) is considered definitive treatment for patients with newly diagnosed brain metastases that are deemed unresectable or not amenable to treatment with stereotactic radiosurgery. Although local control with palliation of symptoms can be achieved in some patients, most patients die (median survival approximately 3 to 4 months) with active intracranial disease despite the use of steroids and whole brain radiotherapy.

Answer 23.35. **The answer is B.**

Extracapsular extension of tumor is an independent adverse prognostic indicator in stage III melanoma, and patients with stage IIIC melanoma are at high risk of recurrence (24% expected 5-year survival). This patient should receive adjuvant therapy and, as mentioned previously, high-dose interferon confers a small but statistically significant relapse free survival (RFS) advantage compared to observation. In the setting of gross extracapsular extension, some experts recommend an abbreviated course of radiation therapy prior to initiation of interferon with the goal of improved local control. Concurrent administration of radiation with interferon at standard doses is discouraged based on severe toxicities reported by investigators. Conventional chemotherapy or high-dose chemotherapy with stem cell transplantation has not been shown to provide a survival benefit to patients with high-risk stage III melanoma and, thus, cannot be advocated. Low-dose regimens of interferon have yet to show a survival benefit in any randomized clinical trial.

Answer 23.36. **The answer is D.**

The toxicities of high-dose interferon α-2b (HDI) given at the recommended dosage and schedule include constitutional symptoms (such as fever, chill, fatigue, malaise, and diaphoresis), myelosuppression, hepatotoxicity, and neurologic, gastrointestinal, and musculoskeletal symptoms. Thyroid dysfunction (hyper- and hypothyroidism) is less common and has been reported in approximately 10% to 20% of patients. Virtually all patients experience fatigue and many experience one (or more) of the remaining constitutional symptoms listed above. The incidence of myelosuppression (92% any grade), hepatotoxicity (63%), neuropsychiatric/depression (40%), nausea/vomiting (66%), and myalgia (75%) is substantial. Accordingly, appropriate management of HDI-related toxicities is essential to successful administration of the 1-year duration of therapy. In the most recently reported randomized clinical trial (E1694/S9512/C509801), 33% of patients required a delay or dose reduction in the induction treatment, while 38% of patients required a delay or dose reduction in the maintenance treatment (for any reason). A three-tiered dose modification guideline based on the dose-limiting toxicities of absolute neutrophil count (<500 cells per mm^3) and hepatic transaminases (elevated SGOT/SGPT >5 times normal) has been proposed by Kirkwood and colleagues. Approximately 75% to 80% of patients are able to complete HDI therapy for 1 year with appropriate medical supervision.

Answer 23.37. **The answer is D.**

The median survival of patients with brain metastasis is 3 to 4 months despite definitive treatment with steroids and whole brain radiotherapy. A recent report from the Sidney Melanoma Unit documents the outcome of patients with cerebral metastases treated by various approaches from 1952 through 2000. The authors conclude that the median survival was dependent on treatment approach with patients undergoing surgery followed by radiation therapy as having the best outcome (median survival 8.9 months). Patient selection for metastasectomy is an essential step in providing optimal care for melanoma patients with one or several metastases confined to a single organ or site. Historic data from multiple institutions support the notion that complete resection of isolated distant metastases confers a survival advantage to some patients. In the case presented, referral to a neurosurgeon for craniotomy is the optimal approach. An acceptable alternative would be stereotactic radiosurgery; however, it is unclear if radiosurgery is equivalent to craniotomy with complete resection, and randomized clinical trials are needed to address this question. A recent report evaluating temozolomide as initial therapy for newly diagnosed brain metastases shows a 7% radiologic response rate with 29% of patients with stable disease recorded after 2 months of treatment; median survival was 3.2 months for the entire cohort of 151 patients.

Answer 23.38. **The answer is A.**

All of the therapies listed except IL-2 are investigational agents and are currently under study for melanoma. High dose IL-2 was approved by the United States FDA for treatment of metastatic melanoma in 1998.

Answer 23.39. **The answer is A.**

A retrospective analysis (n = 374 patients) concludes that the presence of metastases only to subcutaneous and/or cutaneous sites, lymphocytosis immediately after treatment, and long-term immunologic side effects, especially vitiligo, were associated with antitumor response to high dose IL-2 therapy.

Answer 23.40. **The answer is C.**

This is the same patient as in Question 23.39. CNS relapse is a significant problem in patients who respond to DTIC-based regimens of biochemotherapy. As noted in one study, 11 of 19 (58%) responding patients developed a recurrence in the CNS as the initial site relapse. Interestingly, temozolomide-based biochemotherapy resulted in fewer CNS relapses (36% of responders) with no improvement in overall survival. A series of randomized clinical trials evaluating biochemotherapy failed to show a survival advantage compared to combination chemotherapy alone.

Answer 23.41. **The answer is D.**

Despite the expression of *C-KIT* on approximately 50% of cutaneous melanomas, imatinib appears to have minimal to no single agent activity in metastatic melanoma as reported.

Answer 23.42. **The answer is C.**

This patient has recurrent stage IIIC melanoma with in-transit metastases. High-dose interferon is approved as adjuvant therapy for resected stage III disease and, thus, is not optimal. External beam radiotherapy would have a limited role as an initial approach in this patient. A series of reports document response rates of approximately 60% to 90% in patients treated by therapeutic limb perfusion with melphalan. In general, complete response rates of 40% to 60% have been published with 9- to 12-month duration of response. Addition of agents such as tumor necrosis factor-α or interferon-α do not appear to be confer benefit if added to melphalan. Resection of in-transit lesions followed by adjuvant limb perfusion is generally not advocated, especially in patients with innumerable or bulky lesions.

Answer 23.43. **The answer is C.**

Merkel cell carcinoma is a rare cutaneous tumor with an estimated 470 cases each year in the United States. The majority of patients present with localized disease, while approximately 20% of cases present with regional involvement at diagnosis. Staging with CT imaging of the chest, abdomen, and pelvis is recommended based on the notion that Merkel cell carcinoma has aggressive behavior and tendency for early metastasis similar to other (more common) small cell neoplasms. Although no randomized clinical trials have been performed, adjuvant radiotherapy to the primary site and the regional nodal area is recommended by most experts. There is no data to support the administration of adjuvant systemic chemotherapy, despite the fact that Merkel cell carcinoma is responsive to standard combinations such as etoposide and cisplatin.

Answer 23.44. **The answer is E.**

SCC and BCC account for the vast majority of skin cancers in organ transplant patients. SCCs are known to be more aggressive in these patients compared to normal individuals not receiving immunosuppressive medications, and recurrent SCC will metastasize in approximately

8% of patients within 2 years. The risk of SCC is proportional to the degree of immunosuppression with an overall relative risk 65 to 250. The relative risk for BCC is approximately 10 in patients receiving immunosuppression. The risk of melanoma is moderately increased, approximately 2- to 4-fold higher compared to normal individuals. Rowe and colleagues found that primary SCCs less than 4 mm in depth were associated with a low (6.7%) recurrence rate; in contrast, tumors greater than 4 mm in depth recurred at a much higher rate (45%). Mohs micrographic surgery is the optimal approach for resection and allows for normal tissue conservation in most cases. Most importantly, recurrence rates are significantly lower in patients treated by Mohs technique compared to standard excisional approaches. Palliative chemotherapy is often administered to patients with metatstatic SCC.

Answer 23.45. **The answer is B.**

Dermatofibrosarcoma protuberans (DFSP) is a low-grade cutaneous sarcoma and is associated with high (approximately 50%) local recurrence rates. Although metastases are uncommon, the lung is the preferred site for distant disease. Recent discoveries suggest that PDGF-beta is dysregulated in DFSP by virtue of a chromosomal rearrangement involving collagen type I alpha1, which creates a novel fusion protein capable of signaling through the PDGF receptor. It is CD34 positive consistent with a neural origin and carries the t(17;22) (q22;q13), resulting in the (over)expression of PDGF beta. Imatinib is a selective small molecule inhibitor of protein tyrosine kinases *C-KIT*, PDGF receptor, and bcr-abl. A case report presents a 25-year-old patient with unresectable metastatic DFSP treated with imatinib. The patient had a dramatic response to treatment after 4 months of imatinib and the mass was surgically resected with no residual tumor present. Karyotypic analysis failed to reveal the classic t(17;22), but a cryptic translocation involving chromosome 22q13 was discovered.

Answer 23.46. **The answer is D.**

Extrascleral extension into the orbit is observed in about 15% of ocular melanomas, mainly large tumors. Optic nerve invasion is relatively rare. Lymphatic spread has not been demonstrated, consistent with the absence of lymphatics in the eye (this is in contrast to cutaneous melanoma). Hematogenous dissemination to the liver is the most frequent form of metastatic spread, occurring in about 90% of metastasis cases. Metastasis to other sites (e.g., lung, heart, gastrointestinal tract, lymph nodes, pancreas, skin, central nervous system, bone, spleen, adrenal, kidney, ovary, and thyroid) generally occur in association with liver metastases.

Answer 23.47. **The answer is A.**

Atypical moles and cutaneous melanomas associated with dysplastic nevus syndrome have clearly been linked to ocular melanoma. However, isolated sporadic cutaneous melanoma has not been associated with an increased risk of ocular melanoma. Oculo (dermal) melanocytosis, or nevus of Ota, significantly increases the risk of ocular melanoma in the ipsilateral eye. Light iris color and light skin color have been linked to increased ocular melanoma risk, although a role for ultraviolet light overexposure remains controversial.

Answer 23.48. **The answer is C.**

Loss of chromosome 3 and gain of chromosome 8 are associated with increased metastatic risk in ocular melanoma. Hypermethylation of the p16INK4a gene promoter and amplification of *c-Myc* occur in up to 32% and 43%, respectively, of primary ocular melanomas. *BRAF* mutations are common in cutaneous melanomas but are extremely rare in ocular melanomas.

Answer 23.49. **The answer is C.**

Spindle cell tumors (comprising about 30% of ocular melanomas) have the best prognosis, and epithelioid tumors (comprising about 5% of ocular melanomas) have the worst prognosis. Mixed cell melanomas account for the majority of ocular melanomas, but these three cytologic categories form a spectrum rather than discrete stages. The extracellular matrix patterns called *networks* and *parallel with cross-linking* show a strong correlation with epithelioid cell type and metastatic disease.

Answer 23.50. **The answer is E.**

The diagnosis of choroidal and ciliary body melanomas has reached a high degree of accuracy at ocular oncology centers with modern ancillary testing facilities. A noninvasive diagnostic accuracy rate of 99.7% was achieved in the Collaborative Ocular Melanoma Study, based on clinical examination with indirect ophthalmoscopy and standardized ultrasonography. Fine needle aspiration biopsy is required only in a minority of cases in which the clinical and ultrasonographic features are not completely consistent with melanoma. CT and MRI may identify a rare case with gross orbital tumor extension. MRI can be useful to confirm a rare case suspected of having optic nerve invasion. However, neither CT nor MRI is as accurate as indirect ophthalmoscopy and ultrasonography for determining tumor size and location. Fluorescein angiography can be helpful in distinguishing ocular melanoma from a hemorrhagic lesion simulating a melanoma. However, no angiographic pattern has been shown to be pathognomonic of ocular melanoma. By far, the most important ancillary diagnostic test in the evaluation of a potential ocular melanoma is ultrasonography. Using the A-scan ultrasound mode, most melanomas exhibit low to medium internal reflectivity, whereas almost every other choroidal tumor (e.g., hemangioma, metastasis, and granuloma) demonstrates medium to high reflectivity.

Answer 23.51. **The answer is C.**

Even though only about 1% of ocular melanoma patients will have evidence of systemic metastasis at the time of ocular diagnosis, all patients should undergo systemic workup prior to ocular treatment to rule out metastatic disease. This workup should include a physical examination.

Since about 90% of patients with metastatic disease will have liver involvement, this workup should also include liver function studies (especially lactate dehydrogenase, alkaline phosphatase, and gamma-glutamyltransferase). Liver function studies are possibly the most important component of the routine metastatic screening workup, but they lack both specificity (other liver diseases can result in elevated liver enzymes) and sensitivity (micrometastatic disease is often undetected). The sensitivity of the metastatic workup may be slightly increased by addition of abdominal ultrasonography or CT. Since about 10% of metastatic patients will have pulmonary involvement, many centers will also perform a chest x-ray or CT, although the percentage of patients that will have positive findings on these studies yet have negative liver functions studies is extremely low. There is no evidence that screening PET scans or bone marrow biopsies add significantly to the sensitivity of metastatic testing in the absence of localizing signs or symptoms. The mean survival following diagnosis of systemic metastasis is about 7 months.

Answer 23.52. **The answer is D.**

Most patients with very small ocular melanomas (<2.5 mm height and <10 mm in largest basal dimension) should be observed for tumor growth before treatment. Small melanomas are candidates for plaque therapy if there is documented growth. Patients with medium-sized tumors (between 2.5 and 10 mm in height and <16 mm basal diameter) are candidates for episcleral plaque radiotherapy if the patient is otherwise healthy and without metastatic disease. Histopathologic verification is not required for plaque therapy. Some patients with large melanomas (>10 mm height or >16 mm basal diameter) may also be candidates for plaque therapy. Patients with gross extrascleral extension, ring melanoma, and tumor involvement of more than half of the ciliary body are not suitable for plaque therapy. The minimum recommended radiation dose to the tumor apex is 85 Gy at a dose rate of 0.60 to 1.05 Gy per h using AAPM TG-43 formalism for the calculation of dose. This dose is much higher than that required to treat lymphoma and metastatic carcinoma. Enucleation is advised if the tumor shows evidence of optic nerve invasion. Other considerations, including loss of central vision, failure of previous conservative treatment, and the patient's desire for complete surgical removal of the tumor, may make enucleation a reasonable choice.

Answer 23.53. **The answer is E.**

It is generally advisable to treat large melanomas by enucleation. Possible exceptions include patients with only one sighted eye, rare patients in whom vision can be salvaged, and patients who refuse enucleation. The noninvasive accuracy rate for diagnosing ocular melanoma is over 99%, so fine needle biopsy is not required in cases with clinical features highly consistent with ocular melanoma. External beam radiation therapy prior to enucleation was evaluated in the Collaborative Ocular Melanoma Study and was found to confer no survival advantage. Increasing age and tumor location anterior to the ocular equator are risk factors for metastatic disease.

Answer 23.54. **The answer is A.**

Tumor location anterior to the equator (which includes the ciliary body) is a risk factor for metastasis. Endoresection is an experimental therapy that has not been widely accepted. Plaque radiotherapy would be a good treatment option in this patient, but the Bragg peak effect is seen with charged particle radiotherapy. The Collaborative Ocular Melanoma Study showed that survival in patients with medium-sized melanomas treated with plaque radiotherapy was not significantly different from patients treated with enucleation. Because this tumor is medium-sized (thickness >2.5 mm), most experts would recommend prompt treatment. The present of subretinal fluid is a risk factor for tumor growth and malignant change.

Answer 23.55. **The answer is A.**

A predominance of epithelioid cells (not spindle cells), the presence of *networks* and *parallel with cross-linking* extracellular matrix patterns, involvement of the ciliary body, extraocular tumor extension, and mitotic figures are all risk factors for metastatic death.

Answer 23.56. **The answer is A.**

It is important to understand that survival has never been compared between untreated ocular melanoma patients and those treated by enucleation or any other modality. Therefore, it has not been formally proven that any treatment affects patient survival. The Collaborative Ocular Melanoma Study has shown that the 5-year survival of patients with medium-sized ocular melanomas treated with enucleation is not significantly different than those treated with plaque radiotherapy. There is an extensive retrospective literature comparing enucleation, charged particle radiotherapy, and plaque radiotherapy, and no significant differences in survival have been reported. Therefore, currently available information suggests that enucleation, plaque radiotherapy, and charged particle therapy are equivalent in their survival benefit. The statistical quality of the literature on laser photocoagulation, transpupillary thermotherapy, and local tumor resection is inadequate to assess the survival benefit of these less established procedures compared to enucleation and plaque radiotherapy.

Answer 23.57. **The answer is B.**

Radiation retinopathy, ocular inflammation, dryness, and cataract in the treated eye are all common complications of plaque radiotherapy. However, plaque radiotherapy causes virtually no side effects or complications in the contralateral eye.

Answer 23.58. **The answer is E.**

Increased tumor thickness, increased radiation dose rate, and close tumor proximity to the fovea and optic disc are associated with poor visual outcome following plaque or charged particle radiotherapy. Close tumor proximity to the lens may increase the risk of cataract, but this can usually be addressed with cataract surgery. A study comparing treatment doses of 50 CGE versus 70 CGE in patients treated with charged particle radiotherapy showed no significant difference in visual outcomes.

Answer 23.59. **The answer is C.**

Co-60 was one of the early isotopes used for plaque radiotherapy and has been replaced in most centers by I-125, Pd-103, or Ru-106. Helium ions have been used with charged particle radiotherapy but not plaque radiotherapy.

Answer 23.60. **The answer is C.**

An ocular melanoma abutting the optic disc and invading the optic nerve has a very low risk of extension into the brain but an increased risk of hematogenous metastasis compared to a similar tumor located away from the optic disc. Such a tumor should usually be treated by enucleation of the globe with a long optic nerve stump. Exenteration is only required if substantial tumor extension into the orbit is encountered. In an only sighted eye, charged particle radiotherapy may be a reasonable alternative, although profound vision loss should be expected. Transpupillary thermotherapy and other laser techniques have no role in this setting.

CHAPTER 24

Neoplasms of the Central Nervous System

ROGER STUPP

Directions Each of the numbered items below is followed by lettered answers. Select the ONE lettered answer that is BEST in each case unless instructed otherwise.

QUESTIONS

Question 24.1. **Hereditary syndromes/risk factors predisposing to central nervous system (CNS) tumors are**

A. Turcot syndrome
B. cell phones
C. ionizing radiation
D. neurofibromatosis type 1
E. all of the above

Question 24.2. **Which genetic aberration(s) are linked to secondary glioblastoma?**

A. PTEN.
B. p53.
C. 1p/19q loss of heterozygosity (LOH) on chromosomes.
D. Epidermal growth factor receptor (EGFR).

Question 24.3. **Contrast enhancement on magnetic resonance imaging (MRI) of the brain is not seen in which of the following?**

A. Glioblastoma astrocytoma [World Health Organization (WHO) grade IV].
B. Anaplastic astrocytoma (WHO grade III).
C. Pilocytic astrocytoma (WHO grade I).
D. Fibrillary astrocytoma (WHO grade II).
E. Necrosis (e.g., after prior radiotherapy).

Corresponding Chapters in *Cancer: Principles & Practice of Oncology*, Seventh Edition: 39 (Neoplasms of the Central Nervous System).

Question 24.4. **A 53-year-old man, exsmoker, presents with a seizure. Subsequent brain MRI shows a multilobular, contrast-enhancing mass in the left temporal lobe, associated with a moderate edema. The radiologist describes the findings suggestive of brain metastases. Further workup includes a complete blood cell count (CBC) and chemistry as well as a computed tomography (CT) scan of the chest and abdomen, which were all within normal limits. What should be the next diagnostic tests?**

A. Lumbar puncture.
B. Gastroscopy and colonoscopy.
C. Excisional biopsy.
D. Electroencephalogram (EEG).
E. Symptomatic therapy and repeat imaging in 4 weeks.

Question 24.5. **A 55-year-old obese woman presents with an inaugural epileptic grand mal seizure. An MRI is performed showing a large contrast-enhancing tumor with associated edema. Subsequent gross total tumor resection confirms the suspected diagnosis of glioblastoma. Which of the following statements is INCORRECT?**

A. The extent of resection needs to be determined by a postoperative contrast-enhanced MRI or CT within 24 hours.
B. At initial diagnosis, high-doses of dexamethasone of typically 12 to 16 mg daily should be administered. The patient should then remain on a maintenance dose of dexamethasone until the end of radiotherapy.
C. Antiseizure prophylaxis with phenytoin can be discontinued after tumor resection.
D. These patients are frequently also diagnosed with diabetes.
E. Drug interactions of the antiseizure medications should be evaluated.

Question 24.6. **A 33-year-old man presents with recurrent seizures, which are currently controlled with standard antiepileptic treatment. Workup reveals a 5-cm left temporal mass, hypointense on T1-weighted MRI and without contrast enhancement or mass effect. Stereotactic biopsy is performed and histology is showing an oligoastrocytoma WHO grade II. What is the most appropriate treatment?**

A. Watchful waiting.
B. Fractionated focal radiotherapy up to 64 Gy.
C. Chemotherapy [e.g., procarbazine, lomustine, vincristine (PCV) or temozolomide].
D. Radiotherapy followed by adjuvant chemotherapy (e.g., PCV).
E. Additional molecular typing; in case of loss of heterozygosity on chromosomes 1p and 19q, chemotherapy should be the first choice.

Question 24.7. **All of the following factors are considered as higher risk and worse prognosis in patients with proven low-grade glioma EXCEPT**

A. age less than 40 years
B. tumor size greater than 6 cm
C. tumor crossing the midline
D. contrast enhancement
E. incomplete tumor resection

Question 24.8. **All the following factors limit the interpretation of results from phase II and phase III studies in malignant glioma EXCEPT**

A. combined analysis of anaplastic astrocytoma and glioblastoma
B. imbalances in known prognostic factors
C. inadequate and variable response definitions
D. variations in contrast enhancement due to corticosteroid administration
E. time to progression at 6 months not reported in many trials

Question 24.9. **Chemotherapy in conjunction with and after radiotherapy has been shown to be an effective treatment in patients with newly diagnosed glioblastoma, based on**

A. phase II trials
B. phase III randomized trials
C. meta-analysis

Question 24.10. **Which of the following statements on oligodendroglioma is/are correct?**

A. Oligodendroglioma has a more favorable prognosis compared to astrocytoma.
B. Primary therapy for oligodendroglioma should be chemotherapy because these tumors have a particular chemosensitivity.
C. Chemotherapy is only indicated in patients with loss of genetic information on chromosomes 1p and 19q (LOH 1p/19q).
D. For patients with progressive oligodendroglioma, radiotherapy should be considered.
E. Neoadjuvant chemotherapy with PCV has been shown to improve survival in patients with oligodendroglioma and mixed oligoastrocytoma.
F. A and D are correct.

Question 24.11. **Which of the following statements regarding ependymoma are correct?**

A. Calcifications of a fourth ventricular tumor are very suggestive of ependymoma.
B. Transformation from a lower grade to a higher grade ependymoma is uncommon.
C. The majority of ependymomas are infratentorial.
D. Cerebrospinal fluid (CSF) seeding is frequent in ependymomas, and workup should always include CSF cytologic examination.
E. Ependymomas are primitive neuroectodermal tumors which are very sensitive to chemotherapy.

Question 24.12. **Which of the following tumor types is/are not considered a PNET (primitive neuroepithelial tumor)?**

A. Medulloblastoma.
B. Pinealoblastoma.
C. Germ cell tumors.
D. Neuroblastoma.
E. Chordoma.
F. C and E.

Question 24.13. **A 43-year-old woman has been diagnosed with a left frontal meningioma extending to the cavernous sinus. A macroscopically complete resection was performed; however, the dura and bone could not be excised due to the extension to the cavernous sinus. The pathology report describes a tumor with only one mitosis per 10 high power fields, but with a high cellularity and occasional necrosis; the diagnosis is meningioma grade I. What is the appropriate next treatment?**

A. Repeat surgery and complete resection.
B. Observation with regular imaging follow-up.
C. Adjuvant radiotherapy.
D. Stereotactic radiotherapy (radiosurgery).
E. Adjuvant chemotherapy.

ANSWERS

Answer 24.1. **The answers are A, C, and D.**

Genetic predisposition accounts only for a very small percentage of CNS tumors. Neurofibromatosis type 1, a neurocutaneous condition with a mutation of the NF1 gene located on chromosome 17, is associated with optic nerve glioma, brainstem glioma, and other astrocytomas, while acoustic neurinomas (schwannomas), meningiomas, and ependymomas occur in NF2 patients (a rare defect on chromosome 22). Hereditary glioma and an increased frequency of medulloblastoma has been described in patients with Turcot syndrome [mutation of the adenomatous polyposis coli (APC) gene]. Prior radiotherapy (e.g., for skin hemangioma during childhood) has been associated with an increased incidence of meningioma, glioma, and nerve sheet tumors. For other potential risk factors like head trauma, occupational exposure in petroleum refining and vinyl chloride (PVC) production, and electromagnetic exposure from mobile phones, such an association has not been clearly demonstrated.

Answer 24.2. **The answer is B.**

Although primary and secondary glioblastoma are indistinguishable based on histopathologic appearance and clinical outcome, these tumors are genetically distinct. Mutations of the tumor suppressor gene coding for p53 and overexpression of PDGFR (platelet derived growth factor receptor) are hallmarks of low-grade gliomas, which may subsequently progress to (WHO) grade III and IV astrocytic tumors. PTEN mutations and EGFR (epidermal growth factor receptor) overexpression are common features of *de novo* (primary) glioblastoma. Loss of heterozygosity on chromosomes 1p and 19q are typical of oligodendroglial differentiation and carry a more favorable prognosis.

Answer 24.3. **The answer is D.**

The open or fenestrated endothelial cells in pilocytic astrocytoma, a WHO grade I tumor occurring mainly in children and young adults, allow for profound contrast enhancement, while other low-grade gliomas usually do not show contrast enhancement. However, the absence of contrast uptake does not always imply a benign histology. WHO grade III astrocytoma and WHO grade IV astrocytoma usually display diffuse and heterogeneous contrast uptake. Necrosis after prior radiation injury with localized contrast enhancement on MRI may be difficult to distinguish from recurrent tumors. MR spectroscopy based on tumor metabolism is increasingly used to distinguish necrosis, low-grade, and high-grade tumors.

Answer 24.4. **The answer is C.**

The most frequent primary tumor site is in the lung. In women, an occult breast cancer can present with a primary brain metastasis. Melanoma may present with brain metastases; frequently, only a detailed history will reveal resection of a cutaneous nevus many years earlier. For an efficient workup and in particular in the presence of a single lesion, excisional biopsy will rapidly allow for a correct diagnosis and give indications on where to look for a primary tumor. A spinal tap may be contraindicated due to increased intracranial pressure. Further, resection of a single metastasis (usually followed by radiotherapy) is superior to radiotherapy alone. In the particular patient described, the final histology revealed glioblastoma, underlining that a histologic confirmation should always be attempted.

Answer 24.5. **The answer is B.**

Determination of the completeness of resection needs assessment by imaging within 24 to 48 hours. After longer intervals, contrast uptake may be due to postoperative changes and minor bleeding and cannot be distinguished from residual tumor tissue. Dexamethasone is the treatment of choice in order to achieve immediate reduction of increased intracranial pressure. After tumor resection, the corticosteroids should be quickly tapered and discontinued. Occasional patients with residual tumors may require steroids during radiotherapy. Secondary diabetes due to high-dose corticosteroid therapy may require additional therapy or surveillance. As the seizure was due to the tumor and its associated edema, antiepileptic drugs can be discontinued after resection. Many commonly used antiepileptic drugs (e.g., phenytoin, carbamazepin, and phenobarbital) are inducing increased hepatic cytochrome 450 dependent metabolism, and thus decrease the bioavailability of many drugs (e.g., coumadin, digoxin, oral contraceptives, and many chemotherapy agents).

Answer 24.6. **The answer is A.**

This patient has a low-grade glioma. In the absence of other symptoms, watchful waiting is appropriate. In a large randomized trial by the European Organization for Research and Treatment of Cancer (EORTC), no improvement in survival was demonstrated for immediate irradiation as compared to radiotherapy at the time of progression. Two thirds of the patients with deferred therapy subsequently received radiotherapy at progression. The dose of radiotherapy was examined in two randomized trials showing no advantage for doses beyond 45 Gy to 50 Gy. Chemotherapy with procarbazine, CCNU (lomustine), vincristine (PCV) or temozolomide has demonstrated activity in patients with recurrent oligodendroglioma or, to a lesser extent, mixed oligoastrocytoma, after prior radiotherapy. The value of first-line chemotherapy compared to primary radiotherapy is the subject of an ongoing randomized EORTC/NCIC (National Cancer Institute of Canada) Intergroup trial. Adjuvant PCV-chemotherapy after radiation has been examined in two randomized trials by the EORTC and by the RTOG (Radiation Therapy Oncology Group); initial results are expected in 2005. Concomitant radiochemotherapy has been proven an effective therapy in glioblastoma only. Although 1p/19q LOH has been associated with increased sensitivity to chemotherapy in patients with recurrent oligodendrogliomas, no such association could be demonstrated in a trial with neoadjuvant PCV-chemotherapy. Currently, the knowledge of the molecular status does not allow us to make rational treatment decisions, and this association needs to be tested in a prospective trial.

Answer 24.7. **The answer is A.**

Patients older than 40 years and patients with residual tumor are considered at a higher risk for progression. The RTOG used these criteria to define high-risk patients in a clinical trial evaluating radiotherapy with or without chemotherapy. The EORTC established a score of greater than or equal to three risk factors as high risk: age greater than or equal to 40 years, tumor diameter greater than or equal to 6 cm, tumor crossing the midline, pure astrocytic histology, and impaired neurologic function.

Answer 24.8. **The answer is E.**

Indeed, most trials conducted before the 1990s usually included both glioblastoma and anaplastic astrocytoma, the latter having a better prognosis and also higher response rate to chemotherapy. Further, histopathologic definitions have changed over the last three decades. In particular, oligodendrogliomas are more commonly diagnosed based on the latest classification. MRI has largely replaced CT as the preferred imaging method. MRI has a better resolution and allows for more accurate diagnosis and evaluation of the extent of the disease. Favorable prognostic factors like young age, complete tumor resection, and performance status may have a stronger influence on patient survival than the tested treatment itself. Response with two-dimensional tumor measurements according to the standard WHO criteria is particularly difficult to assess in the brain. Measurement of only the contrast-enhancing lesion may underestimate the tumor extension. Further, dexamethasone administration will reduce permeability of the blood-brain barrier, and, thus, decreased contrast uptake may be solely due to the corticosteroids. In neurooncology, response definitions commonly also include the assessment on the use of steroids (McDonald's criteria). As progression seems an easier measure, progression-free survival (PFS) at 6 months (% of patients free of progression after 6 months) has been proposed as an alternative endpoint. Many recent trials in recurrent glioblastoma and anaplastic astrocytoma used this endpoint in comparison to a database of historic controls.

Answer 24.9. **The answer is B.**

Efficacy of new treatments should be demonstrated in phase III trials. Several large randomized trials failed to demonstrate unequivocally a benefit for chemotherapy in patients with glioblastoma. However, in a large meta-analysis based on individual patient data from 12 randomized trials with over 3,000 patients, a small but significant benefit for chemotherapy has been found. The EORTC/NCIC reported in 2004 a significant improvement in survival in a large phase III trial comparing standard radiotherapy alone with the same radiotherapy with concomitant and adjuvant temozolomide chemotherapy. Temozolomide has been approved for the treatment of recurrent anaplastic astrocytoma based on a high response rate in a single phase II study. BCNU wafers (Gliadel) have shown a small survival advantage in selected patients undergoing resection for recurrent or newly diagnosed malignant glioma (glioblastoma and anaplastic astrocytoma).

Answer 24.10. **The answer is F.**

Oligodendrogliomas have a better prognosis than pure astrocytomas. Histologically differentiated (WHO grade II) oligodendroglioma is distinguished from anaplastic oligodendroglioma (WHO grade III); the presence of necrosis in the latter can be a source of misdiagnosis as a glioblastoma. Although oligodendroglioma is felt to be more chemosensitive than pure astrocytoma, the role of primary chemotherapy needs to be assessed in clinical trials first. In a recent report, no association between response to neoadjuvant PCV-chemotherapy and 1p/19q status was found. In patients with anaplastic and progressive low-grade oligodendroglioma or mixed oligoastrocytoma, radiotherapy remains the standard of care. At the 2004 ASCO meetings, the disappointing results of a randomized phase III trial evaluating the role of neoadjuvant PCV-chemotherapy were reported. There was no improvement in overall survival with the addition of chemotherapy, although progression-free survival may be prolonged. This trial was not designed to evaluate whether primary chemotherapy allows replacing or deferring radiotherapy.

Answer 24.11. **The answer is E.**

A tumor lesion that is in connection with the ventricle system with or without contrast enhancement and with some calicification is suggestive of an ependymoma. Although possible, malignant transformation of ependymoma is much less frequent than in astrocytic tumors. About 60% of all ependymomas are infratentorial. Ependymomas are a subgroup of gliomas. Although radiation is commonly administered, there are no comparative trials between the different treatment modalities. Chemotherapy is usually administered after recurrence; however, no standard regimen has been established.

Answer 24.12. **The answer is F.**

Undifferentiated tumors with small round cells arising in different areas of the CNS are considered PNETs. The most common primary brain tumor in children is medulloblastoma, always arising in the posterior fossa. Pinealoblastoma is the designation for an aggressive and rapidly disseminating PNET in the pineal gland. These are all distinct entities within the larger subgroup of embryonal tumors. Common features are the high proliferation rate and the propensity to spread throughout the neuraxis. Diagnostic workup always also includes lumbar puncture (to be performed before surgery) with CSF cytologic examination. If a germ cell tumor is suspected, dosing of beta-human chorion gonadotropin (HCG) and alpha-fetoprotein (AFP) is helpful. Germ cell tumors (germinoma, yolk sac tumors, choriocarcinoma, and teratoma) can occur anywhere in the organism and also rarely in the CNS. Chordomas are mesenchymal tumors of the bone arising from remnants of the embryonal notochord. These extradural tumors should be completely resected whenever possible. For unresectable, incompletely resected, or recurrent tumors, proton irradiation should be considered.

Answer 24.13. **The answer is B.**

In symptomatic patients, complete surgical excision is the treatment of choice; however, patients who are asymptomatic or have a fortuitously found meningioma may be observed with imaging every 6 months. The extent of resection is graded according to definitions based on a seminal description by Simpson: macroscopically complete resections are considered Simpson grades I to III and incomplete resections or biopsy only are Simpson grades IV and V, respectively. For this patient, the resection was a Simpson grade III due to the inability to resect the cavernous sinus. This translates into a risk of recurrence of 20% to 25% at 10 years. For resected meningiomas (Simpson grades I to III) observation remains the standard of care, while for incompletely resected patients, adjuvant fractionated radiotherapy should be considered. The EORTC and NCIC are conducting a randomized trial evaluating the value of adjuvant radiotherapy in patients with resected benign meningioma (Simpson grades II to IV). For patients with unresectable or incompletely resected meningioma, radiosurgery may be an option. For a diagnosis of atypical (WHO grade II) or the rare malignant (WHO grade III) meningioma, greater than 4 or greater than 20 mitoses per 10 high power fields, respectively, should be observed. Necrosis, high cellularity, sheeting, a high nuclear/cytoplasmatic ratio, and prominent nucleoli are other features suggesting WHO grade II meningioma. Chemotherapy has no established role in the management of meningioma. Initial reports on efficacy of antiestrogens (tamoxifen) and antigestagens (mifepristone), interferon-alpha, and hydroxyurea could not be confirmed in well-designed prospective trials.

CHAPTER 25

Cancers of Childhood

SHALINI SHENOY

Directions Each of the numbered items below is followed by lettered answers. Select the ONE lettered answer that is BEST in each case unless instructed otherwise.

QUESTIONS

Question 25.1. **Pediatric malignancies exhibit all the following characteristics EXCEPT**

A. aggressive, rapid growth
B. short latency period
C. associated with exposure to carcinogens
D. responsive to standard treatment modalities
E. familial association in 10% to 15% of cases

Question 25.2. **Genetic abnormalities predispose to malignant disorders in children due to**

A. abnormal mechanisms of genomic DNA repair
B. constitutional activation of molecular pathways of deregulated cellular growth and proliferation
C. increased function of oncogenes
D. inactivation of tumor suppressor genes
E. all of the above

Question 25.3. **Which of the following hereditary disorders is most often diagnosed in children and may cause pediatric cancer?**

A. Beckwith–Wiedemann syndrome.
B. Familial adenomatous polyposis coli.
C. Li–Fraumeni syndrome.
D. Multiple endocrine neoplasias.

Question 25.4. **Retinoblastoma, a rare pediatric retinal tumor, is characterized by abnormalities in the long arm of chromosome 13. Which of these statements regarding tumorigenesis in retinoblastoma is true?**

A. There is deletion of the long arm of chromosome 13.
B. Acquired genetic material results in overexpression of tumor oncogenes.
C. A deletion or mutation results in loss of tumor suppressor gene activity.
D. There is duplication of the long arm of chromosome 13 resulting in cellular growth dysregulation.

Corresponding Chapters in *Cancer: Principles & Practice of Oncology*, Seventh Edition: 40 (Cancers of Childhood).

Question 25.5. **Which of the following pediatric conditions is NOT associated with known genetic events that predispose to tumor development?**

A. Retinoblastoma.
B. Neuroblastoma.
C. Neurofibromatosis.
D. Ewing sarcoma.
E. Glioma.

Question 25.6. **Which of the following statements about the retinoblastoma susceptibility locus (RB1) is NOT true?**

A. Mutations in the RB1 gene result in overexpression and increased function supporting the development and growth of retinoblastoma.
B. Loss of the wild-type RB1 allele in retinal cells is a feature in retinoblastoma.
C. Germline mutations of RB1 are characteristic in heritable retinoblastoma.
D. RB1 is altered in osteosarcoma, small cell lung carcinoma, bladder, breast, and prostate cancers.

Question 25.7. **Which of the following tumors is typically NOT seen in the pediatric age group?**

A. Retinoblastoma.
B. Neuroblastoma.
C. Wilms tumor.
D. Colon carcinoma.
E. Rhabdomyosarcoma.

Question 25.8. **Which of the following statements about nephrogenic rests is true?**

A. It may persist, regress, or grow into a mass lesion.
B. It is associated with Wilms tumor.
C. It consists of foci of primitive nonmalignant cells, a developmental aberration.
D. All the above.

Question 25.9. **WAGR, a syndrome complex with deletions at chromosome 11q13, the locus of the WT1 gene, predisposes to Wilms tumor and also affects which of the following.**

A. Iris, genitourinary system, and IQ.
B. Ovaries, gut, and central nervous system(CNS).
C. CNS, heart, and kidneys.
D. None of the above.

Question 25.10. **Strong correlations are present between all of the following EXCEPT**

A. Wilms tumor, intersex disorders, and progressive renal failure
B. macroglossia, hyperinsulinemia, and Wilms tumor
C. neurofibromas, café au lait spots, and optic glioma
D. mental retardation, spinal abnormalities, and neuroblastoma

Question 25.11. **The NF1 gene**

A. encodes a ubiquitously expressed protein, neurofibromin
B. facilitates the hydrolysis of guanosine triphosphate (GTP) to guanosine diphosphate (GDP) by ras oncoprotein
C. sends inhibitory signals to cell division
D. maps to chromosome 17
E. all of the above

Question 25.12. **N-myc oncogene amplification is most likely to be detected in**

A. neuroblastoma
B. ganglioneuroblastoma
C. ganglioneuroma
D. all of the above

Question 25.13. **Which of the following is a good prognostic feature in neuroblastoma?**

A. N-myc amplification.
B. Trk A expression.
C. Trk B expression.
D. Multidrug resistance-associated protein (MRP) expression.
E. None of the above.

Question 25.14. **The fusion transcript associated with t(11;22) EWS-ETS interacts with p53 and can be associated with all the following tumors EXCEPT**

A. osteosarcoma
B. Ewing sarcoma
C. Askin tumor
D. peripheral primitive neuroectodermal tumor (pPNET)
E. soft tissue Ewing sarcoma

Question 25.15. **Which of the following statements regarding the molecular basis for the development of embryonal rhabdomyosarcoma is NOT true?**

A. They are characterized by loss of heterozygosity (LOH) at the 11p15 locus.
B. IGF-2 gene activity is increased.
C. LOH is associated with loss of tumor suppressor gene activity.
D. There is paternal duplication or loss of maternal imprinting of IGF-2.

Question 25.16. **Alveolar rhabdomyosarcoma has all the following molecular characteristics EXCEPT**

A. t(2;13) or t(1;13) translocation
B. PAX-3-FKHR or PAX-7-FKHR fusion
C. increased c-met expression
D. increased hepatocyte growth factor (HGF) expression
E. increased expression of myoblast growth factor (MGF)

Question 25.17. **The Li–Fraumeni syndrome is characterized by which of the following.**

A. Germline mutations in the tumor suppressor gene p53.
B. Expression of a stabilized mutant protein in affected cells.
C. Mutation or deletion of the second wild-type p53 allele in tumors.
D. Early tumors including sarcomas, breast and brain cancers, leukemia, and adrenocortical carcinoma.
E. All of the above.

Question 25.18. **Therapeutic interventions targeted at known molecular abnormalities and pathways are being tested using which of the following intervention strategies.**

A. Farnesyl transferase inhibitors–ras pathway blockers.
B. Agents targeting mutant transcription factors.
C. Agents blocking growth hormone IGF-1 pathways.
D. Agents targeting tyrosine kinase enzymes that transduce growth factor signals.
E. All of the above.

Questions 25.19–25.21.

A 4-year-old boy presents at his pediatrician's office after his mother notices a hard lump in his abdomen. He is otherwise well. On physical examination, it is noted that he has left-sided hemihypertrophy. A large (6 cm by 6 cm) hard nontender mass is palpable in the left flank. The remainder of his examination is normal. Laboratory evaluation of blood counts, serum electrolytes, calcium, liver and renal function tests, and urinalysis is normal. An initial ultrasound reveals the presence of a mass involving the superior pole of the left kidney and evidence of a thrombus involving the left renal vein. A computed tomography (CT) scan confirms the presence of the left renal mass; the opposite kidney and liver are normal.

Question 25.19. **Which of the tests listed below is necessary to correctly stage this tumor?**

A. Head CT.
B. Bone scan.
C. Plain chest radiograph.
D. Skeletal survey.

Question 25.20. **The patient is taken to surgery. Which of the following is the ideal surgical approach for accurate diagnosis and staging?**

A. Biopsy of the mass.
B. Biopsy the mass and sample draining lymph nodes.
C. Resect the mass and renal vein if involved.
D. Resect the mass with renal vein if involved, explore the opposite kidney, and sample drain lymph nodes.
E. Start preoperative chemotherapy followed by resection at a later date.

Question 25.21. **Following surgical resection and staging, the tumor is confirmed to be consistent with stage III favorable histology Wilms tumor. Treatment should include which of the following.**

A. Surgical resection only.
B. Surgery and radiation therapy to kidney.
C. Radiation and chemotherapy.
D. Surgery, radiation, and chemotherapy.

Question 25.22. **Factors associated with good prognosis during the evaluation of Wilms tumor include which of the following.**

A. Tumor size (<550 gm).
B. Favorable histology with no anaplasia.
C. Absent metastases.
D. Absence of locally invasive features.
E. All of the above.

Questions 25.23–25.24.

A 2-year-old child is brought to the emergency room with low-grade fever, pallor, lethargy, extensive bruising, and "raccoon" eyes (periorbital hematomas). On examination, it is noted that the child appears ill and has a left-sided abdominal mass that is firm and nontender. He also has involuntary rapid eye movements, noticed over 2 to 3 weeks. A biopsy of the mass confirms the presence of a neuroblastoma.

Question 25.23. **Further staging and workup of this patient should include all of the following EXCEPT**

A. CT scan of the chest and abdomen, bone scan, skeletal survey
B. splenectomy and liver biopsy
C. biopsy of local lymph nodes
D. bone marrow aspiration and biopsy
E. determination of histology and biology of the tumor
F. measurement of urine catecholamines

Question 25.24. **Staging workup reveals disseminated stage IV neuroblastoma. Treatment modalities used include all of the following EXCEPT**

A. combination chemotherapy: carboplatinum, cyclophosphamide, doxorubicin, and etoposide
B. high-dose chemotherapy and autologous stem cell rescue
C. allogeneic stem cell transplant
D. radiation to areas of residual disease and involved lymph nodes
E. 13-*cis* retinoic acid

Question 25.25. **Which of the following statements about the genetics of retinoblastoma transmission is NOT true?**

A. It is transmitted as a highly penetrant autosomal dominant trait and is the most common pediatric ocular tumor.
B. The majority of retinoblastomas are hereditary, bilateral, and caused by germline mutations of 13q14; only 10% to 15% are sporadic and unilateral.
C. All sporadic bilateral retinoblastomas also have a germline mutation transmitted in an identical manner as familial retinoblastoma.
D. The parents and siblings of all patients with retinoblastoma should have a thorough ophthalmoscopic evaluation whether or not there is family history of the disease.

Questions 25.26–25.28.

An 11-month-old boy who has just learned to walk is noticed to consistently bump into objects in his path. There is no previous history of major medical illness in this healthy child. The parents report a "white-looking" eye on the right side that was not observed during a regular pediatric checkup at 6 months of age. There is no family history of ophthalmic disease or tumors. On examination, he has a white pupillary reflex on the right side. In addition, mild proptosis and a sixth nerve palsy are noticed in the right eye. The remainder of the physical examination is normal. A biopsy confirms the presence of retinoblastoma.

Question 25.26. **Staging studies should include**

A. CT or magnetic resonance imaging (MRI) of the orbits and head
B. diagnostic lumbar puncture with cerebrospinal fluid (CSF) cytology
C. bone scan
D. bone marrow aspiration and biopsy
E. all of the above

Question 25.27. **Further staging studies reveal complete visual loss in the affected eye and tumor involving the right orbit and optic nerve. The left eye is normal. CSF, bone, and bone marrow studies are normal. Therapy should include**

A. cryotherapy or hyperthermia
B. plaque radiotherapy and chemotherapy
C. enucleation with a sufficient length of the affected optic nerve
D. enucleation with a sufficient length of the affected optic nerve and local radiation
E. chemotherapy only

Question 25.28. **The potential side effects of therapy for this patient include all of the following EXCEPT**

A. second cancers
B. orbital hypoplasia
C. cataract formation in the contralateral eye
D. recurrent disease

Question 25.29. **The most common site(s) of origin of rhabdomyosarcoma is/are**

A. head and neck
B. extremities and trunk
C. abdomen and genitourinary tract
D. spinal canal

Question 25.30. **Staging studies for rhabdomyosarcoma should include all the following EXCEPT**

A. CT or MRI of the primary site
B. chest CT
C. bone scan
D. bilateral bone marrow sampling
E. lymph node sampling
F. (123)I-metaiodobenzylguanidine (MIBG) scan

Question 25.31. **A 6-year-old boy presents with a soft tissue mass involving the right cheek, noticed by his mother to cause facial asymmetry and proptosis, worsening over 3 to 4 weeks. He has no other systemic symptoms. Physical examination reveals a large hard right lower orbital mass. An upper cervical lymph node is also palpable on the right side of his neck, measuring 2 cm in diameter. CT scan of the face and neck confirm the presence of a large tumor involving the right orbit and maxillary sinus. An incisional biopsy confirms the presence of embryonal rhabdomyosarcoma, and the lymph node is positive for tumor. Which of the following would NOT be appropriate therapy for this child?**

A. Gross total resection of tumor with facial reconstruction at initial diagnosis.
B. Chemotherapy: vincristine, dactinomycin, and cyclophosphamide.
C. Radiation therapy to the site of tumor and lymph node metastasis.

Question 25.32. **All of the following statements about treatment of rhabdomyosarcoma are true EXCEPT**

A. treatment for parameningeal rhabdomyosarcoma with intracranial extension should include radiation
B. local radiation should be used for all patients with microscopic or gross residual rhabdomyosarcoma
C. hyperfractionated radiotherapy is better than conventional fractionated radiation for control of local, regional, or metastatic rhabdomyosarcoma
D. surgical intervention in rhabdomyosarcoma should aim for complete tumor resection with negative margins whenever possible
E. vincristine, actinomycin D, and cyclophosphamide (VAC) remains the chemotherapy of choice for rhabdomyosarcoma

Question 25.33. **Small round blue cell tumors of childhood include all of the following EXCEPT**

A. Ewing sarcoma
B. neuroblastoma
C. rhabdomyosarcoma
D. Burkitt lymphoma
E. Wilms tumor

Question 25.34. **The most frequent site of metastasis in Ewing sarcoma is**

A. liver
B. lung
C. spleen
D. gut
E. lymph nodes

Question 25.35. **All of the following are good prognostic factors in the outcome of Ewing sarcoma EXCEPT**

A. localized tumor less than 8 cm in diameter and volume less than 100 mL
B. primary pelvic tumors
C. low serum lactate dehydrogenase level
D. radiographic and histologic response to initial chemotherapy
E. type 1 EWS-FLI1 fusion transcripts

Questions 25.36–25.38.

A 12-month-old boy who had hemihypertrophy at birth presents with abdominal distension and a right-sided abdominal mass. The mass is confirmed to be arising from the right lobe of the liver by ultrasound of the abdomen. No calcification is identified. The serum alpha fetoprotein (AFP) level is increased markedly.

Question 25.36. **The most likely histologic diagnosis of this mass is**

A. hepatoblastoma
B. neuroblastoma
C. hepatocellular carcinoma
D. Wilms tumor
E. choriocarcinoma

Question 25.37. **Family history in this patient can include all of the following EXCEPT**

A. Beckwith–Wiedemann syndrome
B. adenomatous polyposis coli
C. extreme low birth weight
D. Meckel diverticulum
E. hepatitis B infection

Question 25.38. **Staging workup for this patient should include the following EXCEPT**

A. liver and renal function tests
B. chest radiograph or chest CT
C. MRI of the head
D. CT and/or MRI with magnetic resonance (MR) angiography of the abdomen

Question 25.39. **The most important treatment for hepatoblastoma is**

A. adjuvant chemotherapy
B. concomitant radiation
C. cryoablation or radiofrequency ablation of tumor
D. complete resection of tumor

Question 25.40. **Which of the following statements is NOT true?**

A. Gonadal tumors are commonly germ cell tumors in adults.
B. Extragonadal germ cell tumors are more frequent in adults than in children.
C. The sacrococcygeal region is the commonest site for extragonadal germ cell tumors in children.
D. Extragonadal germ cell tumors may involve the pineal gland, mediastinum, vagina, or retroperitoneum.

Question 25.41. **Which of the following is NOT a variety of germ cell tumor?**

A. Teratoma or teratocarcinoma.
B. Yolk sac or endodermal sinus tumor.
C. Choriocarcinoma.
D. Cholangiocarcinoma.
E. Embryonal carcinoma.
F. Seminomas or dysgerminomas.

Question 25.42. **Which of the following statements about germ cell tumors is NOT true?**

A. Staging should include CT or MRI scans of the mass and the lymph node region involved, the chest for metastatic disease, a bone scan, and tumor markers.
B. A transscrotal biopsy of a testicular mass should be performed to confirm the diagnosis of a germ cell tumor.
C. Cisplatinum-based chemotherapy [cisplatin, vinblastine, and bleomycin (PVB) or cisplatin, etoposide, and bleomycin (PEB)] has resulted in excellent survival, even in advanced-stage disease in children.
D. Radiation therapy is indicated as second-line therapy for patients who have relapsed following surgery and chemotherapy.
E. Completely resected pediatric testicular germ cell tumors do not need further chemotherapy if tumor markers such as AFP levels return to normal suggesting no occult disease.

ANSWERS

Answer 25.1. **The answer is C.**

Pediatric malignancies generally cannot be traced to long-term exposure to known carcinogens as they occur in the young, without time for prolonged exposure and transition to a malignant change.

Answer 25.2. **The answer is E.**

The mechanisms listed above are some of the known pathways of carcinogenesis in the pediatric age group and predispose to specific groups of malignant disorders.

Answer 25.3. **The answer is A.**

Many hereditary premalignant disorders such as familial adenomatous polyposis coli manifest with tumors only in adulthood due to prolonged latency until tumor evolution. Other conditions such as Li–Fraumeni syndrome are detected or suspected only after the development of a malignant disorder as nonmalignant characteristics in syndromic form are virtually absent.

Answer 25.4. **The answer is C.**

The deletion or mutation of genetic material on the long arm of chromosome 13 results in down regulation of growth limiting tumor suppressor genes in retinoblastoma.

Answer 25.5. **The answer is E.**

Retinoblastoma is associated with deletions or mutations of RB1. In neuroblastoma, there are deletions or mutations in the short arm of chromosome 1 and, rarely, in chromosomes 10, 14, 17, and 19; neuroblastoma is also associated with amplification of the N-myc oncogene. Neurofibromatosis develops secondary to mutations in NF1 and NF2 genes. Ewing sarcoma is characterized by a reciprocal t(11;22) translocation, fusing a transcription factor FLI-1 with oncogene EWS.

Answer 25.6. **The answer is A.**

The RB1 gene product is ubiquitous and functions as a growth regulator by control of cell cycle genes determining cell transition from G1 to S (DNA synthesis) phase in all cell types. Loss of function is necessary and sufficient for tumor formation in the retina. In the other tumors, it is often one of multiple genetic events resulting in tumor development.

Answer 25.7. **The answer is D.**

Multiple genetic events are necessary for the development of colon cancer, resulting in tumor formation predominantly in adults. All others are common pediatric malignancies.

Answer 25.8. **The answer is D.**

Nephrogenic rests are benign and are incidentally found either on their own or in association with Wilms tumor. They may persist, regress, or grow into large masses that simulate a true Wilms tumor and often present a diagnostic challenge for the pathologist.

Answer 25.9. **The answer is A.**

Three hereditary syndromes genetically predispose to Wilms tumor. WAGR manifests with aniridia, genitourinary (GU) abnormalities, and mental retardation. Denys-Drash syndrome manifests with intersex disorders and progressive renal failure. Beckwith–Wiedemann syndrome, the most common, is a hereditary overgrowth syndrome characterized by macroglossia, visceromegaly, and hyperinsulinemia. The gene for familial Wilms tumor is thought to be distinct from WT1 and WT2 genes that cause the above syndromes but may interact with them.

Answer 25.10. **The answer is D.**

Wilms tumor and neurofibromatosis are often associated with syndromic manifestations that are easy to recognize. No association is described between neurologic abnormalities and neuroblastoma.

Answer 25.11. **The answer is E.**

Loss of neurofibromin activity (on both alleles) due to mutations in NF1 results in elevated levels of GTP-bound ras oncoprotein that transduces signals for cell division. This is one of the mechanisms of tumor development in neurofibromatosis type 1. The NF2 gene located on chromosome 22 has been implicated in tumor genesis in neurofibromatosis type 2, but the exact mechanism is unclear.

Answer 25.12. **The answer is A.**

N-myc amplification is associated with rapid tumor progression, advanced clinical stage, and an aggressive course in neuroblastoma, the least differentiated of this neuroectodermal group of tumors.

Answer 25.13. **The answer is B.**

Nerve growth factor (NGF) receptor Trk A can be terminally differentiated by NGF resulting in ganglionic differentiation. Tumors that demonstrate this feature have favorable prognosis in contrast to tumors that express increased Trk B or MRP. N-myc oncogene amplification is also a poor prognostic feature. These features are associated with an aggressive course and resistance to chemotherapy.

Answer 25.14. **The answer is A.**

EWS-ETS fusion transcripts or related variants can be found in more than 90% of the peripheral PNET group of tumors by RT-PCR or fluorescence *in situ* hybridization.

Answer 25.15. **The answer is C.**

Paternal gene duplication or loss of imprinting (LOI) of the normally transcriptionally silent maternal allele results in over-expression of IGF-2 in embryonal rhabdomyosarcoma.

Answer 25.16. **The answer is E.**

Except for MGF, all other statements regarding alveolar rhabdomyosarcoma are true. Additional mutations on p53, amongst others, are also described. Interestingly, the mouse model with overexpression of PAX-3-FKHR develops no tumors, but mice expressing an HGF transgene develop embryonal RMS.

Answer 25.17. **The answer is E.**

Between 60% and 80% of Li–Fraumeni families have detectable germline mutations in p53. The others may be associated with modifier genes, promoter defects, or involvement of other as yet known candidate genes involved in the p53 tumor suppressor pathway. A checkpoint kinase, hCHK2, is a potential candidate.

Answer 25.18. **The answer is E.**

The identification of disruption in molecular signaling pathways has led to the development of a variety of strategies to combat tumor cells using approaches that are directly targeted to particular tumors based on their etiology and developmental pathways.

Answer 25.19. **The answer is C.**

The presentation described is typical for Wilms tumor. The common pathologic variety is termed "favorable histology Wilms tumor." Pulmonary metastasis is the most common site of distant dissemination. The need for a chest CT in addition to a chest radiograph is controversial as nodules identified by CT scans are often negative on biopsy. Pulmonary nodules should be biopsied to prove tumor dissemination. Brain and bone imaging are necessary if the diagnosis includes rare subtypes of renal tumors such as clear cell sarcoma or rhabdoid tumor.

Answer 25.20. **The answer is D.**

The NWTSG (National Wilms Tumor Study Group) supports tumor resection. There is a 19.8% operative complication rate that includes intestinal obstruction and hemorrhage. Though the SIOP has promoted the use of preoperative chemotherapy prior to biopsy, there is a 7.6% to 9.9% rate of benign or other malignant disorders involving the kidney in children. The risk of rupture of the tumor during surgery is 14% and is associated with an increased risk of local recurrence. Preoperative chemotherapy following a biopsy is recommended for solitary kidneys, bilateral renal tumors, tumor in a horseshoe kidney, or if the patient is an anesthesia risk due to extensive lung involvement. Exploring the opposite kidney is also recommended by the NWTSG as there is a small chance that involvement of the opposite kidney may be missed by all other imaging studies.

Answer 25.21. **The answer is D.**

Surgical resection of the tumor is combined with lymph node sampling and examination of the contralateral kidney (bilateral tumor is present in 5% of patients) to complete staging. Stage III disease involves the presence of residual nonhematogenous tumor confined to the abdomen. The chemotherapy combination used through serial NWTSG trials is vincristine and dactinomycin for low stage patients (I and II); doxorubicin with or without cyclophosphamide for higher stage patients and those with unfavorable histology such as anaplastic Wilms tumor or clear cell sarcoma.

Answer 25.22. **The answer is E.**

Some of these prognostic factors no longer pertain due to the development of effective therapy via the NWSTG (trials 1 through 5) and other international trials. Histology and lymph node involvement remain the most important prognostic factors. Survival for most children with favorable histology Wilms tumor now approaches 90%.

Answer 25.23. **The answer is B.**

Neuroblastoma, a tumor of the sympathetic nervous system, disseminates to the bone, bone marrow, and lymph nodes. Hematogenous dissemination is evident in 62% of patients at diagnosis. Undifferentiated tumor (Shimada histology), low DNA ploidy, N-myc amplification, and disseminated disease are associated with poor prognosis. Other poor prognostic markers include low Trk A and high Trk B expression, chromosome 1p deletion, and chromosome 17q gains. Clinical symptoms depend on the location of the tumor and may include Horner syndrome, spinal cord compression, and others. In a unique small group of infants, small primary tumors and metastatic disease restricted to the liver, skin, and bone marrow without bone involvement (stage IV S) have favorable prognosis. Tumors in infants often have the capacity to regress spontaneously.

Answer 25.24. **The answer is C.**

Intense chemotherapy alone achieves a remission rate of 22% ± 4% in disseminated neuroblastoma and can be improved to 34% ± 4% with autologous BMT. The addition of 13-*cis* retinoic acid improves the 3-year relapse free survival rate to 46% ± 6% in these patients. Those with residual disease or positive lymph nodes have better control with local radiation therapy (24 to 30 Gy) to involved areas. Studies are underway to determine the efficacy of anti-GD2 monoclonal antibody 3F8 and metaiodobenzylguanidine (MIBG) conjugated to iodine-131 for minimal residual disease or disease refractory to frontline therapy. Low-risk patients (stage I, stage II with N-myc amplification <10, or >10 with favorable Shimada histology, stage IVS, and hyperdiploidy) often require no treatment and should be observed for progression. Allogeneic transplants have not demonstrated a definite benefit to date.

Answer 25.25. **The answer is B.**

The majority of retinoblastomas are sporadic and unilateral (70% to 75%). Median age at diagnosis is 1 to 2 years. Between 10% and 15% of unilateral retinoblastoma patients have germline mutations of chromosome 13q14. Between 25% and 30% of children with sporadic retinoblastoma have bilateral disease and carry germline mutations of 13q14. Median age at diagnosis is younger than 12 months.

Answer 25.26. **The answer is E.**

The risk of dissemination of retinoblastoma is determined by the extent of ocular tumor and is increased by involvement of the choroid, optic nerve, anterior chamber, ciliary body, and orbit. Radionuclide bone scans should be obtained only for patients with extensive ocular involvement or presence of symptoms suggesting bone, bone marrow, or CNS involvement.

Answer 25.27. **The answer is D.**

Cryotherapy, hyperthermia, and photocoagulation can be used instead of enucleation for unilateral or bilateral localized disease that does not involve the globe or the anterior chamber to preserve vision. Enucleation, where indicated, should include a 10- to 15-mm length of optic nerve to obtain a tumor-free margin. External beam radiation including the entire orbit and optic nerve up to the optic chiasm (44-50 Gy) is indicated for orbital involvement. For intraocular disease, or recurrent disease, chemotherapy agents (vincristine, etoposide, cyclophosphamide, doxorubicin, cisplatinum, and cyclosporin A as an MDR reversing agent) are used in combination with other modalities to preserve vision, avoid enucleation, or as salvage. They are most useful on group I to IV tumors.

Answer 25.28. **The answer is D.**

Radiation therapy increases the risk of second malignancies, especially bone tumors in the area of radiation, and interferes with normal development of the orbit.

Answer 25.29. **The answer is A.**

In the head and neck area, orbital tumors are the most common, accounting for 13% of all rhabdomyosarcomas diagnosed. The second common site includes the abdomen and GU tract and tends to affect younger children, sometimes in infancy. Tumors at both these sites tend to be embryonal in histology. Genital tumors (cervical, vaginal) are likely to be of botryoid histology with excellent prognosis (6%). Trunk and extremity tumors are likely to be diagnosed in the second decade of life. These tumors are more likely to have an alveolar histology. Twenty-five percent of all newly diagnosed cases are metastatic at initial presentation. Embryonal histology rhabdomyosarcoma has better prognosis than alveolar histology tumors.

Answer 25.30. **The answer is F.**

MIBG scans are indicated for neuroblastoma and not rhabdomyosarcoma. The other scans and bone marrow samples are necessary in view of dissemination patterns of rhabdomyosarcoma that include both hematogenous spread as well as lymphatic spread to the draining lymph nodes. Treatment decisions are based on TNM staging, and clinical group is based on extent of resection. Prognosis depends on stage, age, clinical group, histology, and primary site. Orbital, vaginal, and paratesticular tumors have the best prognosis, whereas extremity and parameningeal tumors are unfavorable. Tumors that are more than 5 cm, and presenting in children less than 10 years of age, have a worse prognosis.

Answer 25.31. **The answer is A.**

Orbital tumors are usually of embryonal histology and have excellent response to radiation and chemotherapy. Surgical resection is only indicated for recurrent disease. The dose of radiation is 45 to 55 Gy over 5 to 6 weeks. Children with group II or III RMS of the orbit have a 5-year progression-free survival rate of 90%. Parameningeal disease (usually group III) has a 5-year progression free survival rate of 78% without CNS involvement and 70% with CNS involvement.

Answer 25.32. **The answer is C.**

Radiation therapy for rhabdomyosarcoma is indicated only for gross or microscopic residual disease or regional and metastatic extension. The dose for microscopic residual disease is 41 to 50 Gy. Tested in IRS IV, hyperfractionated radiation had no added benefit over conventional fractionated radiation. Surgical resection should be attempted in the place of an incisional biopsy upfront only if the tumor is completely resectable. No radiation is necessary in the event of complete resection of the tumor without microscopic residual or regional extension.

Answer 25.33. **The answer is E.**

All the other tumors have similar light microscopy features that group them into this category.

Answer 25.34. **The answer is B.**

The lung, bones, and bone marrow are the most common sites of hematogenous spread of Ewing sarcoma. Lesions that originate in long bones characteristically involve the diaphysis. Parallel lamellated periosteal new bone formation frequently presents with an "onion skin" appearance. Radionuclide scans determine the presence of bone metastases. CT or MRI scans detect the presence of associated soft tissue masses and lung lesions.

Answer 25.35. **The answer is B.**

Pelvic tumors even when nonmetastatic herald a poor prognosis. This may be due to poor resectability at this location. Patients with type 1 fusion transcripts of EWS-FLI1 have a 5-year event-free survival (EFS) of

70% in contrast to 20% for all other types of fusion transcripts. Low lactate dehydrogenase levels and good response to therapy are other predictors of a better prognosis in Ewing sarcoma.

Answer 25.36. **The answer is A.**

Hepatoblastoma is the most common primary hepatic tumor in the young with a median age at presentation of 1 year. In contrast, the median age at which hepatocellular carcinoma (HCC) presents is 12 years. Both demonstrate a male predominance. Hepatoblastoma patients frequently have additional abnormalities such as hemihypertrophy, congenital absence of the kidney or adrenal gland, and umbilical hernia. AFP levels are increased in 90% of patients with hepatoblastoma and in 78% of adult patients with HCC. HCC is associated with hepatitis B, biliary atresia, galactosemia, Fanconi anemia, and α_1-antitrypsin deficiency. Malignant tumors of the liver are rarely calcified.

Answer 25.37. **The answer is E.**

Familial adenomatous polyposis coli has been identified in mothers and maternal relatives of several patients with hepatoblastoma. The risk of hepatoblastoma arising in children from kindreds with the APC gene on the long arm of chromosome 5 is 1,000 to 2,000 times higher than in sporadic cases. In Japanese children, hepatoblastoma accounted for 58% of cancer diagnoses in children with extremely low birth weight (<1,000 g). Hepatocellular carcinoma (HCC) is strongly associated with hepatitis B infection, acquired either by vertical transmission from infected mothers or via contaminated blood products. HCC is also associated with other disorders such as tyrosinemia, galactosemia, biliary atresia, giant cell hepatitis of infancy, and Fanconi anemia.

Answer 25.38. **The answer is C.**

Intracranial metastasis is not a common feature of malignant hepatic tumors. The grouping system employed in therapeutic studies segregates patients according to resectability and lymph node or hematogenous metastases. Laboratory tests are not useful for a differential diagnosis of malignant hepatic tumors in children. Pulmonary metastases are identified on a plain chest radiograph in approximately 10% of patients with hepatic tumors. The PRETEXT staging system by the European liver study group divides the liver into four sectors and characterizes tumors by the sectors involved; it was devised to facilitate the assessment of neoadjuvant chemotherapy in rendering tumors resectable and appears to have prognostic value.

Answer 25.39. **The answer is D.**

Resection is the primary treatment for hepatoblastoma and HCC. Long-term survival is rare in the absence of successful resection. Hepatoblastoma is generally unifocal and approximately one half of all hepatoblastomas are resectable at initial presentation. HCC has an invasive pattern of spread across anatomic planes and is unresponsive to current forms of chemotherapy. Complete resection of HCC is frequently difficult due to multifocality and invasiveness. Only 30% of HCC tumors can be fully resected at diagnosis.

Answer 25.40. **The answer is B.**

Only 5% to 10% of germ cell tumors are extragonadal in adults whereas 60% are extragonadal in children. Forty percent of all childhood germ cell tumors involve the sacrococcygeal region. Germ cell tumors are relatively rare in children and account for 3% of pediatric malignancies.

Answer 25.41. **The answer is D.**

All the others are varieties of germ cell tumors, each with characteristic histologic features. High AFP levels are common in pediatric patients with testicular, ovarian, presacral, and vaginal primary yolk sac tumors. AFP is a glycoprotein produced in the liver, gastrointestinal tract, and yolk sac of the human fetus. It has a long half-life of 7 days. HCG is a glycoprotein secreted by the placenta. Patients with non-yolk sac tumors such as embryonal carcinoma, choriocarcinoma, and malignant germ cell tumors of the ovary have elevated HCG levels. HCG has a short half-life of 24 to 36 hours.

Answer 25.42. **The answer is B.**

A transscrotal biopsy contaminates the scrotum and the lymphatic drainage to the inguinal lymph nodes and prevents high ligation of the spermatic cord. All scrotal masses should be explored through an inguinal incision. If the tumor is malignant, high ligation of the spermatic cord should be performed at the internal ring. With adjuvant chemotherapy consisting of platinum, vinblastine, and bleomycin (PVB) or platinum, etoposide, and bleomycin (PEB), 5-year survival rates for germ cell tumors are over 80%, even for advanced stage disease. Radiation is reserved only for recurrent or refractory disease.

CHAPTER **26**

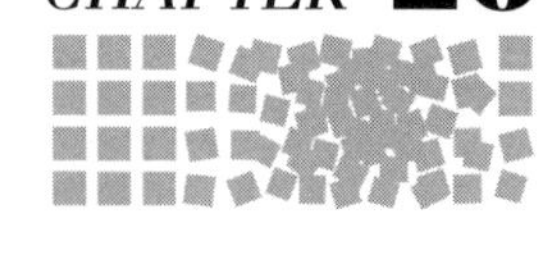

Hodgkin Disease and Non-Hodgkin Lymphomas

WILLIAM T. LESLIE AND PARAMESWARAN VENUGOPAL

Directions Each of the numbered items below is followed by lettered answers. Select the ONE lettered answer that is BEST in each case unless instructed otherwise.

QUESTIONS

Question 26.1. **In the United States, non-Hodgkin lymphomas (NHL)**

A. represent 10% of all new cancer cases
B. are the fifth leading cause of cancer death
C. are the fastest growing cancer in terms of mortality
D. have lower incidence rates than those reported from Europe and Asia

Question 26.2. **Which of the following statements is NOT true regarding the etiology of non-Hodgkin lymphoma?**

A. The incidence of follicular lymphoma is lower in the Asian immigrants to the United States as compared with later generations.
B. Inherited immunodeficiency states account for majority of lymphoma.
C. It is associated with a 25% risk of developing lymphoma.
D. Immunodeficiency-related lymphomas are often associated with Epstein-Barr virus (EBV) and vary from polyclonal B-cell hyperplasia to monoclonal lymphomas.
E. The risk of developing NHL in patients with Sjögren syndrome is increased approximately 30- to 40-fold.
F. Celiac disease associated enteropathy type intestinal T-cell lymphomas have a better prognosis than extranodal B-cell lymphomas.

Question 26.3. **There is a well-documented association between EBV and all of the following lymphomas EXCEPT**

A. endemic Burkitt lymphoma
B. posttransplant lymphoproliferative disorder (PTLD)
C. acquired immunodeficiency syndrome (AIDS)-associated primary central nervous system (CNS) non-Hodgkin lymphoma
D. enteropathy-type intestinal T-cell lymphoma
E. primary effusion lymphoma, in association with human herpesvirus-8 (HHV-8)

Corresponding Chapters in *Cancer: Principles & Practice of Oncology*, Seventh Edition: 41 (Lymphomas).

Question 26.4. **Which of the following statement(s) about bone marrow plasma cells is/are true?**

A. They lack surface immunoglobulin.
B. They lack pan B cell antigens other than CD79.
C. They lack CD40, CD45, and HLADR.
D. They contain cytoplasmic IgG or IgA.
E. All of the above.

Question 26.5. **Most translocations in lymphoid neoplasms place a gene that is normally silent under the influence of a promoter associated with an immunoglobulin. Examples of these include all the following EXCEPT**

A. t(8;14)(q24;q32) in Burkitt lymphoma
B. t(14;18)(q32;q32) in follicular lymphoma
C. t(11;18)(q21;q21) in mucosa-associated lymphoid tissue (MALT) lymphoma
D. t(11;14)(q13;q32) in mantle cell lymphoma

Question 26.6. **A diagnostic cerebrospinal fluid (CSF) study is recommended in patients with large cell lymphoma in all of the following situations EXCEPT**

A. paranasal sinus involvement
B. tonsillar involvement
C. testicular involvement
D. epidural involvement
E. bone marrow involvement

Question 26.7. **Regarding the utility of the fluorodeoxyglucose (FDG) positron emission tomographic (PET) scan in the staging workup of non-Hodgkin lymphomas, which one of the following statements is true?**

A. Most of the studies evaluating FDG-PET in non-Hodgkin lymphoma include only patients with low grade histology.
B. The FDG-PET scan is less reliable in detecting extranodal marginal zone lymphoma.
C. The sensitivity of the FDG-PET scan is similar to the gallium scan in patients with intermediate grade lymphomas.
D. The FDG-PET scan is not useful in the evaluation of splenic involvement.
E. Several studies suggest that a persistently positive FDG-PET scan is more informative than a negative result in the evaluation of a residual mass after the completion of chemotherapy of non-Hodgkin lymphoma.

Question 26.8. **All of the following principles apply to the treatment of early stage (stages I to II) follicular grades I to II lymphoma EXCEPT**

A. the median radiation dose in most series is in the range of 30 to 40 Gy
B. recurrences within the radiation field range from 0% to 11%, with higher percentages in patients with bulky disease
C. there are no large prospective randomized studies evaluating the dose and field size of the radiation therapy in patients with stages I to II follicular lymphoma
D. dose reduction is not beneficial in decreasing morbidity from xerostomia secondary to irradiation of the salivary glands in an elderly patient

Question 26.9. **All of the following are true about mantle cell lymphoma EXCEPT**

A. tumor cells strongly express sIgM and IgD (often of lambda light chain type) and B cell associated antigens
B. most tumor cells coexpress CD5 and are usually CD23 negative
C. t(11;14)(q13;q32) can be demonstrated in the majority of the tumors
D. overexpression of the cyclin D1 gene is seen
E. less than 10% of patients have genetic abnormalities in addition to the t(11;14) detectable by classic cytogenetics or comparative genomic hybridization (CGH)

Question 26.10. **Regarding diffuse large B-cell lymphoma (DLBCL), which of the following statements is NOT correct?**

A. Abbreviated cytoxan, hydroxydoxorubicin, oncovin, prednisone (CHOP) chemotherapy plus involved field radiation therapy is excellent therapy for patients with low-risk, nonbulky, early stage DLBCL.
B. Standard initial treatment for advanced stage DLBCL is CHOP plus rituximab.
C. Rituximab appears to benefit the subset of DLBCL patients with lymphoma that do not express bcl2 on immunocytochemistry.
D. Autologous stem cell transplantation is the treatment of choice for patients with relapsed DLBCL that is shown to be chemosensitive.
E. Allogeneic stem cell transplantation in lymphoma leads to lower recurrence rates and increased transplant-related mortality.

Question 26.11. **A 60-year-old physician is seen by her gastroenterologist because of persistent upper abdominal pain that is not relieved with antacids. The physical examination is unremarkable. The complete blood cell count (CBC) shows a Hb 10 g, MCV 82, white blood cell count (WBC) 5,000, and**

platelet count 500,000. Upper gastrointestinal (GI) endoscopy reveals several superficial raised lesions in the gastric antrum. Biopsy of the lesions show features consistent with low grade MALT lymphoma. *Helicobacter pylori* is present in the biopsy specimen. A computed tomography (CT) scan of the chest, abdomen, and pelvis does not show lymphadenopathy or hepatosplenomegaly. Bone marrow examination reveals no evidence of lymphoma. You recommend

A. antibiotic therapy
B. chemotherapy with CHOP
C. rituximab at 375 mg per m^2 intravenously (IV) weekly for four doses
D. radiation therapy
E. surgical consult for gastrectomy

Question 26.12. **A 26-year-old college student complaints of a sore throat for 4 weeks associated with pain on swallowing. Examination reveals a 3.5-cm mass in the left tonsil. A biopsy reveals diffuse large B-cell lymphoma. Further staging reveals no other adenopathy or hepatosplenomegaly. CT scan of the neck, chest, and abdomen reveals no further abnormality. The patient is ECOG PS 0. A bone marrow biopsy did not reveal evidence of lymphoma involvement. The CBC and lactic dehydrogenase (LDH) are normal. You recommend**

A. CHOP every 3 weeks for 8 cycles
B. CHOP and rituximab every 3 weeks for 8 cycles
C. CHOP for 3 cycles followed by radiotherapy
D. CHOP and rituximab for 3 cycles followed by radiotherapy
E. involved field radiotherapy

Question 26.13. **A 53-year-old college basketball coach is diagnosed with stage IV follicular small lymphocytic lymphoma with "B" symptoms. He has generalized lymphadenopathy and splenomegaly. He is treated with CHOP for 8 cycles and achieves a complete remission. Two years later, he returns to his physician with increasing fatigue and worsening lymphadenopathy and splenomegaly. He is treated with 4 doses of rituximab and achieves a complete remission. A year later the patient presents to the physician again with B symptoms and progressive lymphadenopathy. Biopsy of a cervical lymph node shows the same histology as the original tumor. A CBC reveals Hb 11 g, WBC 5,400 with 2,300 neutrophils, and platelets 160,000. A bone marrow biopsy reveals less than 10% involvement with lymphoma. Retreatment with rituximab produces no response. The patient has expressed his desire to continue working. What would you recommend at this time?**

A. CHOP chemotherapy for 8 cycles.
B. CHOP plus rituximab for 8 cycles.
C. Fludarabine-based chemotherapy with rituximab.
D. Stem cell transplantation.
E. Radioimmunotherapy.

Question 26.14. **A 32-year-old female patient presents with enlarged cervical lymph nodes 18 months after initial therapy with CHOP chemotherapy for diffuse large B-cell lymphoma, stage IVB. She now has no "B" symptoms and her physical examination is unremarkable except for multiple enlarged left cervical lymph nodes, the largest being 3.0 by 2.5 cm. A CBC shows Hb 11g, WBC 4,300 with absolute neutrophil count (ANC) 3,000, and platelets 300,000. LDH is normal. The patient is ECOG PS 0. A biopsy of a left cervical lymph node reveals diffuse large B-cell lymphoma. A CT scan of the chest, abdomen, and pelvis and PET scan do not reveal evidence of disease elsewhere. A bone marrow biopsy does not reveal evidence of lymphoma. What would you recommend?**

A. CHOP for 3 cycles followed by radiotherapy.
B. CHOP and rituximab for 8 cycles.
C. Two cycles of ICE (ifosfamide, cisplatin, and etoposide) chemotherapy followed by autologous peripheral blood stem cell transplantation.
D. Radioimmunotherapy.
E. Allogeneic stem cell transplantation.

Question 26.15. **A 25-year-old man with stage IIA nodular sclerosing Hodgkin disease was treated with total nodal radiation therapy 3 years ago. The patient now presents with a new enlarged lymph node in the groin. A biopsy of the node confirms a diagnosis of recurrent Hodgkin disease, nodular sclerosing type. The patient has no "B" symptoms. A restaging workup includes a CT scan of the chest, abdomen, and pelvis and PET scanning. Recurrent disease is found in nodes above and below the diaphragm. A bone marrow biopsy is negative for Hodgkin disease. The patient is clinical stage IIIA. Which of the following statements is true?**

A. Since the patient has recurrent disease following initial curative therapy, he should be treated with high-dose chemotherapy (HDCT) or autologous stem cell transplant (ASCT).
B. Patients who relapse following therapy for early stage Hodgkin disease and are then treated with conventional chemotherapy have a lower survival rate than patients who have an identical stage of disease and are treated with chemotherapy initially. It appears that treatment with radiation therapy can confer drug resistance and may compromise chemotherapy dose intensity.
C. Treatment with adriamycin, bleomycin, vinblastine, dacarbazine (ABVD) chemotherapy results in superior disease-free survival compared to nitrogen mustard, oncovin, procarbazine, prednisone (MOPP) regimen in patients with recurrent Hodgkin disease following radiation therapy.
D. Patients who relapse with stage IV disease or "B" symptoms following prior radiation therapy and are then treated with conventional salvage chemotherapy have a low 10-year disease-free survival of less than 10%. They should be considered for ASCT as initial therapy rather than conventional chemotherapy.

Question 26.16. **All of the following statements about the possible etiology of Hodgkin disease are true EXCEPT**

A. EBV DNA has been detected in lymph nodes affected by Hodgkin disease using Southern blotting
B. the transcription factor NFkB has been shown to be constitutively active in cultured as well as primary H–RS (Hodgkin–Reed Sternberg) cells
C. chromosomal translocations have been identified in up to two thirds of cases of Hodgkin disease, and specific chromosomal markers for Hodgkin disease have been identified
D. the t(14:18) translocation, which results in overexpression of the bcl-2 protein, has been found in some cases of Hodgkin disease, but the translocation has been localized to nonmalignant bystander B cells

Question 26.17. **A number of studies have suggested a possible genetic predisposition for Hodgkin disease. All of the following statements are true and support this hypotheses EXCEPT**

A. slightly more women develop Hodgkin disease than men, in a ratio of 1.4:1.0
B. Hodgkin disease has been linked to certain human leukocyte antigens (HLA)
C. there is an increased risk of Hodgkin disease among parent–child pairs, but not among spouses
D. siblings of patients with Hodgkin disease have an increased risk of developing the disease, and the risk is increased further if the siblings are of the same sex

Question 26.18. **Which of the following statements about the cell of origin of the H–RS cell is NOT true?**

A. Micromanipulation of single H–RS cells from cases of classic Hodgkin disease have allowed the amplification of rearranged Ig heavy chain genes. Sequence analysis shows that the H–RS cells have a clonal B-cell origin.
B. There is evidence that a substantial proportion of cases of lymphocyte-predominant Hodgkin disease represent monoclonal B cell derived disorders.
C. Rare cases of clonal rearranged T-cell receptor genes in classical Hodgkin disease, with a lack of Ig gene rearrangements, prove that in some rare instances, Hodgkin disease is a T-cell derived lymphoma.
D. The transplantation of biopsy material into severe combined immunodeficiency (SCID) mice allows the growth of primary H–RS cells to be studied *in vivo,* and the model can be used for pre-clinical testing. The cells grown in the SCID mice are CD30 (ki-1) positive and express B-cell markers.

Question 26.19. **Nodular lymphocyte predominant Hodgkin disease (NLPHD) differs in several ways from the subtypes of classic Hodgkin disease, nodular sclerosing, mixed cellularity, and lymphocyte depleted. All of the following statements about NLPHD are true EXCEPT**

A. most patients with NLPHD present with stage III or IV disease at the time of diagnosis
B. the atypical cells are CD45+ and express B-cell associated antigens
C. NLPHD and classic Hodgkin disease both have a small number of neoplastic cells in a reactive background, which distinguishes them both from most B-cell non-Hodgkin lymphomas
D. the RS cell variants in NLPHD differ morphologically from "classic" RS cells; they have vesicular, polylobulated nuclei and distinct, small, usually peripheral nucleoli without perinuclear halos

Question 26.20. **The term lymphocyte rich classic Hodgkin disease (LRCHD) has been proposed in the Revised European–American Lymphoma (REAL) classification for cases of Hodgkin disease with RS cells that appear classic by morphology and immunophenotype and have a background infiltrate consisting predominantly of lymphocytes, with rare or no eosinophils. True statements about LRCHD include all of the following EXCEPT**

A. LRCHD can closely resemble NLPHD morphologically, and immunophenotyping may be required to differentiate the two entities
B. cases of LRCHD have the immunophenotype of classic Hodgkin disease with expression of CD15 and CD30 by the RS cells
C. the overall survival of LRCHD is slightly better than that of NLPHD in the German Hodgkin Study Group studies
D. patients with LRCHD usually lack bulky disease or B symptoms and tend to present with early stage disease; the clinical features at presentation seem to be intermediate between those of NLPHD and classic Hodgkin disease

Question 26.21. **Anaplastic large cell lymphoma (ALCL) is a T-cell lymphoma with large malignant cells containing prominent nucleoli and abundant cytoplasm. Although the cells may resemble Reed-Sternberg cell variants, the tumor cells grow in cohesive sheets and frequently involve lymph node sinuses, which is unusual in Hodgkin disease. However, a subtype of ALCL, called Hodgkin-related or Hodgkin-like in the REAL classification, has been described. All of the following statements about ALCL-Hodgkin-like are true EXCEPT**

A. this entity has cytologic features similar to common ALCL such as confluent sheets of tumor and sinusoidal infiltration; it also has morphologic features that resemble nodular sclerosis type Hodgkin disease
B. the t(2;5) translocation associated with ALCL is absent in cases of typical Hodgkin disease. The ALK protein or the p80 fusion product of the t(2;5) translocation has been found in a subset of ALCL, but cases of ALCL-Hodgkin-like typically lack the ALK protein
C. the currently available data suggest that there is no true borderline between ALCL and Hodgkin disease; for this reason, the category "ALCL-Hodgkin–like" will remain a provisional entity in the World Health Organization (WHO) classification
D. most hematopathologists believe that the cases of ALCL-Hodgkin-like reported in literature are a heterogeneous group of disorders

Question 26.22. **Staging procedures for Hodgkin disease have become simpler and less invasive with the advent of new staging modalities. Which of the following statements is true?**

A. Patients with large mediastinal adenopathy (LMA) have an increased risk of relapsing in nodal and extranodal sites above the diaphragm following treatment with radiation therapy alone. LMA has been defined as mediastinal disease greater than 50% of the thoracic diameter at T5-6 or a ratio of greater than 50% between the largest transverse diameter of the mediastinal mass over the transverse diameter of the thorax at the diaphragm in a staging posterior-anterior (PA) chest x-ray.
B. In a patient with early-stage Hodgkin disease treated initially with chemotherapy, if a PET scan is subsequently negative, there is good evidence that the patient does not need adjuvant involved field radiation therapy after the chemotherapy.
C. Staging laparotomy remains an important part of the routine staging in Hodgkin disease. It should be used in all cases where it is thought that the patient has stage I or II disease above the diaphragm.
D. Although involvement of the central nervous system is rare, invasion of the epidural space can occur by extension from the paraaortic region through the intervertebral foramina.

Question 26.23. **In the treatment of early stage Hodgkin disease, radiation therapy remains a standard approach, and excellent results have been achieved with careful delineation of the disease. Which one of the following statements about radiation therapy in the treatment of Hodgkin disease is not true?**

A. in patients with supradiaphragmatic disease treated with radiation therapy alone, a total dose of 3,000 cGy to the entire mantle field is sufficient. Areas of initial involvement should receive a total dose of 3,600 to 4,000 cGy by the addition of a cone down field
B. patients with infradiaphragmatic stage I or II Hodgkin disease can be treated with pelvic irradiation. The inguinal and femoral nodes should be irradiated, and iliac wing blocks can be used to spare the bone marrow
C. in patients who receive pelvic irradiation for subdiaphragmatic Hodgkin disease, men have a high risk of loss of fertility. The risk of loss of fertility in women is minimal, however, particularly in women less than age 25 at the time of treatment. The risk of infertility increases in women over the age of 25, however, and precautions must be undertaken to reduce the risk of infertility in older women
D. proper use of megavoltage energies is needed to ensure that superficial nodes are not underdosed in the "build-up region." A 4 to 6 MeV linear accelerator should be used for mantle and pelvic fields while higher energies (10 to 15 MeV) can be used for paraaortic nodes

Question 26.24. **Hodgkin disease is the fourth most common cancer diagnosed during pregnancy and has been reported as occurring once in every 1,000 to 6,000 deliveries. All of the following statements about Hodgkin disease during pregnancy are true EXCEPT**

A. CT scanning should be avoided because it exposes the fetus to ionizing radiation, but magnetic resonance imaging (MRI) can be used for staging because it appears to be nonteratogenic
B. chemotherapy drugs that act as antimetabolites, such as methotrexate, have a high risk of causing teratogenesis. The long-term survival of women with Hodgkin disease who were pregnant at the time of initial presentation is worse than that of nonpregnant women with similar stages of disease
C. in the second or third trimester of pregnancy, if there is rapid progression of supradiaphragmatic lymphadenopathy, radiotherapy alone can be used. If involved field or mantle radiation is used with abdominal shielding, the risk of adverse sequelae for the fetus is low
D. if Hodgkin disease is diagnosed in the first trimester of pregnancy, a therapeutic abortion should be encouraged since therapeutic options in early pregnancy are limited. If the woman wants to continue the pregnancy, treatment should be deferred until at least the second trimester

Question 26.25. **Patients with Hodgkin disease treated with chemotherapy and radiation therapy have an increased risk of secondary malignancies including acute leukemia, non-Hodgkin lymphomas, and solid tumors. All of the following statements about secondary malignancies are true EXCEPT**

A. topoisomerase II inhibitors such as etoposide have been implicated in the development of a clinically and cytogenetically distinct form of secondary acute myelogenous leukemia (AML)
B. the occurrence of acute nonlymphocytic leukemia appears to be related to the exposure to alkylating agents; the risk of secondary leukemia is reduced in patients treated with ABVD regimen, compared to patients treated with MOPP
C. treatment-related leukemia has a long latency period of 3 to 5 years and most cases occur within 10 years of the initial treatment
D. most cases of non-Hodgkin lymphoma occurring after Hodgkin disease have a low-grade histology
E. solid tumors tend to occur in the second decade following treatment; breast cancer is seen in women who received radiation therapy at an early age, and lung cancer is seen mostly in smokers

Question 26.26. **Several long-term complications can be seen in patients treated for Hodgkin disease. All of the following statements about these complications are true EXCEPT**

A. paresthesias radiating down the dorsal part of the extremities when the neck is flexed, called the *L'hermitte sign*, can be seen in 10% to 15% of patients following mantle irradiation
B. in men, the incidence of persistent azoospermia following chemotherapy with MOPP/ABVD can be decreased significantly by using gonadotropin-releasing hormone analogues prior to chemotherapy
C. hypothyroidism following mantle radiation therapy can be detected by finding an elevated TSH (thyroid stimulating hormone) level
D. following MOPP chemotherapy, women develop an age-dependent premature ovarian failure and about half of women become amenorrheic
E. the risk of postsplenectomy sepsis can be minimized by immunization with pneumococcal vaccine; recently, vaccines have also been developed against *Neisseria* and *Haemophilus*, which are also associated with postsplenectomy sepsis

Question 26.27. **The German Hodgkin Study Group (GHSG) has recently conducted a series of clinical trials to look at the role of dose intensification in advanced Hodgkin disease. The BEACOPP regimen (bleomycin, etoposide, doxorubicin, cyclophosphamide, vincristine, procarbazine, and prednisone) was used as a standard combination for dose escalation. The GHSG designed a three-arm study comparing COPP/ABVD, standard BEACOPP, and escalated BEACOPP in patients with advanced Hodgkin disease. About two thirds of the patients also received consolidation radiation therapy. In 1996, at an interim analysis, the COPP/ABVD arm was closed to accrual because it was inferior to the BEACOPP arm. All of the following statements about the GHSG trial are true EXCEPT**

A. at a median of 5 years, the freedom from treatment failure rate was 69% for COPP/ABVD, 76% for standard BEACOPP, and 87% for the escalated BEACOPP
B. in the escalated BEACOPP arm, there were nine cases of AML/MDS while there were 2 cases in the standard BEACOPP arm; also, the total rate of second neoplasms was highest in the escalated BEACOPP arm
C. escalated BEACOPP was associated with greater hematologic toxicity, requiring more red cell and platelet transfusions, but there were no differences in hematologic toxicity between the standard BEACOPP arm and the COPP/ABVD arm
D. rates of early progression were significantly lower with the escalated BEACOPP compared to standard BEACOPP and COPP/ABVD

Question 26.28. **Several trials have looked at the use of less toxic chemotherapy combined with radiation therapy. These combinations would allow a reduction in the amount and toxicity of chemotherapy and the use of smaller radiation volumes. Which of the following statements is not true?**

A. at Stanford, Horning and colleagues developed a less toxic chemotherapy regimen, VBM (vinblastine, bleomycin, and methotrexate). A trial treating patients with PS IA to IIB and IIIA patients compared subtotal nodal/total nodal irradiation to involved field irradiation followed by VBM. The difference in overall survival was not statistically significant ($p = 0.09$)
B. the British National Lymphoma Investigation (BNLI) trial found that the combination of VBM with involved field irradiation produced unacceptable pulmonary and hematologic toxicity
C. in a follow-up Stanford trial, patients with CS IA-IIIA Hodgkin disease received either subtotal nodal and splenic irradiation or 2 cycles of VBM, followed by regional mantle irradiation followed by 4 additional cycles of VBM with a reduction in the bleomycin dose. No differences were seen in survival or freedom from disease progression
D. the German Hodgkin Lymphoma Study Group (GHSG) HD7 (1994 to 1998) trial randomized 643 CS IA-IIB patients to either subtotal nodal and splenic irradiation alone, or to 2 courses of ABVD and the same radiation therapy regimen. No difference was seen in the freedom from treatment failure between the two groups

ANSWERS

Answer 26.1. **The answer is B.**

Lymphomas, both Hodgkin and non-Hodgkin together, represent 4% to 5% of all new cancer cases and are the fifth leading cause of cancer deaths in the United States.

Answer 26.2. **The answer is E.**

Patients with celiac disease associated enteropathy type intestinal T-cell lymphoma have a poor prognosis compared to other extranodal non-Hodgkin lymphomas.

Answer 26.3. **The answer is D.**

EBV DNA is detectable in 95% of endemic Burkitt lymphomas. EBV is also linked to PTLD. Virtually all AIDS-associated primary CNS lymphomas have detectable EBV DNA in the tumor. EBV is also seen in association with human herpesvirus-8 in primary effusion lymphoma. There is no well-described association between enteropathy type intestinal T-cell lymphoma and EBV infection.

Answer 26.4. **The answer is E.**

All of the statements are correct regarding bone marrow plasma cells.

Answer 26.5. **The answer is C.**

The t(8;14) (q24;q32) in Burkitt lymphoma places the c-Myc gene under the Ig promoter. t(14;18)(q32;q32) of follicular lymphoma places the bcl2 gene on chromosome 18 under the Ig promoter. t(11;14)(q13;q32) in mantle cell lymphoma places cyclin D1 gene associated with BCL1 breakpoint on chromosome 11 under the Ig promoter. In MALT lymphoma, the (11;18)(q21;q21) translocation produces an API2-MLT fusion protein, which is activated as a consequence of the fusion.

Answer 26.6. **The answer is B.**

Patients with paranasal sinus, testicular involvement, epidural lymphoma, and possibly bone marrow involvement with large cells are especially prone to meningeal spread and should have a diagnostic lumbar puncture. In addition, a lumbar puncture is often recommended for highly aggressive histologies and lymphoma in the setting of immunocompromise, including human immunodeficiency virus (HIV) infection.

Answer 26.7. **The answer is B.**

The majority of studies evaluating FDG-PET in non-Hodgkin lymphoma (NHL) include patients with intermediate grade large cell NHL. Only limited data are available on the role of the FDG-PET scan in other NHL histologic subtypes. Many groups have confirmed the lack of reliability in detecting marginal zone lymphoma, particularly the extranodal marginal type. The available data strongly demonstrate increased sensitivity of FDG-PET compared to the gallium scan in the staging of NHL. The FDG-PET scan is useful in the evaluation of splenic involvement. Because of the high incidence of false-positive rates, a negative PET scan is more informative than a positive result in the evaluation of a residual mass after therapy for non-Hodgkin lymphoma. Although some patients with a persistently positive FDG-PET scan after therapy may remain in prolonged remission, close follow-up is warranted.

Answer 26.8. **The answer is D.**

When there is a possibility of significant morbidity from treatment, such as long-term xerostomia from irradiation of the salivary glands in an elderly patient, lower doses are beneficial in reducing the treatment related morbidity (i.e., 25 to 30 Gy).

Answer 26.9. **The answer is E.**

Over 90% of cases have genetic abnormalities in addition to the t(11;14) detectable by classic cytogenetics or CGH.

Answer 26.10. **The answer is C.**

Based largely on the GELA study, the addition of rituximab to CHOP chemotherapy has become the standard for patients with advanced stage diffuse large cell lymphoma in the United States. In a subset analysis of the GELA study on DLBCL in patients over 60 years of age, rituximab appeared to result in a significant benefit in patients whose lymphoma expressed bcl-2 compared to those that did not express it, when the antibody was added to CHOP chemotherapy.

Answer 26.11. **The answer is A.**

The standard treatment of low-grade MALT lymphoma of the stomach associated with *H. pylori* is antibiotic therapy and follow-up with endoscopy 3 to 6 months later. *H. pylori* eradication can result in lymphoma regression in more than 50% of patients with low grade MALT lymphoma of the stomach. Patients who have complete response should be followed without further treatment. Patients who have a partial response and remain *H. pylori* positive should receive a second course of antibiotics before proceeding to more definitive treatment. Patients who are negative for *H. pylori* are unlikely to respond to antibiotics. These patients should be considered for radiotherapy or chemotherapy.

Answer 26.12. **The answer is C.**

The Southwest Oncology Group Trial randomized 401 patients with stage I and nonbulky stage II diffuse large B cell lymphoma to receive either 3 cycles of CHOP and involved field radiotherapy (40 to 55 Gy) or 8 cycles of CHOP alone. The 5-year progression free-survival and overall survival results favored the CHOP and involved field radiotherapy treatment arm, although after longer follow-up this survival benefit was less apparent. Patients in the lower risk category group (0 or 1 risk factor, as in the patient under discussion) had a higher progression-free and overall survival compared to patients with two or three risk factors. As a result of this study, combination chemotherapy and adjuvant radiation therapy have become the standard of care for patients with stages I to II diffuse large B cell lymphoma.

Answer 26.13. **The answer is E.**

This patient's lymphoma returned after standard chemotherapy and rituximab and he is now resistant to rituximab. Retreatment with CHOP is unlikely to give long duration of remission in this patient. Since he has already received 400 mg per m^2 of doxorubicin, his cardiac function could become compromised if he gets another 8 cycles of CHOP. Fludarabine-based therapy has not been evaluated prospectively in CHOP failures. Stem cell transplantation is investigational in low-grade lymphoma; the bone marrow disease needs to be eradicated before considering an autologous stem cell transplantation. Radioimmunotherapy is an attractive option. It is shown to be very active in patients refractory to rituximab. It is also a one-time treatment and the patient can continue with his current activities.

Answer 26.14. **The answer is C.**

Abbreviated chemotherapy followed by radiotherapy has been shown to be superior to a full course of chemotherapy in patients with untreated limited stage DLBCL, but this has not been shown to be beneficial in patients relapsing following chemotherapy. The role of chemoimmunotherapy combinations in the treatment of relapsed aggressive lymphoma following chemotherapy alone has not been studied. On the basis of the Parma trial, this patient would benefit from cytoreductive chemotherapy followed by autologous stem cell transplantation if her lymphoma is still chemosensitive. Radioimmunotherapy is active in large cell lymphoma, but its role as a single agent in this disease has not been studied prospectively. The results with allogeneic stem cell transplantation are superior to autologous transplantation in this group of patients.

Answer 26.15. **The answer is C.**

Patients who relapse following radiation therapy alone for conventional Hodgkin disease have satisfactory results with conventional combination chemotherapy. Prior radiation therapy does not cause drug resistance or a clinically significant compromise of chemotherapy dose intensity. Patients who relapse with stage IV disease or "B" symptoms have a 10-year disease-free survival as high as 34% and should be treated initially with conventional chemotherapy. It does appear that ABVD gives a better disease-free survival when compared to MOPP in patients with recurrence after radiation (81% with ABVD versus 54% with MOPP).

Answer 26.16. **The answer is C.**

Abnormal karyotypes are seen in 22% to 83% of cases of Hodgkin disease, but a specific chromosomal marker of Hodgkin disease has not been identified. Aneuploidy with hyperdiploidy is the most frequent observed abnormality.

Answer 26.17. **The answer is A.**

Hodgkin disease is slightly more common in men than in women (1.4:1.0). There is a bimodal incidence pattern in the developed countries, the first peak occurring in the third decade and the second smaller peak occurring after age 50.

Answer 26.18. **The answer is D.**

No reproducible growth of primary H–RS cells has been observed after the transplantation of biopsy material into SCID mice.

Answer 26.19. **The answer is A.**

Most patients with NLPHD present with stage I or II disease. The complete response rate following initial therapy is over 90%. The immunophenotype is an important part of the definition of NLPHD. Unlike typical B cell lymphomas, however, they are usually immunoglobulin negative by routine techniques.

Answer 26.20. **The answer is C.**

In the German Hodgkin Study Group, the overall survival of LRCHD was significantly worse than that of NLPHD.

Answer 26.21. **The answer is C.**

The category "ALCL-Hodgkin-like" will be eliminated from the proposed WHO classification.

Answer 26.22. **The answer is D.**

LMA has been defined as mediastinal disease greater than 35% of the thoracic diameter at T5-6 or a ratio from the chest x-ray greater than 33%, not 50%. FDG-PET scan is not an absolute indicator of cure after chemotherapy alone, and there is no information supporting the use of PET scanning to decide whether to proceed with adjuvant involved field radiation therapy. Staging laparotomy is no longer considered a routine staging procedure and it should be reserved for patients with limited stage disease who may be treated with radiation therapy alone.

Answer 26.23. **The answer is C.**

Women also have a high risk of loss of fertility with pelvic irradiation. The risk of loss of fertility is less in women younger than age 25 who are treated with *chemotherapy,* not radiotherapy.

Answer 26.24. **The answer is B.**

Several studies have shown that pregnancy does not worsen the clinical course of Hodgkin disease, and the long-term survival of pregnant women with Hodgkin disease is not different from that of nonpregnant women.

Answer 26.25. **The answer is D.**

Most of the cases of non-Hodgkin lymphoma are of intermediate-grade or high-grade histology.

Answer 26.26. **The answer is B.**

The usefulness of gonadotropin-releasing hormone analogues to prevent sterility has not been proven.

Answer 26.27. **The answer is B.**

The total rate of secondary neoplasms was highest in the COPP/ABVD arm.

Answer 26.28. **The answer is D.**

In the GHSG HD7 trial, the patients who received 2 cycles of ABVD had a statistically significant improvement in freedom from treatment failure (91% versus 75% for irradiation alone, $p < 0.0001$). This study raised several questions. Is the benefit in freedom from treatment failure worth the risk of long-term toxicity from the exposure to doxorubicin and bleomycin? Will it be more difficult to salvage the patients who relapse after the irradiation if they have already received 2 cycles of ABVD? Only longer follow-up will answer these questions.

CHAPTER 27

Acute Leukemias

BRUNO NERVI AND JOHN F. DIPERSIO

Directions Each of the numbered items below is followed by lettered answers. Select the ONE lettered answer that is BEST in each case unless instructed otherwise.

QUESTIONS

Question 27.1. **Which of the following statements is the most accurate concerning secondary leukemias?**

A. A clear cause of secondary leukemia can be found in the majority of patients.
B. Secondary leukemias are frequently associated with use of an epipodophyllotoxin (etoposide or teniposide), anthracyclines, or alkylating agents.
C. Incidence of secondary acute myeloid leukemia (AML) and acute lymphoid leukemia (ALL) are similar.
D. The treatment response is similar to other acute leukemias.
E. All secondary leukemias are preceded by myelodysplastic syndromes.

Question 27.2. **Risk factors for the development of AML include all of the following EXCEPT**

A. exposure to gamma irradiation
B. genetic syndromes like Down syndrome
C. cigarette smoke
D. some chemotherapeutic drugs
E. electromagnetic fields

Question 27.3. **Favorable cytogenetic abnormalities of AML include**

A. t(15;17)
B. inv 16
C. t(16;16)
D. t(8;21)
E. t(15;17) and del 7
F. t(16;16) and 5q-
G. all of the above

Corresponding Chapters in *Cancer: Principles & Practice of Oncology*, Seventh Edition: 42 (Acute Leukemias).

Question 27.4. **Favorable cytogenetic abnormalities of ALL include**

A. t(1;19)/E2A-PBX1 fusion
B. t(12;21)/TEL-AML1
C. hyperdiploidy (modal chromosomal number >50)
D. trisomies of chromosomes 4, 10, and 17
E. all of the above

Question 27.5. **Poor prognostic features of AML include**

A. del 5, 5q-
B. del 7, 7q-
C. +8, +11, +13, +21
D. 11q23
E. inv (3)
F. complex cytogenetics
G. all of the above

Question 27.6. **Which of the following statements is true concerning induction remission therapy in AML?**

A. Age is not associated with the ability to achieve remission.
B. "7+3" regimen is the standard induction therapy in AML.
C. Patients with AML benefit from the administration of hematopoietic growth factors.
D. The early evaluation of bone marrow (BM) on day 14 after induction has no prognostic value.
E. The addition of etoposide to "7+3" induction regime increases overall survival.

Question 27.7. **Which of the following statements is true concerning postremission therapy in AML?**

A. The major cause of failure after autologous stem cell transplantation (SCT) is treatment related mortality (TRM).
B. The major cause of failure after allogeneic SCT is AML relapse.
C. All AML patients require maintenance therapy after consolidation therapy.
D. Allogeneic SCT is recommended for high-risk patients in first complete remission (CR).
E. All AML patients benefit from allogeneic SCT in first CR.

Question 27.8. **What statement is true concerning relapsed AML?**

A. High-dose cytarabine cures 20% of patients with AML in relapse.
B. Before allo-SCT for relapsed AML, it is necessary to achieve a second CR.
C. Allo-SCT is the best chance of cure for a patient with relapsed AML.
D. Auto-SCT offers a better overall survival than allo-SCT.

Question 27.9. **Which of the following statements describes the best treatment for a patient with acute promyelocytic leukemia (APL) in relapse?**

A. These patients are incurable with conventional chemotherapy, all trans-retinoic acid (ATRA) therapy, or arsenic trioxide therapy.
B. Arsenic trioxide achieves CR in 85% of patients as second-line therapy.
C. Allo-SCT may prolong overall survival.
D. Auto-SCT may prolong overall survival.
E. All of the above.

Question 27.10. **Poor prognostic factors in ALL include all of the following EXCEPT**

A. Philadelphia chromosome positive (Ph+) disease
B. white blood cell count (WBC) greater than 10,000 per mm^3
C. age older than 16
D. greater than 4 weeks to achieve CR
E. translocations involving rearrangement of the MLL gene on chromosome 11q23
F. ALL associated with t(12;21)

ANSWERS

Answer 27.1. **The answer is B.**

Secondary AML should refer to AML secondary to prior existing myelodysplastic syndrome (MDS), myeloproliferative disorder, or the development of AML secondary to proven leukemogenic exposure. A clear cause of leukemia can be found in the minority of patients. Such secondary leukemias, 90% of which are myeloid, are notoriously difficult to treat. The chromosomal abnormalities often observed (del 5, del 7, 5q-, trisomy 8, 11q23 rearrangements) in these secondary leukemias are associated with a poor prognosis, even when there is no history of prior therapy or toxic exposure. Chemotherapeutic agents that interfere with DNA-topoisomerase II, such as epidophyllotoxins (etoposide or teniposide) or anthracyclines, can result in the balanced translocations involving the MLL gene on 11q23 and are, with the exception of t(9;11), associated with an unfavorable prognosis and often appear 1 to 3 years after chemotherapy. In contrast, exposure to alkylating agents more typically result in del 5, del 7, and complex chromosomal abnormalities, which frequently begin as myelodysplastic syndromes, have a particularly poor prognosis, and occur 2 to 9 years after initiation of alkylator-based chemotherapy.

Answer 27.2. **The answer is E.**

Although electromagnetic fields have received considerable recent attention as a possible carcinogen, the actual risk of leukemia from exposure to commercial and residential power fields remains controversial. There are a large number of conflicting reports but there is a lack of clear dose-response relationship and a causal relationship, either as a consequence of occupational exposure or residential power use. Risk of developing both AML and ALL are associated with exposure to gamma irradiation. Risks associated with occupational exposure to low-dose radiation are controversial. As much as 20% of AML may be attributable to smoking. Several genetic syndromes are associated with increased risk of leukemias including Down syndrome, Fanconi anemia, Bloom syndrome, and ataxia telangiectasia. Down syndrome is associated with a 20-fold increased risk of leukemia. This is typically a megakaryoblastic leukemia in children younger than 4 years of age and is often preceded by a benign myeloproliferative disease. Those children who develop acute leukemia have been shown to have mutations in one allele of the GATA-1 gene and involve small deletions or insertions in sequences encoding exon 2 of GATA-1. These mutations result in a disruption of the normal reading frame of GATA-1 and in the introduction of a premature stop codon. Down syndrome is also associated in older children with pre-B ALL.

Answer 27.3. **The answer is G.**

All of the translocations mentioned are associated with favorable outcomes [60% to 70% disease free survival (DFS) after modern therapy]. Favorable cytogenetic abnormalities [t(15;17), inv 16, and t(8;21)] maintain a dominant effect on prognosis even when associated with additional pour cytogenetic abnormalities (such as del 7, 7q-, del 5, 5q-). Favorable outcomes of t(15;17) APL patients depend upon the coadministration of ATRA with anthracyclines during induction, anthracycline based consolidation, followed by maintenance therapy with oral ATRA with or without 6-MP and MTX. Favorable outcomes in patients with "core binding factor" AMLs [t(8;21) and inv16] depend upon the administration of 3 to 4 cycles of high-dose cytarabine (3 g per m^2) consolidation chemotherapy after routine 7+3 cytarabine and anthracycline induction-remission therapy.

Answer 27.4. **The answer is E.**

Patients with t(1;19)/E2A-PBX1 fusion, t(12;21)/TEL-AML1 fusion, hyperdiploidy (modal chromosomal number >50), or trisomies are all associated with favorable treatment outcomes with disease-free survival rates approaching 80% to 90%. Different clinical outcomes associated with these abnormalities are related to drug sensitivity or resistance of leukemic blasts harboring specific genetic abnormalities. ALL associated with the t(1:19)/E2A-PBX1 fusion was classified as a high-risk subtype of leukemia when treated with standard antimetabolite-based regimens, but the use of intensified chemotherapy substantially improved the prognosis. Cases of ALL expressing the t(12;21)/TEL-AML1 fusion protein have a favorable outcome if they are treated with intensive chemotherapy, especially with asparaginase. Patients with hyperdiploid ALL have a favorable prognosis when they are treated with an antimetabolite-based regimen.

Answer 27.5. **The answer is G.**

Patients with AML that is characterized by deletions of the long arms or monosomies of chromosomes 5 or 7; by trisomy of chromosomes 8, 11, 13, or 21; by translocations or inversions of chromosome 3, t(6;9), t(9;22); or by abnormalities of chromosome 11q23 [with questionably the exception of t(9;11)] have particularly poor prognoses after treatment with standard chemotherapy. These cytogenetic subgroups predict poor clinical outcome in elderly patients with AML as well as in younger patients. It should be noted, however, that all patients over the age of 55 to 60, regardless of cytogenetics, experience limited leukemia-free and overall survival 0% to 20% after standard AML chemotherapy. Allogeneic transplant is the only therapy associated with improved outcome when performed in CR1 for those patients with high risk cytogenetics.

Answer 27.6. **The answer is B.**

Age is inversely associated with the ability to achieve remission in AML. Standard chemotherapy results in CR in 30% to 50% of patients older than 60 years of age, compared with 65% to 80% CR in younger patients. The standard induction treatment for AML, referred to as "7+3" regimen, includes cytarabine 100 mg/m^2/d for 7 days administered as a continuous infusion with daunorrubicin 45 mg/m^2/d for 3 days infused over 30 to 45 minutes. Idarrubicin 12 to 13 mg per m^2 is an alternative to daunorrubicin. No significant difference in remission induction has been noted in patients induced with either daunorrubicin or mitoxantrone. The inclusion of etoposide does not increase rates of remission-induction. The prognostic significance of day 14 to 16 blasts in the BM is independent of pretherapeutic parameters and predicts outcome even in patients achieving a CR. There is no consensus about the indication of hematopoietic growth factors (G-CSF or GM-CSF) concomitant or following induction chemotherapy. Although some studies have shown a decrease in the number of days of neutropenia and fever and an increase in the leukemic response to cytarabine, the benefit has been variable across patient populations, and economic data supporting their use has been sparse. *In vitro*, the simultaneous exposure of leukemic cells to chemotherapy and growth factors such as G-CSF, referred to as growth-factor priming, increases the susceptibility of the cells to killing by chemotherapy. Clinical studies with G-CSF given concurrently with induction chemotherapy suggest that growth factors may have a role enhancing the efficacy of chemotherapy.

Answer 27.7. **The answer is D.**

Most patients with AML in first remission will relapse without additional consolidation therapy. The options for postremission therapy include repeated cycles of high-dose cytarabine-based chemotherapy [cytarabine 3 g per m^2 intravenously (IV) over 3 hours twice daily on days 1, 3, and 5 for 3 to 4 cycles] and autologous or allogeneic stem cell transplantation (auto-SCT or allo-SCT). Chemotherapy alone has the highest risk of relapse with the lowest treatment related mortality (TRM). Allo-SCT has the lowest risk of relapse with the highest TRM, while auto-SCT has an intermediate risk of relapse and TRM. The good, intermediate, and unfavorable AML risk groups have a 4-year overall survival of 70%, 45%, and less than 20%, respectively, with standard chemotherapy. In the favorable risk group, allo-SCT is not generally recommended due to relatively low relapse rates with standard therapy and TRM of 15% to 30% after allo-SCT. With chemotherapy alone, only 0% to 20% of patients in the unfavorable group are likely to achieve long-term DFS, thus an allo-SCT would be considered acceptable in an effort to improve DFS. This was indeed shown in a large randomized study of AML patients in which patients who achieved a CR1 were assigned to either an allo-SCT or continued consolidation chemotherapy based on the presence of a human leukocyte antigen (HLA)-compatible sibling. The intermediate-risk group is more heterogeneous in response and there appears to be no consensus for recommending allo-SCT in CR1 in this group at the present time. There is no benefit to follow the consolidation with maintenance therapy. The only subgroup of AML that benefits from maintenance therapy is promyelocytic leukemia AML-M3.

Answer 27.8. **The answer is C.**

Chemotherapy alone is not curative in the relapsed setting. Both auto- and allo-SCT provide prolonged DFS in approximately 20% to 30% of patients treated either early in first relapse or in second remission. Allo-SCT (sibling or unrelated donor) offers the important benefit of the graft versus leukemia (GVL) effect compared with auto-SCT, which can salvage some patients whose disease fails to go into remission with intensive chemotherapy and offers the best chance of cure for a patient with relapsed AML. The outcomes of patients receiving an allograft in second CR are similar to those of patients transplanted in untreated first relapse. Therefore, in a patient with relapsed AML with moderately or minimal disease burden, an allo-SCT is recommended in early first relapse to avoid the toxic effect of reinduction chemotherapy. Other alternatives for relapsed AML included high-dose cytarabine (2 to 3 g per m^2 twice daily times 8 to 12 doses) with second remissions in approximately 20% to 50% of patients but with short DFS.

Answer 27.9. **The answer is E.**

Despite the good results with ATRA plus conventional chemotherapy, 30% of patients relapse. These patients are incurable with conventional chemotherapy alone or after treatment with ATRA or arsenic trioxide. Arsenic trioxide induces molecular CR (negative FISH and RT-PCR for PML-RARα) in approximately 85% of patients as a second-line therapy. Despite this result, the ability of arsenic trioxide to sustain prolonged remissions and cure is limited at best. For relapsed patients who are able to achieve remission, both allo- and auto-SCT have been reported to result in long-term survival. Long-term DFS after auto-SCT is dependent on the presence of minimal residual disease prior to auto-SCT since

75% of the patients who are RT-PCR negative prior to undergoing auto-SCT remain in clinical and molecular remission with a median follow-up of 28 months, and all patients who are RT-PCR positive prior to auto-SCT relapse at a median time of 5 months. Prolonged DFS after auto-SCT is seen especially in those patients who experience CR1 at greater than 18 to 24 months. Allo-SCT therapy remains the only curative therapy for relapsed APL patients, especially those that are RT-PCR positive for PML/RARα after salvage therapy with either arsenic trioxide or chemotherapy.

Answer 27.10. **The answer is F.**

Cure rates (defined by the absence of evidence of disease for at least 10 years) for ALL are currently about 80% for children and 40% for adults. The t(12;21)/TEL-AML1 fusion is associated with a favorable treatment outcome (90%). Patients with (Ph+) ALL are rarely cured with chemotherapy (only children who present with a low WBC/μL can be cured with standard ALL therapy). Some (40% to 50%) of these patients may be cured if they undergo allogeneic transplant in first CR. Leukocytosis at presentation (WBC counts >10,000/μL) is associated with a worse prognosis as is older age, which may in part be related to the increased incidence of the Philadelphia chromosome (Ph+) in older ALL patients. Time to achieve a CR during induction therapy carries significant prognostic implications. Patients requiring more than 4 to 5 weeks to achieve a complete response have a lower likelihood of being cured. An additional chromosomal abnormality associated with a poor prognosis is t(4;11), which is characterized by rearrangements of the MLL gene on chromosome 11q23. These patients should also be referred for allo-SCT in first remission.

CHAPTER **28**

Chronic Leukemias

SUSAN O'BRIEN

Directions Each of the numbered items below is followed by lettered answers. Select the ONE lettered answer that is BEST in each case unless instructed otherwise.

QUESTIONS

Question 28.1. **A 60-year-old man with Rai stage IV chronic lymphocytic leukemia (CLL) did not respond to therapy with chlorambucil, prednisone, and fludarabine. He is receiving therapy with alemtuzumab. At 4 weeks he is responding to treatment and the plan is to continue for another 4 weeks. One week later, he develops spiking fevers without any localizing signs. Broad-spectrum antibiotic therapy is initiated, and cultures and chest x-ray are negative. The patient is not responding to antibiotics. The most likely cause of this fever is**

A. transformation to large cell lymphoma (Richter)
B. fungal infection
C. herpes infection
D. Cytomegalovirus (CMV) reactivation

Question 28.2. **Which of the following factors is associated with a better prognosis in CLL?**

A. 11q deletion.
B. Unmutated immunoglobulin genes.
C. Mutated immunoglobulin genes.
D. 17p deletion.

Question 28.3. **A 50-year-old woman was referred for management of recently diagnosed chronic lymphocytic leukemia. The patient was asymptomatic except for concern about cervical, axillary, and inguinal lymph nodes. Physical examination showed only 2- to 3-cm nodes in each area but no hepatomegaly or splenomegaly. A complete blood cell count (CBC) showed a white count of 19.1 with 71% lymphs, a hemoglobin of 13.9, and a platelet count of 210,000 per µl. Review of the peripheral smear showed atypical, clefted lymphocytes. Flow cytometry revealed the cells**

Corresponding Chapters in *Cancer: Principles & Practice of Oncology*, Seventh Edition: 43 (Chronic Leukemias).

to be CD20+, CD5−, CD10+, and CD23+. The bone marrow was positive with tumor cells showing a paratrabecular pattern. The most likely diagnosis is

A. CLL
B. lymphoplasmacytic lymphoma
C. mantle cell lymphoma
D. follicular lymphoma

Question 28.4. **A 55-year-old man is found to have lymphocytosis after a routine physical examination. White blood cell (WBC) is 65,000 with 77% lymphocytes. Hemoglobin and platelet count are normal. B-2 microglobulin is 3.0. Which of the following approaches should be taken for this patient?**

A. Watch and wait.
B. Chlorambucil treatment.
C. Fludarabine treatment.
D. Fludarabine and rituximab treatment.

Question 28.5. **A 67-year-old man with CLL develops hemolytic anemia. Which of the following would be the best therapeutic option?**

A. Prednisone +/− cyclosporine.
B. Fludarabine.
C. Rituximab.
D. Alemtuzumab.

Question 28.6. **A 67-year-old man notices an enlarged lymph node in his neck while shaving and goes to the doctor. The physical exam reveals 1- to 2-cm nodes in the cervical, axillary, and inguinal regions. There is no palpable splenomegaly. White blood cell count is 150,000 with 69% mature lymphocytes, hemoglobin is 12.2, and platelet count is 170,000. Computed tomographic (CT) scan reveals abdominal adenopathy and an enlarged spleen. The correct Rai stage for this patient is**

A. 1
B. 2
C. 3
D. 4

Question 28.7. **A patient presents with adenopathy, splenomegaly, anemia, and thrombocytopenia and is diagnosed with CLL. Cytogenetic analysis reveals two abnormalities, including 17p-. Which of the following statements is true?**

A. This chromosomal abnormality is associated with Bcl-2 deficiency.
B. Multiple cytogenetic abnormalities confer a better prognosis than a single abnormality.
C. 17p- is associated with a poor survival.
D. The median survival for this patient is approximately 5 years.

Question 28.8. **Which of the following statements is true regarding untreated patients with CLL?**

A. Fludarabine produces lower overall response rates than chlorambucil.
B. Fludarabine and chlorambucil produce similar complete remission (CR) rates.
C. Fludarabine therapy results in longer remission duration.
D. Fludarabine-treated patients have superior survival to those treated with chlorambucil.

Question 28.9. **A 63-year-old woman presents with lymphocytosis, adenopathy, splenomegaly, and anemia. Workup is consistent with CLL and she receives fludarabine for 6 cycles and achieves a partial remission. Twelve months later she has progressive disease and receives 3 cycles of fludarabine without a response. Physical examination at this time reveals 1- to 2-cm lymph nodes, a 5-cm palpable spleen, WBC count of 60,000 with mild anemia, and thrombocytopenia. The best treatment option at this time would be**

A. rituximab
B. alemtuzumab
C. unrelated allogenic stem cell transplant
D. chlorambucil

ANSWERS

Answer 28.1. **The answer is D.**

Although all choices above could be responsible for a fever in a patient with CLL, the most common etiology for a fever occurring a few weeks into treatment with alemtuzumab would be reactivation of CMV. Typically, this is diagnosed by sending blood for a CMV antigen test, or PCR. The important point about this is that CMV reactivation will not be diagnosed unless the physician thinks to look for it. Once the diagnosis is made, therapy can be initiated with ganciclovir given intravenously, valganciclovir, the oral pro drug of ganciclovir, or foscarnet. Patients who are stable do not necessarily need to be admitted to the hospital but can be treated with the oral drug on an outpatient basis. Foscarnet may be chosen in a patient who has pancytopenia because the main side effect of ganciclovir is myelosuppression. However, foscarnet can result in renal insufficiency, and patients need to be well hydrated and have their creatine monitored if that agent is to be used. In addition, foscarnet is only available as an intravenous therapy. Most patients will respond promptly, often within 24 hours of initiation of an anti-CMV antibiotic. Unlike in the setting of bone marrow transplant, where organ involvement is frequent after CMV reactivation and carries a high mortality rate, organ involvement is uncommon in patients with CLL, although it has been reported. If the patient defervesces quickly and looks well, alemtuzumab treatment can be restarted, but CMV therapy should be continued; if CMV therapy is complete and alemtuzumab is ongoing, then prophylaxis should be used to prevent subsequent reactivation. Transformation to large cell lymphoma occurs in about 5% of patients with CLL and is usually seen in the setting of advanced stage disease after failure of multiple prior therapies. This is usually associated with progressive adenopathy and occasionally rapid enlargement of one lymph node site. B symptoms are also frequent, which is why fever can herald Richter transformation. A test on the chemistry panel that can suggest transformation is a markedly elevated lactate dehydrogenase (LDH), which is otherwise uncommon in patients with CLL. Fungal infection and herpes infection can also cause fever but would be less common as a source of fever in a patient receiving alemtuzumab therapy.

Answer 28.2. **The answer is C.**

Mutated immunoglobulin genes confer a favorable prognosis in CLL. While traditionally it was felt that CLL was a disease of naïve B cells that had not traversed the lymph node and encountered antigen, recent evidence disputes this assumption. Somatic mutation occurs as a way of increasing B-cell diversity with the endpoint being generation of memory B-cells that will respond later to rechallenge with antigen. Diversity in the formation of a B-cell initially occurs with the juxtaposition of the J, V, and D segments of the immunoglobulin gene; there are a number of possible germline genes that can combine. This occurs early in the development of the B-cell in the bone marrow. Further diversity occurs when the lymphocyte enters the lymph node and encounters antigen. Subsequently, multiple point mutations occur. The definition of somatic mutation is when the gene of interest has less than 98% homology to the germline gene. Small changes (i.e., those that cause differences from the germline gene of 1.0% to 1.9%) represent polymorphisms rather than somatic mutation. Patients with CLL can be divided into 2 groups, roughly 50:50, depending on whether or not they have unmutated or mutated immunoglobin genes. Although it was assumed that the 50% of patients who do not have mutated immunoglobin genes may have disease that has arisen from naïve B-cells, this conflicts with microarray data which suggest that many proteins expressed in CLL are consistent with an activated B-cell. There are emerging data that CLL cells containing unmutated immunoglobin genes may have traversed the lymph node, but that the somatic mutation machinery or enzymes necessary to accomplish this process are defective in such cells. The reason for the varying prognosis related to the mutation status of the immunoglobin gene is uncertain. Recent data have shown that patients with unmutated immunoglobin genes have a high likelihood of expressing a protein, ZAP70, that is normally found in T-cells and transmits downstream messages after ligation of the T-cell receptor. The group at University of California at San Diego (UCSD) recently showed that patients with CLL whose cells express ZAP70 have markedly increased phosphorylation of downstream proteins after ligation of the B-cell receptor, so that the ZAP70 protein appears to be functioning in these B-cells as it does in T-cells. This suggests that ongoing stimulation through the B-cell receptor may be delivering a signal for survival and is hypothetically a reason why patients with unmutated immunoglobin genes may have a worse prognosis.

Cytogenetic or molecular abnormalities also have prognostic significance in CLL. Both 11q deletions and 17p deletions are associated with a poor prognosis, with the latter being the worst single molecular abnormality in terms of survival. Patients with 11q deletions are usually younger men with bulky adenopathy. 17p deletion is uncommon at diagnosis, but occurs frequently in patients with refractory disease. Of note is that patients with p53 deletions (at the site of 17p deletion) have no response to nucleoside analogs, agents which rely on an intact p53 system to affect cell kill. This may be part of the reason for the poor prognosis in patients with 17p deletions.

Answer 28.3. **The answer is D.**

Although uncommon, patients with follicular lymphoma may present with a leukemic phase and thus be confused with patients with CLL. The physical findings may be identical as in this case where the patient has peripheral adenopathy and elevated white blood cell count with lymphocytosis. The peripheral smear can be helpful in differentiating these two diseases, as CLL lymphocytes appear relatively normal whereas follicular lymphoma cells are atypical with clefted nuclei. The pattern of involvement in the bone marrow can also be helpful, as the paratrabecular pattern is uncommon in CLL but typical for follicular lymphoma. The most important test in making the differential diagnosis is the immunophenotyping. B-CLL cells, as well as follicular lymphoma cells, are CD20 positive, reflecting the B-cell origin, as well as CD23 positive. However, CLL cells express CD5, which is not found in follicular lymphoma, and follicular lymphoma cells express CD10, which is not found on the surface of CLL cells. Patients with mantle cell lymphoma may also present with a leukemic phase. Like CLL, these cells also express CD5, but they do not express CD23 and they do not express CD10. Lymphoplasmacytic lymphoma also rarely presents with a leukemic phase, but again these cells are not CD10 positive and not CD23 positive and do not express CD5.

Answer 28.4. **The answer is A.**

This patient has Rai stage 0 CLL. This is the earliest stage of CLL. The diagnosis is based on the fact that the patient has an elevated white blood cell count with lymphocytosis, but no evidence of adenopathy or splenomegaly, and no cytopenias. Approximately one third of patients with Rai stage 0 CLL have very indolent disease and may never require treatment. Thus, the approach to patients with early stage disease is to watch and wait. Of some concern is the fact that the B-2 microglobulin is elevated at 3.0 and the patient is young at 55 years old. The elevated B-2 microglobulin suggests that this patient may not have very indolent disease and will be likely to progress. Nevertheless, the current approach would be to monitor this patient a bit more carefully than in a similar patient with a low B-2 microglobulin, but to delay treatment until clearly required. Several randomized studies were conducted in the 1980s wherein patients with early stage disease were randomized to a watch and wait approach versus early treatment with chlorambucil. All of these large studies had the same finding, which was that early treatment with chlorambucil did not improve survival. Although one can convincingly argue that in the year 2005 there are much better therapies available for CLL, it would likely not be productive to repeat such randomized trials. The reason is, as noted above, that about one third of patients will never require treatment for their disease and so randomizing those patients to early therapy is unlikely to show a benefit and dilute the potential benefit in the other patients. However, new prognostic factors may be able to identify patients with early stage disease who are at high risk for progression. Some of these prognostic factors include 11q or 17p deletions, unmutated immunoglobin gene, CD38 expression, and expression of ZAP70. Randomized trials are now beginning in patients with early-stage disease and multiple high-risk factors to examine whether early treatment with a fludarabine-based regimen would benefit these patients in terms of survival. Nevertheless, it will be some time before data from these trials are available.

Answer 28.5. **The answer is A.**

Hemolytic anemia may develop in about 10% of patients with CLL, although Coombs positivity indicating antibody presence on the surface of the red cell is even more common. Typically, these patients have a low hemoglobin and are diagnosed because of symptoms of anemia. LDH is often elevated, as is bilirubin. Reticulocyte count is not that reliable in the setting of CLL because the packed marrow may interfere with the ability to respond to the hemolysis, and thus the reticulocyte count may be lower than expected. Some patients may have Coombs negative hemolytic anemia; this can be established by a low haptoglobin. The traditional approach to hemolytic anemia is prednisone, which is effective in about 50% to 60% of patients. The other oral agent which has been shown to be quite effective is low-dose cyclosporine, typically given at 100 mg t.i.d. That low dosing does not require monitoring of cyclosporine levels, but does require monitoring of serum magnesium levels. Serum creatinine and bilirubin should also be monitored periodically with the use of cyclosporine. Recent anecdotal reports have suggested that rituximab may be effective in the setting of hemolytic anemia and CLL. However, all of the data are in the form of case reports and so it is difficult to know what percentage of patients would actually respond. Ongoing trials are using rituximab in patients failing initial therapy for hemolytic anemia, and data from these trials will give a better idea of the efficacy of rituximab in this setting. Alemtuzumab has also been used in Europe to treat autoimmune complications of CLL and can be effective. However, fludarabine is a drug that some people avoid the use of in the setting of hemolytic anemia because patients can occasionally have hemolytic anemia that occurs on rechallenge with fludarabine. The early trials with fludarabine in the 1980s indicated that patients with refractory hemolytic anemia could respond to treatment with this agent. Thus, this is not an absolute contraindication in patients with hemolytic anemia but would not be the initial approach; it would be reserved for patients who do not respond to standard therapy.

Answer 28.6. **The answer is A.**

The Rai staging system is a simple and prognostically relevant staging system that has been available for almost 30 years. It relies only on a physical exam and a complete blood count. The Rai staging system was not formulated based on CT scans. Nevertheless, it has clear prognostic significance with worsening survival as the stage increases. The original Rai staging system encompassed five stages, Rai stage 0 with lymphocytosis as the only manifestation of disease, Rai stage I where patients had adenopathy, and Rai stage II indicating the presence of splenomegaly or hepatomegaly. Rai stages III and IV are associated with anemia (hemoglobin <11.0/g/dL) and thrombocytopenia (platelet count <100,000 per μL) respectively. The modified Rai staging system grouped patients into early stage, Rai 0 to I; intermediate stage, Rai II; and advanced stage, Rai III to IV. Although patients with Rai stage III to IV disease have a poor prognosis on the basis of extensive marrow involvement causing cytopenias, it is uncommon for newly diagnosed patients to present with advanced stage disease, and at least two thirds of patients will present with early or intermediate stage disease.

Answer 28.7. **The answer is C.**

Cytogenetics reveal important prognostic information in CLL. However, the yield on cytogenetic analysis overall is low, probably partly because CLL is an indolent disease with a low proliferative index so metaphases are not easily discernable. Nevertheless, if cytogenetic analysis reveals abnormalities, this clearly gives prognostic information. As noted previously, the worst abnormality in terms of prognosis is the 17p deletion, which is associated with p53 deficiency. This is uncommon as a single abnormality, particularly in newly diagnosed patients, but very frequent in refractory patients, often as part of a complex karyotype. In CLL, as in other leukemias, the more abnormalities seen, the worse the prognosis. Median survival for this patient would be approximately 2 years. The likelihood of discovering molecular abnormalities with interphase fluorescent *in situ* hybridization (FISH) is slightly higher than with cytogenetics because, as noted above, there is often a lack of metaphases. However, there is one abnormality where the detection rate is dramatically different between cytogenetics and FISH and that is the 13q deletion. Because of the small size of the deletion, this molecular abnormality is usually not detected with standard cytogenetics; thus, all patients with CLL should have a FISH test to look for, among other abnormalities, 13q deletion. When present as a sole abnormality the 13q deletion is the one molecular aberration in CLL that appears to confer a favorable prognosis in terms of survival when outcome is compared to patients with no abnormalities.

Answer 28.8. **The answer is C.**

The large Intergroup trial published several years ago in the *New England Journal of Medicine* randomized patients with previously untreated CLL to receive pulse chlorambucil, fludarabine given at the standard dose for 5 days per month, or a combination of chlorambucil and fludarabine together. The combination arm of the trial was closed early because of increased myelosuppression and infections. The results from this trial in over 500 patients showed that fludarabine produced a higher overall response rate than chlorambucil and a higher complete remission rate at 20% versus 4% with chlorambucil. Not only were CR and overall response rates higher with fludarabine, but the remission duration was significantly longer. Nevertheless, there was no difference in survival between the two arms. There are several potential explanations for this. One reason for the lack of survival advantage is the crossover design. Patients failing to respond to either agent could be crossed over to the other one. Thus, in the long run, essentially all patients were treated with fludarabine. Another important point is that although fludarabine produces a significantly higher complete remission rate of 20%, this means that fully 80% of newly diagnosed patients with CLL will not achieve a complete remission with the most active single agent. Complete remission is defined by normalization of the blood counts, resolution of organomegaly or adenopathy, and a bone marrow showing fewer than 30% lymphocytes on the aspirate with no evidence of disease on the biopsy. It would be naïve to believe that if 80% of patients being treated with the most effective single agent could not achieve a complete remission that the overall survival of the group would be improved. This has led investigators to combine agents to try and improve the CR rates in CLL. The hypothesis is that only by increasing the CR rate will survival be affected.

Answer 28.9. **The answer is B.**

Alemtuzumab was approved by the Food and Drug Administration (FDA) for the treatment of fludarabine-refractory CLL based on data from the pivotal trial showing a 33% response rate in this population. Progressive disease during therapy with alemtuzumab was unusual, and approximately 55% of the patients had stable disease. Some of these patients with stable disease were of interest because they actually achieved a complete remission in the blood and the bone marrow but failed to qualify overall even as a partial remitter secondary to a bulky lymph node site that did not decrease by 50%. The vast majority of the patients who did respond achieved partial remissions, and yet 50% of the responders had completely normal blood and bone marrow. The reason for the discrepancy in the site of activity of this agent is under investigation. Nevertheless, this patient would be a good candidate for treatment with alemtuzumab because the disease is primarily in the blood and bone marrow with moderate splenomegaly and small lymph nodes. This patient would be expected to have a good response to therapy with alemtuzumab. The use of chlorambucil in patients who are refractory to fludarabine is not effective. Rituximab at the standard dose of 375 mg per m^2 weekly times 4 produces response rates in 10% to 15% of patients with relapsed CLL. The response rate may be even lower in those who are truly refractory to fludarabine. Two trials examined dose intensification of rituximab in patients with CLL. In one trial the standard dose was given 3 times a week for 4 weeks, and in the other trial the dose was escalated in cohorts of patients. Response rates on those trials were 35% to 45%, significantly better than what was seen with standard dose rituximab. In all these trials, the responses are partial remissions. Rituximab shrinks lymph nodes and lowers the white blood cell count but has almost no effect on the bone marrow; even in the study with escalated doses of rituximab, up to 2,250 mg per m^2, little effect was seen on the bone marrow except at the highest dose. It would be reasonable to consider allogeneic transplant in a 63-year-old with refractory CLL since the expected survival, even with effective alemtuzumab therapy, is not long. Most of the data in this age range is with nonmyelobative transplants and this would still be considered investigational and should only be done as part of a clinical trial. However, in this case the patient would need an unrelated donor transplant, and the data regarding unrelated donor nonmyelobative transplants is almost nonexistent. This would be a reasonable approach on a clinical trial. Nevertheless, because a nonmyelobative transplant relies heavily on the graft versus leukemia effect to control disease, it is preferable to debulk the patient prior to transplant. Thus proceeding directly to transplant at this point, even if there was an available donor, would not be the best option.

CHAPTER 29

Plasma Cell Neoplasms

RAVI VIJ

Directions Each of the numbered items below is followed by lettered answers. Select the ONE lettered answer that is BEST in each case unless instructed otherwise.

QUESTIONS

Question 29.1. **A 36-year-old female presents with abdominal pain for the last 2 weeks. She has been taking ibuprofen several times a day for the last few weeks on account of persistent back pain. On admission she is anemic with a hemoglobin (Hb) of 9 g per dL and a creatinine of 2.6 g per dL. Imaging studies reveal several lytic lesions in the thoracolumbar spine. Serum protein electropheresis (SPEP)/immunofixation reveals an IgA kappa monoclonal protein of 5.7 g per dL. Bone marrow biopsy is hypercellular with 70% plasma cells. She undergoes an upper endoscopy, which shows a large gastric ulcer with evidence of recent bleeding. The most appropriate initial therapy would be**

A. thalidomide and dexamethasone
B. melphalan and prednisone
C. pegylated liposomal doxorubicin in combination with vincristine and dexamethasone
D. bortezomib

Question 29.2. **A 62-year-old patient with stage IIA multiple myeloma achieves a partial response following 6 cycles of chemotherapy with vincristine, adriamycin, and dexamethasone. You subsequently discuss high-dose chemotherapy and autologous stem cell transplantation with the patient. Appropriate strategies include all the following EXCEPT**

A. tandem autologous transplantation with melphalan 140 mg per m^2 prior to the first transplant and melphalan 140 mg per m^2 plus 8 Gy total body irradiation (TBI) in four fractions over 4 days prior to the second transplant
B. single autologous transplant using melphalan 200 mg per m^2 as the conditioning regimen
C. single autologous transplant using melphalan 140 mg per m^2 plus 8 Gy TBI in four fractions over 4 days as conditioning
D. delay autologous stem cell transplant till relapse of disease

Corresponding Chapters in *Cancer: Principles & Practice of Oncology*, Seventh Edition: 44 (Plasma Cell Neoplasms).

Question 29.3. **A 59-year-old white man with stage IIIA IGG kappa multiple myeloma undergoes an autologous stem cell transplant. He attains a complete remission and five years later has no evidence of disease progression. Flourescent *in situ* hybridization (FISH) studies on his bone marrow at time of diagnosis would most likely have shown which of the following abnormalities?**

A. del 13q.
B. Translocation (11,14).
C. Translocation (4,14).
D. Translocation (14,16).

Question 29.4. **A 67-year-old African American was diagnosed with stage IIIA multiple myeloma 5 months ago. SPEP showed a small monoclonal peak, and he was noted to have free kappa light chains on serum immunofixation. A 24-hour urine collection showed 12.5 g of light chain excretion. He was started on thalidomide/dexamethasone and monthly doses of zolendronate. He last received a dose of zolendronate 2 weeks ago, and a full staging workup at that time showed him to be in complete remission with a creatinine of 1.8 g per dL. On a routine follow-up visit today, his creatinine is found to be elevated to 4.2 g per dL. A kidney biopsy is performed. This will most likely show**

A. nodular sclerosing glomerulopathy with positive glomerular basement membrane and/or tubular basement membrane immunofixation with anti-kappa anti-sera
B. apple-green birefringence on staining with congo red
C. tubular casts staining positive with anti-kappa anti-sera
D. marked tubular degenerative changes

ANSWERS

Answer 29.1. **The answer is C.**

Pegylated liposomal doxorubicin in combination with vincristine and decadron (DVD) has been shown to provide equivalent response rates to the regimen of vincristine, adriamycin, and decadron (VAD) in a randomized trial. DVD avoids the need for protracted infusions of adriamycin and vincristine and is associated with a lower risk for alopecia and severe neutropenia. The incidence of hand-foot syndrome is higher, however. Thalidomide and dexamethasone, too, is an accepted first-line regimen with response rates similar to VAD. However, due to the teratogenic potential of thalidomide, it needs to be administered with extreme caution to women of childbearing age. Also, there is a 12% to 15% risk for deep venous thrombosis (DVT) (risks are even higher when thalidomide is administered concurrently with an anthracycline-containing regimen), and most practitioners recommend concurrent administration of coumadin and/or aspirin. Both coumadin and aspirin would be contraindicated in this patient with a recent upper gastrointestinal bleed from a gastric ulcer. Response rates with melphalan and prednisone are lower. Also, melphalan, being an alkylating agent, has the potential to damage bone-marrow stem cells and make future stem cell mobilization for autologous transplantation problematic. Bortezomib, a novel proteosome inhibitor, has shown impressive response rates of 35% in trials for patients with heavily pretreated myeloma. In the future, it is expected to become part of the up-front therapy for myeloma. However, it is currently licensed only for the treatment of refractory disease.

Answer 29.2. **The answer is C.**

A prospective randomized trial of autologous bone marrow transplantation and chemotherapy by the French group *Intergoupe Francais Du Myelome (IFM)* established autologous transplantation as standard of care for patients with multiple myeloma. In this trial, the 5-year event-free and overall survival rates were 28% and 52% in the high-dose arm and 10% and 12% in the conventional-therapy arm. A subsequent trial by the Medical Research Council of the United Kingdom confirmed the superiority of high-dose chemotherapy. A comparison of 200 mg per m^2 melphalan and 8 Gy total body irradiation plus 140 mg per m^2 melphalan as conditioning regimen for peripheral blood stem cell transplantation by the *IFM* group showed that hematologic recovery was significantly faster, transfusion requirements and incidence of severe mucositis was significantly lower, and survival was longer in the chemotherapy-alone arm of the trial. In a randomized trial, the French group *Myeloma Autogreffe* showed that autologous transplantation obtained a median overall survival exceeding 5 years in young patients with symptomatic myeloma whether performed early, as first-line therapy, or late, as rescue treatment. Early transplant was associated with a shorter period of chemotherapy. In another *IFM* trial, as compared with a single autologous stem-cell transplant after high-dose chemotherapy, double transplantation improved overall survival, especially in those who did not have a very good partial response after undergoing one transplant. However, three other randomized trials, albeit with shorter follow-up, have so far failed to show a benefit to tandem autologous transplantation.

Answer 29.3. **The answer is B.**

With the development of techniques to circumvent the low proliferative potential of plasma cells, especially fluorescence *in situ* hybridization (FISH), it is possible to assess the impact of specific recurrent chromosomal changes on response to therapy and survival. Deletions of 13q14 are detectable in up to 45% of patients with myeloma and predict a decreased overall survival (in one series 24.2 months versus 88.1 months for those in whom this abnormality was not detectable). Translocations involving the immunoglobin heavy chain (IgH) are detectable by interphase FISH in 60% to 70% of patients with multiple myeloma. Also, t(4,14) observed in about 10% to 15% and t(14, 16) in 5% to 10% of patients with myeloma both predict a poor prognosis with median survivals of 2 years or less. On the other hand, t(11,14) present in about 15% of patients with myeloma is characterized by cyclin D1 upregulation and a favorable outcome with median survival of 4 years. Patients with 17p13 deletions have a median survival of less than 2 years.

Answer 29.4. **The answer is D.**

Bisphosphonate use has been associated with renal toxicity. Pamidronate can cause a collapsing focal segmental glomerulosclerosis. By contrast, in zolendronate-associated renal failure, there is toxic tubulopathy without associated glomerular injury characterized by the absence of significant proteinuria. The incidence appears to be dependent on the dose and rate of infusion. For myeloma patients with lytic destruction of bone, intravenous pamidronate 90 mg delivered over at least 2 hours or zolendronate 4 mg over 15 minutes every 3 to 4 weeks are recommended. In patients with preexisting renal disease and a serum creatinine less than 3 mg per dL, no change in dosage, infusion time, or interval is required. Evaluation for the presence of albuminuria (>500 mg per 24 h) and azotemia (increase of ≥0.5 mg per dL in serum creatinine or absolute value >1.4 mg per dL among patients with normal baseline serum creatinine) every 3 to 6 months is recommended. These patients should have their bisphosphonates discontinued until the problem has resolved. Tubular casts are common in patients with renal insufficiency secondary to myeloma with Bence Jones proteinuria. This is unlikely to be the cause of renal insufficiency in this patient who was found to be in complete remission 2 weeks ago. Renal insufficiency characterized by a nodular sclerosing glomerulopathy is a common feature of light chain deposition disease. This is a systemic disorder characterized by the deposition of monotypical immunoglobulin light chains (usually kappa) in various organs. It can occur in the absence of any detectable hematologic disorder. Apple-green birefringence on staining with congo red is a feature of amyloidosis.

CHAPTER 30

Paraneoplastic Syndromes

PHILIP C. HOFFMAN

Directions Each of the numbered items below is followed by lettered answers. Select the ONE lettered answer that is BEST in each case unless instructed otherwise.

QUESTIONS

Question 30.1. **A 57-year-old woman with recent diagnosis of metastatic ovarian cancer complains of gradual onset of problems maintaining her balance while walking over 2 months. More recently, she has noted slurred speech and double vision. This has progressed to the point that she cannot walk without considerable assistance. She otherwise has felt well, without other systemic complaints. There is no lymphadenopathy or organomegaly on examination. Magnetic resonance imaging (MRI) of the brain revealed no evidence of brain metastasis. The most likely diagnosis is**

A. carcinomatous meningitis
B. encephalopathy secondary to chemotherapy
C. paraneoplastic cerebellar degeneration
D. occult brain metastasis

Question 30.2. **The syndrome exhibited in Question 30.1 is commonly associated with which of the following abnormalities.**

A. Presence of anti-Yo antibodies in the serum.
B. Presence of anti-Hu antibodies in the serum.
C. Loss of cerebellar Purkinje cells.
D. Antibodies to acetylcholinesterase.
E. A and C.
F. B and D.

Question 30.3. **A 26-year-old man notes bilateral gynecomastia for a few months. Physical examination is unremarkable, including examination of the testes. Blood studies might be expected to show which of the following.**

A. Increased adrenocorticotropin hormone (ACTH) level.
B. Elevated follicle-stimulating hormone (FSH) level.
C. Elevated alpha-fetoprotein level.
D. Elevated beta-human chorionic gonadotropin (HCG) level.
E. Low fibrinogen level.

Corresponding Chapters in *Cancer: Principles & Practice of Oncology*, Seventh Edition: 45 (Paraneoplastic Syndromes).

Question 30.4. **The patient mentioned in Question 30.3 had a normal testicular ultrasound. Which of the following imaging tests may give the best yield as to the primary tumor?**

A. Computed tomography (CT) scan of the chest.
B. Positron emission tomography (PET) scan.
C. Octreotide scan.
D. MRI scan of the brain.
E. Pelvic ultrasound.

Question 30.5. **A 66-year-old man has a long history of alcohol abuse and alcoholic cirrhosis. For many years, he has been mildly anemic, hemoglobin around 11 g per dL, mean corpuscular volume (MCV) 79, red cell distribution width (RDW) 13%. Which of the following laboratory findings is he likely to have?**

A. Normal serum iron and normal total iron binding capacity (TIBC).
B. Low serum iron and high TIBC.
C. Low serum iron and low TIBC.
D. Low serum ferritin.

Question 30.6. **After being lost to follow-up for 2 years, the patient in Question 30.5 presents for evaluation, and he is found to be plethoric. Hemoglobin is 18.4 g per dL. Platelet and white blood cell (WBC) counts are normal. What other blood abnormality might you expect at this time?**

A. Elevated alpha-fetoprotein level.
B. Presence of anti-Hu.
C. Low serum ferritin.
D. Undetectable serum erythropoietin level.
E. Elevated beta-HCG level.

Question 30.7. **Which of the following paraneoplastic syndromes is NOT likely to improve with successful therapy of the underlying cancer?**

A. Syndrome of inappropriate secretion of antidiuretic hormone (ADH).
B. Hypertrophic pulmonary osteoarthropathy.
C. Anorexia-cachexia syndrome.
D. Subacute sensorimotor neuropathy.

Question 30.8. **All of the following are classically associated with small cell lung cancer EXCEPT**

A. syndrome of inappropriate ADH secretion
B. Eaton-Lambert myasthenic syndrome
C. hypertrophic pulmonary osteoarthropathy
D. ectopic ACTH production
E. limbic encephalitis associated with anti-Hu antibodies

Question 30.9. **Which of the following paraneoplastic syndromes is NOT immunologically mediated?**

A. Polycythemia related to renal cell cancer.
B. Progressive cerebellar degeneration.
C. Nephrotic syndrome from membranous nephropathy.
D. Eaton-Lambert myasthenic syndrome.

Question 30.10. **Which of the following drugs should be considered for treating ectopic ACTH production?**

A. Dexamethasone.
B. Cosyntropin.
C. Ketoconazole.
D. Epoetin.
E. Demeclocycline.

Question 30.11. **Which of the following associations is INCORRECT?**

A. Hypoglycemia and large abdominal sarcoma.
B. Acanthosis nigricans and Hodgkin disease.
C. Ichthyosis and Hodgkin disease.
D. Sweet syndrome and myelodysplastic syndrome.
E. Thrombophlebitis and pancreatic cancer.

Question 30.12. **Which of the following associations is INCORRECT?**

A. Warm-autoantibody hemolytic anemia and chronic lymphocytic leukemia.
B. Polycythemia and renal cell carcinoma.
C. Normochromic, normocytic anemia and lung cancer.
D. Microangiopathic hemolytic anemia and chronic lymphocytic leukemia.
E. Thrombocytosis and lung cancer.

Question 30.13. **All of the following are true of opsoclonus-myoclonus EXCEPT**

A. in children, it is usually associated with Wilms tumor
B. antineuronal antibodies are frequently detected
C. major neurologic recovery, with successful cancer therapy, is not typical
D. in women with gynecologic cancers, anti-Ri antibodies have been found

Question 30.14. **Progressive sensorimotor neuropathy is commonly associated with which of the following.**

A. Osteosclerotic myeloma.
B. Typical osteolytic myeloma.
C. Amyloidosis.
D. A and B.
E. A and C.

Question 30.15. **With respect to the Lambert-Eaton myasthenic syndrome, all of the following are true EXCEPT**

A. the syndrome appears to be mediated by antibodies directed against a component of the presynaptic neuron
B. therapy with plasma exchange and immunosuppressives may be beneficial
C. most patients will have a thymoma with further evaluation
D. electromyography can distinguish it from typical myasthenia gravis

Question 30.16. **Which of the following associations is INCORRECT?**

A. Pemphigus and large B-cell lymphoma.
B. Necrolytic migratory erythema and glucagonoma.
C. Dermatomyositis and colorectal cancer.
D. Fever and urothelial cancer.
E. Retinopathy and melanoma.

Question 30.17. **Gastric cancer is associated with which of the following syndromes.**

A. Rapid development of seborrheic keratoses.
B. Acanthosis nigricans.
C. Peutz-Jeghers syndrome.
D. Disseminated intravascular coagulation.
E. All of the above.

Question 30.18. **Which of the following is NOT characteristic of the syndrome of ectopic ACTH production?**

A. Nonsuppressibility by dexamethasone.
B. Weakness and hypokalemia.
C. Buffalo hump and striae.
D. No effect on ACTH production by metyrapone stimulation.
E. No effect on ACTH production by corticotropin-releasing hormone (CRH).

ANSWERS

Answer 30.1. **The answer is C.**

The patient is manifesting progressive cerebellar degeneration, the most common cause of which is ovarian cancer.

Answer 30.2. **The answer is E.**

The anti-Yo antibodies presumably cause cerebellar Purkinje cell loss.

Answer 30.3. **The answer is D.**

Gynecomastia results from elevated beta-HCG levels.

Answer 30.4. **The answer is A.**

If the testicles are normal, extragonadal germ cell tumors in the mediastinum must be considered.

Answer 30.5. **The answer is C.**

This is the anemia of chronic disease, usually normocytic or minimally microcytic. The serum iron is always low, and the TIBC is also low, with a normal to high ferritin level.

Answer 30.6. **The answer is A.**

Over time, the cirrhosis has led to hepatocellular carcinoma, which is associated with polycythemia as a paraneoplastic syndrome. Alpha-fetoprotein level is markedly elevated in most cases of hepatocellular carcinoma.

Answer 30.7. **The answer is D.**

The humorally mediated syndromes commonly improve with therapy, whereas the immunologically mediated ones (e.g., neuropathies) are less prone to improve.

Answer 30.8. **The answer is C.**

Hypertrophic pulmonary osteoarthropathy (HPOA) is generally associated with non-small cell carcinoma.

Answer 30.9. **The answer is A.**

Polycythemia related to renal cell cancer is related to excessive epoetin production.

Answer 30.10. **The answer is C.**

Ketoconazole has been used to suppress ACTH production. Dexamethasone suppression is used as a test and does not suppress steroid production in ectopic ACTH syndrome. Cosyntropin is a form of ACTH. Demeclocycline may be used to treat inappropriate antidiuretic hormone secretion.

Answer 30.11. **The answer is B.**

Acanthosis nigricans is associated with gastrointestinal cancers, especially gastric cancer.

Answer 30.12. **The answer is D.**

Chronic lymphocytic leukemia is associated with an antibody-mediated spherocytic hemolytic anemia, not a microangiopathic hemolytic anemia, which would imply red cell fragmentation [such as seen in thrombotic thrombocytopenic pupura (TTP) or disseminated intravascular coagulation (DIC)].

Answer 30.13. **The answer is A.**

Opsoclonus-myoclonus is typically associated with neuroblastoma in children.

Answer 30.14. **The answer is E.**

Progressive sensorimotor neuropathy is often severe with amyloidosis and is part of the unusual syndrome of osteosclerotic myeloma [associated with syndrome of polyneuropathy, organomegaly, endocrinopathy, monoclonal gammopathy, skin changes (POEMS)].

Answer 30.15. **The answer is C.**

Typical myasthenia gravis is commonly associated with a thymoma. The Lambert-Eaton myasthenic syndrome has different electromyographic (EMG) characteristics and is associated with small cell lung cancer.

Answer 30.16. **The answer is D.**

Fever may be a paraneoplastic syndrome associated with renal cell carcinoma but not with urothelial cancers (i.e., transitional cell cancers of the renal pelvis, ureter, and bladder).

Answer 30.17. **The answer is E.**

Gastric cancer can be associated with a wide variety of paraneoplastic syndromes such as acanthosis nigricans, disseminated intravascular coagulation and sudden onset of multiple seborroheic keratosis.

Answer 30.18. **The answer is C.**

Patients with ectopic ACTH syndrome may have the metabolic and constitutional manifestations of hypercortisolism but not usually the body habitus changes.

CHAPTER **31**

Cancer of Unknown Primary Site

GAURI R. VARADHACHARY AND JORDAN D. BERLIN

Directions Each of the numbered items below is followed by lettered answers. Select the ONE lettered answer that is BEST in each case unless instructed otherwise.

QUESTIONS

Question 31.1. **A 58-year-old man comes to your office for evaluation of a metastatic poorly differentiated squamous cell carcinoma found on excisional biopsy of a 2.5-cm subdigastric lymph node. Patient reports that the "lump" on the right side of his neck (near the angle of the mandible) had been growing slowly for 4 months. The patient did chew tobacco for 10 years and quit 5 years ago. He has minimal alcohol intake and is currently asymptomatic. Physical examination of the oral cavity reveals no lesions and that of the neck reveals a well-healed scar with no evidence of lymphadenopathy. What is the next step in his evaluation?**

A. Computed tomography (CT) of the head and neck.
B. Upper endoscopy.
C. CT of the abdomen and liver.
D. All of the above.

Question 31.2. **The patient in Question 31.1 undergoes a CT scan of the neck, which shows subtle postoperative changes at and beneath the right parotid tail and lateral to the sternocleidomastoid muscle. Positron emission tomography (PET) scan is essentially negative. Biopsies of inconspicuous sites as well as tonsillectomy are negative for pathology. What would be the most appropriate therapy for this patient now?**

A. Radical neck dissection.
B. Definitive radiation therapy.
C. Radical neck dissection followed by radiation therapy.
D. All of the above.

Question 31.3. **The chances of achieving a long-term, disease-free state for the patient described in Questions 31.1 and 31.2 are**

A. 0%
B. 5%
C. 25%
D. 40%

Corresponding Chapters in *Cancer: Principles & Practice of Oncology*, Seventh Edition: 46 (Cancer of Unknown Primary Site) and 47 (Peritoneal Carcinomatosis).

Question 31.4. **A 36-year-old man, nonsmoker, presents with an 8-cm mediastinal mass, chest pain, and constitutional symptoms. Biopsy of this mass reveals "poorly differentiated carcinoma," and immunohistochemistry is negative for thyroid transcription factor-1 (TTF-1) stain. A CT scan of the abdomen is essentially negative, and testicular ultrasound is negative. Serum alpha fetoprotein (AFP) is 3 ng per dL and β-HCG is 85 mIU per mL. This patient has been referred to the unknown primary cancer clinic. What is the most appropriate treatment for him?**

A. Cisplatin-based therapy for presumed extragonadal germ cell tumor.
B. Taxane-based therapy for presumed non-small cell lung cancer.
C. Anthracycline-based therapy for presumed thymoma.

Question 31.5. **A 62-year-old white woman presents with left-sided isolated axillary adenopathy. Biopsy is positive for a well-differentiated adenocarcinoma. Chest x-ray, bilateral mammogram, and breast ultrasound are negative for any masses. CT scan of the chest and abdomen are within normal limits with no evidence of metastasis. What is the next step in her evaluation and what is the most appropriate treatment?**

A. Random breast biopsies.
B. Magnetic resonance imaging (MRI) of the breast.
C. PET scan.

Question 31.6. **Which of the following immunohistochemical stains are considered relatively specific for diagnosing the appropriate primary site?**

A. Prostate specific antigen (PSA) and common leukocyte antigen (CLA).
B. S-100 and HMB-45.
C. Chromogranin and synaptophysin.
D. Vimentin and factor VIII antigen.

Question 31.7. **A 72-year-old man with hypertension undergoes a renal ultrasound for a creatinine of 2.1 mg per dL. Incidental note is made of possible hypodensities in the liver, and a dedicated imaging study of the liver is recommended. Given the inability to take contrast, an MRI of the abdomen is ordered, which shows multiple hypodensities in the right lobe of the liver, the smallest measuring about 1.5 cm and the largest about 3 cm. The patient is asymptomatic. Biopsy of one of these masses shows "low grade neuroendocrine carcinoma." Workup with endoscopies, small bowel follow through (SBFT), and octreotide scan does not reveal a primary. Which of the following is the most appropriate treatment option for this patient at the present time?**

A. Immediate right hepatectomy.
B. Chemoembolization.
C. Liver transplant to improve chances of long-term disease-free survival.
D. Observation with close follow-up and serial CT scans; hormonal therapy versus surgery versus chemotherapy at a later date if indicated.

Question 31.8. **A 58-year-old woman is evaluated for abdominal pain and increase in abdominal girth noticed over 3 months. She complains of constitutional symptoms including lethargy and anorexia. CT scan of the abdomen and pelvis shows peritoneal nodules and loculated ascites between bowel loops. There is no obvious ovarian mass or abnormality seen on the pelvic scan. Liver, kidneys, spleen, and adrenals appear normal. Laboratory tests reveal mild anemia and tumor marker Ca-125 is elevated at 758 U per mL. CT-guided biopsy of one of the superficial peritoneal nodules reveals "adenocarcinoma, favoring papillary serous type." What is the best treatment?**

A. Surgery.
B. Chemotherapy.
C. Radiation.
D. Optimal debulking surgery followed by chemotherapy.

Question 31.9. **Ms. ED is a 72-year-old female smoker, diagnosed with a left adrenal mass on a CT scan done for recent onset severe abdominal and back discomfort. Patient denies shortness of breath, chest pain, or cough. She has lost 7 pounds in the last 2 months. The adrenal mass is 5.2 by 4.5 by 3.0 cm and abuts the abdominal aorta, left side of the celiac artery, and partially encases left the renal artery. Metastatic lymphadenopathy is noted in the retroperitoneal region and extends to about the level of the inferior mesenteric artery. CT scan also reveals lytic bone lesions suspicious for metastatic disease in the ribs and pelvis, and this is confirmed by a bone scan and plain x-rays. CT scan of the chest is essentially negative. CT-guided left adrenal biopsy reveals metastatic moderately differentiated adenocarcinoma. What other test is required for the search of a primary site?**

A. Careful review of the pathology and additional immunostains.
B. PET imaging.
C. Bronchoscopy.
D. Colonoscopy.

Question 31.10. **What percentage of unknown primary cancer is squamous cell carcinoma on light microscopy?**

A. 15%.
B. 5%.
C. 50%.
D. 25%.

Question 31.11. **What would the management of a woman who presents with isolated pleural effusion involve?**

A. Cytologic evaluation of pleural effusion.
B. Bronchoscopy.
C. PET imaging.

ANSWERS

Answer 31.1. **The answer is A.**

This patient belongs to the category of cervical lymphadenopathy and unknown primary. Most patients who have a high cervical lymph node presentation have head and neck primary in some inconspicuous site. The workup includes a CT scan of the head and neck region, a pan endoscopy with tonsillectomy; a PET scan is optional but recommended.

A CT scan of the head and neck region is usually sufficient and an MRI scan is not indicated unless there is a contraindication for a CT scan. Pan endoscopy includes a direct laryngoscopy, bronchoscopy, and esophagoscopy, and most institutions include a bilateral tonsillectomy to look for occult cancer. Beside imaging and invasive procedures, this is one situation in the cancer of unknown primary (CUP) setting in which an 18F-fluorodeoxyglucose-PET scan is useful. There have been several small studies evaluating the role of PET scans in cervical CUP, and a primary tumor has been identified in about 21% to 30% of these patients. This is important because a suspected primary on a PET scan can help direct biopsy and determine the extent of disease, as well as help with planning the radiation treatment.

Answer 31.2. **The answer is D.**

The same patient as in Question 31.1 has a level II left-sided node, which showed metastatic poorly differentiated squamous cell carcinoma without an identifiable primary on detailed workup. Radiotherapy is indicated to control his neck disease as well as suspected primary mucosal sites. Results using high-dose radiation therapy alone, radical neck dissection, or a combination of these treatments have been similar. Most authorities prefer radiation therapy alone, and long-term disease-free survival can be achieved by this modality.

Answer 31.3. **The answer is D.**

The same patient as in Question 31.1 should be aggressively treated because he has a very favorable presentation and high chance of a long-term remission.

Compared to patients with CUP who present with disseminated metastases, patients who present with cervical CUP have a better prognosis, and up to 40% of the patients can achieve a long-term disease-free survival. Patients with N1 or N2 disease do better than patients with N3 disease or very bulky neck adenopathy. Patients with low cervical and supraclavicular node(s) presentation may not do as well as high cervical node presentation because a substantial number of these patients may have an occult lung primary instead of a head and neck primary. Patients who have bulky adenopathy may benefit from a combination of chemotherapy and radiation.

Answer 31.4. **The answer is A.**

A small group of patients with poorly differentiated carcinoma have favorable clinical features, which identify them as being chemoresponsive. This young man with no history of smoking and an elevated serum beta human chorionic gonadotropin (HCG) should be treated with a cisplatin-based chemotherapy regimen used to treat extragonadal germ cell tumor. Genetic analysis of these tumors may show abnormalities of chromosome 12 [i(12)p; del (12p); multiple copies of 12p], which is diagnostic of germ cell malignancies.

Answer 31.5. **The answer is B.**

In a woman presenting with isolated axillary adenopathy, occult breast cancer should be suspected. Most authorities would get an MRI of the breast if the mammogram and ultrasound are negative, and in two small studies, in 70% of patients a primary was found on an MRI using a dedicated breast coil. If the MRI is negative, mastectomy is not indicated, and radiation therapy is often used for the breast and the axilla. This patient should be treated as a stage II breast cancer after the pathologic tissue is checked for estrogen receptor, progesterone receptor, and Her2-neu status.

Answer 31.6. **The answer is A.**

Prostate specific antigen (PSA) and common leukocyte antigen (CLA) are quite specific for the diagnosis of prostate cancer and hematologic malignancies respectively. It is important to be aware, though, that no stain is 100% specific including PSA, which can rarely be positive in salivary gland carcinoma. Technical expertise is required for accurately performing and interpreting these stains. The other stains mentioned are used to support the diagnosis of melanoma (B), neuroendocrine carcinoma/differentiation (C), and sarcoma (D), but are not specific for those entities.

Answer 31.7. **The answer is D.**

This 72-year-old man is currently asymptomatic from his low-grade neuroendocrine carcinoma. This pathologic entity can remain indolent for several years with very slow progression and not require any therapy for a long time (hormonal or other). Pathology may show features suggestive of carcinoid and urine 5-HIAA and/or serum chromogranin may be elevated and can be followed as markers. Often, the patient is treated with endocrine therapy alone for hormone-related symptoms (diarrhea, flushing, nausea) with somatostatin analogs. Specific local therapies such as right hepatectomy, chemoembolization, or systemic therapies, such as chemotherapy with a streptozotocin + adriamycin ± 5-fluorouracil (5FU) based regimen would only be indicated if the patient is symptomatic with local pain secondary to significant growth of the metastasis, or the hormone-related symptoms are not controlled with endocrine therapy.

Answer 31.8. **The answer is D.**

Diffuse peritoneal involvement is typical of ovarian carcinoma, although gastrointestinal carcinomas, especially signet ring cell gastric cancer, as well as lung or breast cancer can present in this manner. The term "primary peritoneal papillary serous carcinoma" has been described in women who present with carcinomatosis in whom the pathologic and laboratory (elevated Ca-125 antigen) characteristics of the cancer are that of ovarian cancer but no ovarian primary is identified on transvaginal ultrasound or even on laparotomy. Patients with BRCA1 mutations are at risk for primary peritoneal carcinoma along with breast and ovarian cancer. Ovarian and primary peritoneal carcinomas are both thought to have a "Mullerian" origin, and studies suggest that they have similar gene expression profiles. In one retrospective study evaluating 258 women with peritoneal carcinomatosis who had undergone cytoreductive surgery and chemotherapy, 22% of all patients had a complete response to chemotherapy; the median survival was 18 months (range 11 to 24 months).

This patient should be managed as advanced ovarian cancer, including aggressive surgical cytoreduction followed by postoperative chemotherapy with a taxane in combination with carboplatin.

Answer 31.9. **The answer is A.**

Given her pattern of metastases involving adrenal glands and bones and with a history of smoking, suspicion for lung cancer is high. Most authorities would request a mammogram if one was not done in the last year. The role of invasive studies is controversial, and the yield with bronchoscopy is low given she has no pulmonary symptoms and has a negative CT scan of the chest. The role of PET scan is also not defined in unknown primary cancer except in the setting of cervical lymphadenopathy presentation and would not be indicated. Effort should be spent on requesting the pathologist to provide immunohistochemistry staining to further define the lineage of the tumor. Thyroid transcription factor-1 (TTF-1) immunohistochemical stain is positive in approximately 75% of patients with lung adenocarcinoma and, if positive, would favor a lung primary. Estrogen receptor and progesterone receptor studies can also be requested if TTF-1 is negative.

Answer 31.10. **The answer is B.**

Approximately 5% of patients with CUP are reported to have squamous cell carcinoma on light microscopy. Sixty percent of the cases are adenocarcinoma, and in 35% of the cases the light microscopy reports the tumor as poorly differentiated adenocarcinoma, poorly differentiated carcinoma, or poorly differentiated neoplasm.

Answer 31.11. **The answer is A.**

Isolated pleural effusions are usually adenocarcinomas. The possible primaries usually include a lung carcinoma, a mesothelioma, or metastatic tumor from other sites, especially breast cancer in a woman. The primary may not be apparent even after significant drainage of the fluid, and usually pleurodesis is pursued either at the time of presentation (if chest tube is placed) or with reaccumulation. Diagnosis may be difficult; a pleural biopsy may be necessary if cytology specimens are insufficient or nondiagnostic. Immunohistochemical stains may help (including TTF-1, ER, PR, calretinin), and electron microscopy may reveal ultrastructural features diagnostic of mesothelioma. In a series of 42 patients, a primary lung cancer was eventually found in 15 patients (36%). In patients with good performance status, a trial of chemotherapy for unknown primary carcinoma should be considered. Symptomatic improvement can be seen in a subset of patients, and in one small series of 37 patients, chemotherapy produced symptomatic improvement in 78% of patients and their median survival was 12 months (3 to 60 or more months).

CHAPTER 32

Immunosuppression-related Malignancies

BENJAMIN R. TAN AND LEE RATNER

Directions Each of the numbered items below is followed by lettered answers. Select the ONE lettered answer that is BEST in each case unless instructed otherwise.

QUESTIONS

Question 32.1. **A 45-year-old man who has recently been diagnosed with human immunodeficiency virus (HIV) infection was found to have a CD4 count of 60 and high viral load. He complains of headache, slurred speech, and blurred vision. A brain magnetic resonance imaging (MRI) revealed three ring-enhancing lesions in the parietal and occipital lobes. The locations of these lesions preclude a brain biopsy. Appropriate diagnostic and therapeutic options for this patient include the following EXCEPT**

A. obtain serum antitoxoplasma antibody and, if positive, treat empirically with anti-toxoplasmosis therapy
B. send cerebrospinal fluid (CSF) for cytology and Epstein-Barr virus (EBV)-DNA
C. institute highly active antiretroviral therapy (HAART)
D. surgical resection

Question 32.2. **Which feature is more common in patients with HIV-associated Hodgkin lymphoma compared to non-HIV-related primary Hodgkin lymphoma?**

A. Mixed cellularity type.
B. Mediastinal involvement.
C. Extranodal disease.
D. EBV positivity.
E. Advanced stage.

Corresponding Chapters in *Cancer: Principles & Practice of Oncology*, Seventh Edition: 48 (Immunosuppression-related Malignancies).

Question 32.3. **A 39-year-old HIV-infected man presented with anal pain and was found to have a 2-cm anal lesion with several anal warts. Biopsy confirmed squamous cell carcinoma. All of the following statements about anogenital cancers associated with HIV infection are true EXCEPT**

A. anal cancer is not considered an acquired immunodeficiency syndrome (AIDS)-defining illness
B. similar to Kaposi sarcoma, the institution of HAART usually results in the regression of anal squamous intraepithelial lesions
C. the Centers for Disease Control (CDC) recommends periodic Papanicolau testing in women with HIV infection; if initial or follow-up smears shows squamous intraepithelial lesions, the patient should be referred for colposcopy
D. after proper staging, the recommended therapy for the patient above with anal cancer would include both chemotherapy and radiation

Question 32.4. **Which of the following statements regarding epidemic Kaposi sarcoma is NOT true?**

A. Coinfection with both Kaposi sarcoma associated herpesvirus (KSHV) and HIV dramatically increases risk for the development of Kaposi sarcoma compared to infection with KSHV alone.
B. KSHV transmission may occur through both sexual and nonsexual means.
C. Hyperproliferation of endothelial-derived spindle cells appears to be directly or indirectly induced by KSHV.
D. In the era of HAART, the goal for therapy is cure.

Question 32.5. **Which of the following is not considered "Poor Risk" in the Revised AIDS Clinical Trials Group (ACTG) Staging for Kaposi sarcoma?**

A. Pulmonary Kaposi sarcoma.
B. CD4 count of 170 per μL.
C. Fever and night sweats.
D. Previously treated *Pneumocystis jiroveci* (previously *P. carinii*) pneumonia.

Question 32.6. **Comparing the HIV-associated lymphomas, which statement is true?**

A. Both primary central nervous system (CNS) diffuse large B-cell lymphoma and Burkitt lymphoma are associated with EBV infection and expression of bcl-2.
B. C-myc expression is associated with Burkitt lymphoma and primary effusion lymphoma (PEL).
C. KSHV infection occurs in virtually all primary effusion lymphoma cases.
D. CD4 counts are usually well preserved in patients with HIV-associated primary CNS lymphoma.

Question 32.7. **An HIV-infected man developed an enlarging neck mass associated with night sweats, fevers, and weight loss. Biopsy confirmed diffuse large B-cell lymphoma. Appropriate workup and therapy for this patient include which of the following.**

A. Staging CT scans, including brain with bilateral bone marrow biopsies.
B. Routine labs with lactate dehydrogenase (LDH), HIV viral load, CD4 count, and CSF examination.
C. CNS prophylaxis with intrathecal methotrexate or Ara-C.
D. Combination chemotherapy.
E. All of the above.

Question 32.8. **Risk factors for developing posttransplant lymphoproliferative disorder (PTLD) include all of the following EXCEPT**

A. unrelated donor hematopoietic stem cell transplant
B. T-cell depleted allogeneic stem cell transplant
C. anti-graft versus host disease (GVHD) medications including cyclosporine
D. autologous bone marrow transplant

ANSWERS

Answer 32.1. **The answer is D.**

As it may be difficult to distinguish toxoplasma opportunistic CNS infection with PCNSL, many centers have empirically treated HIV-infected patients with focal brain lesions and positive antitoxoplasma antibodies with antitoxoplasmosis therapy. CSF EBV DNA, when combined with ^{201}Tl SPECT, has a 100% sensitivity and positive predictive value for diagnosing PCNSL. Rapid immune reconstitution with HAART has been associated with prolonged remissions and survivals in patients with PCNSL. Once PCNSL is confirmed, radiation should commence immediately. Surgical interventions have no role in the treatment of PCNSL.

Answer 32.2. **The answer is B.**

Although not considered an AIDS-defining illness, Hodgkin lymphoma risk for HIV-infected individuals is increased by 8-fold over that of the risk in the general population. The mixed cellularity subtype and lymphocyte-predominant subtypes are more common in AIDS-related Hodgkin lymphoma, whereas the nodular sclerosing subtype is more common in primary Hodgkin lymphoma. The latent membrane protein (LMP-1) is expressed in virtually all cases of AIDS-Hodgkin disease, suggesting the etiologic role of EBV in its development. As AIDS-Hodgkin lymphoma is clinically more aggressive, most patients are diagnosed in more advanced stages with more widespread extranodal involvements compared to patients with primary Hodgkin lymphoma.

Answer 32.3. **The answer is B.**

The relative risk for an HIV-infected individual compared to the general population to develop anal cancer is 31-fold higher. The relative risk for an HIV-infected woman to develop cervical cancer is 2.9 compared to the general population. Both cancers are associated with the human papilloma virus (HPV). However, cervical cancer is designated by the CDC as AIDS-defining, whereas anal cancer is not. HIV-infected patients appear to develop more aggressive and advanced anogenital cancers compared to non-HIV-infected anal cancer patients. Greater immunosuppression is associated with greater incidence of squamous intraepithelial lesions among HIV-infected patients. However, the use of HAART generally does not cause regression of these lesions. The incidence of cervical cancer appears unchanged since the advent of HAART. A Pap smear is recommended as part of the initial evaluation when HIV seropositivity occurs in a woman. If normal, another Pap smear is recommended within 6 months, and if follow-up Pap smear is normal, an annual exam is recommended. For those with reactive epithelial changes, a repeat Pap smear should be done within 3 months. If any Pap smear shows squamous epithelial lesions or atypical cells, a colposcopy is recommended. A similar recommendation has been suggested for cytologic examination in anal cancer screening of homosexual or bisexual men. The case presented above requires staging including a chest x-ray and pelvic computed tomography (CT) or MRI to assess for nodal or distant metastases. Complete blood counts with CD4 counts and HIV viral load should also be done. As in patients without HIV infection, standard chemoradiation is recommended. Fluorouracil-based chemotherapy with concurrent external beam radiation to the anal and inguinal areas is recommended.

Answer 32.4. **The answer is D.**

Coinfection with both HIV and KSHV increases the risk for developing Kaposi sarcoma by 500- to 10,000-fold compared to infection with KSHV alone. The 10-year probability of developing Kaposi sarcoma in this situation is 33% to 50%. Transmission of Kaposi sarcoma could occur in either sexual or nonsexual means. Blood, semen, saliva, mother to child, and organ donor to recipient transmissions can occur. The pathogenesis of Kaposi sarcoma is complex. KSHV is present in virtually all cases of Kaposi sarcoma, whether HIV-related or non-HIV related, as in endemic, Mediterranean, or transplant-related Kaposi sarcoma. A model for the pathogenesis of Kaposi sarcoma proposes the creation of an inflammatory-angiogenic environment induced directly or indirectly by KSHV and the HIV tat protein through a cascade of cytokines such as IL-6. Although maximal reductions of HIV viral load consequent to the use of HAART can cause regression and disappearance of cutaneous and visceral Kaposi sarcoma, treatment remains palliative and attempts to only prolong survival. Epidemic Kaposi sarcoma remains incurable.

Answer 32.5. **The answer is B.**

The revised ACTG staging for Kaposi sarcoma classifies patients into good-risk or poor-risk based on tumor (T), immune status (I), and systemic illness (S) parameters. Patients are staged good-risk if all the following are present: tumor confined to the skin or lymph nodes or with minimal mucosal disease, CD4 greater than or equal to 150 per µL, performance status of greater than or equal to 70%, and no B symptoms or opportunistic infections. Poor-risk Kaposi sarcoma patients have any of the following: visceral Kaposi sarcoma or extensive mucocutaneous involvement, CD4 less than 150 per µL, poor performance status, B symptoms, and history of any opportunistic infections.

Answer 32.6. **The answer is C.**

Almost all of the HIV-associated lymphomas are associated with EBV. Bcl-2 is expressed in 90% of PCNSL but not in Burkitt lymphoma. C-myc expression occurs in Burkitt lymphoma but not in PEL. PEL is associated with KSHV infection. Generally, CD4 counts are depressed in patients who develop HIV-associated PCNSL.

Answer 32.7. **The answer is E.**

Once HIV-associated lymphoma is diagnosed, proper staging studies including CT scans of the chest, abdomen, and pelvis with brain scans are appropriate. Bone marrow biopsies and CSF cytology with routine labs are also appropriate. CD4 counts and HIV load may be done to assess the patient's immune status. Since a high percentage of HIV-associated lymphomas are associated with CNS involvement at presentation, routine CNS prophylaxis with intrathecal chemotherapy is standard. Systemic chemotherapy remains the standard therapy for HIV-associated peripheral lymphomas.

Answer 32.8. **The answer is D.**

The risk for developing PTLD is increased by 3.7-fold with the use of unrelated or mismatched donors and 9-fold with the use of T-cell depletion from stem cell grafts and the use of anti-GVHD regimens including cyclosporine, FK506, and anti-T-cell monoclonal antibodies. PTLD is rarely associated with autologous stem cell transplantation.

CHAPTER 33

Oncologic Emergencies

JOANNE E. MORTIMER AND MARY-ELLEN MAZURYK

Directions Each of the numbered items below is followed by lettered answers. Select the ONE lettered answer that is BEST in each case unless instructed otherwise.

QUESTIONS

Questions 33.1–33.5.

A 48-year-old woman is brought to the emergency department by her family because of headache, nausea, and vomiting. Two years ago, she was diagnosed with a T1cN0 infiltrative ductal carcinoma of the breast that was estrogen and progesterone receptor negative and Her-2 neu positive by fluorescence *in situ* hybridization (FISH). She underwent a lumpectomy followed by 4 cycles of doxorubicin and cyclophosphamide and adjuvant breast irradiation. Six months ago, she complained of right upper quadrant pain and was found to have hepatic metastases. She was treated with paclitaxel and trastuzumab, and recent follow-up scans have documented an excellent partial response. She has been clinically stable until now. She denies any symptoms of abdominal pain. On physical exam, she is noted to be somewhat drowsy but arousable. Her vital signs are stable. She is oriented to self but is not oriented to time or place. Funduscopic exam is normal. Neurologic exam is normal. There is no lymphadenopathy. Chest is clear. Abdominal examination is normal with no hepatomegaly noted.

Question 33.1. **The diagnostic test(s) most likely to confirm her symptoms is/are**

A. contrast enhanced magnetic resonance imaging (MRI) study
B. spinal tap with spinal fluid submitted for protein, glucose, cell count, and cytology
C. serum calcium
D. serum ammonia level
E. all of the above

Question 33.2. **Which of the following space-occupying lesions with edema is the most common clinical sign in a patient with brain metastases?**

A. Hemiparesis.
B. Papilledema.
C. Altered mental status exam.
D. Gait ataxia.
E. Focal numbness.

Corresponding Chapters in *Cancer: Principles & Practice of Oncology*, Seventh Edition: 49 (Oncologic Emergencies).

Question 33.3. **You tell the patient and her family that**

A. dexamethasone will decrease the need for radiation therapy
B. resection of the tumor will decrease the likelihood of recurrence and improve the patient's quality of life
C. radiation therapy after removal of the tumor will not prolong survival
D. phenytoin (Dilantin) should be prescribed to decrease the risk of seizures
E. none of the above

Question 33.4. **Resection of the solitary tumor followed by radiation (when compared with radiation alone) will**

A. decrease the likelihood of recurrence
B. improve the quality of life
C. increase the likelihood of survival
D. all of the above

Question 33.5. **The family is concerned that systemic treatment will be discontinued as a result of the treatment required for the central nervous system (CNS) metastasis. Your response is**

A. the brain may act as a sanctuary site in breast cancer
B. Her-2 positive breast cancer is associated with a higher incidence of brain metastasis
C. chemotherapy does not penetrate the CNS in a high enough concentration to treat the disease
D. her systemic disease may still be under control
E. all of the above

Questions 33.6–33.7.

A 76-year-old man is evaluated in the emergency department because of progressive worsening of cough, the development of facial swelling, and difficulty sleeping over the past 2 weeks. He has a history of smoking 2 packs of cigarettes per day for 45 years, but quit 6 months ago at the insistence of his daughter. He notes that his weight has decreased by 65 pounds over the past 6 months. His only active medical problem is hypertension that is well controlled by metoprolol. Physical exam is remarkable for mild facial swelling. His oral mucosa is moist and sublingual varicosities are noted. A left supraclavicular node measuring 3 cm by 3 cm is appreciated. Across the right anterior chest, dilated superficial vessels are identified. Breath sounds are diffusely decreased bilaterally consistent with preexisting chronic obstructive pulmonary disease (COPD). Scattered wheezes are noted but are nonfocal. Abdominal and neurologic exams are unremarkable.

Question 33.6. **The most common symptom for patients with superior vena caval (SVC) obstruction is**

A. headache
B. dyspnea
C. dysphagia
D. arm swelling
E. cough

Question 33.7. **Which of the following is true about SVC syndrome?**

A. Without emergent therapy, the incidence of stroke is high.
B. Anticoagulation will increase the probability that the vena cava will recanalize.
C. Lung cancer is the most common cause of SVC obstruction.
D. A venogram should be performed to document the degree of vascular obstruction.
E. Biopsy of mediastinal lymph nodes is associated with an unacceptably high rate of complication.

Question 33.8. **A 45-year-old man presents with cough, dyspnea, and right-sided hilar and mediastinal mass. Physical examination reveals a palpable enlarged supraclavicular adenopathy. A biopsy of the supraclavicular node confirms a diagnosis of diffuse large cell lymphoma of B-cell origin (CD20 positive). You recommend**

A. computed tomographic (CT) scans of the chest, abdomen, and pelvis
B. initial chemotherapy using an anthracycline-based regimen
C. pretreatment hydration and allopurinol
D. bilateral bone marrow biopsies
E. all of the above

Questions 33.9–33.12.

A 75-year-old man is brought to the emergency department with progressive dyspnea. He was diagnosed with non-small cell lung cancer 3 months ago, with documented metastases to the bones and the liver. He received palliative radiation to the primary lung mass to relieve bronchial obstruction. Combination chemotherapy with docetaxel and carboplatinum was initiated 2 weeks ago. As per protocol, he received dexamethasone 8 mg b.i.d. for 3 days, starting the day prior to chemotherapy.

The patient has a history of smoking 2.5 packs per day for 50 years. His present medications include bronchodilators and extended release morphine for pain.

On exam he is alert but somewhat agitated and tachypneic. He appears thin and has obvious temporal wasting. He is markedly hypotensive with a blood pressure of 60/40 mm Hg. Peripheral pulse is difficult to palpate, but heart rate by auscultation is 100 beats per minute. Oxygen saturation is 88% on room air. His neck is supple and jugular veins are distended bilaterally. A right supraclavicular node measuring 3 cm by 3 cm is appreciated. Breath sounds are decreased bilaterally, consistent with obstructive airway disease. Heart sounds are distant and no pericardial rubs or murmurs are noted. Abdominal examination is remarkable for an enlarged, nonpulsatile liver which is palpable 3 cm below the costal margin.

Question 33.9. **The presentation is most consistent with**

A. pericardial sclerosis from radiation therapy
B. impending pericardial tamponade
C. collapse lung secondary to progressive tumor
D. pericardial effusion secondary to docetaxel
E. pericarditis

Question 33.10. **Appropriate measures at this time include**

A. provision of supplemental oxygen
B. electrocardiogram
C. transfer the patient to the intensive care unit
D. chest x-ray
E. all of the above

Question 33.11. **The patient becomes increasingly dyspneic and hypotensive. You place a needle into the pericardial sac and aspirate 500 cc of serosanguinous fluid. Blood pressure increases and he is transferred to the intensive care unit for further cardiac monitoring. The most appropriate management of the pericardial fluid includes**

A. placement of a catheter in the pericardial sac for drainage of fluid as needed
B. pericardial sclerosis with bleomycin
C. radiation to the heart
D. subxiphoid pericardial window
E. none of the above

Question 33.12. **The patient's condition has stabilized after a drainage catheter is placed. The family wants to know what to expect in the future. You tell them**

A. it is likely the fluid will reaccumulate
B. radiation therapy will be necessary to ensure that the disease remains under control
C. docetaxel may have precipitated this event
D. the median survival for someone with a malignant pericardial effusion from non-small cell lung cancer is 8 to 12 weeks
E. none of the above

Questions 33.13–33.14.

A 68-year-old man has been treated with Lupron and Casodex for the past 2 years for prostate cancer with widespread bone metastases. His disease has been stable both clinically and radiologically. He last received Lupron 2 weeks ago. For the past week, he notes increasing pain in the region of T9-12 and over the past 3 days, he also notes bilateral leg weakness. His wife brings him to see you because of these complaints. His only other medical problem is diabetes that is managed by diet and oral hypoglycemic agents.

On physical examination the patient is alert and oriented and vital signs are stable. He rates his pain as 6/10 on a visual analogue scale. Abdominal examination is remarkable for a mass in the lower abdomen, presumed to be a distended bladder. Neurologic examination is significant for decreased sensation and weakness in the legs bilaterally at the level of L1. He is hyporeflexic and sphincter tone is decreased.

Question 33.13. **The diagnostic test that will provide the most valuable information is**

A. myelogram
B. MRI of the whole spine
C. CT scan of thoracic and lumbar spine
D. bone scan
E. plain film radiographs of thoracic and lumbar spine

Question 33.14. **MRI demonstrates lytic disease at T12 to L1 with additional epidural disease involving T9, with spinal cord compression. The patient is started on dexamethasone and opioid analgesic. A Foley catheter is inserted and 1,800 cc of clear urine is drained. Neurosurgery recommends that the patient undergoes an immediate decompression and stabilization of the spine prior to radiation therapy. Which of the following statements is true?**

A. Aggressive surgical removal of the cancer prior to radiation therapy results in improved neurologic recovery.
B. High-dose dexamethasone (100 mg) is superior to conventional dose (10 mg) in preserving neurologic function.
C. Because the patient's symptoms developed rapidly, he is likely to experience full neurologic recovery.
D. Treatment with a radiopharmaceutical (e.g., strontium-89) will relieve the patient's symptoms.
E. Surgery should be performed to confirm the diagnosis of metastatic prostate cancer.

Questions 33.15–33.16.

A 48-year-old man comes in to see you regarding treatment of newly diagnosed non-Hodgkin lymphoma, stage IIIB. Four months ago, he developed left upper quadrant discomfort. A CT scan demonstrated diffuse, bulky retroperitoneal adenopathy. Within the next 2 weeks, a left anterior cervical node became enlarged, and biopsy confirmed a diagnosis of diffuse large cell lymphoma of B-cell origin, CD20 positive. He elected to go on a business trip for 10 days prior to consulting with you. He notes that over the past week, he has been getting up hourly to urinate. He denies any fevers or night sweats. However, he has lost 35 pounds over the past 3 months and attributes this to decreased food intake secondary to nausea. He also complains of constipation, with his last bowel movement occurring 5 days prior.

On physical examination, he is an alert man who is oriented and in no obvious distress. Matted nodes in the left anterior cervical region are noted. A nontender abdominal mass is palpable in the midabdomen. Testicular exam is unremarkable. The prostate feels smooth and of normal size with no nodularity. His stool is guaiac negative. Neurologic examination is unremarkable.

Question 33.15. **The most likely diagnosis is**

A. bilateral ureteral obstruction from lymphoma
B. hypercalcemia
C. CNS involvement with lymphoma
D. sepsis
E. prostatism

Question 33.16. **You send urine and peripheral blood for routine laboratory. Bilateral bone marrow biopsies are also obtained to complete the staging workup. The following laboratory values are obtained.**

white blood cell count (WBC): 2.2 (25% granulocytes)
hemoglobin (Hb): 13.9
platelets: 296,000
calcium (Ca): 15.7
albumin (Alb): 4.1
total protein (TP): 6.7
lactic dehydrogenase (LDH): 213
blood urea nitrogen (BUN) and creatinine are normal
urinalysis is unremarkable

You recommend

A. cyclophosphamide, doxorubicin, vincristine, and prednisone (CHOP) chemotherapy
B. rituximab
C. bisphosphonate
D. hydration
E. all of the above

Questions 33.17–33.18.

A 58-year-old man presents with increased shortness of breath over the past 3 days. He also notes fatigue, nausea, and a decrease in urine production over the past week. He has noted a slow decrease in urine output for the past several days and has had no urine output for the past 24 hours. He has a history of smoking three packs per day for 40 years. He is presently on no medications and has no active medical problems. On physical examination, he is alert and oriented. He is afebrile with normal vital signs. Crackles are heard in both lung bases and the patient has moderate pedal edema, which is new. Prostate and rectal examination are normal. A straight catheterization results in 50 cc of clear urine. Laboratory examination is significant for a BUN of 82 mg per dL, serum creatinine of 7.1 mg per dL, and potassium of 6.2 mg per dL.

Question 33.17. **The most appropriate diagnostic study would be**

A. cystoscopy
B. intravenous pyelogram
C. CT scan with contrast
D. retrograde pyelogram
E. abdominal ultrasound

Question 33.18. **The patient is admitted to the intensive care unit for monitoring and stabilization. On ultrasound, a mass is seen arising from the bladder and causing obstruction of both ureters. Cystoscopy and biopsy confirms transitional cell carcinoma of the bladder. The urologist attempted to place ureteral stents but was unable to do so because of obstruction of ureteral orifices by tumor. The most appropriate treatment would be**

A. initiate neoadjuvant chemotherapy
B. external beam radiation to the bladder
C. percutaneous nephrostomy tube placement
D. exploratory laparotomy
E. renal scan to assess the function of the kidneys

ANSWERS

Answer 33.1. **The answer is A.**

Brain metastases represent a common problem, developing in up to 20% to 40% of all patients with cancer. The highest incidence (approximately 20%) occurs in patients with lung cancer, but 5% of breast cancer patients develop brain metastases over their lifetime. A contrast enhanced MRI is the most sensitive test for identifying brain metastasis. MRI also identifies a higher frequency of multiple metastases than described in CT-based studies. In addition, it is more accurate than CT scan in the diagnosis of leptomeningeal disease. In cases where a lumbar puncture is considered, either an MRI or CT scan should be obtained to rule out evidence of increased intracranial pressure.

Hypercalcemia is a possibility, given this patient's presentation with nausea and depressed level of consciousness. Hypercalcemia is seen in breast cancer, usually in conjunction with release of parathyroid hormone-related protein and/or bone metastases. However, this would not explain the patient's complaint of headache. Hepatic failure, as documented by an elevation in serum ammonia level, is also considered unlikely in this patient with a recent radiologic confirmation of regression of hepatic metastases.

Based on the information provided, it is most likely that the patient has developed progressive disease in the brain. This can occur despite the response of other metastatic sites to therapy since few antineoplastic agents cross the blood-brain barrier in high enough concentrations to effectively control disease in the brain. Brain metastases may be more common in women whose breast cancers overexpress Her-2 neu.

Answer 33.2. **The answer is A.**

The most common presenting signs in a patient with brain metastases include hemiparesis, altered mental status exam, and gait ataxia. Papilledema and focal numbness are reported in less than 10% of patients. Additional neurologic findings may relate to the location of metastatic foci; however, the localization of brain metastasis by clinical examination is especially difficult since the majority of patients present with multiple lesions. Headache can occur in up to 50% of patients and is most common in patients with multiple metastases or metastases involving the posterior fossa. It is most commonly bifrontal in location, often resembling a tension-type headache. Suggestive characteristics include headache that is present first thing in the morning. It is important to ask about symptoms suggestive of increased intracranial pressure, such as worsening of headache with position change or Valsalva maneuver, nausea and vomiting, and syncope. The opportunity for tumor emboli to implant in the brain is related to relative blood flow to the different areas of the brain. As a result, 80% of metastases occur in the cerebral hemispheres, 15% in the cerebellum, and 5% in the brainstem.

Answer 33.3. **The answer is B.**

Resection of the tumor will decrease the likelihood of recurrence and improve the patient's quality of life.

Answer 33.4. **The answer is D.**

Dexamethasone has been shown to provide palliation of neurologic symptoms, especially when significant edema has been documented by imaging. It does not obviate the need for whole brain irradiation. However, dexamethasone should be used with caution in patients suspected of having a CNS lymphoma as small doses of corticosteroids may cause tumor regression and alter the histology.

A solitary lesion will be identified in 25% to 30% of patients with brain metastasis. Candidacy for surgical resection should be determined according to the location of the brain lesion, status of the systemic cancer, performance status of the patient, and underlying cancer. Patients with treatable cancers and a good performance status should be considered for surgical resection. Neither surgical excision alone nor whole brain irradiation alone is as effective as the combination. Resection of a "solitary" lesion followed by whole brain irradiation is superior to whole brain irradiation alone. In clinical trials, surgery followed by irradiation therapy decreased the "distant" disease in the brain, decreased the incidence of death from CNS metastasis, and improved both the patient's quality of life and survival compared with radiation therapy alone.

Patients who receive prophylactic anticonvulsants are more likely to experience allergic reactions. More importantly, the use of anticonvulsants in this setting does not clearly reduce seizure risk. Therefore, anticonvulsants such as phenytoin should be reserved for patients experiencing seizures and have no role as prophylaxis.

Answer 33.5. **The answer is E.**

The most common primary tumor sites associated with brain metastasis are lung (60%) and breast (30%) cancers. Although a less common cancer, melanomas commonly spread to the CNS. Brain metastases from breast cancer are more likely to be estrogen receptor negative. Recent data suggest a high incidence of brain metastases in women whose breast cancers overexpress the Her-2 protein. Brain metastases develop in the setting on systemic control with trastuzumab and chemotherapy. To minimize the risk of radiosensitization, systemic therapy is generally withheld until the course of radiation has been completed.

Answer 33.6. **The answer is B.**

The most common presentation for patients with SVC obstruction is dyspnea, which occurs in 65% of patients. Other symptoms reported from three combined series include head fullness and facial swelling in 50%, cough in 24%, arm swelling in 18%, chest pain in 15%, and dysphagia in 9%. SVC is largely a clinical diagnosis. The most common physical findings include dilated veins in the neck in 66%, dilated veins of the chest wall in 54%, facial edema in 46%, cyanosis in 19%, and facial plethora in 19%.

Answer 33.7. **The answer is C.**

Historically, SVC syndrome was considered to be an oncologic emergency. Within the past two decades, a better understanding of the pathophysiology has significantly changed the urgency with which these patients are treated. Obstruction of the SVC is not acutely life threatening. Animal models and human experience support the lack of need for emergent therapy. Acute ligature of the vena cava in dogs results in engorgement of collateral circulation and not acute cardiovascular collapse. In a review of almost 2,000 patients with SVC obstruction reported in the literature, only one patient died. The patient's death was attributed to bleeding resulting from a head and neck cancer invading the tracheal wall and not as a result of venous obstruction. Thus, SVC obstruction is no longer considered an emergent medical problem.

The diagnosis of SVC obstruction is largely clinical and is further supported by the finding of a mass on chest radiograph or CT in 84% of patients. Venography is not required for confirmation and, in fact, may be patent in as many as 41% of patients.

Cancer is responsible for SVC obstruction in approximately 85% of cases. Yet, only 42% of the patients who present with SVC syndrome have been previously diagnosed with cancer. Lung cancer (especially small cell lung cancer), non-Hodgkin lymphoma, and germ cell tumors account for the majority of all cases of SVC obstruction. Because these are potentially curable diseases, it is essential that adequate diagnostic and staging information be obtained before determining a treatment plan. Physicians have argued that an increase in venous pressure from SVC obstruction might result in excessive complications when invasive procedures are performed. That has not been substantiated in the literature. In one review,

843 patients underwent a diagnostic procedure such as bronchoscopy, mediastinoscopy, lymph node biopsy, or thoracotomy without an obvious increase in surgical complications. Patients whose cancers initially present with SVC obstruction should undergo biopsy to confirm the diagnosis of cancer, and adequate staging information should be obtained before determining the treatment plan.

Answer 33.8. **The answer is E.**

As many as 4% of newly diagnosed patients with non-Hodgkin lymphoma present with obstruction of the SVC. It is essential that the patient be treated appropriately, and staging should be completed before institution of therapy. Thus, CT and marrow biopsy are indicated. The patient has at least stage II disease clinically and would be treated with chemotherapy and radiation therapy. Because non-Hodgkin lymphoma tends to be a relatively chemosensitive disease, chemotherapy would be the initial treatment of choice.

Answer 33.9. **The answer is B.**

The findings of dilated neck veins, hypotension, and distant heart sounds are most consistent with impending pericardial tamponade. Pulsus paradoxus refers to an accentuation of the normal decrease in systolic arterial pressure which occurs during inspiration. Clinically, the peripheral pulse may disappear completely during inspiration. The presence of pulsus paradoxus is worrisome for hemodynamically significant pericardial tamponade.

Radiation-induced pericardial sclerosis is an uncommon complication of chest irradiation and generally develops 3 to 12 months after completion of radiation therapy. This patient has only recently completed radiation therapy, making this diagnosis unlikely. Idiopathic pericarditis is also unlikely in the absence of a pericardial friction rub.

Third-space fluid collection is a recognized toxicity of docetaxel and may develop in peripheral tissues, the pleura, or pericardium. However, fluid retention is generally a cumulative effect of docetaxel, developing after several cycles of the drug and delayed by the use of dexamethasone as a premedication. This patient recently received his first cycle of docetaxel with dexamethasone, making docetaxel an unlikely cause of his effusion.

Answer 33.10. **The answer is E.**

The patient is in severe distress and clinically has impending cardiovascular collapse. Most patients with malignant pericardial effusions are only recognized when they are acutely ill and at risk for acute decompensation. The patient should be made comfortable with oxygen. An electrocardiogram may demonstrate decreased voltage and electrical alternans. As a result of excessive fluid, the heart size is enlarged and appears like a "water bottle" on chest radiograph. A two-dimensional echocardiogram will demonstrate collapse of the right atrial and ventricular chambers as a result of fluid accumulation.

Answer 33.11. **The answer is A.**

Malignant pericardial effusion generally develops as a late complication of advanced cancer. The median survival for all patients with a malignant pericardial effusion is less than 6 months, although patients with chemotherapy-sensitive disease may survive longer. Therefore, the chronic management of the effusion should be directed by the patient's performance status and underlying disease-specific prognosis.

A drainage catheter may safely be placed in the pericardial sac under local anesthesia with conscious sedation and used for repeated drainage of fluid that reaccumulates. Extended catheter drainage is an effective palliative measure, especially in patients with a limited prognosis. Given that this patient appears to have progressive non-small cell lung cancer, such an approach is effective and relatively noninvasive. Patients with a more favorable outcome should be considered for pericardial sclerosis or placement of a pericardial window. The instillation of sclerosing agents such as bleomycin through a pericardial catheter may prevent the reaccumulation of fluid. This procedure is usually performed with cardiac monitoring, is accompanied by pain, and may have to be repeated to prevent reaccumulation of fluid.

Alternatively, subxiphoid pericardiotomy, video-assisted thoracic surgery (VATS)–assisted pericardiectomy, and balloon pericardial window may also control reaccumulation of fluid without the need for chronic catheter drainage. Radiation therapy is seldom used to control malignant pericardial effusions because the dose of radiation required to control most epithelial tumors may be high enough to produce myocardial damage. Furthermore, the efficacy of radiation is not immediately appreciated in this acute clinical emergency.

Answer 33.12. **The answer is D.**

Pericardial tamponade generally occurs in the setting of extensive lung cancer and, therefore, patients have a limited survival. In non-small cell lung cancer, median survival in this setting is less than 3 months, and fewer than 10% are alive after 1 year.

Answer 33.13. **The answer is B.**

The differential diagnosis of back pain in a patient with cancer is broad and includes not only malignancy but degenerative changes and infection as well. This patient's clinical examination is most consistent with an acute spinal cord compression. Spinal cord compression may be due to growth of cancer from the vertebral body into the epidural space or vertebral collapse secondary to bone metastasis. Cancer may also involve nerve roots and foramina. Back pain is the most common symptom of spinal cord metastasis and may precede cord compression by days to months. Typically, the pain is worse when the patient is supine, a symptom that may help distinguish epidural metastasis from disc disease. The thoracic spine is involved in 65% of patients. Weakness generally occurs before autonomic instability. Bladder symptoms of hesitance or urinary retention are relatively common symptoms of spinal cord compression. Almost half of patients are incontinent or require bladder drainage.

MRI of the spine is the most sensitive test in this setting. It will accurately identify the location of symptomatic and asymptomatic lesions and will help the radiation oncologist to plan the treatment field. Furthermore, MRI may provide additional information about the presence of meningeal carcinomatosis, paraspinal masses, or inflammatory/infectious myelitis. If MRI is not available, CT scan of the spine with CT myelogram is recommended.

Answer 33.14. **The answer is A.**

A recent controlled trial compared surgical decompression followed by radiation with radiation therapy alone in patients with isolated epidural metastasis presenting with acute spinal cord damage. Patients in the surgery and radiation arm were more likely to recover neurology function, experienced an improvement in quality of life, and required lower doses of dexamethasone than those treated with radiation therapy. This approach is considered the standard of care. In a patient without a previous diagnosis of cancer, surgery can also be important for confirmation of the diagnosis. However, in contrast to SVC syndrome, most patients who present with spinal cord compression are already known to have cancer.

In controlled trials, high-dose dexamethasone has been found to be equivalent to conventional low dose in terms of rates of neurologic recovery. There may be some differences in the degree of pain control. Historically, those patients with slow development of neurologic symptoms tend to recover neurologic function more fully than those who experience a rapid neurologic deterioration.

Relief of associated bone pain is often achieved with dexamethasone, surgery, and external beam radiation. Strontium-89 may play a role in pain management in selected patients but is not expected to reverse the neurologic symptoms.

Answer 33.15. **The answer is B.**

Hypercalcemia is the most common metabolic emergency in cancer patients, and the production of parathyroid hormone-related peptide (PTHrP) by the tumor is the most common mechanism. It can also occur as a result of focal bone destruction secondary to bone metastases. Hypercalcemia is the most common paraneoplastic syndrome and is most frequently seen in association with multiple myeloma and cancers of the breast, lung, kidney, and head and neck. It is relatively uncommon in non-Hodgkin lymphoma, where both excess production of calcitriol and cytokines that promote osteolysis have been proposed as the mechanism. PTHrP has not been identified in lymphoma patients.

Answer 33.16. **The answer is E.**

In this instance, the patient's polyuria, nausea, and constipation are most likely caused by hypercalcemia and associated dehydration. Vigorous intravenous hydration and administration of a bisphosphonate are appropriate to increase urinary excretion of calcium and decrease bone absorption of calcium. In malignant hypercalcemia, the rapidity of response and duration of benefit favor zolendronic acid over pamidronate.

The patient should also receive therapy to prevent tumor lysis syndrome. The metabolic abnormalities that can result from treatment-associated cancer cell death include hyperkalemia, hypocalcemia, hyperphosphatemia, and hyperuricemia and may occur within hours or days of instituting therapy. Although it is most likely to occur with high grade lymphomas, tumor lysis may develop after treatment of any non-Hodgkin lymphoma. It is also frequently reported in other rapidly growing, chemosensitive hematologic malignancies such as myeloproliferative diseases and acute leukemias. It is less commonly associated with solid tumors, due to comparatively lower tumor doubling times and chemosensitivities. The best medical approach is to recognize its possible development and to treat the patient in a prophylactic manner with aggressive hydration and allopurinol, beginning prior to the administration of chemotherapy.

Although this patient is relatively young, he has a number of poor prognostic factors including weight loss and bulky nodal disease. The data suggest a higher response rate and improved survival when rituximab is added to CHOP chemotherapy.

Three days after institution of aggressive hydration, zolendronate, CHOP, and rituximab, the WBC rose to 5.0 (61% granulocytes). Hemoglobin decreased to 11.9 (possibly as a result of rehydration), and serum calcium decreased to 10.9. After 6 cycles of chemotherapy and rituximab, the patient achieves a complete remission, both clinically and by fluorodeoxyglucose (FDG)-PET imaging.

Answer 33.17. **The answer is E.**

The patient has signs of volume overload most likely secondary to acute renal failure. Abdominal ultrasound will provide information about the potential cause of renal failure, particularly with regards to urinary tract obstruction.

Answer 33.18. **The answer is C.**

Malignant ureteral obstruction may be the initial presentation of cancer, particularly those arising from the genitourinary tract, rectum, or cervix. Obtaining tissue confirmation of cancer is essential in determining disease-specific treatment. To protect renal function, it is critical that urine flow resume. Cystoscopy placement of stents may be difficult when the ureters are obstructed by tumor or bleeding. In this case, percutaneous nephrostomy tubes should be placed to relieve obstruction to renal flow. Antegrade placement of ureteral stents can be delayed until the patient's condition has stabilized.

CHAPTER 34

Interventional Radiology

DANIEL B. BROWN

Directions Each of the numbered items below is followed by lettered answers. Select the ONE lettered answer that is BEST in each case unless instructed otherwise.

QUESTIONS

Question 34.1. **Which of the following types of catheters is NOT tunneled?**

A. Subcutaneous portacatheter.
B. Hickman.
C. Peripherally inserted central catheter (PICC).

Question 34.2. **Which of the following statements is true regarding the Groshong catheter tip?**

A. It is designed to function as a one-way valve to prevent infection.
B. It is only used for portacatheters.
C. It does not require regular heparin flushing to prevent thrombosis.

Question 34.3. **All of the following statements regarding chest-wall implantable portacatheters are true EXCEPT**

A. they need to be accessed by noncoring needles
B. little differences in infectious complications have been identified between portacatheters and externalized infusion catheters
C. a skilled catheter care team is important in maintaining long-term catheter integrity
D. intraoperative placement is always required

Question 34.4. **Which of the following catheter types is appropriate for infusion of chemotherapy once weekly for several months?**

A. PICC.
B. Subcutaneous infusion port.
C. Externalized large-bore tunneled catheter.

Corresponding Chapters in *Cancer: Principles & Practice of Oncology*, Seventh Edition: 50 (Specialized Techniques in Cancer Management).

Question 34.5. **Which of the following catheter types is appropriate for administration of 2 weeks of antibiotics therapy administered once a day?**

A. PICC.
B. Subcutaneous infusion port.
C. Externalized large-bore tunneled catheter.

Question 34.6. **Which of the following catheter types is appropriate for stem cell transplant?**

A. PICC.
B. Subcutaneous infusion port.
C. Externalized large-bore tunneled catheter.

Question 34.7. **Factors to consider when selecting a venous access device include all of the following EXCEPT**

A. immune status
B. frequency of blood draws
C. patient size
D. presence of an inferior vena cava filter
E. history of previous access

Question 34.8. **Which of the following access routes has the highest percentage of procedural success?**

A. Internal jugular vein for portacatheter.
B. Subclavian vein for portacatheter.
C. Subclavian vein for external tunneled catheter.
D. Peripheral arm vein for PICC.
E. All of the above.

Question 34.9. **Which of the following complications has a greater than 3% incidence during central venous catheter placement?**

A. Pneumothorax.
B. Hematoma.
C. Air embolism.
D. Procedure-induced sepsis.
E. None of the above.

Question 34.10. **A patient had a subcutaneous portacatheter placed using the left internal jugular vein as an access. He has colon carcinoma with metastatic disease confined to the liver. Two weeks after portacatheter placement, the patient experiences left neck and arm swelling. He is afebrile and his neurologic examination is normal. The next appropriate management step is**

A. anticoagulation
B. immediate port removal
C. placement of an inferior vena caval filter
D. systemic injection of thrombolytic agents

Question 34.11. **Which of the following routes is most likely to result in symptomatic venous thrombosis following placement of a large-bore external infusion catheter?**

A. Subclavian vein.
B. Jugular vein.

Question 34.12. **Which of the following infectious pathogens is most likely to be successfully eradicated without removal of a central venous catheter?**

A. *Candida albicans.*
B. *Staphylococcus aureus.*
C. *Staphylococcus epidermidis.*
D. *Klebsiella pneumonia.*

Question 34.13. **Which of the following scenarios is typical for infection with *S. epidermidis*?**

A. Redness and purulence at the catheter exit site.
B. Treatment with total parenteral nutrition.
C. Endocarditis.

Question 34.14. **All of the following vessels are used for arterial access for isolated limb perfusion EXCEPT**

A. external iliac artery
B. internal iliac artery
C. brachial artery
D. axillary artery
E. popliteal artery

Question 34.15. **All of the following are true regarding the perfusate EXCEPT**

A. total volume is approximately 1 liter
B. 700 cc of saline solution are used
C. 1,500 units of heparin are added
D. an ideal hematocrit is 35%

Question 34.16. **Which of the following statements regarding hyperthermia for isolated perfusion is true?**

A. Tumor microvessels dilate more than normal tissue microvessels at temperatures up to 46°C.
B. Initial research with hyperthermic perfusates demonstrated an increase in antitumor efficacy and fewer complications.
C. Tissue temperatures of 40°C to 41°C maximize safety and efficacy of hyperthermic perfusion.
D. Tissue temperature is the only determinant of adverse events following isolated perfusion.

Question 34.17. **Which of the following statements regarding tumor necrosis factor (TNF) is NOT true?**

A. Maximally tolerated systemic administration has little antitumor effect.
B. The combination of TNF and hyperthermia significantly improves outcomes from isolated limb perfusion.
C. TNF has procoagulant activity against tumor vascularity.
D. TNF increases vascular permeability.

Question 34.18. **Which one of the following statements regarding the current status of isolated limb perfusion is true?**

A. Addition of TNF is a standard of practice.
B. Prophylactic isolated limb perfusion to treat in-transit melanoma greater than 1.5 mm in depth increases patient survival.
C. It may be useful in treating unresectable extremity sarcoma.

Question 34.19. **Which of the following statements regarding the current status of isolated liver perfusion is NOT true?**

A. In experienced centers, radiographic response may be as high as 74%.
B. Percutaneous techniques have been reported with the potential benefit of easy retreatment.
C. Survival following isolated liver perfusion for unresectable metastases from colorectal cancer may be greater than 12 months.
D. Isolated liver perfusion needs to be disseminated to the community to improve survival from metastases from colorectal cancer.

ANSWERS

Answer 34.1. **The answer is C.**

Both portacatheters and Hickman catheters are inserted on the chest wall, and a tunnel is made from the pocket site to the venous access site. PICC lines typically exit the skin immediately adjacent to the entry site into the vein. Tunneling a portacatheter from a chest wall site allows a more comfortable position for a patient in the subclavicular region if the internal jugular vein is used for access. Hickman and other central externalized catheters are tunneled from the chest wall to allow placement of the Dacron cuff in the tract. This cuff decreases the risk of infection.

Answer 34.2. **The answer is A.**

Groshong catheter tips have a slit valve that is designed to stay closed unless positive (injection) or negative (aspiration) pressure is being exerted. Ideally, this catheter would maintain the heparin flush that is infused at the end of each session of use. Unfortunately, this valve often fatigues and, therefore, regular flushing is still required.

Answer 34.3. **The answer is D.**

Placement of any central venous catheter should be done with strict aseptic technique. By doing so, performance and infectious outcomes have been shown to be similar to or better than those done intraoperatively.

Answer 34.4. **The answer is A.**

Portacatheters maintain a lower risk of infection when they are used intermittently. Patients are also allowed greater modesty with a subcutaneous device.

Answer 34.5. **The answer is B.**

A PICC line is ideal for the short-term administration of medications.

Answer 34.6. **The answer is C.**

Stem cell transplant often requires a tunneled catheter with multiple large-bore lumens.

Answer 34.7. **The answer is C.**

The presence of an inferior vena cava filter adds a level of complexity to the placement of any central venous access catheter. Guide wires, especially those with a J-shaped tip, may become ensnared in the filter and require removal by interventional radiology. Placement of central catheters in patients with inferior vena cava filters should be done with fluoroscopic assistance if possible.

Answer 34.8. **The answer is E.**

In its *Quality Improvement Guidelines for Central Venous Access,* the Society of Interventional Radiology reviewed success rates for all the above-described approaches in over two dozen peer-reviewed publications. All access routes had a sum success rate of approximately 95%.

Answer 34.9. **The answer is E.**

In its *Quality Improvement Guidelines for Central Venous Access,* the Society of Interventional Radiology reviewed and reported incidence rates of the above outcomes. Only pneumothorax was as high as 2%. The remainder was 1% or less. A higher incidence should lead to a performance review of the operator placing central venous access.

Answer 34.10. **The answer is A.**

Patients with venous thrombosis are usually symptomatic secondary to a lack of collateral blood vessels. However, these usually develop quickly, and anticoagulation can prevent further propagation of thrombus. Catheter removal will eliminate the left jugular and likely the left subclavian vein from future use if other venous access is required and is not guaranteed to maintain venous patency. Placement of an inferior vena caval filter will have no effect on thrombus in the upper extremity.

Catheter-directed thrombolysis at the site of thrombus might provide symptomatic relief and maintain venous patency in carefully selected patients. However, systemic administration of thrombolytic agents has no role in the management of this patient.

Answer 34.11. **The answer is A.**

Trerotola et al. studied outcomes of 279 Hickman catheters ranging from 9.0 to 12.5 French. Subclavian (n = 166) and jugular (n = 113) routes were used. Catheters were managed identically no matter which vein was used for access. Symptomatic venous thrombosis occurred in 13% of patients with subclavian catheters versus 3% in those with jugular catheters ($p = 0.018$). This difference was maintained after adjustment for catheter size and side of placement.

Answer 34.12. **The answer is C.**

S. epidermidis is a common contaminant in blood cultures. Treatment for infection with *S. epidermidis* is usually only initiated following two positive cultures. Successful treatment of this infection is more common than with the other infectious pathogens listed above, although treatment times may need to be lengthened if the catheter is removed.

Answer 34.13. **The answer is A.**

S. epidermidis typically affects the exit site of externalized catheters. Endocarditis is an uncommon but feared complication of catheter infection with *S. aureus*. Catheter infection during administration of total parenteral nutrition is associated with infection with fungal species, especially *Candida parapsilosis*.

Answer 34.14. **The answer is B.**

The internal iliac (hypogastric) artery is temporarily occluded during isolated limb perfusion. Distal branches of the internal iliac artery may be ligated to prevent systemic spillage of perfusate via cross-pelvic collateral branches.

Answer 34.15. **The answer is D.**

The ideal hematocrit for isolated limb perfusion is 25%. No benefit has been identified with higher hematocrits.

Answer 34.16. **The answer is C.**

The lack of vasodilatation of tumor vessels when compared to normal microvessels leads to relative stasis of flow. The antineoplastic agents perfused then have longer contact time with tumor cells. Initial experiments with hyperthermic perfusion had high complication rates until the ideal tissue temperature of 40 to 41°C was determined. Decreases in perfusate pH and female gender have also been identified as risk factors from isolated perfusion.

Answer 34.17. **The answer is B.**

TNF is highly toxic when administered systemically, and it is ideally suited for closed-circuit administration. However, when used as the sole antineoplastic agent for isolated perfusion, results have been poor. TNF works by a combination of increasing vascular permeability that allows better penetration of chemotherapeutic agents and procoagulant activity that may promote tumor vessel thrombosis.

Answer 34.18. **The answer is C.**

There is evidence from European trials that isolated limb perfusion results in an 80% clinical response and limb salvage rate. Outcomes with and without TNF have been mixed, and there is no definitive evidence that it is of clinical benefit. There was no difference in patient survival when isolated limb perfusion was performed prophylactically to treat in-transit melanoma.

Answer 34.19. **The answer is D.**

Radiographic response rates from isolated liver perfusion have been reported as high as 74% in two separate trials, one of which also included hepatic artery chemotherapy following surgery. These trials reported survivals of 14.5 and 16.5 months. Unfortunately, this rate is less than that of two recent publications with intravenous chemotherapy. Isolated liver perfusion has a very high toxicity, morbidity, and potential mortality when initially performed. Until significantly enhanced survival is demonstrated and procedure complications are limited, isolated liver perfusion will remain a study procedure at highly advanced tertiary care centers. Percutaneous techniques have been described to perform isolated liver perfusion. These may eventually simplify the procedure but are far from becoming a standard of practice.

CHAPTER **35**

Treatment of Metastatic Cancer

ALEX E. DENES

Directions Each of the numbered items below is followed by lettered answers. Select the ONE lettered answer that is BEST in each case unless instructed otherwise.

QUESTIONS

Question 35.1. **In patients with breast cancer, lung cancer, renal cancer, and prostate cancer, which of the following is the most common site of bone metastases?**

A. Femur.
B. Pelvis.
C. Spine.
D. Skull.

Question 35.2. **Which of the currently available imaging techniques for the detection of bone metastases is the least useful in monitoring response to therapy?**

A. Plain radiography.
B. Technetium bone scan.
C. Magnetic resonance imaging (MRI).
D. Positron emission tomography (PET).

Question 35.3. **The mechanism of action of bisphosphonates in the treatment of bone metastases in patients with breast cancer is thought to involve**

A. induction of apoptosis in the tumor cells
B. increased recruitment of osteoblasts
C. interference with osteoclast recruitment and activation
D. reduction of parathyroid related protein (PTHRP) activity

Question 35.4. **A 48-year-old housewife with metastatic breast cancer develops left shoulder pain. X-rays confirm a lytic lesion in the distal left clavicle. She is referred for external beam radiation. What is the likelihood that she will derive symptomatic benefit from radiation?**

A. 25%.
B. 40%.
C. 65%.
D. 85%.

Corresponding Chapters in *Cancer: Principles & Practice of Oncology*, Seventh Edition: 51 (Treatment of Metastatic Cancer).

Question 35.5. **The most extensively studied radionuclide in management of skeletal metastases is**

A. strontium-85
B. strontium-89
C. samarium-153
D. rhenium-188

Question 35.6. **A patient with known breast cancer develops increasing left hip pain especially with weight bearing. Plain radiographs are obtained and confirm a 4.5-cm area of cortical destruction in the proximal left humerus. Which is the most appropriate course of action?**

A. Initiation of external beam irradiation.
B. Surgical stabilization followed by external beam irradiation.
C. Surgical stabilization followed by systemic therapy.
D. Placing the patient nonweight bearing and initiating systemic chemotherapy.

Question 35.7. **The surgical management of epiphyseal fractures is most successful with**

A. open reduction and internal fixation
B. intramedullary nailing
C. plate fixation
D. prosthetic joint replacement

Question 35.8. **Which of the following primary cancers is LEAST likely to be complicated by the development of brain metastases?**

A. Malignant melanoma.
B. Carcinoma of the lung.
C. Carcinoma of the prostate.
D. Carcinoma of the breast.

Question 35.9. **Which area of the brain is the most common site of involvement by metastatic carcinoma?**

A. Cerebral hemispheres.
B. Cerebellum.
C. Brainstem.
D. Midbrain.

Question 35.10. **A patient with non-small cell lung cancer (NSCLC) presents with headaches and lethargy. A contrast-enhanced computed tomographic (CT) scan demonstrates a solitary metastatic lesion in the right temporal/parietal region. What is the likelihood that a gadolinium enhanced MRI scan will reveal additional brain metastases?**

A. 10%.
B. 20%.
C. 40%.
D. 60%.
E. 75%.

Question 35.11. **Which of the following statements regarding the use of anticonvulsants in patients with brain metastases is true?**

A. Patients with asymptomatic brain metastases from lung cancer should not receive prophylactic antiseizure medication.
B. Prophylactic antiseizure medication prolongs the survival of patients with brain metastases from breast cancer.
C. Patients with deep intracerebral metastases are at high risk for seizures.
D. The majority of patients with brain metastases will develop seizures unless they are given prophylactic antiseizure medication.

Question 35.12. **Which of the following is NOT a commonly used fractionation schedule for whole brain radiation therapy (WBRT) in patients with brain metastases?**

A. 30 Gy in 10 fractions.
B. 37.5 Gy in 15 fractions.
C. 40 Gy in 10 fractions.
D. 40 Gy in 20 fractions.

Question 35.13. **A patient presents with solitary brain metastasis from NSCLC. His systemic disease is controlled and he is referred for neurosurgical evaluation. Metastases in which of the following locations can be considered for surgical resection?**

A. Thalamus.
B. Brainstem.
C. Cerebellar hemispheres.
D. Basal ganglia.

Question 35.14. **A 55-year-old engineer with NSCLC presents with a solitary right frontal lobe brain metastasis. His performance status is 1 and his systemic disease is controlled. He is started on dexamethasone. You now recommend**

A. needle biopsy followed by WBRT and taper steroids after radiation is completed
B. complete surgical resection followed by observation with periodic MRI scans
C. complete surgical resection followed by WBRT
D. needle biopsy followed by chemotherapy with temazolamide

Question 35.15. **What percentage of patients with carcinomatous meningitis will have negative cerebrospinal fluid (CSF) cytology on initial lumbar puncture?**

A. 5% to 10%.
B. 20% to 30%.
C. 40% to 50%.
D. 60% to 70%.

Question 35.16. **Repeated administration of intrathecal chemotherapy in patients with carcinomatous meningitis is usually accomplished using which of the following devices or techniques.**

A. Infusaport reservoir.
B. Ommaya reservoir.
C. Groshong catheter.
D. Repeated lumbar puncture.

Question 35.17. **Patients with which of the following cancers are most likely to benefit from resection of hepatic metastases?**

A. Breast cancer.
B. Ocular melanoma.
C. Neuroendocrine carcinoma of the pancreas.
D. Adenocarcinoma of the pancreas.

Question 35.18. **Randomized clinical trials comparing hepatic artery infusion of floxuridine (FUDR) to systemic intravenous infusion of FUDR have consistently shown superior results with hepatic artery infusion of FUDR in all of the following end points EXCEPT**

A. overall response rates
B. disease-free survival
C. time to hepatic progression
D. overall survival

Question 35.19. **The most common toxicity of protracted hepatic artery infusion (HAI) with FUDR is**

A. stomatitis
B. hepatic toxicity
C. diarrhea
D. thrombocytopenia

Question 35.20. **Liver metastases from which of the following neoplasms are most commonly treated with hepatic artery chemoembolization?**

A. Ocular melanoma.
B. Carcinoma of the pancreas.
C. Colorectal cancer.
D. Malignant carcinoid of the appendix.

Question 35.21. **A patient with multiple hepatic metastases from an islet cell carcinoma of the pancreas is being evaluated for hepatic artery chemoembolization. Which of the following findings is a contraindication to chemoembolization?**

A. Periportal lymphadenopathy.
B. Serum bilirubin of 2.5.
C. Portal vein occlusion.
D. Serum albumin of 1.9.

Question 35.22. **Three years after his initial diagnosis a healthy 55-year-old man with stage III colon cancer is found to have an elevated carcinoembryonic antigen (CEA). His hepatic enzymes are normal but CT scans confirm three hepatic metastases with the largest being 2.5 cm in diameter. If the lesions are confirmed to be surgically resectable, which of the following approaches would have the highest likelihood of improving his disease-free survival and possibly his overall survival?**

A. Systemic 5-fluorouracil (5FU) based chemotherapy and bevacizumab.
B. Hepatic artery chemoembolization.
C. Hepatic artery infusion with FUDR.
D. Surgical resection followed by adjuvant HAI using FUDR and systemic chemotherapy.

Question 35.23. **A patient with malignant carcinoid develops recurrent flushing and episodes of diarrhea. CT scans confirm multiple metastases in both hepatic lobes and occlusion of the portal vein. Which of the following local ablative techniques can be considered as therapeutic options?**

A. Cryotherapy.
B. Percutaneous ethanol injection with transcatheter arterial embolization.
C. Whole liver irradiation.
D. Whole liver irradiation with HAI using FUDR.

Question 35.24. **A 54-year-old man is found to have malignant ascites without an obvious source. Which of the following procedures is most likely to identify the underlying neoplasm?**

A. Repeated paracentesis for cytologic examination.
B. Fluorodeoxyglucose (FDG)-PET scan.
C. Laparoscopy.
D. Laparoscopy with peritoneal biopsy.

Question 35.25. **A 62-year-old woman presents with increasing abdominal girth. CT scans confirm generalized ascites but no other abnormalities. Cytology is positive for adenocarcinoma. What is the most likely source of her malignant ascites?**

A. Adenocarcinoma of the pancreas.
B. Clinically occult breast cancer.
C. Ovarian or primary peritoneal carcinoma.
D. Gastric adenocarcinoma.

Question 35.26. **A 72-year-old housewife with pancreatic cancer develops recurrent malignant ascites. Which of the following conditions would make a peritoneovenous shunt unlikely to successfully control her ascites?**

A. High ascites fluid total protein level.
B. Chylous ascites.
C. Bloody ascites.
D. High peritoneal fluid lactate dehydrogenase (LDH)/serum LDH ratio.

Question 35.27. **A patient with gastric carcinoma develops increasing abdominal distension and early satiety. Abdominal x-rays are ordered. All of the following are signs of abdominal ascites EXCEPT**

A. central displacement of the small bowel loops
B. ground-glass appearance of the abdomen
C. multiple air-fluid levels in the small bowel
D. loss of the psoas shadow

Question 35.28. **Risks associated with rapid drainage of large volume malignant ascites by peritoneovenous shunting include all of the following EXCEPT**

A. disseminated intravascular coagulation (DIC)
B. volume overload
C. pulmonary edema
D. pulmonary tumor embolization

Question 35.29. **The sensitivity of helical CT scanning with the single breath-hold technique to detect pulmonary nodules smaller than 6 mm is**

A. 25%
B. 45%
C. 65%
D. 85%

Question 35.30. **In patients undergoing surgical resection of pulmonary metastases, the most important determinant of long-term prognosis is**

A. histology
B. complete surgical resection
C. disease-free interval
D. number of pulmonary nodules

Question 35.31. **In patients who are being considered for surgical resection of pulmonary metastases, each of the following criteria must be present EXCEPT**

A. metastases limited to one lung
B. controlled primary tumor
C. no extrapulmonary metastases
D. All pulmonary metastases are resectable.

Question 35.32. **Which of the following patients with soft tissue sarcoma has the best long-term prognosis following resection of pulmonary metastases?**

A. A patient found to have five bilateral pulmonary nodules 6 months after completing adjuvant chemotherapy for an intermediate-grade leiomyosarcoma of the right shoulder.
B. A patient with a 10-mm solitary pulmonary nodule detected 3 years after undergoing resection of a lower extremity high-grade liposarcoma.
C. A patient with a solitary 1.8-cm left lung nodule detected 4 years after resection of a low-grade malignant fibrous histiocytoma of the thigh.
D. A patient with two pulmonary nodules noted 1.5 years after resection of a high-grade leiomyosarcoma of the thigh.

Question 35.33. **A 63-year-old man with colon cancer is found to have pulmonary metastases on screening chest x-rays. Which of the following factors would NOT adversely influence the likelihood of successful long-term outcome following resection?**

A. Previous resection of hepatic metastases.
B. Incomplete resection of pulmonary metastases.
C. Synchronous liver and lung metastases.
D. Involvement of the mediastinal lymph nodes.

Question 35.34. **A 22-year-old college athlete undergoes orchiectomy for a stage I non-seminomatous germ cell tumor (NSGCT). Eighteen months following surgery, his beta-human chorionic gonadotropin (HCG) is elevated and chest x-rays reveal a total of three bilateral pulmonary nodules. There is no mediastinal or retroperitoneal adenopathy on CT scans. Which of the following do you now recommend?**

A. Resection of all pulmonary nodules and mediastinal exploration through median sternotomy.
B. Resection of all pulmonary nodules by sequential bilateral thoracotomies.
C. Initiation of platinum-based chemotherapy and resection of any residual nodules.
D. Resection of pulmonary nodules followed by platinum-based chemotherapy.

Question 35.35. **A patient with NSGCT is found to have multiple bilateral pulmonary metastases. His beta HCG is 180,000 u per ml. Following 4 cycles of PEB (cisplatin, etoposide, bleomycin) chemotherapy, the beta HCG is less than 3 and there are two small (<10 mm) residual pulmonary nodules. At 6 months follow-up, one of the nodules is noted to have enlarged to 2.5 cm. His tumor markers remain normal. You now recommend**

A. to begin chemotherapy with VIP (vinblastine, iphosphamide, cisplatin)
B. to continue observation and initiate chemotherapy with VIP when the tumor markers become elevated
C. surgical resection of the 2.5-cm nodule as well as the smaller nodule (if accessible)
D. surgical resection followed by VIP chemotherapy

Question 35.36. **A patient with a large (>50% of pleural cavity) pleural effusion undergoes a therapeutic thoracentesis. Slow, gradual drainage of the effusion is recommended to avoid**

A. hemoptysis
B. pneumothorax
C. postexpansion pulmonary edema
D. pulmonary embolism

Question 35.37. **A 66-year-old carpenter presents with increasing dyspnea. Chest x-rays reveal a large, free-flowing right pleural effusion. He has no prior history of cardiac or pulmonary disease but has smoked two packs of filtered cigarettes daily since age 20. A diagnostic/therapeutic thoracentesis is performed. The fluid sample should be evaluated for all of the following EXCEPT**

A. cell count
B. cytologic examination
C. alkaline phosphatase
D. LDH

Question 35.38. **A patient presents with a moderate right pleural effusion. He undergoes a diagnostic/therapeutic thoracentesis and pleural fluid cytology is positive for adenocarcinoma. What is the likelihood that the effusion will recur within 30 days of initial thoracentesis?**

A. 25%.
B. 50%.
C. 75%.
D. 95%.

Question 35.39. **Commonly used sclerosing agents in the management of malignant pleural effusions include all of the following EXCEPT**

A. bleomycin
B. adriamycin
C. doxycycline
D. talc

Question 35.40. **Malignant pleural effusions can be drained by indwelling catheters such as the Pleurx catheter. Advantages of chronic pleural catheter drainage include all of the following EXCEPT**

A. outpatient placement of the pleural catheter
B. ease of catheter insertion
C. daily or every other day drainage of effusion
D. ability to control effusion in patients with a trapped lung

Question 35.41. **Patients presenting with a malignant pleural effusion can sometimes be successfully treated by thoracentesis followed by initiating systemic therapy for the primary malignancy. Patients with which of the following diagnoses are most likely to be successfully managed by this approach without requiring pleurodesis or chronic pleural drainage?**

A. Renal cell carcinoma.
B. Pancreatic carcinoma.
C. Malignant lymphoma.
D. Malignant melanoma.

Question 35.42. **A 55-year-old man with a history of NSCLC presents to an emergency department with symptoms of progressive exertional dyspnea, orthopnea, and edema. He denies chest pain. Auscultation of the heart reveals a prominent friction rub. Chest x-rays confirm an enlarged pericardial silhouette. Which of the following findings on electrocardiogram (ECG) suggest the presence of a pericardial effusion?**

A. Narrow complex tachycardia.
B. Sinus bradycardia.
C. T wave inversion.
D. Electrical alternans.

Question 35.43. **A 38-year-old woman with a history of stage II breast cancer reports increasing fatigue and exertional dyspnea. Chest x-rays reveal an enlarged globular cardiac silhouette but no pleural or parenchymal abnormalities. Which of the following imaging modalities is recommended as the next procedure to investigate the cause of her symptoms?**

A. Contrast-enhanced CT of the chest.
B. Contrast-enhanced MRI of the chest.
C. Echocardiography.
D. FDG-PET scan.

Question 35.44. **Among the surgical techniques available to manage malignant pericardial effusion, currently the most commonly employed method is**

A. pericardial sclerotherapy
B. percutaneous balloon tube pericardiostomy
C. subxyphoid pericardiostomy
D. transthoracic partial pericardiectomy

ANSWERS

Answer 35.1. **The answer is C.**

Breast, prostate, lung, and renal cancers are the most common solid tumors which metastasize to bone. In these patients, the spine is the most common site of skeletal metastases and may be complicated by compression fracture, instability, and spinal cord compression. Early intervention in patients with spinal cord compression is imperative to prevent devastating neurologic complications.

Answer 35.2. **The answer is B.**

Technetium bone scans identify foci of active bone mineralization rather than tumor activity and are not helpful in evaluating response to treatment. The development of new lesions is, however, generally indicative of disease progression. Plain radiography, PET, and MRI can be useful in following response of bone metastases to treatment. MRI does not provide information on the structural integrity of skeletal lesions and requires correlation with plain radiography.

Answer 35.3. **The answer is C.**

The primary mechanism of action of bisphosphonates involves inhibition of osteoclast recruitment and activation. All of the bisphosphonates have been shown to induce osteoclast apoptosis *in vitro.* Large randomized clinical trials of bisphosphonates in a variety of solid tumors as well as multiple myeloma have demonstrated decreased skeletal morbidity in patients receiving these agents. The main toxicity has been impairment of renal function; therefore, close monitoring of renal function is recommended in patients receiving intravenous bisphosphonates.

Answer 35.4. **The answer is D.**

Approximately 80% to 90% of patients with skeletal metastases from breast cancer will obtain symptomatic benefit form external beam irradiation and 50% to 85% will obtain complete pain relief. The time course of response is quite variable and some patients may require 5 to 6 weeks to derive maximum symptomatic benefit from radiation.

Answer 35.5. **The answer is B.**

The radionuclides represent focused delivery of radioisotope to areas of accelerated bone turnover. The most widely studied of the radionuclides is strontium-89. This agent has been extensively evaluated in both breast and prostate cancer where it has shown a clinical benefit rate of greater than 80%. The most common toxicity of these agents is myelosuppression, so patients receiving these agents should be closely monitored with periodic complete blood counts.

Answer 35.6. **The answer is B.**

Patients with endosteal cortical destruction of greater than 50% or a cortical defect greater than 2.5 cm are at increased risk of pathologic fracture, especially when the lesion involves a weight-bearing bone. These patients should be managed by surgical stabilization in the hope of preventing a pathologic fracture followed by external beam irradiation. The decision to initiate systemic therapy should be based on multiple factors including hormone receptor status, extent of metastatic disease, presence of visceral metastases, and prior therapy.

Answer 35.7. **The answer is D.**

Pathologic epiphyseal fractures heal poorly, and, therefore, operative reduction and internal fixation are usually unsuccessful. Cemented prosthetic joint replacement followed by external beam irradiation is the accepted treatment of choice. Medullary rod placement is the treatment of choice in diaphyseal fractures but is not indicated in epiphyseal lesions.

Answer 35.8. **The answer is C.**

Malignant melanoma has been reported to metastasize to the brain in as many as 25%, breast cancer in 21%, and lung cancer (combined small cell and non-small cell) in 65% of patients. Prostate cancer and non-melanoma skin cancers rarely lead to parenchymal brain metastases.

Answer 35.9. **The answer is A.**

The vast majority of brain metastases from solid tumors result from hematogenous spread. The distribution of brain metastases reflects cerebral blood flow: 80% of CNS metastases are found in the cerebral hemispheres, 15% in the cerebellum, and 5% in the brainstem. Posterior fossa metastases may be more common with primary pelvic or abdominal cancers because malignant cells may gain access to the posterior fossa through Batson vertebral venous plexus.

Answer 35.10. **The answer is B.**

During the CT era, approximately 50% of brain metastases appeared to be solitary lesions. With contrast-enhanced MRI scanning, studies have found multiple metastases in 20% to 25% of patients thought to have a solitary metastasis on CT scan. Triple-dose gadoteridol MRI appears to be superior to conventional dose gadopentate dimeglumine MRI in detecting small metastatic lesions. The two main characteristics of brain metastases missed by CT are smaller diameter and frontotemporal location.

Answer 35.11. **The answer is A.**

Patients with brain metastases who present with or develop seizures should be given antiseizure medication, but controlled clinical trials have not demonstrated a benefit in asymptomatic patients. Possible exceptions are patients with brain metastases in highly epileptogenic areas of the cortex and melanoma, which often involves the cerebral cortex. Metastases deep in the brain parenchyma are less likely to result in seizures than cortical lesions. Randomized studies have not demonstrated a survival benefit in patients given prophylactic antiseizure medication.

Answer 35.12. **The answer is C.**

WBRT results in symptomatic improvement in 60% to 90% of patients and also extends survival. Several fractionation schedules are acceptable, but daily fractions much greater than 3 Gy are associated with an increased risk of developing cognitive impairment and dementia in patients surviving beyond 6 months and should be avoided.

Answer 35.13. **The answer is C.**

Lesions in the cerebellar hemispheres, especially peripheral lesions, can be resected with minimal morbidity and should be considered for resection. Lesions in the thalamus, brainstem, or basal ganglia are generally not considered resectable due to the significant mortality and/or morbidity associated with surgical resection in these locations. These lesions are usually treated with radiosurgery or WBRT.

Answer 35.14. **The answer is C.**

WBRT following complete surgical resection of solitary brain metastases results in long-term local control rates of 80% to 90%, whereas local control with WBRT without resection is successful in 40% to 50% of patients. Similarly, patients who undergo resection without postoperative WBRT have higher rates of local failure, in-brain failure, and higher risk of neurologic deaths than patients receiving postoperative WBRT. While there are no studies comparing chemotherapy with WBRT in patients with brain metastases, chemotherapy is usually reserved for patients who have highly chemosensitive tumors, especially in the salvage setting after failing surgery and/or WBRT.

Answer 35.15. **The answer is C.**

Cytologic examination of the CSF has high specificity but low sensitivity. Approximately 40% to 50% of patients with carcinomatous meningitis will have negative CSF cytology. The sensitivity increases with repeated examinations but does not exceed 80%. In patients with negative cytology, MRI imaging may be of benefit. As many as 50% of patients with neoplastic meningitis have abnormal imaging using gadolinium-enhanced MRI. Findings may include abnormal enhancement of the meninges or hydrocephalus without an identifiable mass lesion.

Answer 35.16. **The answer is B.**

The most reliable and practical administration of intrathecal chemotherapy is through an implanted subcutaneous reservoir and ventricular catheter (Ommaya reservoir). Chemotherapeutic agents administered into the lateral ventricles disseminate through the neuroaxis. If obstruction of CSF flow is suspected, the patients should undergo radionuclide ventriculography and receive local radiation to sites of obstruction before continuing intrathecal therapy.

Answer 35.17. **The answer is C.**

Resection of hepatic metastases in patients with neuroendocrine carcinomas of the pancreas has been reported to produce 5-year survival in as many as 50% of patients. Hepatic resection in patients with breast cancer and carcinoma of the pancreas are generally much less successful in achieving long-term benefit. Patients with ocular melanoma may benefit from resection of hepatic metastases, but the long-term prognosis is guarded with 5-year survival rates approximately 30% in carefully selected patients.

Answer 35.18. **The answer is D.**

HAI infusion of FUDR has consistently demonstrated superior response rates, disease-free survival, and time to hepatic progression compared to intravenous FUDR or intravenous 5FU. The impact of HAI FUDR on survival has been inconsistent. This may be a result of study design in that in several trials patients who were initially assigned to receive intravenous therapy were allowed to cross over and receive HAI FUDR at time of disease progression.

Answer 35.19. **The answer is B.**

The most common toxicities with HAI are hepatic toxicity and ulceration of the stomach and duodenum. Myelosuppression, stomatitis, and diarrhea rarely occur with HAI using FUDR. Hepatotoxicity is usually characterized by elevations of aspartate aminotransferase (AST), alkaline phosphatase, and bilirubin. These enzymes must be monitored closely in patients receiving HAI to prevent the development of sclerosing cholangitis. Ulceration of the proximal gastrointestinal (GI) tract results from inadvertent perfusion of the stomach and/or duodenum through small collateral branches of the common hepatic artery.

Answer 35.20. **The answer is D.**

Hepatic artery chemoembolization has been widely used in the treatment of unresectable hepatocellular carcinoma. It is also successful in controlling metastases from carcinoid or islet cell carcinomas with response rates as high as 50%. This approach has been much less successful in the treatment of more aggressive cancers such as melanoma or colorectal cancer.

Answer 35.21. **The answer is C.**

The efficacy of chemoembolization for isolated hepatic metastases is based on the principle that hepatic metastases derive their blood supply from the hepatic artery, whereas the portal vein supplies blood and oxygen to normal hepatocytes. Therefore, occlusion or thrombosis of the portal vein is an absolute contraindication to hepatic artery chemoembolization. Although patients with severely impaired liver function are not ideal candidates for chemoembolization, there are no clear guidelines as to the degree of hepatic functional impairment that constitute a contraindication to the procedure, and, in these patients, the decision is generally made on a case-by-case basis.

Answer 35.22. **The answer is D.**

Systemic chemotherapy, hepatic artery chemoembolization, and HAI are generally reserved for patients who are not candidates for surgical resection. Complete resection of hepatic metastases results in 5-year disease-free and overall survival of 20% to 50% in carefully selected patients. A limited number of randomized clinical trials have reported improved long-term outcome with adjuvant chemotherapy following resection of hepatic metastases, especially in those patients who receive both HAI and systemic treatment.

Answer 35.23. **The answer is A.**

Improvements in cryotherapy including intraoperative ultrasound to guide probe placement and the development of vacuum-insulated cryoprobes have improved the efficacy and reduced the morbidity of cryotherapy. Results in patients with metastatic neuroendocrine carcinomas have been particularly encouraging with greater than 90% reduction in 5-hydroxyindolacetic acid levels in almost all treated patients.

Whole liver irradiation offers only temporary symptomatic benefit and is associated with high incidence of radiation hepatitis. Attempts to decrease the radiation dose to the liver by combining radiation with chemotherapy have been reported with mixed success. This approach remains clearly investigational. Percutaneous ethanol injection has been most commonly studied in patients with unresectable hepatocellular carcinoma. Attempts to improve the outcome by addition of hepatic artery chemoembolization have also been reported, but this technique is contraindicated in this patient with occlusion of the portal vein.

Answer 35.24. **The answer is D.**

While repeated (large volume) paracentesis increases the cytologic detection of malignant ascites, if the initial cytology is positive, repeated paracentesis is unlikely to further identify the source. FDG-PET can be helpful in localizing sites of involvement but is usually not diagnostic. Laparoscopy identifies the cause of malignant ascites in approximately 60% of patients, while the addition of peritoneal biopsy identifies the cause in 85% of patients with malignant ascites of unknown source.

Answer 35.25. **The answer is C.**

In 50% to 75% of women presenting with malignant ascites, the cause is ultimately identified as a gynecologic neoplasm, most commonly ovarian carcinoma. Unless another source is clearly identified, these patients should be treated as ovarian cancer. These patients often have high response rates to platinum-based chemotherapy and 15% to 20% achieve results in long-term remission.

Answer 35.26. **The answer is C.**

High peritoneal fluid protein and LDH levels are diagnostic of malignant ascites. Chylous ascites is usually seen with obstruction or injury of the retroperitoneal lymphatic channels. Patients with bloody peritoneal fluid often encounter difficulties with peritoneovenous shunting due to clotting of the limbs of the shunt, which lead to occlusion and malfunction.

Answer 35.27. **The answer is C.**

Multiple small bowel air fluid levels usually indicate the presence of mechanical intestinal obstruction. Each of the other findings are common signs of abdominal ascites.

Answer 35.28. **The answer is D.**

Rapid drainage of large volume peritoneal fluid may be associated with volume overload, pulmonary edema, and, less frequently, with DIC. In the absence of underlying hepatic insufficiency, DIC is not a frequent complication of shunt placement but should be anticipated. Pulmonary tumor embolization is a rare complication of peritoneovenous shunt placement.

Answer 35.29. **The answer is C.**

Helical CT with the single breath-hold technique is more sensitive than conventional CT to detect small pulmonary nodules; however, the number of pulmonary nodules found at surgery is underestimated by both techniques. While the sensitivity of helical CT scanning to detect nodules greater than 6 mm is 95%, the sensitivity to detect smaller nodules drops to 60% to 70%.

Answer 35.30. **The answer is B.**

Recent surgical series have demonstrated that histology, disease-free interval, and number of pulmonary nodules influence prognosis. However, the most consistent predictor of survival is complete resection of all pulmonary nodules.

Answer 35.31. **The answer is A.**

Although some studies have indicated that metastases to both lungs have an adverse influence on prognosis, the presence of bilateral pulmonary metastases is not a contraindication to surgical resection as long as the other criteria listed above are met. Reresection of pulmonary nodules may be considered in patients who present with recurrent nodules, as long as the above criteria are fulfilled.

Answer 35.32. **The answer is C.**

Metastases from soft tissue sarcomas are usually limited to the lungs, making these patients especially attractive candidates for metastasectomy. Histology and disease-free interval as well as the number of metastatic lesions influence prognosis. Patients with liposarcoma, high-grade histology, disease free interval (DFI) less than 12 months, and multiple lesions have a less favorable prognosis and have a higher probability of relapse following surgical resection. Patients presenting with favorable features are reported to have 5-year survival rates of 35% to 45% with complete resection of pulmonary metastases.

Answer 35.33. **The answer is A.**

The 5-year survival of patients with colorectal cancer who are found to have hilar or mediastinal lymph node involvement at surgery is less than 10%. Resection of synchronous liver and lung metastases is also associated with a poor prognosis. Patients with incomplete resection of pulmonary metastases are destined to relapse even with current chemotherapy regimens. Interestingly, successful prior resection of hepatic metastases is not an adverse prognostic factor in patients with colorectal cancer undergoing resection of lung metastases.

Answer 35.34. **The answer is C.**

The lung is the most common site of metastases from NSGCT. However, these tumors are highly sensitive to platinum-based chemotherapy and are often curable with chemotherapy, even with advanced metastases. Surgical resection of residual pulmonary nodules following chemotherapy is recommended in patients whose tumor markers return to normal levels. These patients are at risk of having mature teratoma, which is not responsive to chemotherapy and may undergo degeneration into sarcoma or poorly differentiated carcinoma.

Answer 35.35. **The answer is C.**

In this patient with an enlarging pulmonary nodule without elevation of tumor markers, one has to suspect a teratoma. Because these tumors are not sensitive to chemotherapy and may undergo malignant degeneration, surgical resection is recommended. Additional chemotherapy is recommended if viable residual NSGCT is found at surgery.

Answer 35.36. **The answer is C.**

Postexpansion unilateral pulmonary edema is a serious complication of thoracentesis. It usually occurs in the setting of a large effusion and rapid drainage of the pleural space. When using vacuum bottles to collect the pleural fluid, it is advisable to clamp the drainage tube periodically to avoid this complication.

Answer 35.37. **The answer is C.**

Malignant pleural effusions are usually exudative. The criteria for exudative effusions are based on the fluid/serum protein ratio and/or LDH ratio. If at least one of the following three criteria are present, the fluid is almost always an exudate; if none is present, the fluid is virtually always a transudate:

- Pleural fluid protein/serum protein ratio greater than 0.5
- Pleural fluid LDH/serum LDH ratio greater than 0.6
- Pleural fluid LDH greater than two thirds of the upper limits of normal of the serum LDH

The fluid nucleated cell count is rarely diagnostic but can be helpful in certain settings, such as empyema. Cytologic evaluation is essential in the diagnosis of malignant pleural effusion.

Answer 35.38. **The answer is D.**

In the absence of effective systemic therapy, almost all malignant effusions will recur within 30 days of initial thoracentesis. Repeated thoracentesis can be performed but is usually reserved for patients who are debilitated and have a short predicted survival. Methods which obliterate the pleural space or chronic drainage procedures are more effective and practical in preventing recurrence of malignant pleural effusions.

Answer 35.39. **The answer is B.**

A variety of agents are currently in use to sclerose the pleural space. The most commonly used agents are talc, bleomycin, and doxycycline. In uncontrolled trials, talc appears to be the most effective agent with reported response rates of 72% to 100%. Doxycycline usually requires repeated instillations for pleurodesis. Bleomycin appears to be less effective than talc or doxycycline and is by far the most expensive of the three compounds. Adriamycin is an intense vesicant and has not been successful as a sclerosing agent due to poor efficacy and significant toxicities (e.g., pain, fever, emesis).

Answer 35.40. **The answer is C.**

The Pleurx indwelling intrapleural catheter is usually inserted under local anesthesia in an outpatient setting. Prospective randomized studies demonstrated treatment success in 92% of patients and spontaneous pleurodesis in 46% of patients. It is also particularly helpful in the situation of recurrent effusion and a trapped lung since it does not require obliteration of the pleural space to be effective. One disadvantage is the necessity of daily or every other day drainage, especially during the first few weeks after insertion of the catheter.

Answer 35.41. **The answer is C.**

Systemic chemotherapy is generally disappointing for the control of malignant pleural effusions. However, systemic therapy can be successful in controlling pleural effusions in patients with chemotherapy or hormone-therapy responsive diseases such as malignant lymphoma, Hodgkin disease, small cell lung cancer, germ cell tumors, and breast cancer. It is reasonable to offer a trial of systemic therapy to these patients before performing a chemical pleurodesis or placing a pleural catheter for chronic pleural drainage.

Answer 35.42. **The answer is D.**

Electrical alternans is recognized by the alternating lower and higher amplitude of the QRS complexes with every other heartbeat. This is thought to result from a pendulum motion of the heart as it swings from beat to beat within the fluid-distended pericardial sac. The most common cause of electrical alternans is a pericardial effusion.

Answer 35.43. **The answer is C.**

Echocardiography is the diagnostic procedure of choice when a pericardial effusion is suspected because of its high sensitivity and specificity. The procedure is rapid and does not require patient preparation or venous access. More importantly, echocardiography can also provide information regarding the hemodynamic significance of the effusion. Finally, echocardiography can be helpful to image the effusion during pericardiocentesis. Contrast-enhanced CT and MRI scans are also effective in imaging pericardial effusion but are more time consuming and costly than echocardiography.

Answer 35.44. **The answer is C.**

Subxyphoid pericardiostomy is now the most commonly performed surgical procedure for benign as well as malignant pericardial effusions. Following this procedure, the recurrence rate is less than 5%, and the overall morbidity and mortality rates are 1.5% and 0.5% respectively. Balloon-tube pericardiostomy can be considered in patients who are too frail for surgical pericardiostomy and can be performed at the bedside. It is, however, more painful than subxyphoid pericardiostomy and is associated with a higher risk of significant complications. Sclerotherapy is less effective than surgical pericardiostomy, usually requires multiple instillations, and can be very painful, especially if using tetracycline or doxycycline.

CHAPTER **36**

Hematopoietic Therapy

GIANCARLO PILLOT, JANAKIRAMAN SUBRAMANIAN, KRISTIN L. HENNENFENT, AND RAMASWAMY GOVINDAN

Directions Each of the numbered items below is followed by lettered answers. Select the ONE lettered answer that is BEST in each case unless instructed otherwise.

QUESTIONS

Question 36.1. **In computer cross-matching for blood products, all of the following tests are done EXCEPT**

A. antibody screening
B. ABO typing
C. Rh typing
D. conventional cross-matching

Question 36.2. **For patients requiring platelet transfusions, ABO typing is done to avoid**

A. acute intravascular hemolytic transfusion reactions
B. immunization of Rh-negative recipients
C. reduction by 10% to 20% in posttransfusion platelet increment
D. A, B, and C
E. B and C

Question 36.3. **The following are indications for fresh frozen plasma (FFP) transfusions EXCEPT**

A. hemophilia A
B. rapid reversal of warfarin therapy
C. disseminated intravascular coagulation (DIC)
D. bleeding diatheses secondary to liver disease
E. hypofibrinogenemia

Question 36.4. **Cryoprecipitate is not used alone in the treatment of DIC because it is deficient in**

A. factor V
B. fibronectin
C. factor VIII
D. von Willebrand factor (VWF)
E. fibrinogen

Corresponding Chapters in *Cancer: Principles & Practice of Oncology*, Seventh Edition: 52 (Hematopoietic Therapy).

Question 36.5. **Leukoreduction in blood transfusion products has all of the following benefits EXCEPT**

A. decreasing the incidence of febrile transfusion reactions
B. reducing cytomegalovirus (CMV) transmission
C. decreasing the risk of human leukocyte antigen (HLA) alloimmunization
D. delaying platelet refractoriness
E. preventing graft versus host disease (GVHD)

Question 36.6. **All of the following are adverse reactions seen in granulocyte donors due to apheresis EXCEPT**

A. anaphylaxis
B. fluid retention
C. hypercalcemia
D. hypotension

Question 36.7. **Albumin transfusions are used for all of the following indications EXCEPT**

A. volume expansion
B. to replace plasma removed during apheresis
C. nutritional source in chronic protein deficiency states
D. after large volume paracentesis hypoalbuminemia due to liver disease

Question 36.8. **The following can be seen in both delayed extravascular hemolytic reactions (DHTRs) and acute intravascular hemolytic reactions (AIHTRs) EXCEPT**

A. antibodies against red blood cell antigens
B. elevated lactate dehydrogenase (LDH)
C. cytokine storm
D. positive direct *Coombs* test

Question 36.9. **A 75-year-old woman presents at the emergency department with diffuse petechial rash and nosebleed. She otherwise feels well. She has a platelet count of 7K, normal creatinine, normal mental status, and no fever. She received a red blood cell (RBC) transfusion 8 days prior, complicated by a mild fever but otherwise uneventful, and she had been sent home after a period of observation. She has not used any heparin products. Which of the following statements about this case is NOT true?**

A. The patient has developed an antiplatelet antibody, typically anti-PLA1.
B. Treatment may include corticosteroids.
C. Treatment may include intravenous immunoglobin (IVIg).
D. This condition will resolve when the patient clears the transfused cells.
E. This condition only occurs after transfusion of platelets.

Question 36.10. **A 56-year-old white man diagnosed with non-Hodgkin lymphoma receives a RBC transfusion for anemia secondary to his malignancy. Within 1-hour posttransfusion, the patient is complaining of chills, cough, shortness of breath, and fatigue. His vital signs are temp 37.5°C, heart rate (HR) 98, respiratory rate (RR) 24, blood pressure (BP) 96/60, and saturation 82%. On physical examination, the patient is found to be in distress and is tachypneic. On auscultation, diffuse rales are heard in all lung fields. A chest x-ray shows diffuse bilateral fluffy infiltrates. Review of his transfused blood and patient armband confirm the correct unit was given to the correct patient. Which of the following is true regarding this condition?**

A. Corticosteroids are indicated for this condition.
B. Immediate broad-spectrum antibiotics improve mortality.
C. The likelihood of reoccurrence is high during future transfusions.
D. The clinical picture is compatible with transfusion-associated acute lung injury.

Question 36.11. **A 67-year-old white woman diagnosed with non-small cell lung cancer receives a unit of RBCs for her anemia. Within a few minutes post-transfusion, the patient develops fever, chills, and severe rigors. Her vital signs are temp 38.6°C, HR 86, RR 20, BP 88/56, and saturation 89%. Physical examination is insignificant except for diffuse warmth and flushing. Review of her transfused blood and patient armband confirm the correct unit was given to the correct patient. All of the following statements are true EXCEPT**

A. immediate broad-spectrum antibiotics are indicated
B. gram stain is not a very sensitive test for this condition
C. most likely the cause is a gram-negative organism
D. platelet transfusions are associated with higher incidence rates for this condition
E. patient's blood culture is sufficient to make the diagnosis

Question 36.12. **A 26-year-old white postpartum woman received two units of packed RBCs for excessive intrapartum blood loss. Posttransfusion, the patient's hemoglobin and hematocrit were 11.6 g per dL and 33 respectively. Four days later, the patient had hemoglobin and hematocrit of 9.1 g per dL and 28. The patient denied any symptoms and her vital signs were temp 37°C, HR 86, RR 16, BP 110/72, and saturation 96%. Further examination did not indicate any evidence of hemorrhage. The laboratory tests revealed elevated lactate dehydrogenase, unconjugated bilirubin, and positive direct Coombs test. You would**

A. start intravenous (IV) fluids to maintain a urine output of 100 mL per hr
B. begin prednisone at a dose of 1 mg per kg
C. follow her without any intervention
D. begin intravenous cyclophosphamide

Question 36.13. **A 76-year-old white man with stage IV colon carcinoma and iron deficiency anemia is given a unit of RBCs. Immediately after commencing the transfusion, the patient develops low-grade fever, pruritus, and diffuse rash. On physical exam, the patient has diffuse erythema and maculopapular rash. Subsequently, the patient continues to develop similar reactions to RBC transfusions, which are extremely uncomfortable for him. The best step in the management of this patient's anemia is to**

A. irradiate future RBC transfusions
B. transfuse washed RBCs in which the donor plasma has been removed
C. identify the antibody and perform plasmapheresis
D. give IVIg infusions
E. administer corticosteroids prior to transfusions

Question 36.14. **All units of blood collected in the United States are tested for all of the following EXCEPT**

A. human immunodeficiency virus (HIV)
B. hepatitis B virus (HBV)
C. hepatitis C virus (HCV)
D. human T-lymphotrophic virus (HTLV) I/II
E. CMV

Question 36.15. **Patients with immunoglobulin A (IgA) deficiency should not receive IVIG because of the risk of developing**

A. severe and extensive skin rash
B. anaphylaxis
C. infection
D. development of renal failure

Question 36.16. **For which blood product did the American Association of Blood Banks (AABB) require pretransfusion bacterial testing from 2004 onward?**

A. Granulocytes.
B. Platelets.
C. RBCs.
D. Fresh frozen plasma (FFP).
E. Cryoprecipitate.

Question 36.17. **Which of the following statements regarding CD34+ cells is true?**

A. CD34 is present on nearly all colony-forming progenitor units.
B. CD34 is a marker for pluripotent as well as more committed progenitor cells.
C. The CD34 cell count of stem cell product is the most reliable marker of rapidity of engraftment after high-dose chemotherapy.
D. CD34 cells can be rapidly measured by flow cytometric techniques.
E. All of the above.

Question 36.18. **Which of the following regarding CD34+ cells in the setting of autologous stem cell transplant is correct?**

A. A CD34 cell count of 2.5×10^6 per kg is generally considered to be an adequate stem cell dose for engraftment after high-dose therapy (HDT).
B. A CD34 dose greater than 5.0×10^6 per kg is associated with more rapid neutrophil recovery than a dose between 2.5×10^6 per kg and 5.0×10^6 per kg.
C. CD34 doses of less than 2.5×10^6 per kg are not associated with delayed platelet engraftment.
D. Peripheral blood CD34 cells may not be mobilized immediately after the use of most chemotherapy due to its cytotoxic effect.
E. None of the above.

Question 36.19. **Which of the following factors is associated with poor stem cell mobilization?**

A. Prior use of fludarabine.
B. Prior use of melphalan.
C. Number of prior regimens.
D. C and B.
E. All of the above.

Question 36.20. **A 45-year-old patient with non-Hodgkin lymphoma in remission for whom high-dose chemotherapy with autologous stem cell rescue is planned has undergone stem cell mobilization with G-CSF alone; a stem cell dose of 1.1 CD34+ cells per kg has been collected. Which of the following is/are appropriate?**

A. Proceed with high-dose chemotherapy, using G-CSF to speed engraftment after stem cells have been infused.
B. Recollect stem cells after another mobilization, but this time use a higher dose of G-CSF.
C. Recollect stem cells after another mobilization, but this time use chemo mobilization followed by G-CSF.
D. Recollect stem cells after another mobilization, but this time use GM-CSF and G-CSF.
E. B or C.

Question 36.21. **Which of the following statements is true about the use of hematopoietic growth factors after autologous stem cell infusion?**

A. G-CSF is necessary for engraftment of the stem cells and count recovery.
B. Most studies do not reveal a shortening of the period of neutropenia.
C. There is a clear benefit to initiating G-CSF immediately after stem cell infusion.
D. There is an advantage in terms of time to neutrophil recovery with higher G-CSF doses, albeit at a cost of a greater number and intensity of side effects.
E. Use of G-CSF after stem cell infusion is associated with a small but statistically significant shortened duration of hospital stay.

Question 36.22. **Which of the following toxicities may complicate allogeneic but not autologous stem cell transplant?**

A. Mucositis.
B. Febrile neutropenia.
C. Venoocclusive disease (VOD) of the liver.
D. GVHD.
E. C and D.

Question 36.23. **Strategies undergoing evaluation that may improve the therapeutic effect of autologous stem cell transplant include which of the following.**

A. Purging of tumor cells from the stem cell product.
B. Increase intensity via the addition of more agents to conditioning.
C. Perform sequential courses of high-dose chemotherapy with stem cell rescue.
D. Perform a reduced-intensity allogeneic transplant after the autologous transplant.
E. All of the above.

Question 36.24. **Which of the following statements regarding conditioning regimens for allogeneic stem cell transplant is NOT true?**

A. Chemotherapy-based conditioning regimens are typically associated with greater risk of secondary malignancies, cataracts, and growth retardation than total-body irradiation (TBI)-based regimens.
B. Higher doses of TBI or chemotherapy-based conditioning regimens are associated with decreased rates of relapse.
C. Conditioning regimens are intended to eradicate as many malignant cells as possible.
D. Conditioning regimens are intended to cause immunosuppression.
E. Busulfan conditioning is associated with a risk of VOD.

Question 36.25. **Which of the following is evidence of a graft versus leukemia (GVL) effect?**

A. There is an increased recurrence rate of leukemia in matched sibling transplants as opposed to twin transplants.
B. Lack of GVHD is associated with decreased relapse rates.
C. T-cell depleted stem cell sources are associated with decreased GVHD and increased recurrence rates.
D. Withdrawal of immunosuppression in the setting of cytogenetic relapse has not been associated with cases of reinduction of cytogenetic remission in CML.
E. All of the above.

Question 36.26. **Which of the following statements is NOT true regarding chemotherapy-induced complications of transplant?**

A. Late hemorrhagic cystitis (occurring after 72 hours) from high-dose cyclophosphamide administration can be prevented by use of mesna, hydration, and maintenance of adequate urine output.
B. Hemorrhagic cystitis in the first 72 hours of high-dose cyclophosphamide is typically related to viral infection such as BK virus or adenovirus.
C. High-dose busulfan is associated with a risk of seizure, which may be decreased by prophylactic use of antiepileptic drugs such as Dilantin.
D. High-dose busulfan is associated with a risk of VOD.
E. A and B.

Question 36.27. **A 45-year-old patient has undergone cytoxan and TBI conditioning for her matched sibling allogeneic transplant. During the infusion of her stem cell product, she becomes flushed, rigorous, hypoxic, and mildly hypotensive; she continues to mentate well and complains only of wheezing. She stabilizes with IV fluids and supplemental oxygen by nasal cannula. Which of the following is true?**

A. She is experiencing acute GVHD.
B. She is experiencing acute interstitial pneumonitis (IP) related to her conditioning.
C. She is experiencing CMV reactivation from donor lymphocytes.
D. The incidence and severity of this reaction is decreased by red blood cell reduction of the stem cell product and pretreating the patient with steroids and antihistamines prior to infusion.
E. Her stem cell product infusion should be stopped and sent to the lab for testing in the morning.

Question 36.28. **Which of the following statement(s) is/are true regarding infections in the neutropenic period after conditioning for stem cell transplant?**

A. Fluconazole fungal prophylaxis decreases the incidence of candidal and aspergillus infections.
B. Prophylactic oral quinolones decrease the incidence of gram-negative infections but may be associated with an increased risk of gram-positive infections.
C. Voriconazole is not as effective as amphotericin B in the treatment of acute invasive aspergillosis.
D. Patient contact during conditioning-induced neutropenia should be limited to decrease spread of bacteria and fungal infections from visitors to the patient, which is the most common source of opportunistic infections.
E. B and D.

Question 36.29. **A 32-year-old woman is 10 days postconditioning for allogeneic stem cell transplant with a busulfan-based regimen. She develops right upper quadrant abdominal pain, mild jaundice, and her weight has increased 6 kilograms in the last 2 days. Which of the following is true?**

A. Her condition could have been effectively prevented by use of heparin post-conditioning.
B. Her condition is more likely associated with the busulfan-containing regimen.
C. The course of her condition is typically benign, with a less than 2% mortality rate.
D. Acute GVHD is not a risk factor for her condition.
E. Broad-spectrum antibiotics should be immediately initiated for this condition.

Question 36.30. **All of the following interventions may reduce the incidence of interstitial pneumonitis EXCEPT**

A. early detection and treatment of CMV
B. using a conditioning regimen that reduces or eliminates radiation dose to the lung parenchyma
C. use of a busulfan-conditioning regimen
D. hyperfractionation of TBI in the conditioning regimen
E. none of the above

Question 36.31. **Which of the following statements is true regarding secondary malignancies associated with allogeneic stem cell transplant?**

A. Patients who have received an allogeneic transplant are at no higher risk for malignancy than age-matched controls.
B. Most secondary solid tumor malignancies occur within the first year of transplant.
C. Secondary lymphomas are typically not Epstein-Barr virus (EBV) related.
D. Chronic skin GVHD is associated with increased risk of squamous cell carcinoma of the skin.

Question 36.32. **Which of the following statements are manifestations of GVHD related to stem cell transplant?**

A. Skin rash.
B. Hyperbilirubinemia and transaminitis.
C. Diarrhea.
D. Crampy abdominal pain.
E. All of the above.

Question 36.33. **T-cell depletion of the allograft is associated with which of the following.**

A. Decreased risk of graft rejection.
B. Decreased risk of GVHD.
C. Decreased risk of opportunistic viral infection.
D. Decreased risk of leukemia relapse posttransplant.

Question 36.34. **Which of the following statements is NOT true regarding the treatment of acute GVHD in the posttransplant setting?**

A. Approximately 50% of patients respond to corticosteroid/cyclosporine therapy.
B. Response of GVHD to steroids predicts survival from GVHD.
C. Antithymocyte globulin (ATG) clearly improves survival in the steroid refractory GVHD setting.
D. The high mortality rate in steroid-refractory GVHD is partially related to chronic immunosuppression and infectious complications.
E. The majority of steroid refractory GVHD patients die as a consequence of their GVHD.

Question 36.35. **Which of the following patients is at greatest risk of morbidity from CMV reactivation in the postallogeneic stem cell transplant setting?**

A. A CMV(−) host receiving CMV negative blood products.
B. A CMV(−) host receiving leuko-filtered blood products.
C. A CMV(+) host receiving CMV(−) stem cell donor.
D. A CMV(+) host receiving CMV(+) stem cell donor and receiving ganciclovir prophylaxis.

Question 36.36. **Which of the following statements regarding the role of allogeneic transplant is true in the setting of CML treatment?**

A. There is no longer a role for stem cell transplant now that imatinib is an available therapy.
B. Patients in chronic phase transplanted within a year of diagnosis have the best long-term outcomes.
C. CML is subject to a significant graft versus leukemia effect.
D. B and C.
E. A, B, and C.

Question 36.37. **Which of the following statements is NOT true regarding nonmyeloablative conditioning for stem cell transplant?**

A. Donor and recipient lymphoid and myeloid elements are often both present at the time of engraftment.
B. Donor lymphocyte infusions may be a part of a nonmyeloablative transplant regimen to enhance graft versus tumor effect.
C. Acute toxicity and early transplant-related mortality is relatively low in the nonmyeloablative transplant setting.
D. Due to decreased degree and duration of neutropenia, patients who have undergone nonmyeloablative transplant rarely suffer from opportunistic fungal infections.
E. Graft rejection occurs more frequently in the setting of nonmyeloablative transplant.

Question 36.38. **Which of the following factors does NOT contribute to chronic anemia in cancer patients?**

A. Marrow progenitor cell impaired response to erythropoietin (EPO).
B. Treatment-related bone marrow toxicity.
C. Elevated endogenous EPO levels.
D. Impaired iron utilization.
E. Tumor infiltration of bone marrow.

Question 36.39. **Which of the following statement(s) is/are correct?**

I. Darbepoetin alpha is identical to endogenous human erythropoietin.
II. Following initiation of recombinant human erythropoietins, rise in red cell count does not begin until 2 weeks of continuous dosing.
III. Recombinant human erythropoietins should be routinely considered in cancer patients with Hgb less than or equal to 10 mg per dL.

A. I only.
B. III only.
C. I and II.
D. II and III.
E. I, II, and III.

Question 36.40. **JL is a 52-year-old white woman who presents to the clinic for follow-up after 3 courses of CHOP chemotherapy for treatment of non-Hodgkin lymphoma. The patient received the last cycle of chemotherapy 4 weeks ago. Routine laboratory evaluation reveals Hgb/Hct 8.1/24.4. The patient weighs 62 kg. Which of the following are appropriate initial dosing recommendations for epoetin alpha?**

A. Epoetin alpha 9,300 units subcutaneous (SC) 3 times per week or epoetin alpha 40,000 units weekly times 4 weeks.
B. Epoetin alpha 18,600 units SC 3 times per week times 2 weeks.
C. Epoetin alpha 40,000 units SC once weekly times 2 weeks.
D. Epoetin alpha 60,000 units SC once weekly times 4 weeks.

Question 36.41. **JL returns to clinic 4 weeks after initiation of epoetin alpha. Laboratory evaluation reveals Hgb 9.8 mg per dL. Which of the following recommendations would be indicated at this time?**

A. Discontinue therapy due to absence of response.
B. Continue initial dosing recommendation indefinitely.
C. Switch patient to darbepoetin alpha.
D. Increase dose of epoetin alpha.
E. Continue treatment with epoetin alpha until Hgb normalizes near 12 mg per dL.

Question 36.42. **Which of the following clinical situations justifies primary prophylaxis of a colony stimulating factor?**

A. Receiving chemotherapy regimen associated with incidence of febrile neutropenia greater than or equal to 20%.
B. Receiving palliative chemotherapy.
C. Maintaining treatment intensity that is associated with prolonged disease-free survival.
D. A and B.
E. A and C.

Question 36.43. **JT is a 61-year-old white woman who presents following a first cycle of sequential doxorubicin and cyclophosphamide (AC) followed by paclitaxel (T) adjuvant chemotherapy for treatment of lymph-node positive breast cancer. Treatment was planned on an every 21-day schedule. On day 11, JT presented to the emergency department with temperature of 101.7°F and activated neutrophil count (ANC) of 0.3. Patient was admitted to the hospital and received intravenous antibiotic therapy. Routine laboratory evaluation reveals WBC 1.8, ANC 0.6, Hg 12.3, and Hct 31. Treatment is delayed 1 week to await neutrophil recovery. Which of the following treatment options would be viable as secondary prophylaxis for JT after a second cycle of adjuvant chemotherapy?**

A. Filgrastim 10 μg per kg SC daily until ANC 1,000 cells per mm^3.
B. Pegfilgrastim 6 mg SC times 1 dose immediately following chemotherapy administration.
C. Sargramostim 500 μg per m^2 SC daily until ANC 1,000 cells per mm^3.
D. Sargramostim 250 μg per m^2 SC times 1 dose 24 hours after chemotherapy administration.
E. Filgrastim 5 μg per kg SC daily until ANC 1,000 cells per mm^3.

Question 36.44. **Which of the following statement(s) is/are correct?**

I. Exogenous administration of rHu G-CSF increases level of circulating neutrophils.
II. Serum clearance of pegfilgrastim is directly related to blood neutrophil concentrations.
III. GM-CSF stimulates macrophage as well as granulocyte lineages.

A. I only.
B. III only.
C. I and II.
D. II and III.
E. I, II, and III.

Question 36.45. **Which of the following toxicities is/are associated with administration of rHu IL-11?**

A. Fluid retention.
B. Bone pain.
C. Dyspnea.
D. A and C.
E. B and C.

Question 36.46. **Which of the following statement(s) is/are true?**

I. Secondary prophylaxis with filgrastim at doses higher than recommended may provide additional clinical benefit for prevention of febrile neutropenia.
II. rHu IL-11 has demonstrated a reduction in platelet transfusions following chemotherapy.
III. Pegfilgrastim must not be administered fewer than or equal to 14 days prior to chemotherapy administration.

A. I only.
B. III only.
C. I and II.
D. II and III.
E. I, II, and III.

ANSWERS

Answer 36.1. **The answer is D.**

Computer cross-matching is a recently introduced method that does not require a true serologic cross-matching. Patients of known ABO and Rh types and who already have a documented negative antibody screen are provided computer-selected ABO and Rh-compatible blood while omitting the cross-match step. This method is safe if appropriate measures are taken to avoid clerical errors and proper patient identification.

Answer 36.2. **The answer is E.**

Acute intravascular hemolytic transfusion reactions do not occur in platelet transfusions because the transfusion product has very few red cells as contaminants. Immunization of Rh-negative patients can occur if they are transfused Rh-positive platelets; this is especially important in female patients of childbearing age to prevent future hemolytic disease of the newborn. This can be avoided by transfusing Rh-negative platelets or by administration of Rh immune globulin within 72 hours of transfusion. Transfusion of ABO compatible platelets is a level IIA recommendation. Transfusing ABO incompatible platelets may not have a large effect on the post-transfusion platelet count or the effectiveness of the transfused platelets (which is probably due to the low density of the antigens on the platelets). However, destruction of platelets and reduction in the posttransfusion levels has been observed in patients, particularly in those who have high Anti-A/Anti-B titers. This can be an especially significant problem in children.

Answer 36.3. **The answer is A.**

FFP transfusions are not indicated for individual coagulation factor deficiencies due to the large volume of FFP required to achieve the desired level of the factor in the plasma. Such large volumes can result in volume overload, pulmonary edema, and congestive failure. Hence, it is recommended that whenever individual coagulation factors are available they should be used for coagulation factor deficiency. Bleeding secondary to warfarin therapy is an indication for FFP. It is also indicated in DIC and bleeding diatheses secondary to multiple clotting factor deficiencies. It can also be used in hypofibrinogenemia although cryoprecipitate is preferred.

Answer 36.4. **The answer is A.**

A single 10- to 15-mL unit of cryoprecipitate contains fibrinogen (100 to 350 mg per bag), factor VIII (at least 80 IU per bag), some von Willebrand factor, factor XIII, and fibronectin. It does not have factor V; hence, it should not be used alone in DIC. In acute decompensated DIC, there is consumption of factor V along with factor VII, prothrombin, fibrinogen, and platelets, and thus cryoprecipitate is lacking in many plasma components consumed in this process. In chronic compensated DIC, usual factor levels are normal and transfusion of platelets and FFP is not useful unless the patient is bleeding or is at a high risk for bleeding.

Answer 36.5. **The answer is E.**

In oncology patients requiring multiple transfusions, leukoreduced blood products are used to delay the onset and reduce the incidence of developing HLA alloantibodies. Leukocytes in blood components can provoke febrile nonhemolytic reactions, induce HLA alloimmunization, and transmit CMV to both immunocompetent and immunosuppressed recipients. Leukoreduction reduces the incidence and severity of febrile transfusion reactions (but does not completely prevent it) and decreases the risk of HLA alloimmunization. Specifically, leukoreduced products are less likely to stimulate the HLA alloantibodies implicated in both febrile transfusion reactions and antibody-mediated platelet reactions. Other generally accepted benefits of white cell reduction include delaying platelet refractoriness and decreasing the risk of transmitting white cell-related infectious agents including CMV and HTLV-I/II. GVHD has been described in the setting of leukoreduced (and not irradiated) blood products, and, therefore, leukoreduction without irradiation is inadequate to prevent GVHD.

Answer 36.6. **The answer is C.**

The collection of granulocytes by apheresis is associated with complications to the donor related to the collection process. The donor can develop allergic reactions to FFP or any other plasma replacement agent, which can be severe enough to result in anaphylaxis. They can develop volume retention due to hydroxyethyl starch, which is used as a sedimenting agent to maximize granulocyte yields. They can develop hypocalcemia due to the use of citrate as an anticoagulant, which acts by binding calcium. Hypotension can occur as a result of volume shifts during the pheresis process. Hypercalcemia is not typically caused by the pheresis procedures nor chemicals used during the process.

Answer 36.7. **The answer is C.**

An albumin transfusion can be used for volume expansion even though it has been replaced by others. It is used as a replacement for plasma in apheresis and rarely to replace albumin in hypoalbuminemia. But it is not sufficient as a nutritional source for patients with chronic protein deficiency.

Answer 36.8. **The answer is C.**

Both DHTRs and AIHTRs have features in common. The pathogenesis of both involves development of antibodies to red cell antigens. Elevation of LDH is seen in both of these causes of hemolysis. Both display a positive direct *Coombs* test due to antibodies adhering to the transfused cells. However, the cytokine storm seen in patients with AIHTRs is not seen in DHTRs so that patients with DHTRs do not usually display hemodynamic instability. Patients with DHTRs are typically asymptomatic and a fall in hematocrit may be the only clinical feature.

Answer 36.9. **The answer is D.**

This patient has developed posttransfusion purpura, a rare complication of transfusion with any blood product. It typically occurs when a PLA-1 negative patient develops anti-PLA-1 antibodies; this antibody then attacks the patient's own platelets via an "innocent bystander" mechanism. Treatment may involve corticosteroids, IVIG, or even plasma exchange.

Answer 36.10. **The answer is D.**

This patient has developed respiratory distress following a transfusion. He is hypoxemic and chest x-ray finding is consistent with pulmonary edema; the diagnosis is transfusion-related acute lung injury (TRALI). In this condition, corticosteroids may be helpful; however, there have been no prospective randomized studies that prove the benefit of steroids for TRALI. Antibiotics have no role in the initial management. Up to 80% to 90% survive with supportive respiratory care, which may include oxygen supplementation or mechanical ventilation.

Answer 36.11. **The answer is E.**

This patient has a high fever, hypotension with diffuse warmth, and flushing, all of which are signs indicating septic shock. The cause is septic transfusion reaction (STR) due to contaminated blood product. Bacterial contamination is more common than viral or fungal contamination of blood products. Antibiotics have to be started immediately without waiting for blood culture results. Gram stain may be positive for the causative organism; however, it is not sensitive enough and blood culture is required to confirm the diagnosis. In red blood cell transfusions, *Yersinia enterocolitica* is common because it can withstand refrigeration and can use hemoglobin as a substrate to survive. Refrigeration of red blood cells markedly diminishes the growth of most bacteria, with bacterial contamination rate at 1 in 30,000 units. The risk of septic transfusion reactions (STRs) is higher for platelet transfusions than for other blood components because platelets are stored at room temperature, with bacteria contamination rate of 1 in 2,000 to 3,000 units. When STR is suspected, both the recipient's blood as well as the blood component being transfused has to be cultured.

Answer 36.12. **The answer is C.**

This young woman has developed an unexplained drop in hematocrit, with no signs of hemorrhage. She has an elevated lactate dehydrogenase, unconjugated bilirubin, and direct Coombs test is positive. This evidence of hemolysis with a newly positive direct Coombs several days after the transfusion is typical of delayed extravascular hemolytic reactions (DHTRs). This condition is usually self-limited and manifested only by a drop in hematocrit that resolves after the hemolysis stops. IV fluids are not needed in this patient since her vital signs are stable and her volume status appears to be normal. Prednisone is not indicated for this self-limiting condition. Even though this condition is caused by antibodies to Rh, Duffy, Kidd, and Kell blood group antigens and testing for them confirms diagnosis, it has no role in immediate management. However, the offending antigen is best identified so that the hemolytic reaction can be avoided in future transfusions. These patients do not need any acute intervention except for follow-up until the hemolysis resolves.

Answer 36.13. **The answer is B.**

This patient has developed an allergic reaction to the transfusion. He continues to have repeated allergic reactions to RBC transfusions, which are clinically bothersome. The use of irradiated blood products is unlikely to prevent these reactions as they are typically to plasma components. Plasmapheresis and IVIG are not the treatment options for such allergic reactions. Corticosteroids prior to transfusion may help suppress these reactions, but in patients with repeated or severe reactions, their usefulness is limited. Washed red blood cells in which the residual donor plasma has been removed and replaced by saline may benefit patients with repeated or severe allergic reactions.

Answer 36.14. **The answer is E.**

Transfusion transmitted disease (TTD) testing in the United States includes screening for syphilis; hepatitis B (HBsAg, anti-Hbc); hepatitis C (anti-HCV, HCV NAT); HIV (anti-HIV-1/2, HIV NAT); HTLV (anti-HTLV-I/II); and West Nile virus (NAT). CMV is not tested for routinely.

Answer 36.15. **The answer is B.**

Patients who have IgA deficiency are at risk of developing anaphylaxis due to formation of anti-IgA immunoglobulin, which is usually a IgG antibody. For these patients, IgA-deficient preparations should be used.

Answer 36.16. **The answer is B.**

Platelets have a higher incidence of bacterial contamination: 1 in 2,000 units to 1 in 3,000 units. This is due to the fact that platelets are typically stored at room temperature to maintain function and shelf life. Refrigeration has reduced the incidence of bacteria contamination rate in red blood cells to 1 in 30,000 units, which is not typically used for platelets. Other products such as granulocytes, FFP, and cryoprecipitate can also be refrigerated. This is the reason for the AABB to require routine pretransfusion bacterial testing.

Answer 36.17. **The answer is E.**

CD34 is a cell surface marker that was found to be present on the surface of colony forming units on *in vitro* assays. It appears to be a marker of early hematopoietic cells, likely both pluripotent cells as well as cells that may be more committed to a certain cell line (i.e., megakaryocytic, granulocytic, or erythropoietic cell lines). The number of CD34+ cells in a collected stem cell product is closely associated with rapidity of cell count recovery, and these cells can be easily measured by flow cytometric techniques.

Answer 36.18. **The answer is A.**

A CD34 dose of greater than 5.0×10^6 is generally considered optimal, with the most rapid recovery of cell counts after HDT. Intermediate doses (between 2.5×10^6 and 5.0×10^6) are felt to have similar neutrophil recovery time, but more patients will have delay of platelet recovery; this dose is felt to be an acceptable amount for recovery after HDT. Lower doses are associated with high rates of either delayed platelet recovery or quite prolonged delay of platelet recovery, and must be used with caution. Mobilization of peripheral blood CD34+ cells may be pursued by use of either G-CSF or chemotherapy followed by G-CSF.

Answer 36.19. **The answer is E.**

The most important factor determining adequacy of stem cell mobilization is how heavily the patient has been pretreated. Alkylating agents are the most notorious for subsequent poor stem cell collection, but fludarabine has also been shown to be associated with poor collection.

Answer 36.20. **The answer is E.**

When faced with an inadequate stem cell collection, there are a few possible courses of action. The collected dose of stem cells can be used for stem cell rescue after high-dose chemotherapy despite low collection numbers, but this must be done with caution using such low collections. Although there is no clearly accepted standard approach, use of higher doses of G-CSF or chemo mobilization and G-CSF are certainly reasonable options. The concomitant use of GM and G-CSF does not appear more effective than the use of higher doses of G-CSF alone.

Answer 36.21. **The answer is E.**

There is considerable controversy regarding the utility of hematopoietic growth factors. Although most studies show a shortening of the period of neutropenia and duration of hospitalization, there is no survival benefit, and its omission will not in any way prevent engraftment. If G-CSF is used posttransplant, most but not all studies suggest that there is little advantage to beginning G-CSF immediately versus delaying 5 to 7 days after stem cell infusion, and there does not appear to be any advantage for using higher doses of G-CSF in the posttransplant period.

Answer 36.22. **The answer is D.**

Toxicities related to conditioning regimens are shared by both autologous and allogeneic stem cell transplant: nausea, vomiting, mucositis, neutropenia, and opportunistic infection all can complicate any chemotherapy. Venoocclusive disease of the liver is no exception, and any conditioning regimen can cause it. Graft versus host disease is unique to allogeneic transplant as a phenomenon of alloreactive donor T-cells recognizing host tissues.

Answer 36.23. **The answer is E.**

There are several limitations to autologous stem cell transplant that prevent it from being a cure for many patients. The intensity of the chemotherapy, while enough to cause myeloablation, may be insufficient to completely kill all residual tumor cells. Increasing the doses of conditioning agents or adding additional agents may increase therapeutic effect, although these strategies have not met with significant success. Performing a "tandem" autologous stem cell transplant is a strategy that may maximize tumor cell kill and has some evidence for its utility in the setting of multiple myeloma, although this is not universally accepted. Contaminating tumor cells in the autologous stem cell product may also contribute to relapse after transplant. Purging of tumor cells is a strategy to minimize this effect; data regarding its utility have been mixed. Finally, after high-dose chemotherapy with stem cell rescue, attempting reduced intensity allogeneic transplant to take advantage of an immunologic graft versus tumor effect during a state of minimal residual disease is being investigated and may have utility in the setting of low-grade lymphoma.

Answer 36.24. **The answer is A.**

Conditioning regimens for allogeneic stem cell transplant serve the dual role of eradicating malignant cells to a minimal level and creating a sufficiently immunosuppressed state to allow for stem cell engraftment. Increasing doses of TBI or chemotherapy in conditioning regimens are typically associated with decreased relapse rate but are limited by excessive toxicity. Busulfan conditioning regimens are particularly associated with VOD. In general, TBI-based regimens are associated with greater risk of secondary malignancies, cataracts, hypothyroidism, and growth retardation, while chemotherapy-based regimens are associated with a greater risk of VOD.

Answer 36.25. **The answer is C.**

Graft versus leukemia effect has been postulated based on the observation that the incidence of GVHD is associated with a decrease in relapse rates in leukemia. Typically, GVHD and GVL are closely linked; twin (as opposed to matched sibling) transplants and T-cell depletion of stem cell product are associated with decreased rates of GVHD but increased relapse rates. Further evidence for a donor immune-related effect of the allograft is reinduction of remission following withdrawal of immunosuppression in the setting of cytogenetic relapse after transplant for CML.

Answer 36.26. **The answer is E.**

There are early and late (occurring after 72 hours) forms of high-dose cyclophosphamide-induced hemorrhagic cystitis. Early hemorrhagic cystitis is the result of a direct toxic effect on the bladder, usually prevented by use of mesna, hydration, and maintenance of adequate urine output. Late hemorrhagic cystitis is typically related to viral infection such as BK virus or adenovirus in the setting of profound immunosuppression. High-dose busulfan-containing regimens are associated with increased risk of seizure, which can be ameliorated by prophylaxis, and with increased risk of VOD.

Answer 36.27. **The answer is D.**

This patient is demonstrating signs and symptoms of a mild hemolytic transfusion reaction. In her case, A+ stem cells from her sibling were infused into the patient, who is O+. This is too early for GVHD, and the acuity argues against IP and CMV reactivation. Steps to reduce this are red blood cell reduction of the stem cell product and premedication. Such transfusion reactions, if they occur at all, are typically mild and self-limited and only require observation. The stem cell product, although it may be paused briefly during evaluation of the patient, should typically never be withheld from the patient as it is the patient's only route to count recovery and avoidance of a cytopenic death.

Answer 36.28. **The answer is B.**

Opportunistic infections during conditioning-induced neutropenia most often originate from the host, rather than person-to-person spread. Prophylactic quinolone antibiotics directed at gram-negative bacteria appear to decrease the incidence of gram-negative opportunistic infection but may be associated with greater risk of gram-positive infection. Fluconazole prophylaxis, while decreasing the incidence of certain *Candida* species infections, is ineffective against *Candida krusei* and *Aspergillus* species. Randomized studies have shown therapeutic equivalence of voriconazole and amphotericin B; voriconazole may have a more favorable side-effect profile.

Answer 36.29. **The answer is B.**

This patient has likely developed VOD of the liver, which is a serious, life-threatening complication of transplant. It is associated with busulfan conditioning, recent Mylotarg use, acute GVH, and intensity of conditioning. It progresses to severe life-threatening disease including liver failure in approximately 25% of those affected. There is some controversy regarding the utility of VOD prophylaxis, with ursodiol possibly having some effect. Heparin has not been definitively shown to prevent it. Broad-spectrum antibiotics, although appropriate in the case of concomitant infection, are not specifically a therapy for VOD.

Answer 36.30. **The answer is C.**

Interstitial pneumonitis is an inflammatory lung disease characterized by pneumonitis, alveolitis, and, occasionally, interstitial fibrosis. It is associated with CMV reactivation, bleomycin exposure, history of GVHD, and radiation dose to the lungs. Lower dose conditioning, reduced or hyperfractionated radiation exposure to the lung, and avoidance of CMV reactivation may all decrease its incidence.

Answer 36.31. **The answer is D.**

Patients who have undergone stem cell transplant are at a 3.8 times increased risk of secondary malignancies when compared to age-matched controls. Median time to secondary leukemia and lymphoma is less than 1 year, while median time to solid tumors is 5 to 6 years. Secondary lymphomas are primarily EBV related. Chronic skin GVHD (or its treatment) is associated with an increased risk of squamous cell carcinoma of the skin.

Answer 36.32. **The answer is E.**

GVHD may manifest as either acute or chronic disease; the major target tissues of GVHD are the skin, liver, and gastrointestinal tract, although other tissues may be involved. Skin manifestations include a "sunburn-like" erythematous maculopapular rash, which often involves the palms and soles, and may be associated with desquamation. Hepatic involvement is characterized by a rise in alkaline phosphatase and total bilirubin often in association with a mild to moderate increase in hepatic transaminases. Gastrointestinal GVHD predominantly involves the distal small bowel and colon and clinically is associated with crampy abdominal pain and watery diarrhea, which may be voluminous and bloody under severe circumstances.

Answer 36.33. **The answer is B.**

In both HLA-identical sibling and unrelated transplants, T-cell depletion [both *in vitro* using CD34 selection or *in vivo* using ATG or alemtuzumab (Campath)] is the most effective method for preventing GVHD but is associated with an increased risk of graft rejection, opportunistic viral infection, and leukemic relapse.

Answer 36.34. **The answer is C.**

The mainstay of therapy for the treatment of acute GVHD is corticosteroid therapy, usually in association with CSA or tacrolimus (FK506). Approximately 40% to 60% of patients with grade II to IV GVHD can be expected to respond to these agents. Response to steroids appears to predict survival, and steroid refractory patients have a dismal prognosis, with 60% to 80% dying from GVHD-related causes; unmitigated GVHD and infectious complications related to prolonged immunosuppression contribute to the high mortality rate observed in these patients. ATG has been used with minimal success (20% to 40% response rate) with no evidence that it improves survival in this setting.

Answer 36.35. **The answer is C.**

While 40% to 60% of patients who are serologically positive for CMV will reactivate this virus following conventional allogeneic transplantation, the risk of reactivation in patients who are serologically negative before transplantation is extremely rare. Effective prevention can be achieved through the use of CMV negative or leukocyte filtered blood products (in seronegative patient-donor pairs) and prophylactic intravenous ganciclovir or foscarnet therapy. Several studies have shown that immunity to CMV after transplantation is mediated through donor CMV-specific T-cells that are transplanted with the allograft. Therefore, for patients at risk for CMV reactivation (i.e., pretransplant CMV serologically positive), a donor who is serologically positive for CMV is actually desirable, as transference of donor immunity against this virus may result in a reduction of CMV-associated morbidity.

Answer 36.36. **The answer is D.**

Although imatinib is associated with an impressive cytogenetic response rate, allogeneic hematopoietic cell transplantation (HCT) remains the only treatment approach with proven curative potential in this leukemia. Patient age, disease status (chronic phase versus accelerated or blastic phase), and the time interval from diagnosis to transplant (i.e., <1 year versus >1 year) are the best predictors for long-term disease-free survival. Patients with chronic phase CML transplanted within 1 year from the time of diagnosis have the best outcome, with long-term disease-free survivals of 75% to 80%. Among hematologic malignancies, CML appears most susceptible to the GVL effect.

Answer 36.37. **The answer is D.**

Nonmyeloablative stem cell transplant is a newer approach in evaluation that attempts to use reduced intensity conditioning prior to transplant. A nonmyeloablative regimen allows for some degree of autologous hematopoietic recovery as a consequence of recipient hematopoietic stem cells surviving the conditioning regimen, but a significantly immunosuppressive regimen is still required to allow for donor engraftment. Graft rejection appears to occur more frequently with the reduced intensity conditioning. Several have reported regimen-related mortality rates of less than 20%. A mixture of both donor and patient myeloid and lymphoid cells is usually detectable at the time of neutrophil recovery; this state is called mixed chimerism. Donor lymphocytes may be employed during the treatment strategy to induce graft-host-host hematopoietic effects that shift chimerism from mixed to complete donor, enhancing a GVT effect. Compared to myeloablative approaches, conditioning-induced toxicity is relatively mild with nonmyeloablative regimens. Although the occurrence of partial autologous hematopoietic recovery shortens the overall depth and duration of neutropenia and reduces platelet and RBC transfusion requirements, 10% to 15% of patients still develop invasive fungal infections.

Answer 36.38. **The answer is C.**

Cancer patients with chronic anemia frequently suffer from an anemia similar to anemia of chronic disease, with impaired marrow progenitor response to erythropoietin and impaired iron utilization. They also may have *decreased* endogenous erythropoietin levels. Tumor infiltration of the bone marrow may also contribute. It should also be appreciated that cancer patients are certainly not immune from other causes of anemia such as nutritional deficiencies (i.e., iron or folate deficiency), chronic renal dysfunction, myelodysplastic syndromes (often related to prior therapy), and others.

Answer 36.39. **The answer is D.**

Darbepoetin-alpha is similar to endogenous human erythropoietin but differs in that there is a change in glycosylation at two sites to produce a longer half-life. There is typically a delay of approximately 2 weeks until a rise in hemoglobin can be appreciated; the delay to rise in hemoglobin may be slightly longer in darbepoetin use as compared to erythropoietin. These agents may be considered in any patient with a hemoglobin less than 10 mg per dL with symptoms of anemia.

Answer 36.40. **The answer is A.**

Epoetin alpha may be dosed either on a 3 times per week weight-based schedule at 150 U per kg, or empirically on a 40,000 U per week once-weekly dosing schedule. A period of 4 weeks is typically pursued before making an evaluation of therapeutic response.

Answer 36.41. **The answer is E.**

The patient in question is responding to epoetin therapy (>1 mg per dL response after 4 weeks of therapy); discontinuation or change of therapy is not indicated at this time. The goal of therapy is stabilization of Hgb at 12 mg per dL, so therapy may be continued until this goal is achieved. Therapy should be modified if there is "overshoot" of 12 mg per dL, as further increases in hemoglobin do not convincingly provide therapeutic benefit, and there is some evidence that this may in fact be harmful.

Answer 36.42. **The answer is E.**

Current guidelines indicate that G-CSF is indicated for *primary* prevention of neutropenia in chemotherapy regimens, with an expected risk of neutropenia of greater than 20% in treatment regimens in which a reduction in treatment intensity may compromise disease-free or overall survival (i.e., dose-dense chemotherapy for adjuvant breast cancer treatment) and in patients older than 65 years of age.

Answer 36.43. **The answer is E.**

The appropriate starting dose of filgrastim when used for secondary prophylaxis is 5 mg per kg daily, maintained until ANC is 1,000 cells per mm^3; a practice often followed is to "round" to the nearest vial size (300 μg or 480 μg). Higher doses of filgrastim (e.g., 10 mg/kg/day) are indicated for peripheral blood stem cell (PBSC) mobilization and do not seem to provide clinical benefit when used for secondary prevention. Pegfilgrastim at a single dose of 6 mg is another reasonable option for secondary prophylaxis; however, it (and filgrastim) administration needs to be delayed at least 24 hours after finishing the chemotherapy administration. The Food and Drug Administration (FDA)-approved labeling for sargramostim includes indications for stem cell mobilization, neutropenia post-stem cell transplant, neutropenia post-AML induction chemotherapy, and after failure of bone marrow transplant, but it is not appropriate for secondary prophylaxis.

Answer 36.44. **The answer is E.**

When exogenously administered, rHu G-CSF increases the level of circulating neutrophils by accelerating production through reducing transit time from stem cell to mature neutrophil and by inhibiting neutrophil apoptosis. The serum clearance of pegfilgrastim is directly related to blood neutrophil concentrations, which extends its half-time from 3.5 hours (rHu G-CSF) to approximately 33 hours when neutrophil counts are low. Administration of rHu GM-CSF increases levels of circulating neutrophils, eosinophils, and, to a lesser extent, macrophages and lymphocytes. Although endogenous GM-CSF is involved in erythropoiesis and megakaryocyte development, other growth factors are required for final maturation of these cell lines, and rHu GM-CSF has no significant clinical effect on erythrocyte or platelet levels.

Answer 36.45. **The answer is D.**

IL-11 has been approved by the FDA for prevention of severe thrombocytopenia following myelosuppressive chemotherapy. At doses indicated for thrombopoiesis, oprelvekin use is associated with several serious toxicities including allergic reactions and anaphylaxis. About two thirds of patients receiving oprelvekin in clinical trials experienced edema, and nearly half experienced dyspnea. Fluid retention has also resulted in exacerbation of existing pleural effusions and atrial arrhythmias. These troublesome side effects have limited the practical use of this agent. Bone pain and myalgias are not typical side effects and are more common with G-CSF and GM-CSF.

Answer 36.46. **The answer is D.**

There is no clear indication that escalating doses of filgrastim provides additional clinical benefit over standard doses in the setting of secondary prophylaxis. IL-11 has been shown to decrease need for platelet transfusions and degree of thrombocytopenia, but side effects limit its use (see Answer 36.45). Given the extended half-life of pegfilgrastim, it should not be given in the period 14 days prior to chemotherapy.

CHAPTER 37

Complications of Cancer Therapy

JULIE R. BRAHMER AND DAVID S. ETTINGER

Directions Each of the numbered items below is followed by lettered answers. Select the ONE lettered answer that is BEST in each case unless instructed otherwise.

QUESTIONS

Question 37.1. **A 45-year-old woman with a history of Hodgkin disease, who was treated at age 26 with a splenectomy as part of the staging, presented with 1 day history of cough progressing to shortness of breath. On evaluation she is febrile, tachycardic, tachypneic, and her blood pressure is 80/42. The infection she most likely has is**

A. *Streptococcus pneumoniae*
B. *Escherichia coli*
C. *Staphylococcus aureus*
D. tuberculosis

Question 37.2. **Why is the patient in Question 37.1 prone to developing increased susceptibility to infections?**

A. Decreased T-cell immunity.
B. Decreased antibody response.
C. Hypogammaglobulinemia.
D. Neutropenia.

Question 37.3. **A 50-year-old man with metastatic small cell lung cancer presents 14 days after receiving etoposide and carboplatin with fever. He does not have an indwelling intravenous (IV) catheter. His neutrophil count is 300. What bacteria should be considered and covered initially with antibiotics?**

A. *Pseudomonas.*
B. *S. aureus.*
C. *Enterococcus.*
D. *Aspergillus.*

Corresponding Chapters in *Cancer: Principles & Practice of Oncology*, Seventh Edition: 54 (Adverse Effects of Treatment).

Question 37.4. **What antibiotic should be started as soon as the patient described in Question 37.3 presents to the hospital?**

A. Cephalexin.
B. Vancomycin.
C. Ceftazidime.
D. Penicillin.

Question 37.5. **What species of *Streptococcus* bacteria is commonly seen in colon cancer patients?**

A. *S. pneumonaie.*
B. *S. pyogenes.*
C. *S. bovis.*
D. *S. monocytogenes.*

Question 37.6. **Within 1 month post-high-dose chemotherapy followed by stem cell transplant, a patient is most prone to what type of immune compromise?**

A. T-cell dysfunction.
B. Decreased humoral immunity.
C. Neutropenia.
D. Phagocyte dysfunction.

Question 37.7. **A 67-year-old man with non-small cell lung cancer is currently undergoing whole brain radiation for brain metastasis. He is currently on dexamethasone 4 mg PO q.i.d. He presents with severe pain on swallowing. On exam you see large white patches with an erythematous base in the back of his throat. He most likely has**

A. *Herpes simplex* virus infection
B. chemotherapy-induced mucositis
C. candidiasis
D. streptococcal infection

Question 37.8. **What medication should be used to treat the infection described in Question 37.7?**

A. Fluconazole.
B. Penicillin.
C. Cephalexin.
D. Gatifloxacin.

Question 37.9. **If the patient in Question 37.7 is diagnosed with *Herpes simplex* virus, what medication should be used to treat the infection?**

A. Penicillin.
B. Fluconazole.
C. Acyclovir.
D. Gancyclovir.

Question 37.10. **A 40-year-old man, 4 months out from an allogenic stem cell transplant, is being treated for graft versus host disease (GVHD). He presents to clinic with a fever, sinus congestion, cough, pleuritic chest pain, and hemoptysis. Chest x-ray reveals bilateral nodular lesions. This patient most likely has what infection?**

A. *S. pneumoniae.*
B. Aspergillosis.
C. Cytomegalovirus (CMV) pneumonia.
D. *Haemophilus influenzae.*

Question 37.11. **What medication should be used to treat the infection described in Question 37.10?**

A. Fluconazole.
B. Amphotericin B.
C. Voriconazole.
D. Gatifloxacin.

Question 37.12. **A 65-year-old man with chronic lymphocytic leukemia (CLL) completed his treatment of fludarabine about 3 months ago and achieved nice cytoreduction. He presents with a fever, severe headache, and confusion. What infection should be considered?**

A. *Listeria monocytogenes* meningitis.
B. *Legionella* pneumonia.
C. *E. coli* urinary tract infection.
D. *Klebsiella* infection.

Question 37.13. **A 67-year-old woman with metastatic breast cancer presents with minimally worsening shortness of breath over the past week. She has been on dexamethasone for the past 2 months for the treatment of brain metastasis. She has not been able to taper completely off of steroids yet. On chest x-ray, she has bilateral infiltrates. Her oxygen saturation is 82%. What infection could be a complication of her steroid use?**

A. *S. pneumoniae.*
B. *S. aureus.*
C. *Candida.*
D. *Pneumocystis jiroveci.*

Question 37.14. **A 35-year-old man with metastatic testicular cancer presents with neutropenia, fever, and severe abdominal pain. Abdominal x-ray shows an abnormal gas pattern in the right lower quadrant. Computed tomographic (CT) scan of the abdomen reveals gas within the abdominal wall. He was diagnosed with typhlitis. The most likely organism is**

A. *S. pneumoniae*
B. *Clostridium perfringens*
C. *H. influenzae*
D. *S. epidermidis*

Question 37.15. **The treatment of choice for the patient described in Question 37.14 is**

A. metronidazole plus ceftazidime
B. penicillin and clindamycin
C. meropenem
D. A and C
E. any of the above

Question 37.16. **Stomatitis is characterized by all of the following EXCEPT**

A. erythema
B. atrophy
C. edema
D. ulceration
E. all of the above

Question 37.17. **The severity of xerostomia depends on**

A. radiation dose
B. chemotherapy
C. volume of exposed salivary glands
D. A and C only
E. all of the above

Question 37.18. **All of the following are validated assessment methods to evaluate oral mucositis EXCEPT**

A. World Health Organization Index
B. Oral Mucositis Rating Scale
C. Oral Mucositis Index
D. Oral Mucositis Assessment Scale
E. Oral Assessment Guide

Question 37.19. **Which of the following chemotherapy agents have a serious risk of stomatitis?**

A. Continuous infusion 5-fluorouracil (5FU).
B. Methotrexate.
C. Etoposide.
D. All of the above.

Question 37.20. **Which cytoprotectant can reduce oral stomatitis in patients receiving 5FU or melphalan?**

A. Silver nitrate.
B. Sucralfate.
C. Cryotherapy.
D. Glutathione.
E. All of the above.

Question 37.21. **Which of the following has been shown in randomized trials to reduce the incidence of xerostomia in patients receiving radiation to the head and neck?**

A. Vitamin E.
B. Artificial saliva.
C. Gum.
D. Capsaicin.
E. Amifostine.

Question 37.22. **Patients with oral cavity GVHD post-BMT (bone marrow transplant) may NOT benefit from which of the following treatments.**

A. Topical steroids.
B. Vitamin E.
C. Cyclosporine oral rinse/swishes.
D. Systemic cyclosporine.

Question 37.23. **A 76-year-old woman with oral cancer presents with severe mouth pain after 5FU and cisplatin concurrent with radiation. On exam, her oral pharynx is erythematous with significant ulcerations. What can she try to control the pain?**

A. Allopurinol.
B. Pilocarpine.
C. Topical morphine.
D. Vitamin E.
E. All of the above.

Question 37.24. **What are the common infections that can contribute to oral stomatitis in cancer patients?**

A. *Candida.*
B. *E. coli.*
C. *Herpes simplex* virus.
D. A and C.
E. All of the above.

Question 37.25. **The mechanisms by which chemotherapy-induced nausea and vomiting occurs is thought to be due to its effect on the**

A. central nervous system
B. gastrointestinal tract
C. A and B
D. none of the above

Question 37.26. **Neurotransmitters involved in chemotherapy-induced nausea and vomiting include**

A. dopamine
B. serotonin
C. histamine
D. substance P
E. all of the above

Question 37.27. **Substance P, which is involved in chemotherapy-induced nausea and vomiting, has which of the following characteristics.**

A. It is a neurotransmitter.
B. Binds to the NK_1 receptor in the midbrain.
C. NK_1 receptor antagonists inhibit both acute and delayed emesis in animal and human studies.
D. Can also bind to the 5-hydroxytryptamine (5HT) receptor.
E. A, B, and C.

Question 37.28. **Types of chemotherapy-induced nausea and vomiting include which of the following.**

A. Acute.
B. Chronic.
C. Delayed.
D. Anticipatory.
E. A, C, and D.

Question 37.29. **The known risk factors for chemotherapy-related acute nausea and vomiting include**

A. gender
B. cisplatin 80 mg per m^2 or higher
C. history of motion sickness
D. history of severe emesis during pregnancy
E. all of the above

Question 37.30. **Antiemetics that are NOT $5HT_3$ receptor antagonists include**

A. phenothiazines
B. butrophenones
C. canabinoids
D. all of the above

Question 37.31. **Which of the following facts about $5HT_3$ receptor antagonists is/are true?**

A. Dolasetron, granisetron, ondansetron, and palonosteron are $5HT_3$ receptor antagonists.
B. Common side effects include mild headaches, mild constipation, and extrapyramidal reactions.
C. They are used in patients receiving high or moderately emetogenic chemotherapy.
D. The addition of corticosteroids does not significantly improve the antiemetic efficacy of the $5HT_3$ receptor antagonists.
E. A and C.

Question 37.32. **Which of the following statement(s) is/are true with regard to palonosteron, the new $5HT_3$ receptor antagonist?**

A. It has higher tissue-binding affinity for $5HT_3$ receptor and significantly longer serum half-life than other $5HT_3$ antagonists.
B. In the United States, it is Food and Drug Administration (FDA) approved for acute nausea and vomiting with the use of both highly and moderately emetogenic chemotherapy; it is also approved for delayed nausea and vomiting associated with moderately emetogenic chemotherapy.
C. It has side effects similar to other $5HT_3$ receptor antagonists.
D. All of the above.

Question 37.33. **Aprepitant, an NK-1 receptor antagonist, has which of the following characteristics.**

A. It is the first NK_1 receptor antagonist approved for use effective in preventing both acute and delayed nausea and vomiting in patients receiving highly emetogenic chemotherapy when given in combination with a $5HT_3$ receptor antagonist and a corticosteroid.
B. It is a moderate inhibitor of CYP3A4.
C. All of the above.

Question 37.34. **A 50-year-old man with mestastatic non-small cell lung cancer with a performance status of 1 is to be treated with gemcitabine plus cisplatin. The perferred antiemetic regimen is**

A. ondansetron + corticosteroid
B. aprepitant + palonosteron + corticosteroid
C. aprepitant + corticosteroids
D. phenothiazine + corticosteroids

ANSWERS

Answer 37.1. **The answer is A.**

She is at increased susceptibility to encapsulated organisms because of her splenectomy.

Answer 37.2. **The answer is B.**

B-cells produce opsonizing antibodies after rapid antigen presentation in the spleen. Splenectomy results in decreased antibody production in response to certain bacterial infections.

Answer 37.3. **The answer is A.**

This man has a neutropenic fever. Neutropenic fever is defined as a single oral temperature of greater than 38.3°C or greater than or equal to 38°C for over 1 hour with associated neutropenia (<500 per µL). A meticulous physical exam, chest x-ray, and at least blood cultures should be done. However, there is usually a lack of significant physical exam findings. Thus, empiric antibacterial therapy should begin immediately to cover gram-negative infections. Empiric coverage for gram-positive infections is required only if there is a strong suspicion of infection involving the indwelling catheter.

Answer 37.4. **The answer is C.**

Ceftazidime was compared to piperacillin combined with tobramycin. The two regimens were similar in regards to infection control and mortality but ceftazidime was associated with less adverse reactions. Cetrazidime is effective empiric therapy in patients with febrile neutropenia. Cefipime, imipenem, and meropenem can also be used as monotherapy for neutropenic fever.

Answer 37.5. **The answer is C.**

Direct invasion through the colonic mucosa is associated with local abscess formation and sepsis by enteric flora. *Streptococcus bovis* bacteremia is highly associated with colon cancer.

Answer 37.6. **The answer is C.**

Neutropenia before engraftment is the immune-compromised state that this patient is most prone to within 1 month of receiving high-dose chemotherapy followed by stem cell transplantation. Neutropenia predisposes a patient to bacterial, fungal, and viral infections. After engraftment, these patients can be prone to the other types of immune compromise.

Answer 37.7. **The answer is C.**

Oral candidiasis is common in patients on steroids. *Herpes simplex* virus infections tend to be characterized by blisters or ulcerations, not white patches.

Answer 37.8. **The answer is A.**

Fluconazole is the only antifungal treatment on this list. Nystatin topical treatment can also be used.

Answer 37.9. **The answer is C.**

Herpes simplex virus esophagitis can be severe. *Herpes simplex* virus should be treated with intravenous acyclovir and then a switch to oral acyclovir when the disease improves. Fluconazole is used to treat oral candidiasis. Penicillin would not be used to treat herpes. Gancyclovir would not be the first choice in treating herpes stomatitis.

Answer 37.10. **The answer is B.**

Systemic aspergillosis can cause bilateral nodular lesions on chest x-ray. Aspergillosis can also cause hemoptysis and pleuritic chest pain since it invades blood vessels, causing lung necrosis as well as bleeding.

Answer 37.11. **The answer is C.**

Voriconazole is the drug of choice for invasive aspergillosis. Patients with invasive aspergillosis were randomized to either voriconazole or conventional amphotericin B. Voriconazole was associated with improved survival at 12 weeks (71% versus 59% with amphotericin B).

Answer 37.12. **The answer is A.**

This patient has symptoms of possible meningitis. Fludarabine is lymphotoxic primarily to CD4+ lymphocytes. Also, patients with CLL can have hypogammaglobulinemia, which can predispose them to infections with encapsulated organisms such as *Listeria.*

Answer 37.13. **The answer is D.**

This patient has *P. jiroveci* (formerly *P. carinii*). This infection is associated with chronic steroid use causing a defective T-cell immunity. Diagnosis is by visualization of the organism microscopically. The treatment of choice is trimethoprim/sulfamethoxazole.

Answer 37.14. **The answer is B.**

Clostridium is associated with necrotizing enterocolitis (typhlitis) in the neutropenic patient. Typhlitis should be thought of when a neutropenic patient presents with diffuse abdominal pain. On gram stain, *Clostridium* appear as large, thick gram-positive rods.

Answer 37.15. **The answer is D.**

For neutropenic patients with enterocolitis, metronidazole or clindamycin plus an antipseudomonal cephalosporin (ceftazidime) or single-agent meropenem can be used. Penicillin should not be used.

Answer 37.16. **The answer is E.**

Stomatitis is defined as inflammation of the mucous membranes of the oral cavity. Stomatitis can present with erythema to desquamative patches to painful ulcerated lesions. Edema is also seen.

Answer 37.17. **The answer is D.**

Xerostomia is a decrease is quality and quantity of saliva. Patients with head and neck cancer treated with radiation can experience xerostomia. The severity depends on radiation dose and location, especially in regards to the volume of the exposed salivary glands. Chemotherapy alone does not affect the degree of xerostomia.

Answer 37.18. **The answer is A.**

The World Health Organization (WHO) Index is a simple overall rating of stomatitis that has yet to be validated. The Oral Assessment Guide is a clinical tool used to assess changes related to effects of therapy on the oral cavity, which has been validated. The Oral Mucositis Rating Scale is an index used in BMT patients for evaluating acute stomatitis. Clinical and research utility has been demonstrated for this scale. The Oral Mucositis Index was developed from the Oral Mucositis Rating Scale, which is validated. The Oral Mucositis Assessment Scale is a system for scoring the anatomic extent and severity of stomatitis and is validated.

Answer 37.19. **The answer is D.**

All of the chemotherapy agents listed above can cause severe stomatitis.

Answer 37.20. **The answer is C.**

Sulcralfate creates a protective barrier, but study results are conflicting as to its benefit for prevention of stomatitis. One study revealed reduction of edema and ulceration but another demonstrated no beneficial reduction. Glutathione, an antioxidant, has been tested in patients receiving chemoradiation but not specifically 5FU. Silver nitrate has been tested in radiotherapy-related stomatitis with mixed results. Studies have evaluated oral cryotherapy and have been favorable when 5FU or melphalan are given as short infusions.

Answer 37.21. **The answer is E.**

While pilocarpine, artificial saliva, and gum may improve salivation in patients with xerostomia, it cannot prevent it. Vitamin E has not been studied to see if it prevents xerostomia. Capsaicin is used for the treatment of oral pain. Amifostine in a randomized trial decreased the incidence of acute and late xerostomia.

Answer 37.22. **The answer is B.**

Patients with extensive chronic GVHD involving the oral cavity may benefit from topical steroids (dexamethasone elixir), cyclosporine swishes, or systemic immunosuppression therapy such as cyclosporine. Psoralens with ultraviolet A (PUVA) therapy can also be used. However, Vitamin E has not been studied for the treatment of oral GVHD.

Answer 37.23. **The answer is C.**

Allopurinal in a randomized, double-blind trial showed no protective effect against 5FU-induced stomatitis. Topical morphine mouthwash showed shortened duration and lower intensity of oral pain than magic mouthwash. Capsaicin can also be used for partial and temporary pain reduction. Pilocarpine can be used to stimulate salivary function in someone with xerostomia but not for pain control. Sucralfate can be used to treat mucosal edema, pain, and dysphagia in patients with stomatitis, but studies have demonstrated mixed results. Vitamin E in combination with vitamin C and glutathione given with azelastine may be useful in the prevention of chemoradiation-induced stomatitis. Vitamin E does not treat the oral pain caused by stomatitis. Oral lidocaine is also used frequently for the treatment of oral pain.

Answer 37.24. **The answer is D.**

E. coli is not a common infection to cause oral stomatitis in cancer patients. *Herpes simplex* virus and *Candida* are common oral infections causing stomatitis. In BMT patients who are seropositive for *Herpes simplex* virus, acyclovir is used for prophylaxis. Fluconazole can be used for prophylaxis of *Candida* oral infections.

Answer 37.25. **The answer is C.**

The emetic process begins when chemotherapy affects the chemoreceptor trigger zone and then releases neurotransmitters that activate the vomiting center within the brainstem. In addition, release of serotonin from enterochromaffin cells of the gastrointestinal (GI) tract by chemotherapy-induced irritation and/or damage to the GI mucosa activates vagal afferent fibers to the vomiting center.

Answer 37.26. **The answer is E.**

The chemoreceptor trigger zone and GI tract contain receptors for these neurotransmitters as well as other endogenous neurotransmitters. When these receptors are activated by chemotherapy, emesis is induced.

Answer 37.27. **The answer is E.**

Substance P belongs to the group of peptides known as neurokinins and exerts its effect by binding to the NK receptor located in the midbrain. It does not bind to other receptors such as the $5HT_3$ receptor. NK_1 receptor antagonists inhibit both acute and delayed emesis induced by cisplatin, both in animal and human studies.

Answer 37.28. **The answer is E.**

Acute nausea and vomiting occurs within the first 24 hours after the administration of chemotherapy. Delayed chemotherapy-induced nausea and vomiting occurs more than 24 hours after chemotherapy. Anticipatory nausea and vomiting is a conditioned response and occurs usually only after a negative past experience with chemotherapy.

Answer 37.29. **The answer is E.**

Apart from the factors outlined above, history of severe emesis with previous chemotherapy coupled with anxiety may increase the chances of developing chemotherapy-related emesis. Chronic and heavy alcohol usage, defined as greater than 100 g of alcohol or five mixed drinks per day, whether in the past or currently, has been shown to decrease the chances of developing chemotherapy-related emesis.

Answer 37.30. **The answer is D.**

These antiemetics are useful in controlling nausea and vomiting in patients with cancer. Commonly used phenothiazines include prochlorperazine and thiethylperazine; the butyropenones include haloperidol and droperiodol; the cannabinoids include dronabinol.

Answer 37.31. **The answer is E.**

Extrapyramidal reactions are not common side effects of the $5HT_3$ receptor antagonists. They are more common with the phenothiazines and dopamine antagonists such as metoclopramide.The use of corticosteroids significantly improves the antiemetic efficacy of the $5HT_3$ receptor antagonists, especially when used in patients receiving cisplatin-containing chemotherapy regimens.

Answer 37.32. **The answer is D.**

In three large phase III clinical trials when compared with currently available $5HT_3$ receptor antagonists, palonosteron provided patients with improved control during the acute and delayed phases. The side effects observed were similar in severity and frequency to the comparator agents. The most common side effects related to palonosteron were headache and constipation.

Answer 37.33. **The answer is C.**

Aprepitant (Emend), in combination with other antiemetic agents, is indicated for the prevention of acute and delayed nausea and vomiting associated with initial and repeat courses of highly emetogenic cancer chemotherapy, including high dose cisplatin. It is a moderate inhibitor of CYP34A. Aprepitant is well tolerated. The recommended dose of aprepitant is 125 mg orally 1 hour prior to chemotherapy treatment on day 1 and 80 mg once a day on days 2 and 3.

Answer 37.34. **The answer is B.**

Cisplatin-containing chemotherapy is classified as highly emetogenic. Such therapy causes both significant acute and delayed nausea and vomiting. Presently, the treatment of choice is aprepitant + a $5HT_3$ receptor antagonist and a corticosteroid.

CHAPTER 38

Supportive Care and Quality of Life

SUSAN B. LEGRAND

Directions Each of the numbered items below is followed by lettered answers. Select the ONE lettered answer that is BEST in each case unless instructed otherwise.

QUESTIONS

Questions 38.1–38.4.

Mary Jane is a 30-year-old woman who presents to your office in referral from her surgeon. She has been diagnosed with inflammatory left breast cancer and is referred to you for primary treatment. She is a single mother of two girls ages 5 and 12. Her mother had a right breast cancer at age 35 and later developed ovarian cancer. She died of this disease 3 years ago. The patient's maternal aunt was also diagnosed with a breast cancer at age 40, and Mary Jane remembers her having a difficult time with her treatments. She expresses fear that she will have similar problems and is not sure she can handle chemotherapy. Her past medical history is notable for an episode of major depression following her mother's death that was treated with antidepressants. She stopped taking them 1 year ago and has been feeling well since.

Question 38.1. **Excluding the immediate treatment choices, the key supportive care issues of concern in this history include**

A. family members with similar illness
B. complicated grief reaction with the loss of her mother
C. single parent
D. all of the above

Question 38.2. **The resources that might be useful for Mary Jane at this phase of her disease include**

A. support group
B. referral to a social worker
C. child support services
D. all of the above

Corresponding Chapters in *Cancer: Principles & Practice of Oncology*, Seventh Edition: 55 (Supportive Care and Quality of Life) and 56 (Rehabilitation of the Cancer Patient).

Question 38.3. **Which of the following efforts would be helpful to prepare Mary Jane for chemotherapy?**

A. Attention to prevention of chemotherapy-induced nausea.
B. Referral for relaxation training.
C. Adequate counseling regarding the treatment of chemotherapy-related side effects.
D. All of the above.

Question 38.4. **Which of the following statements about Mary Jane is true?**

A. She is a candidate for genetic counseling.
B. The knowledge of her genetic status will change her chemotherapy options.
C. A and B.
D. None of the above.

Question 38.5. **Which of the following statements about cancer genetic counseling is true?**

A. It is a benefit provided to all under existing insurance plans.
B. A negative test conclusively rules out hereditary cancer.
C. There are no risks to future insurance coverage.
D. Results of testing cannot be released to other family members at potential risk without permission from the patient.

Question 38.6. **Mary Jane elects to have genetic testing and is found to be BRCA1 positive. With close attention to symptom management, she tolerates her chemotherapy with minimal distress. She has developed a good rapport with the cancer center social worker who has been quite helpful with counseling her as therapy progressed. Her children's teachers are aware of the diagnosis and the school guidance counselors are meeting with them regularly. She has completed all planned chemotherapy and is in your office to discuss her surgical options. The fact that she has BRCA1 mutation implies**

A. she is at risk for bilateral breast cancer
B. she is at risk for ovarian cancer
C. A and B
D. none of the above

Question 38.7. **Mary Jane ultimately has bilateral mastectomies without immediate reconstruction and defers the decision on oophorectomy. She returns to your office 3 weeks after the surgery in extreme distress with severe pain beginning shortly after surgery. The surgeon has reviewed the wounds and feels they are healing well. The pain is both constant (7/10) and episodic with lancinating pains (10/10) frequently during the day. She has been unable to sleep because of pain. On physical exam, she appears uncomfortable. There is pain with light touch in the area of the surgical incisions (allodynia). There are no other significant physical**

findings and nothing to suggest recurrent disease. Which of the following is true regarding her pain?

A. This neuropathic pain is related to postmastectomy syndrome.
B. The incidence of postmastectomy syndrome is less than 5%.
C. Postmastectomy syndrome is seen in older women more commonly than in younger women.
D. This pain does not respond to opioids.

Question 38.8. **You start Mary Jane on 10 mg nortriptyline with PRN oxycodone and see her in follow-up 1 week later. She noticed a 50% improvement in her pain overall with decrease in the burning and lancinating pain. She is sleeping better and rarely uses the oxycodone, taking it primarily at night. She had slight dry mouth with the nortriptyline but it has resolved and does not bother her. On physical exam you note she has significant limitation in range of motion of the left arm. She had been given exercises by the surgeon but has not been able to do them secondary to pain. You would recommend**

A. increasing the dose of nortriptyline
B. physical therapy
C. oxycodone prior to physical therapy
D. all of the above

Question 38.9. **Mary Jane returns to your office for her first follow-up after completing her radiation therapy. All adjuvant therapy is now complete and she is to begin routine follow-up at 3-month intervals. She is hormone negative so no additional medication is required. Her range of motion is improving with therapy and her pain is under adequate control, but she complains of fatigue, is having difficulty in sleeping, has lost some weight, and finds herself worrying constantly about the cancer returning. You would**

A. reassure and counsel her on the warning symptoms of recurrence
B. encourage her to attend a support group
C. talk to her about augmenting social support
D. discuss the role of antidepressants
E. all of the above

Question 38.10. **You start Mary Jane on an antidepressant and she returns every 3 months for follow-up. She is adjusting well and has resumed her normal activities. She developed amenorrhea with her chemotherapy and has not resumed menstrual cycles. She has begun a new relationship but finds she does not have what she considers a normal libido and that sexual intercourse is uncomfortable. The factors contributing to her sexual problems include**

A. vaginal dryness
B. body image issues
C. impact of antidepressant
D. all of the above

Question 38.11. **Several years pass and Mary Jane does well. Three years after her last chemotherapy, she presents to your office off schedule with new complaints of pain. She had stopped taking the nortriptyline after completing physical therapy for her arm several years ago and has not had pain problems since. She describes an aching pain in her lower back that she initially thought was a pulled muscle but seems to be getting worse. Her pain is constant 7/10 with worsening episodes when she gets up to walk (incident pain) that can be 10/10 at times. She has cut back her activity because of the pain and is unable to do her usual household chores. She has taken the past several days off from work and stayed in bed much of the time. The pain is aching with some radiation down the leg and around to her abdomen. Oxycodone 5 mg relieves her baseline pain only 50%, but she has never tried to take more than one. The relief lasts approximately 2 hours. With regard to pain control, your initial step should be**

A. starting her on a long-acting opioid
B. increasing the dose of the short-acting opioid
C. adding stool softeners
D. starting an adjunct nonnarcotic analgesic

Question 38.12. **The side effects of narcotics include**

A. nausea
B. sedation
C. pruritis
D. constipation
E. all of the above

Question 38.13. **Metastatic disease to bone is confirmed with bone scans involving femur, multiple levels in spine, and multiple ribs. There is no spinal cord compression demonstrated on magnetic resonance imaging (MRI), but there is some nerve root impingement from a mass at L1. No visceral disease is identified. She returns to your office to discuss therapy. She is taking sustained release (SR) morphine 15 mg every 12 hours and using her breakthrough 10-mg morphine tablet 6 times a day. She says her pain is not controlled but she does get relief when she takes the extra medication. Which of the following would be an appropriate adjustment to her medication regimen?**

A. Increase her SR morphine to 30 mg every 12 hours.
B. Change to an alternate sustained-release medication.
C. Change her SR morphine to 15 mg every 8 hours.
D. Increase her SR morphine to 45 mg every 12 hours.

Question 38.14. **Which of the following histories is most consistent with end-of-dose failure, that is, inadequate dose at trough levels?**

A. An individual taking SR oxycodone awakens every morning in pain and while adequately controlled during the day needs a breakthrough dose each afternoon before the next SR dose is due.
B. An individual taking transdermal fentanyl who rarely uses breakthrough dosing until the third day and then needs it often.
C. A and B.
D. None of the above.

Question 38.15. **You increase Mary Jane's morphine to 45 mg every 12 hours and see her in 1 week documenting improved pain control with minimal toxicity as long as she maintains her bowel regimen. After completing radiation therapy and 2 weeks after her first dose of chemotherapy, she begins to complain of nausea and vomiting. Her daughter complains that she is always sleeping. Her excessive sedation is likely due to**

A. opioid analgesics
B. brain metastasis
C. hypercalcemia
D. chemotherapy

Question 38.16. **Mary Jane gradually tapers her SR morphine to 15 mg every 12 hours and continues on her chemotherapy with reasonable tolerance. She is also receiving a monthly bisphosphonate infusion. As time passes, she is transitioned from one therapy to another as disease progresses and has now had three regimens since recurrence. She then presents with increasing pain and severe nausea and vomiting. Her current pain medications are SR morphine 100 mg every 12 hours and a breakthrough dose of 30 mg, which she is taking every 3 hours. In the past 24 hours, she has taken eight extra doses of medication without relief. She was unable to keep her sustained medication down this morning and you elect to admit her. You are going to give her an intravenous (IV) infusion of her pain medication. What would be an appropriate starting dose of morphine?**

A. 2 mg per hr.
B. 4 mg per hr.
C. 6 mg per hr.
D. 9 mg per hr.

Question 38.17. **After initial evaluation she is found to have multiple brain metastases and extensive involvement of her liver. Steroids decrease her nausea, and radiation therapy to the brain is recommended and completed. After a brief stay in rehab she returns to the office to discuss further treatment options. The primary treatment options now include**

A. supportive care
B. additional standard chemotherapy
C. phase 1 chemotherapy
D. all of the above

Question 38.18. **Social issues of concern at this time include which of the following questions.**

A. What do her children know of her prognosis?
B. Have arrangements been made for their guardianship after her death?
C. Is there a proxy decision maker established?
D. All of the above.

Question 38.19. **If you were to offer Mary Jane phase 1 chemotherapy, it is important to emphasize**

A. full disclosure regarding the known benefits and risks
B. alternate options for therapy
C. continuation of best supportive care
D. all of the above

Question 38.20. **Mary Jane is not interested in phase 1 chemotherapy. Her goals are to live as long as possible to be with her children, but she also wants to feel well enough to care for them. Her sister has been assisting with her daughters and is in the process of establishing guardianship. She wants to try another standard chemotherapy that you have offered. She has a transient response to the treatment but then presents with progressive pain and fatigue. You do not feel that further chemotherapy is reasonable for her. Which of the following statements might best convey this recommendation?**

A. There is nothing more that I can do.
B. I think it is time for you to go to hospice.
C. There are other chemotherapies we could try but they are unlikely to help you live longer and may make you feel worse.
D. We could try another chemotherapy.

Question 38.21. **Mary Jane enrolls with hospice care and her sister takes family leave and moves in to provide care. She has expressed a desire not to die at home as she thinks this would be difficult for her children and chooses to enter an inpatient hospice unit when she is no longer able to get out of bed. It appears that she is rapidly approaching death when she begins to moan and becomes very restless. No recent medication changes have been made. The most likely cause of her restlessness is terminal delirium. The appropriate therapy includes**

A. benzodiazepines
B. barbiturates
C. neuroleptics
D. any of the above

Question 38.22. **Mary Jane dies peacefully at the inpatient hospice several days later with her family at her bedside. Available services for the families through hospice include**

A. bereavement counseling for 1 month
B. bereavement counseling for 3 months
C. bereavement counseling for 6 months
D. bereavement counseling for 12 months

Question 38.23. **Phillip is a 45-year-old man with a history of ulcerative colitis who developed colon cancer. He had a total colectomy and adjuvant chemotherapy. He developed metastatic disease and has undergone several different regimens of chemotherapy with initial response and then progression. He had begun to decline recently and then presented to the emergency room with nausea and vomiting. He was found to have a small bowel obstruction and went to exploratory laparotomy where he was found to have carcinomatosis. No diversion was possible and a venting gastrostomy was placed for palliation. Options include**

A. no fluids
B. intravenous fluids only
C. total parenteral nutrition
D. all of the above

Question 38.24. **Dysgeusia may be caused by which of the following.**

A. Chemotherapy.
B. Nutritional deficiencies.
C. Depression.
D. All of the above.

Question 38.25. **Which of the following is NOT true of cancer cachexia?**

A. Nutritional support will reverse the weight loss.
B. Cytokines and other inflammatory mediators related to the tumor are thought to cause the syndrome.
C. Loss of lean body mass from skeletal muscle breakdown occurs.
D. Fat and carbohydrate metabolism are disrupted.

Question 38.26. **Which of the following has been shown to increase lean body mass in cancer patients?**

A. Omega-3 fatty acids.
B. Cyproheptadine.
C. Megestrol acetate.
D. Corticosteroids.

Question 38.27. **Risks factors for lymphedema include all of the following EXCEPT**

A. extent of surgery
B. type of chemotherapy
C. obesity
D. radiation

Question 38.28. **Methods to manage lymphedema include all of the following EXCEPT**

A. elevation of the limb
B. specialized wraps
C. massage techniques
D. diuretics

Question 38.29. **Which of the following would disqualify a patient from acute rehabilitation?**

A. Spinal cord compression with paralysis.
B. Recent amputation.
C. Karnovsky performance score of 40.
D. Recent brain tumor resection with right upper extremity paralysis.

Question 38.30. **The dramatic increase in health-care costs are thought to relate to which of the following.**

A. The proliferation and cost of new technology.
B. The increase in the aged population.
C. Government spending for the Medicare and Medicaid programs.
D. Lack of incentive for efficiency and productivity.
E. All of the above.

Question 38.31. **Which of the following is NOT a role of the Food and Drug Administration (FDA) in drug development?**

A. Protection of research subjects.
B. Designing clinical trials.
C. Deciding if drugs should be marketed.
D. Verifying accuracy of marketing applications.

Question 38.32. **Investigational new drug (IND) applications are required in all of the following circumstances EXCEPT**

A. a study seeking FDA approval for adjuvant use of an established medication
B. a study of significantly higher than established doses of an existing medication
C. use of an approved chemotherapy in established doses for "off-label" indications
D. a study the pharmaceutical company will use in advertising an existing medication

Question 38.33. **To qualify for accelerated approval, a new medication must demonstrate all of the following EXCEPT**

A. treat a serious or life-threatening illness
B. show an improvement over existing therapy
C. demonstrate an improvement in survival
D. a plan to continue trials to confirm the benefit

ANSWERS

Answer 38.1. **The answer is D.**

There are several red flags in this history that may affect Mary Jane's adjustment to the diagnosis and therapy:

- She has watched family members cope with the same illness and experienced a relatively recent loss from cancer. These experiences will clearly impact her perceptions of what to expect from her therapy. She enters treatment with fear and trepidation.

- She had a complicated grief reaction to her mother's death with a major depression. This puts her at higher risk of depression with her diagnosis.
- As a single mother, her support system may be somewhat limited. Child care may be difficult to share, and she may risk burdening the older child with adult responsibilities as she manages side effects from treatment.
- Family history of breast and ovarian cancer.

It is your responsibility as her physician to be aware of these concerns, monitor them as treatment proceeds, and make the appropriate referrals.

Answer 38.2. **The answer is D.**

Mary Jane might well benefit from a support group, particularly one for younger women dealing with breast cancer. Some individuals in active therapy may not have the energy to go to support groups, but they are a useful option for others. A referral to a social worker experienced in cancer care would be the best choice. She or he could discuss the options that would be available for her and her children, who may also need counseling to cope with their mother's illness.

Answer 38.3. **The answer is D.**

Given her fear and the experience of her aunt, Mary Jane's expectations put her at greater risk of not only anticipatory symptoms but delayed nausea and vomiting. Young women also tend to have more nausea symptoms than older women. In order for her to successfully complete her therapy, careful attention to prevention of chemotherapy-induced nausea and vomiting (CINV), both immediate and delayed, will be very important. One could consider a referral for relaxation training that would allow her to feel in control and prepared for her first treatment if there were adequate time. You would also want to follow existing guidelines for prevention of delayed nausea and vomiting. Despite published guidelines, studies have shown that less than 50% of physicians followed the recommendations for management of delayed nausea and vomiting with noncisplatin containing regimens.

Answer 38.4. **The answer is A.**

Given Mary Jane's family history with two first-degree relatives with premenopausal breast cancer, one of whom also had ovarian cancer, and her age at diagnosis, she is at risk for BRCA1/2, and genetic counseling could be considered. Referral to a center specializing in cancer genetics counseling would be preferred. The knowledge of her genetic status will not impact your immediate therapeutic recommendations but might impact the surgical choices after her induction chemotherapy.

Answer 38.5. **The answer is D.**

Complete DNA testing costs in excess of $2,500 and, while covered by many insurance companies, it is not covered by all and is restricted to those in whom it is medically necessary. Preauthorization is often required. Tests may be true positive or true negative but may also be uninformative or of uncertain significance. In uninformative tests, no genetic mutation is identified, but there could be an undetectable mutation or a different gene involved. Hereditary cancer may still exist in the family. There may also be changes of undetermined significance. When cancer genetic counseling was starting, there were fears of impact on health and life insurance. The concern regarding health insurance has not materialized, but life insurance may be problematic. This should be discussed prior to testing. The issue of discussing results with family members is complex. Confidentiality rules state that only information approved by the patient can be shared with others. There has also been concern about the potential harm/liability of not notifying an affected family member. To complicate the issue further, extended family may not want the information as it is emotionally charged. At the present time, whether or not to release information remains the patient's decision.

Answer 38.6. **The answer is C.**

Mary Jane has a substantial risk of bilateral breast cancer and also ovarian cancer. You should discuss the options of bilateral mastectomy with/without reconstruction and consideration of oophorectomy.

Answer 38.7. **The answer is A.**

This is neuropathic pain. Postmastectomy syndrome, which had been thought rare, has been described in from 20% to 65% of women, with the higher number seen in younger women. There have not been any controlled trials of management; therefore, standard guidelines for neuropathic pain apply. Treatment choices include

- topical agents such as the lidoderm patch 5% or capsaicin
- tricyclic antidepressants (TCA) such as amitriptyline or nortriptylene; she would be a good candidate for this as she is not sleeping well and it might be helpful for both symptoms
- anticonvulsant medications (AED) such as gabapentin and others
- opioid medications; despite the fact the neuropathic pain is often called "opioid resistant," there are randomized trials that confirm the benefit of these medications in neuropathic pain
- nerve blocks; referral to a pain management specialist for a nerve block which may temporarily relieve the pain

The best choice would be either a TCA or AED first with a PRN opioid and then frequent reassessment. Topical treatments such as the lidoderm patch could also be started and might help with the allodynia but would not address the lancinating pain. If the opioid were needed frequently, then the addition of sustained-release medications could be considered.

Answer 38.8. **The answer is D.**

Since Mary Jane has improved with the nortriptyline and is not having any significant side effects, an increase would be appropriate to see if better control can be obtained. Referral to physical therapy would also be reasonable. She is almost a month from surgery and should have better range of motion. Therapy may also help her with the pain symptoms. She should be encouraged to take her oxycodone prior to the therapy sessions to make them more comfortable and therefore more successful. She should be warned about the potential for constipation and given recommendations for management.

Answer 38.9. **The answer is E.**

The transition time can be difficult for survivors. Mary Jane has been accustomed to very frequent medical care and has the security of knowing her cancer is being treated. She now must learn to move forward with her life with the uncertainty of her prognosis and the intense monitoring of her body that may occur. Discomforts she used to ignore may now carry a different significance. The need for social support may increase. Given her prior history of major depression, these symptoms, while not diagnostic, are of concern. You would want to encourage her continued contact with the social worker, possible involvement in a support group if not already active, and could consider antidepressants now or wait and see if things improve. If you were to start antidepressants, then the one she had success with in the past would be the best choice.

Answer 38.10. **The answer is D.**

There are multiple factors that may be contributing to her sexual problems: (a) vaginal dryness related to menopause, (b) body image issues with bilateral mastectomies, and (c) the impact of an antidepressant on sexual functioning. Intervention will depend on what you think are the causes and can include vaginal lubricants, topical hormone replacement therapy, a change in antidepressant medication, or referral to a therapist experienced in sexual dysfunction after cancer.

Answer 38.11. **The answer is A.**

Since Mary Jane has constant pain she should have constant medication, which is most readily given via SR medication. She is tolerating oxycodone; therefore, SR oxycodone would be one option. Alternatively, one could use SR morphine since it would be less expensive and equally as effective. She is relatively narcotic naïve so starting with the lowest dose would be best. Adjustments can then be made based on the degree of control. A patient prescribed a sustained-release preparation must also have something to take for breakthrough pain. Ideally this should be the same medication in immediate-release form as used in the SR medications. Given the 50% pain relief with 5 mg oxycodone, one could start with 10 mg oxycodone or 10 to 15 mg morphine tablets. Any person taking consistent narcotic medications will become constipated. It is the physician's responsibility to educate and begin preventive medications.

One could also consider the addition of an adjuvant such as acetaminophen or a non-steroidal anti-inflammatory drug (NSAID), but given the severity of her pain, medications of this type should not be the primary treatment.

Answer 38.12. **The answer is E.**

Mary Jane should be prepared for transient nausea, pruritis, and sedation. These side effects will usually resolve in 24 to 48 hours. A person educated to anticipate a problem and armed with medication to treat it is more likely to give the side effect time to resolve and thereby avoid premature termination of an effective program. If they fail to resolve after a week or more, then an alternate medication should be considered.

Answer 38.13. **The answer is D.**

Mary Jane is currently using an additional 60 mg of morphine in a 24-hour period. The 24-hour consumption is totaled, divided by the number of doses desired (2), and then added to the existing regimen. SR morphine (and oxycodone) can almost always be dosed at 12-hour intervals (excluding those products intended for 24-hour dosing). A change in interval has greater impact on the trough levels of a given medication than on the peak. Pain that is uncontrolled all day requires increased peak levels.

Answer 38.14. **The answer is C.**

Both of the above are classic histories of end-of-dose failure and the primary circumstances in which shortening the dosing interval could be considered. Alternatively, the dose can be increased and the interval left unchanged. This will also affect trough levels and result in less inconvenience and cost for the patient. Transdermal fentanyl patches should not be changed more often than 48 hours.

Answer 38.15. **The answer is A.**

While one would be concerned about metabolic causes such as hypercalcemia or metastatic disease to the brain, too much opioid is the likely cause and easily remedied. You have done two things that should have decreased the amount of pain she is experiencing: radiation and her chemotherapy. A decrease in the amount of pain will result in toxicity from previously tolerated doses. Rare need for breakthrough medication or side effects without dose increase merits a trial of dose reduction.

Answer 38.16. **The answer is C.**

Mary Jane is currently taking 200 mg plus an additional 240 mg in breakthrough for a total of 440 mg. To convert to IV, this is divided by the conversion ration (3:1) which equals 146 mg per 24 hours and then by 24 for the hourly rate (6 mg per hour) with an appropriate bolus dose. When one is converting for uncontrolled pain, all of the medication is totaled for the conversion. If you were converting her for nausea and her pain had been controlled, then only the SR dosing would have been used in the calculation: 200 mg/3/24 = 2.7 mg per hr that could be rounded to an even number if desired.

Answer 38.17. **The answer is D.**

At this time in Mary Jane's disease course, supportive care should be routinely included as an appropriate option even if further chemotherapy is planned. Acknowledging this as a legitimate choice, even if you do not recommend it now, can give individuals permission to stop futile therapy in the future. This is a time to explore her hopes and goals for the future. They may well be unrealistic and need to be sensitively refocused. As she becomes more ill, it is time to start discussing her wishes regarding resuscitation if she has not already expressed her wishes. This is not a one-time talk but a gradual discussion over time. In the immediate treatment arena, it is time to discuss "quality of life versus quantity" if this discussion has not already begun. The goals of further treatments need to be clearly outlined and benefit/burden ratio should be discussed.

Answer 38.18. **The answer is D.**

You, as Mary Jane's physician, should encourage her to address these details if not already done.

Answer 38.19. **The answer is D.**

There are significant ethical concerns with phase I trials in advanced disease. Informed consent implies (a) full disclosure including prognosis and the potential risks and benefits of the proposed study, (b) competency, and (c) free choice without undue coercion/inducements. Yet, in a small European study of phase I participants, those who gave consent did so because (a) they hoped it would make them better, (b) they were responding to family pressure, and (c) they felt they had "no choice." Therapeutic benefit was the most commonly identified reason in a similar study at the University of Chicago. Other studies have shown poor understanding of the research purpose and an inability to recall if other alternatives were offered. Therefore, the existing consent process may be less than adequate in this setting. There are many other issues of concern in the advanced disease setting, including but not limited to:

- physician/patient reluctance to discuss prognosis
- problems with decision-making capacity given frequent delirium in this population
- inadequate knowledge of the potential burden of research in advanced disease settings such as fatigue with long questionnaires, time away from home/family when time may be short, discomfort from additional testing, etc.

Answer 38.20. **The answer is C.**

The goal is to sensitively explain that other treatments do exist but that you do not think they are a good idea. If your patient wants to take the risk despite your recommendations, you must decide if you are willing. There is always something else to do to help the person even if there is no longer useful therapy for the cancer. The statement "nothing more to do" can leave a person feeling more hopeless than knowing there is no more disease-specific therapy. The focus should be on what one can offer, such as symptom management and emotional, spiritual, and social support, rather than on what one cannot offer—disease-modifying therapy. One does not "go to" hospice. Hospice generally comes to the individual in their home and should be offered as a benefit to the person and their family. If you do not feel further therapy is of value, then not only is it unethical to offer it but your patient needs to know this honestly rather than being offered futile treatment to avoid "taking away hope."

Answer 38.21. **The answer is D.**

The most likely cause of Mary Jane's restlessness and moaning is terminal delirium. At least 80% of actively dying patients develop delirium that is not reversible and therefore is a symptom to be managed. Symptom assessment can be difficult in the nonverbal. Facial expressions and the feeling of the family and medical personnel involved in care are the best guides. Medical management is directed at easily reversible causes such as urinary retention and/or fecal impaction, and then sedative medications are administered as needed. Opioids given in the absence of pain or dyspnea may contribute to delirium particularly if doses are increased in the setting of declining renal function. Typical medications used are neuroleptics (chlorpromazine), benzodiazepines (midazolam or lorazepam), and barbiturates.

Answer 38.22. **The answer is D.**

Medicare-certified hospices must offer at least 12 months of bereavement services to families in their care. Payment to hospice stops with the death of the patient, but these services are still provided at no cost to families.

Answer 38.23. **The answer is D.**

The value of nutritional support in the setting of bowel obstruction depends on the goals of care, the performance status of the patient, and the life expectancy. Total parenteral nutrition (TPN) would be the only option for nutritional support in this setting and should not be automatically started without appropriate discussion with the patient and the family. A study suggested that a Karnovsky of greater than 60 and normal albumin was somewhat predictive of prolonged survival with TPN. The discussion needs to include three options of care:

1. No fluids or nutrition, which will result in death in a relatively short interval; this option is chosen rarely
2. Fluids only
3. TPN

The value of TPN is controversial. If further chemotherapy is planned, then nutritional support would be indicated. If the patient already has anorexia and evidence of cachexia, he is unlikely to benefit from support (benefit implies weight maintenance/gain, improvement or maintenance of nutritional parameters, improved quality of life, improved survival, etc.).

Answer 38.24. **The answer is D.**

Taste changes are a common problem in cancer patients. Chemotherapy alters taste, with metallic taste as one of the more common presentations. Zinc deficiency has been implicated but replacement has not routinely been effective. Depression has been reported to cause taste changes that can resolve with antidepressants. Medical therapy for dysgeusia is disappointing, with most patients left to trial-and-error approaches to identify the least noxious tastes.

Answer 38.25. **The answer is A.**

Despite the weight loss seen in cancer cachexia, there is substantial evidence that nutritional support alone does not improve nutritional parameters nor promote weight gain. Therefore, attempting to increase caloric intake by percutaneous endoscopic gastrostomy (PEG) placement in the setting of cachexia is inappropriate. Approaches that effect cytokines such as tumor necrosis factor (TNF)-α are being investigated. Cachexia reflects the body's inflammatory response and many cytokines are implicated. It results in loss of lean body mass and disruption of fat and carbohydrate metabolism.

Answer 38.26. **The answer is A.**

Omega-3 fatty acids in several reports have seemed to promote a gain in lean body mass. Megestrol acetate is the best studied agent for anorexia but promotes fat weight rather than lean body mass. Corticosteroids are catabolic agents and may increase muscle breakdown. A placebo-controlled trial of cyproheptadine found continued weight loss comparable to that lost by the placebo patients.

Answer 38.27. **The answer is B.**

There is no evidence that chemotherapy affects the development of lymphedema. The extent of the surgical procedure and the need for subsequent radiation therapy, particularly in the axilla, clearly increases the risk of lymphedema. Newer surgical procedures such as sentinel node biopsy may help prevent future problems. Studies suggest that obese patients are also at increased risk.

Answer 38.28. **The answer is D.**

Physical therapy techniques can improve lymphedema by promoting outflow (exercise, massage, elevation) and decreasing lymph production (compression garments). There is no evidence that diuretics decrease lymphedema.

Answer 38.29. **The answer is C.**

To qualify for acute rehabilitation, a person must be able to participate in therapy for 3 hours per day. Someone with a performance score of 40 will not be able to do this. All of the other circumstances could be appropriate for acute rehabilitation.

Answer 38.30. **The answer is E.**

All of the above are felt to contribute to the increasing costs of medical care. The insulation of those Americans with insurance from the actual costs of care is also felt to be a contributing factor.

Answer 38.31. **The answer is B.**

The FDA is available to offer guidance on clinical trial design and development but does not specifically design a trial. The other answers are key roles for the FDA.

Answer 38.32. **The answer is C.**

Oncologists often use medications in combinations and for diseases not described in the FDA label indications yet supported by existing research of efficacy. When published data exist on the safety of a combination or clinical experience supports the use, then an IND is not required. Any study seeking to change the FDA approved indications or to be used for advertising requires IND. Studies that may significantly increase the risk to a subject either by escalating established doses or changing routes may also require IND.

Answer 38.33. **The answer is C.**

Under the 1992 regulations that permitted accelerated approval (AA), medications for serious or life-threatening illness that could show benefit over existing therapy are eligible for AA. Studies must show improvement in a surrogate endpoint such as overall response rate that, based on other evidence, is likely to predict clinical benefit. Typical studies have shown response rates in refractory disease. Manufacturers must continue the study process to confirm standard benefit criteria such as survival or improvement in quality of life to obtain regular approval. Failure to complete these trials or to demonstrate the expected benefit can result in withdrawal of the medication from the market.

CHAPTER **39**

Newer Approaches in Cancer Treatment

JULIAN R. MOLINA AND ALEX A. ADJEI

Directions Each of the numbered items below is followed by lettered answers. Select the ONE lettered answer that is BEST in each case unless instructed otherwise.

QUESTIONS

Question 39.1. **A 65-year-old white woman who is a current smoker presented to the emergency department with several episodes of hemoptysis. As part of her initial workup, she underwent x-rays of the chest that showed a 5-cm spiculated mass in the left hilum. While in the emergency department, the patient developed massive hemoptysis and required emergent thoracotomy and left lower lobectomy. A 4.6-cm tumor was resected. The final pathology report showed a grade 3 adenocarcinoma, margins of resection were negative, and only one solitary peribronchial node was found to be involved by neoplasia. Further testing ruled out metastatic disease. Three weeks after surgery, the patient comes to your office for recommendations regarding further therapy. Physical examination shows a patient who has recovered well from surgery; her chest scar is completely healed. On auscultation of the chest, some wheezes and basilar crackles are found in the left base. There are no other significant findings on physical exam, and laboratory values are within normal limits. Her performance status is considered to be Eastern Cooperative Oncology Group (ECOG) 1. Your recommendation for this patient is**

A. follow-up in 3 months, no need for further therapy
B. radiation therapy to the left chest and mediastinum
C. pemetrexed
D. gefitinib
E. adjuvant chemotherapy

Corresponding Chapters in *Cancer: Principles & Practice of Oncology*, Seventh Edition:
60 (Gene Therapy), 61 (Cancer Vaccines), 62 (Cell Transfer Therapy), 63 (Antiangiogenesis Agents), 64 (Focused Ultrasounds), and 65 (Antisense Inhibition of Gene Expression).

Question 39.2. **A 61-year-old man, a former smoker, presented to your office complaining of pain radiating down the right arm and weight loss. The patient underwent multiple testing that included a computed tomographic (CT) scan of the chest, which revealed a right chest tumor involving the superior ribs and the brachial plexus. Other testing ruled out distant metastasis. Upon evaluation, you notice a patient whose main complaint is pain in his right arm. Physical examination also reveals pain and tenderness on palpation of the right upper ribs. There are decreased breath sounds in the right chest with occasional crackles. Performance status is considered to be ECOG 1. The remainder of the physical examination is within normal limits. His forced expiratory volume in one second (FEV1) is 1.92 (80% of predicted). Other laboratory values are within normal range. Your recommendation for this patient is**

A. chemotherapy with a platinum-based regimen
B. gefitinib
C. combined modality (chemoradiation) followed by surgery
D. single therapy with pemetrexed
E. hospice care

Question 39.3. **A 61-year-old woman presents to your office with complaints of recent-onset dizziness and difficulty with her gait. She has a history of smoking at least one pack of cigarettes a day for the last 30 years and hypertension that is well controlled with an angiotensin converting enzyme (ACE) inhibitor. There is no other significant medical history. A magnetic resonance image (MRI) of the head reveals a 2.3-cm ring-enhancing mass in the pons. A fused positron emission tomography (PET)/computed tomography (CT) scan shows a 4.0-cm right lower lobe mass and one lymph node in the right hilum. There is no evidence of other metastasis. Fine needle aspiration biopsy confirms the diagnosis of squamous cell lung cancer. Your recommendation for this patient is**

A. chemotherapy with platinum-based regimen
B. temazolamide
C. treatment of the brain metastasis by surgery or radiosurgery followed by complete resection of the primary tumor followed by adjuvant chemotherapy
D. whole brain radiation followed by radiation therapy to the chest
E. no aggressive treatment, only hospice care

Question 39.4. **The patient is a 63-year-old woman, current smoker of one-half pack per day who 1 year prior to presentation was found to have an indeterminate pulmonary nodule in the right lower lobe. This lesion was managed with close observation. At the time of presentation, the patient had a 1.9-cm nodule located in the right lower lobe. PET was positive at the nodule as well as in the hilum. The patient underwent mediastinoscopy with cervical approach and was found to have five nodes in the inferior mediastinum and two nodes in the superior mediastinum compromised by non-small cell lung cancer. Further workup demonstrated an FEV1 of 1.78 (79% of predicted) and no evidence of metastasis to other organs. Her**

performance status was ECOG 1. Final staging was T1N2, M0 (stage IIIA). Your recommendation for this patient is

A. surgery followed by adjuvant chemotherapy
B. radiation therapy as a single modality treatment
C. combined modality of chemotherapy and radiation
D. gefinitib
E. pemetrexed

Question 39.5. **A 66-year-old male former smoker initially consulted his local physician due to cough. Chest x-ray (CXR) done at the time of consultation revealed an infiltrate in the right lower lobe. CT scan of the chest showed a large mass-like opacity in the right lower lobe located posterolaterally. In addition, several small opacities were seen in the right upper and middle lobes. A CT-guided biopsy of the mass demonstrated adenocarcinoma with bronchioloalveolar features. The patient's past medical history was significant for severe coronary artery disease (CAD) that required several angioplasties. PET scan shows increased uptake in the right chest corresponding to areas of mass and ground glass opacities and no increased uptake. The patient is treated with a platinum-based doublet. Reevaluation of the case after 3 cycles of chemotherapy shows progression of the infiltrates and mild pleural effusion. On physical exam, the patient is found to have significant dyspnea and moderate pain in the right side of the chest. Auscultation reveals decreased sound and crackles in the right lung. The patient performance status is considered to be ECOG 3. The patient wants to explore other treatment options. Your recommendation for this patient is**

A. weekly carboplatin
B. trial of gefitinib
C. combined modality treatment with chemotherapy and radiation
D. phase I clinical trial
E. single-modality treatment with radiation therapy

ANSWERS

Answer 39.1. **The answer is E.**

This case introduces two important issues for discussion: (1) severe, (massive) hemoptysis, and (2) adjuvant treatment for completely resected non-small cell lung cancer (NSCLC). Massive hemoptysis requiring emergent surgery of percutaneous embolization is a rare complication of lung cancer. Patients with massive hemoptysis due to lung cancer are better treated with surgical resection. If considered to be unresectable, arterial embolization should be done. Once the diagnosis is established, in the event of lung cancer, the patient requires the same workup for staging and treatment. In this particular case, the patient was staged as a T2N1, M0 (stage IIB) lung cancer and requires adjuvant chemotherapy. Two large adjuvant trials have been reported in the past few years.

The Adjuvant Lung Project of Italy (ALPI) showed no difference in survival between its chemotherapy and control arms. The International Adjuvant Lung Cancer Trial (IALT), presented at the American Society of Clinical Oncology (ASCO) meeting in 2003, showed an absolute survival benefit of 4.1% for those receiving adjuvant therapy. In addition to these two trials, two recent reports also support the use of adjuvant chemotherapy for lung cancer. In one of the trials, led by the National Cancer Institute of Canada (NCIC), there was an absolute survival benefit of 15% after 5 years for patients receiving chemotherapy (69% versus 54%). This trial included patients with stage IB and II disease, whose tumors had been completely removed. Patients were randomly assigned to receive either postsurgical therapy with cisplatin and vinorelbine or to observation. The second trial was done by the Cancer and Leukemia Group B (CALGB) and showed an absolute benefit of 12% after 4 years. The (CALGB 9633) trial included only patients with stage IB disease, and they were randomly assigned to receive either carboplatin and paclitaxel or no chemotherapy. After 4 years, 71% of patients who had received chemotherapy were alive compared with 59% of those who had surgery alone.

Answer 39.2. **The answer is C.**

Superior sulcus tumors or Pancoast tumors are lung cancers that occur in the apex of the chest and invade apical chest wall structures. The textbook description of such patients describes a syndrome of pain radiating down the arm as a manifestation of brachial plexus involvement. Tumors in the apex can be classified as a Pancoast tumor if they invade into the most superior ribs or periostium, the lower nerve roots of the brachial plexus, the sympathetic chain near the apex of the chest, or the subclavian vessels. The available data for patients with Pancoast tumors suggest that the best survival is achieved with preoperative chemoradiotherapy followed by surgical resection in carefully selected patients. Preoperative radiotherapy followed by surgical resection is a reasonable alternative. Several clinical trials have reported the benefit of preoperative chemoradiotherapy followed by surgery for patients with T4 tumors. In a trial of 57 patients with T4 tumors, a 5-year survival of 20% was reported for those cases that completed chemoradiation followed by surgery. In contrast, the 5-year survival for patients with stages IIIA and IIIB ranges from 9% to 14%. Moreover, a retrospective analysis of T4 N0-1, M0 tumors conducted by the Southwest Oncology Group (SWOG) showed a clear benefit in the form of 2-year survival (64% versus 33%) for the group treated with chemoradiation followed by surgery compared to chemoradiation alone.

Answer 39.3. **The answer is C.**

Metastasis to the brain or the adrenal glands occurs in about 25% of patients with stage IV NSCLC. If left untreated, the median survival of patients with a brain metastasis is approximately 2 months, with 4 to 6 months for untreated adrenal metastasis. It is important to consider that there is a group of patients with an isolated brain metastasis as the only site of their stage IV disease. In this group, it is reasonable to consider aggressive therapy of both the primary lesion as well as the isolated metastatic site as a potentially curative therapy. The best treatment for the brain metastasis may involve either surgical resection (if less than three metastases) or ablation of the metastasis by radiosurgery. Patients with a brain metastasis should be selected for curative treatment only after a thorough search for other sites of disease has been negative. It is also important to determine with mediastinoscopy or PET scan the potential involvement of N2 or N3 nodes before recommending this approach. Once a careful search for other sites of metastasis is done, it is possible to consider patients with a solitary brain metastasis, a metastasis to the adrenal, or both for treatment with curative intent. The same applies to patients who have been treated with complete resection of the primary tumor and soon after are found to have a solitary cranial or adrenal metastasis. A 5-year survival rate of 15% to 20% has been reported for those patients who underwent successful complete resections of both the primary tumor and the metastasis. The overall survival for patients with isolated brain metastasis treated with curative intent averages 14% (range 8% to 21%) with a 5-year survival of 21% (range 16% to 30%). In the case of isolated adrenal metastasis, treatment of selected patients has yielded 5-year survival rates of 10% to 23%. Survival after resection of the primary and the adrenal metastasis appears to be good, primarily in patients without nodal involvement.

Answer 39.4. **The answer is C.**

The percentage of NSCLC patients who present with unresectable stage IIIA and IIIB disease is considered to be 30% to 40%. The treatment of patients who present with locally advanced disease has been an area of considerable debate over the last few years. There is currently no official consensus regarding the definitive management of locally advanced stage III NSCLC. A meta-analysis of 14 randomized trials compared survival after radiotherapy (RT) alone or chemoradiotherapy (CRT) in patients with locally advanced stage IIIA/IIIB NSCLC. The study shows that the addition of chemotherapy to RT improved survival but the absolute benefit was relatively small. This finding was later confirmed by two meta-analyses. The larger of them was based on 22 randomized studies involving 3,033 patients. In this study, a platinum-based regimen combined modality approach was associated with a 13% reduction in the risk of death and with the absolute benefit of 4% at 2 years. Further validation of this approach was provided by two recent trials, the West Japan Lung Cancer Study and the Radiation Therapy Oncology Group (RTOG 9410). A 2-year survival difference of 35% versus 16% was shown in the RTOG study ($p = 0.038$). Even at 5 years there was a difference in survival (15.8% versus 8.8%) as shown by the West Japan Lung Study.

Answer 39.5. **The answer is B.**

Gefitinib is an orally active, selective epidermal growth factor receptor tyrosine kinase inhibitor that blocks signal transduction pathways implicated in proliferation and survival of cancer cells. Results from phase I studies demonstrated that gefitinib is well tolerated and active in patients with NSCLC. Two large multicenter, randomized phase II studies (IDEAL 1 and 2) undertaken in Japan and the United States reported response rates of 18.4% and 11.8%, respectively. The median progression-free survival (PFS) was 2.7 and 1.9 months, and the median overall survival was 7.6 and 6.5 months in IDEAL 1 and 2, respectively. Significantly, quality of life and symptom control was reported in the gefitinib arm. This agent and others in its class have shown activity in patients with adenocarcinoma with bronchoalveolar features.

Index

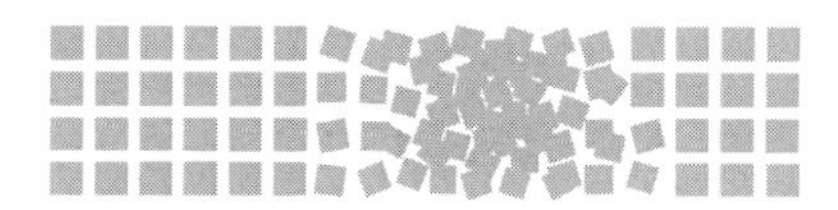

C

D

E

F

M

N

O

R

S

T